THE SOUTH LONDON A[
NHS FOUNDATIOI

D0545618

OXLEAS NHS FOUNDATION TRUST

PRESCRIBING GUIDELINES
9th Edition

The Maudsley

The South London and Maudsley NHS Foundation Trust
&
Oxleas NHS Foundation Trust

PRESCRIBING GUIDELINES

9th Edition

David Taylor
Carol Paton
Robert Kerwin

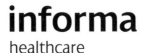

© Taylor, Paton, Kerwin 2007

First published in the United Kingdom in 2007 by Informa Healthcare, Telephone House, 69–77 Paul Street, London EC2A 4LQ. Informa Healthcare is a trading division of Informa UK Ltd. Registered Office, 37/41 Mortimer Street, London W1T 3JH. Registered in England and Wales number 1072954.

Tel: +44 (0)20 7017 5000
Fax: +44 (0)20 7017 6699
Email: info.medicine@tandf.co.uk
Website: www.informahealthcare.com

Although every effort has been made to ensure that all owners of copyright material have been acknowledged in this publication, we would be glad to acknowledge in subsequent reprints or editions any omissions brought to our attention.

Although every effort has been made to ensure that drug doses and other information are presented accurately in this publication, the ultimate responsibility rests with the prescribing physician. Neither the publishers nor the authors can be held responsible for errors or for any consequences arising from the use of information contained herein. For detailed prescribing information or instructions on the use of any product or procedure discussed herein, please consult the prescribing information or instructional material issued by the manufacturer.

A CIP record for this book is available from the British Library.
Library of Congress Cataloging-in-Publication Data

Data available on application

ISBN-10: 0 415 42416 X
ISBN-13: 978 0 415 42416 5

Distributed in North and South America by
Taylor & Francis
6000 Broken Sound Parkway, NW, (Suite 300)
Boca Raton, FL 33487, USA

Within Continental USA
Tel: 1 (800) 272 7737; Fax: 1 (800) 374 3401
Outside Continental USA
Tel: (561) 994 0555; Fax: (561) 361 6018
Email: orders@crcpress.com

Distributed in the rest of the world by
Thomson Publishing Services
Cheriton House
North Way
Andover, Hampshire SP10 5BE, UK
Tel: +44 (0)1264 332424
Email: tps.tandfsalesorder@thomson.com

Composition by Exeter Premedia Services Private Ltd, Chennai, India
Printed and bound in Great Britain by MPG Books, Bodmin, Cornwall, UK

Contents

For Rob

Authors and editors

David Taylor, Editor and Author
Chief Pharmacist, South London and Maudsley NHS Foundation Trust
Honorary Senior Lecturer, Institute of Psychiatry
Visiting Professor, King's College, London

Carol Paton, Editor and Author
Chief Pharmacist, Oxleas NHS Foundation Trust
Honorary Research Fellow, Imperial College, London

Robert Kerwin, Founding Editor
Professor of Clinical Neuropharmacology, Institute of Psychiatry
Consultant Psychiatrist, South London and Maudsley NHS Foundation Trust

Preface

The 9th edition of the *Maudsley Prescribing Guidelines* has been thoroughly revised and updated to include published data available in March 2007. There are, in addition, 20 new sections including reviews and guidance on promoting adherence, the treatment of delirium, SSRIs and bleeding and the use of unlicensed medicines.

During their lifetime, *The Guidelines* have grown in size and scope but gradually contained less and less unequivocal guidance and instruction. This is no bad thing and points to the less than conclusive nature of much of the data in many fields of clinical psychopharmacology. What we hope to provide however, are brief but detailed reviews of subject areas and general guidance based on the data reviewed and current clinical practice. With this in mind, we have continued to provide full reference lists for all sections despite the valuable space taken up by these lists.

The breadth of subjects covered in *The Guidelines* means that we rely upon the generous assistance of a variety of specialists. In this edition, we are particularly grateful to Soraya Mayet for overseeing the writing of the substance misuse chapter; Jennifer Chan and Geoffrey Wolff for the section on eating disorders; Russel Foster for the sections on HIV and on biochemistry; Sally Jones for the section on Multiple Sclerosis; Melinda Sweeting for the section on clozapine in the community; Azizah Attard for the section on delirium and Richard Gray for the section on adherence. These and many others (below) contributed invaluable expert advice without which *The Guidelines* could not have been produced. Special thanks are also due to Maria O'Hagan who typed this edition of *The Guidelines* and who successfully re-formatted the whole book using Reference Manager software.

In February 2007, during the final stages of writing this edition of the Guidelines, Rob Kerwin unexpectedly passed away. It was Rob's idea, in 1993, to produce evidence-based prescribing guidelines for psychiatrists – a fairly radical idea at the time. He tirelessly contributed to all editions of *The Guidelines* and played a major part in their development into an internationally renowned reference text. Around the world, Rob was known for his exceptional intellect and his extraordinary knowledge of the drug treatment of schizophrenia, amongst many other subjects. To those closer to him, Rob was also a generous and loyal friend who sought and expected no credit for the frequent efforts he made on behalf of others. He is sorely missed.

David Taylor
May 2007

Acknowledgements

The Maudsley Prescribing Guidelines are a product of the authors' knowledge and expertise and the helpful contributions of a large number of specialists and experts. The input from these experts not only allows a greater range of subjects to be covered but also provides crucial, if informal, peer review of many sections. We are, therefore, deeply indebted to previous contributors and to the following contributors to the present edition of *The Guidelines*.

Azizah Attard
Sube Banerjee
Chris Ball
David Ball
Elizabeth Bevan
Steve Bleakley
Dan Bressington
Peter Brex
Jennifer Chan
Tony Cleare
Anne Connolly
Vivenne Curtis
Sarah Elliott
Radia Esop
Russel Foster
Richard Gray
Mike Issac
Sally Jones
Shubhra Mace
Jane Marshall
Soraya Mayet
Veronica O'Keane
Banke Olofinjana
Deborah Robson
Eli Silber
John Strang
Guy Sutherland
Melinda Sweeting
Eromona Whiskey
Geoffrey Wolff
Deborah Zador

Special thanks to

Jo Taylor

Notes on using *The Maudsley Prescribing Guidelines*

The main aim of *The Guidelines* is to provide clinicians with practically useful advice on the prescribing of psychotropic agents in commonly encountered clinical situations. The advice contained in this handbook is based on a combination of literature review, clinical experience and expert contribution. We do not claim that this advice is necessarily 'correct' or that it deserves greater prominence than guidance provided by other professional bodies or special interest groups. We hope, however, to have provided guidance that helps to assure the safe, effective and economic use of medicines in mental health. We hope also to have made clear the sources of information used to inform the guidance given.

Please note that many of the recommendations provided here go beyond the licensed or labelled indications of many drugs, both in the UK and elsewhere. Note also that, while we have endeavoured to make sure all quoted doses are correct, clinicians should always consult statutory texts before prescribing. Users of *The Guidelines* should also bear in mind that the contents of this handbook are based on information available to us up to March 2007. Much of the advice contained here will become outdated as more research is conducted and published.

No liability is accepted for any injury, loss or damage, however caused.

Notes on inclusion of drugs

The Guidelines are used in many other countries outside the UK. With this in mind, we have included in this edition those drugs in widespread use throughout the western world in March 2007. Thus, we have included, for example, ziprasidone, even though the drug is not marketed in the UK at this time. Its inclusion gives *The Guidelines* relevance in those countries where ziprasidone is marketed and may also be of benefit to UK readers, since many unlicensed drugs can be obtained through formal pharmaceutical importers. Many older drugs (methotrimeprazine, pericyazine, maprotiline, etc.) are either only briefly mentioned or not included on the basis that these drugs are not in widespread use at the time of writing.

Notes on commonly used abbreviations

Throughout this text we have abbreviated *British National Formulary* to *BNF* and extrapyramidal side-effects to EPSEs. We have also used FGA for first generation antipsychotics and SGA for second generation antipsychotics (broadly speaking, those antipsychotics marketed in the UK since 1990). SPC refers to the UK Summary of Product Characteristics for the drug in question.

All other abbreviations are explained in the text itself.

chapter 1

Plasma level monitoring of psychotropics and anticonvulsants

Introduction

Plasma drug concentration or 'plasma level' monitoring is a process surrounded by some confusion and misunderstanding. Drug level monitoring, when appropriately used, is of considerable help in optimising treatment and assuring adherence. However, in psychiatry, as in other areas of medicine, plasma level determinations are frequently undertaken without good cause and results acted upon inappropriately[1]. In other instances, plasma levels are underused.

Before taking a blood sample for plasma level assay, make sure that the following criteria are satisfied:

- **Is there a clinically useful assay method available?**
  Only a minority of drugs have available assays. The assay must be clinically validated and results available within a clinically useful timescale.

- **Is the drug at 'steady state'?**
  Plasma levels are usually meaningful only when samples are taken after steady-state levels have been achieved. This takes 4–5 drug half-lives.

- **Is the timing of the sample correct?**
  Sampling time is vitally important for many but not all drugs. If the recommended sampling time is 12 hours post-dose, then the sample should be taken 11–13 hours post-dose if possible; 10–14 hours post-dose, if absolutely necessary. For trough or 'pre-dose' samples, take the blood sample immediately before the next dose is due. Do not, under any circumstances, withhold the next dose for more than 1 or (possibly) 2 hours until a sample is taken. Withholding for longer than this will inevitably give a misleading result (it will give a lower result than that ever seen

in the usual, regular dosing), and this may lead to an inappropriate dose increase. Sampling time is less critical with drugs with a long half-life (e.g. olanzapine) but, as an absolute minimum, prescribers should always record the time of sampling and time of last dose.

If a sample is not taken within 1–2 hours of the required time, it has the potential to mislead rather than inform. The only exception to this is if toxicity is suspected – sampling at the time of suspected toxicity is obviously appropriate.

- **Will the level have any inherent meaning?**
  Is there a target range of plasma levels? If so, then plasma levels (from samples taken at the right time) will usefully guide dosing. If there is not an accepted target range, plasma levels can only indicate adherence or potential toxicity. However, if the sample is being used to check compliance, then bear in mind that a plasma level of zero indicates only that the drug has not been taken in the past several days. Plasma levels above zero may indicate erratic compliance, full compliance or even long-standing non-compliance disguised by recent taking of prescribed doses. Note also that target ranges have their limitations: patients may respond to lower levels than the quoted range and tolerate levels above the range; also, ranges quoted by different laboratories vary sometimes widely without explanation.

- **Is there a clear reason for plasma level determination?**
  Only the following reasons are valid:
  – to confirm compliance (but see above)
  – if toxicity is suspected
  – if drug interaction is suspected
  – if clinical response is difficult to assess directly (and where a target range of plasma levels has been established)
  – if the drug has a narrow therapeutic index and toxicity concerns are considerable.

Interpreting sample results

The basic rule for sample level interpretation is to act upon assay results in conjunction with reliable clinical observation ('*treat the patient, not the level*'). For example, if a patient is responding adequately to a drug but has a plasma level below the accepted target range, then the dose should not normally be increased. If a patient has intolerable adverse effects but a plasma level within the target range, then a dose decrease may be appropriate. Of course, where plasma levels above the target range are known to be dangerous (e.g. lithium; clozapine) the dose should usually be reduced even if no effects are apparent.

Where a plasma level result is substantially different from previous results, a repeat sample is usually advised. Check dose, timing of dose and recent compliance but ensure, in particular, the correct timing of the sample. Many anomalous results are the consequence of changes in sample timing.

Table Interpreting sample results

Drug	Target range	Sample timing	Time to steady state	Comments
Carbamazepine[2,3]	>7 mg/l bipolar disorder	Trough	2 weeks	Carbamazepine induces its own metabolism. Time to steady state dependent on autoinduction
Clozapine	350–500 µg/l Upper limit of target range is ill-defined	Trough	2–3 days	See below
Lamotrigine[4–7]	Not established but suggest 2.5–15 mg/l	Trough	5 days Auto-induction is thought to occur, so time to steady state may be longer	Some debate over utility of lamotrigine levels, especially in bipolar disorder. Toxicity may be increased above 15 mg/l
Lithium	0.6–1.0 mmol/l (may be >1.0 mmol/l in mania)	12 hours	5 days post-dose	Well-established target range
Olanzapine	20–40 µg/l	12 hours	1 week	See below
Phenytoin[3]	10–20 mg/l	Trough	Variable	Follows zero-order kinetics. Free levels may be useful
Quetiapine[8–10]	Around 50–150 µg/l	Trough	2–3 days oral	Target range not defined. Plasma level monitoring not recommended
Risperidone	20–60 µg/l (active moiety)	Trough	2–3 days oral 6–8 weeks injection	Plasma level monitoring is not recommended
Tricyclics[11]	Nortriptyline 50–150 µg/l Amitriptyline 100–200 µg/l	Trough	2–3 days	Rarely used and of dubious benefit. Use ECG to assess toxicity
Valproate[2,3,12–15]	50–100 mg/l Epilepsy and bipolar	Trough	2–3 days	Some doubt over value of levels in epilepsy and bipolar disorder. Some evidence that levels up to 125 mg/l are tolerated and more effective than lower levels (in mania)

Clozapine

Clozapine plasma levels are broadly related to daily dose[16], but there is sufficient variation to make impossible any precise prediction of plasma level. Plasma levels are generally lower in younger patients, males[17] and smokers[18], and higher in Asians[19]. A series of algorithms has been developed for the approximate prediction of clozapine levels according to patient factors and are recommended[20]. Algorithms cannot, however, account for other influences on clozapine plasma levels such as changes in adherence, inflammation[21] and infection[22].

The plasma level threshold for acute response to clozapine has been suggested to be 200 μg/l[23], 350 μg/l[24–26], 370 μg/l[27], 420 μg/l[28] and 504 μg/l[29]. Limited data suggest a level of at least 200 μg/l is required to prevent relapse[30].

Despite these varied estimates of response threshold, plasma levels can be useful in optimising treatment. In those not responding to clozapine, dose should be adjusted to give plasma levels in the range **350–500 μg/l**. Those not tolerating clozapine may benefit from a reduction to a dose giving plasma levels in this range. An upper limit to the clozapine target range has not been defined. Plasma levels do seem to predict EEG changes[31] and seizures occur more frequently in patients with levels above 1000 μg/l[32], so levels should probably be kept well below this. Note also that clozapine metabolism may become saturated at higher doses: the ratio of clozapine to norclozapine increases with increasing plasma levels, suggesting saturation[33–35]. The effect of fluvoxamine also suggests that metabolism via CYP1A2 to norclozapine can be overwhelmed[36].

A further consideration is that placing an upper limit on the target range for clozapine levels may discourage potentially worthwhile dose increases within the licensed dose range. Before plasma levels were widely used, clozapine was fairly often dosed to 900 mg/day, with valproate being added when the dose reached 600 mg/day. It remains unclear whether using these high doses can benefit patients with plasma levels already above the accepted threshold. Nonetheless, it is prudent to use valproate as prophylaxis against seizures and myoclonus when plasma levels are above 500–600 μg/l and certainly when levels approach 1000 μg/l.

Olanzapine

Plasma levels of olanzapine are linearly related to daily dose, but there is substantial variation[37], with higher levels seen in women[29], non-smokers[38] and those on enzyme-inhibiting drugs[38,39]. With once-daily dosing, the threshold level for response in schizophrenia has been suggested to be 9.3 μg/l (trough sample)[40], 23.2 μg/l (12-hour post-dose sample)[29] and 23 μg/l at a mean of 13.5 hours post-dose[41]. There is evidence to suggest that levels greater than around 40 μg/l (12-hour sampling) produce no further therapeutic benefit than lower levels[42]. Severe toxicity is uncommon but may be associated with levels above 100 μg/l, and death is occasionally seen at levels above 160 μg/l[43] (albeit when other drugs or physical factors are relevant). A target range for therapeutic use of **20–40 μg/l** (12-hour post-dose sample) has been proposed[44] for schizophrenia; the range for mania is probably similar[45]. Notably, significant weight gain seems most likely to occur in those with plasma levels above 20 μg/l[46].

In practice, the dose of olanzapine should be governed by response and tolerability. Plasma level determinations should be reserved for those suspected of non-adherence or those not responding to the maximum licensed dose. In the latter case, dose may then be adjusted to give 12-hour plasma levels of 20–40 μg/l.

Risperidone

Risperidone plasma levels are rarely measured in the UK and very few laboratories have developed assay methods for the drug's determination. In any case, plasma level monitoring is probably unproductive (dose–response is well described), except where compliance is in doubt, and in such cases measurement of prolactin will give some idea of compliance.

The therapeutic range for risperidone is said to be **20–60 μg/l** of the active moiety (risperidone + 9-OH-risperidone)[47,48]. Plasma levels of this magnitude are usually provided by oral doses of between 3 mg and 6 mg a day[47,49–51]. Occupancy of striatal dopamine D_2 receptors has been shown to be around 65% (the minimum required for therapeutic effect) at plasma levels of approximately 20 μg/l[48].

Risperidone long-acting injection (25 mg/2 weeks) appears to afford plasma levels averaging between 4.4 and 22.7 μg/l[50]. Dopamine D_2 occupancies at this dose have been variously estimated at between 25% and 71%[48,52,53]. There is considerable inter-individual variation around these mean values, with a substantial minority of patients with plasma levels above those shown. Nonetheless, these data do cast doubt on the efficacy of a dose of 25 mg/2 weeks[50], although it is noteworthy that there is some evidence that long-acting preparations are effective despite apparently sub-therapeutic plasma levels and dopamine occupancies[54].

References

1. Mann K et al. Appropriateness of therapeutic drug monitoring for antidepressants in routine psychiatric inpatient care. Ther Drug Monit 2006;28:83–8.
2. Taylor D et al. Doses of carbamazepine and valproate in bipolar affective disorder. Psychiatr Bull 1997; 21:221–3.
3. Eadie MJ. Anticonvulsant drugs. Drugs 1984;27:328–63.
4. Cohen AF et al. Lamotrigine, a new anticonvulsant: pharmacokinetics in normal humans. Clin Pharmacol Ther 1987;42:535–41.
5. Kilpatrick ES et al. Concentration–effect and concentration–toxicity relations with lamotrigine: a prospective study. Epilepsia 1996;37:534–8.
6. Johannessen SI et al. Therapeutic drug monitoring of the newer antiepileptic drugs. Ther Drug Monit 2003;25:347–63.
7. Lardizabal DV et al. Tolerability and pharmacokinetics of oral loading with lamotrigine in epilepsy monitoring units. Epilepsia 2003;44:536–9.
8. Aichhorn W et al. Influence of age, gender, body weight and valproate comedication on quetiapine plasma concentrations. Int Clin Psychopharmacol 2006;21:81–5.
9. Hiemke C et al. Therapeutic monitoring of new antipsychotic drugs. Ther Drug Monit 2004;26:156–60.
10. Degner D et al. Relevance of therapeutic drug monitoring (TDM) in patients with quetiapine administration. http://www.thieme-connect.com DOI: 10.1055/s-2003-825297. 2003.
11. Taylor D et al. Plasma levels of tricyclics and related antidepressants: are they necessary or useful? Psychiatr Bull 1995;19:548–50.
12. Davis R et al. Valproic acid – a reappraisal of its pharmacological properties and clinical efficacy in epilepsy. Drugs 1994;47:332–72.
13. Perucca E. Pharmacological and therapeutic properties of valproate. CNS Drugs 2002;16:695–714.
14. Allen MH et al. Linear relationship of valproate serum concentration to response and optimal serum levels for acute mania. Am J Psychiatry 2006;163:272–5.
15. Bowden CL et al. Relation of serum valproate concentration to response in mania. Am J Psychiatry 1996;153:765–70.
16. Haring C et al. Influence of patient-related variables on clozapine plasma levels. Am J Psychiatry 1990; 147:1471–5.
17. Haring C et al. Dose-related plasma levels of clozapine: influence of smoking behaviour, sex and age. Psychopharmacology 1989;99(Suppl):S38–S40.
18. Taylor D. Pharmacokinetic interactions involving clozapine. Br J Psychiatry 1997;171:109–12.
19. Ng CH et al. An inter-ethnic comparison study of clozapine dosage, clinical response and plasma levels. Int Clin Psychopharmacol 2005;20:163–8.
20. Rostami-Hodjegan A et al. Influence of dose, cigarette smoking, age, sex, and metabolic activity on plasma clozapine concentrations: a predictive model and nomograms to aid clozapine dose adjustment and to assess compliance in individual patients. J Clin Psychopharmacol 2004;24:70–8.
21. Haack MJ et al. Toxic rise of clozapine plasma concentrations in relation to inflammation. Eur Neuropsychopharmacol 2003;13:381–5.
22. de Leon J et al. Serious respiratory infections can increase clozapine levels and contribute to side effects: a case report. Prog Neuropsychopharmacol Biol Psychiatry 2003;27:1059–63.
23. VanderZwaag C et al. Response of patients with treatment-refractory schizophrenia to clozapine within three serum level ranges. Am J Psychiatry 1996;153:1579–84.
24. Perry PJ et al. Clozapine and norclozapine plasma concentrations and clinical response of treatment refractory schizophrenic patients. Am J Psychiatry 1991;148:231–5.
25. Miller DD. Effect of phenytoin on plasma clozapine concentrations in two patients. J Clin Psychiatry 1991;52:23–5.
26. Spina E et al. Relationship between plasma concentrations of clozapine and norclozapine and therapeutic response in patients with schizophrenia resistant to conventional neuroleptics. Psychopharmacology 2000;148:83–9.
27. Hasegawa M et al. Relationship between clinical efficacy and clozapine concentrations in plasma in schizophrenia: effect of smoking. J Clin Psychopharmacol 1993;13:383–90.
28. Potkin SG et al. Plasma clozapine concentrations predict clinical response in treatment-resistant schizophrenia. J Clin Psychiatry 1994;55(Suppl B):133–6.
29. Perry PJ. Therapeutic drug monitoring of antipsychotics. Psychopharmacol Bull 2001;35:19–29.
30. Xiang YQ et al. Serum concentrations of clozapine and norclozapine in the prediction of relapse of patients with schizophrenia. Schizophr Res 2006;83:201–10.
31. Khan AY et al. Examining concentration-dependent toxicity of clozapine: role of therapeutic drug monitoring. J Psychiatr Pract 2005;11:289–301.
32. Greenwood-Smith C et al. Serum clozapine levels: a review of their clinical utility. J Psychopharmacol 2003;17:234–8.
33. Volpicelli SA et al. Determination of clozapine, norclozapine, and clozapine-N-oxide in serum by liquid chromatography. Clin Chem 1993;39:1656–9.
34. Guitton C et al. Clozapine and metabolite concentrations during treatment of patients with chronic schizophrenia. J Clin Pharmacol 1999;39:721–8.
35. Palego L et al. Clozapine, norclozapine plasma levels, their sum and ratio in 50 psychotic patients: influence of patient-related variables. Prog Neuropsychopharmacol Biol Psychiatry 2002;26:473–80.

36. Wang CY et al. The differential effects of steady-state fluvoxamine on the pharmacokinetics of olanzapine and clozapine in healthy volunteers. J Clin Pharmacol 2004;44:785–92.
37. Aravagiri M et al. Plasma level monitoring of olanzapine in patients with schizophrenia: determination by high-performance liquid chromatography with electrochemical detection. Ther Drug Monit 1997;19: 307–13.
38. Gex-Fabry M et al. Therapeutic drug monitoring of olanzapine: the combined effect of age, gender, smoking, and comedication. Ther Drug Monit 2003;25:46–53.
39. Bergemann N et al. Olanzapine plasma concentration, average daily dose, and interaction with co-medication in schizophrenic patients. Pharmacopsychiatry 2004;37:63–8.
40. Perry PJ et al. Olanzapine plasma concentrations and clinical response in acutely ill schizophrenic patients. J Clin Psychopharmacol 1997;6:472–7.
41. Fellows L et al. Investigation of target plasma concentration–effect relationships for olanzapine in schizophrenia. Ther Drug Monit 2003;25:682–9.
42. Mauri MC et al. Clinical outcome and olanzapine plasma levels in acute schizophrenia. Eur Psychiatry 2005;20:55–60.
43. Rao ML et al. [Olanzapine: pharmacology, pharmacokinetics and therapeutic drug monitoring]. Fortschr Neurol Psychiatr 2001;69:510–17.
44. Robertson MD et al. Olanzapine concentrations in clinical serum and postmortem blood specimens – when does therapeutic become toxic? J Forensic Sci 2000;45:418–21.
45. Bech P et al. Olanzapine plasma level in relation to antimanic effect in the acute therapy of manic states. Nord J Psychiatry 2006;60:181–2.
46. Perry PJ et al. The association of weight gain and olanzapine plasma concentrations. J Clin Psychopharmacol 2005;25:250–4.
47. Olesen OV et al. Serum concentrations and side effects in psychiatric patients during risperidone therapy. Ther Drug Monit 1998;20:380–4.
48. Remington G et al. A PET study evaluating dopamine D2 receptor occupancy for long-acting injectable risperidone. Am J Psychiatry 2006;163:396–401.
49. Lane HY et al. Risperidone in acutely exacerbated schizophrenia: dosing strategies and plasma levels. J Clin Psychiatry 2000;61:209–14.
50. Taylor D. Risperidone long-acting injection in practice – more questions than answers? Acta Psychiatr Scand 2006;114:1–2.
51. Nyberg S et al. Suggested minimal effective dose of risperidone based on PET-measured D2 and 5-HT2A receptor occupancy in schizophrenic patients. Am J Psychiatry 1999;156:869–75.
52. Medori R et al. Plasma antipsychotic concentration and receptor occupancy, with special focus on risperidone long-acting injectable. Eur Neuropsychopharmacol 2006;16:233–40.
53. Gefvert O et al. Pharmacokinetics and D2 receptor occupancy of long-acting injectable risperidone (Risperdal Consta™) in patients with schizophrenia. Int J Neuropsychopharmacol 2005;8:27–36.
54. Nyberg S et al. D2 dopamine receptor occupancy during low-dose treatment with haloperidol decanoate. Am J Psychiatry 1995;152:173–8.

chapter 2

Schizophrenia

General introduction to antipsychotics[*]

The class of drugs used to treat schizophrenia and other psychotic illnesses is known as 'antipsychotics' (the terms 'neuroleptics' and 'major tranquillisers' are also sometimes used although neither is strictly correct).

The antipsychotic potency of most antipsychotics is directly proportional to their ability to block dopamine receptors in the brain, although the exact mechanism by which they exert their antipsychotic effect is probably more complicated than this. They vary greatly in their selectivity for dopamine receptors, many also having significant effects on acetylcholine, norepinephrine, histamine and serotonin pathways. A wide range of side-effects is therefore to be expected, the most common of which are listed below.

Extrapyramidal side-effects

- **Dystonic reactions** (such as oculogyric spasm and torticollis) may be treated with oral, im or iv anticholinergics, depending on their severity. Approximately 10% of patients exposed to the older typical drugs develop an acute dystonic reaction[1]. This is more likely in the early stages of treatment or after an increase in dose and can be both painful and very frightening. Adverse early experiences are likely to reduce long-term willingness to take medication. Dystonia may also occur on drug withdrawal. Tardive dystonia can be very difficult to treat.
- **Pseudoparkinsonism** (characterised by tremor, bradykinesia and rigidity) is seen in approximately 20% of patients prescribed typical drugs[2]. It can be

This section contains a brief overview of antipsychotic properties. Many issues are covered in greater depth in later sections.

8

treated with anticholinergic drugs, but not dopamine agonists, as these would obviously diminish the dopamine antagonistic action of the antipsychotics. Anticholinergics should not be prescribed prophylactically with antipsychotics. The majority of patients appear to cope without them in the long term. It is also worth noting that anticholinergics have their own side-effects (dry mouth, blurred vision, constipation, cognitive impairment, etc.) and may exacerbate tardive dyskinesia. They can also be misused for their euphoric effects and have a 'street value'.

- **Akathisia** (a subjectively unpleasant state of motor restlessness) responds poorly to anticholinergics. It is decidedly unpleasant and contributes to anxiety and dysphoria. Approximately 20–25% of patients prescribed the older drugs are affected[3]. If this is severe, it is often best to try a drug with a lower liability for akathisia – usually an atypical (see page 97). Alternatively a non-selective beta-blocker such as propranolol (10–20 mg t.d.s.)[4] is well supported, and the antihistamine cyproheptadine (4–8 mg b.d.)[5,6] may be worth a try. These approaches are probably equally effective[7]. It is important that akathisia is distinguished from agitation secondary to psychosis, as it may have serious consequences if left untreated (akathisia has been linked to violence and suicide)[8]. For further guidance see page 97.

- **Tardive dyskinesia** (TD) has traditionally been thought to be caused by supersensitivity of dopamine receptors, which develops because of prolonged therapy with dopamine-blocking drugs. This denervation supersensitivity theory has been supported by the observation that TD is temporarily improved by increasing the dose of the offending drug (this is the wrong approach clinically, as it can only perpetuate the problem). Undoubtedly, the aetiology of TD is more complex, probably involving GABA pathways to a significant extent. In the present state of our knowledge, TD is best dealt with by:
  - reducing and discontinuing anticholinergics
  - reducing the antipsychotic dose to the minimum that is effective
  - substituting older drugs with second-generation antipsychotics[9]
  - trying clozapine if appropriate (may actually treat TD as well as psychosis)[10].

If the above fail to control the abnormal movements, various other options (tetrabenazine, sodium valproate, etc.) may be worth pursuing depending on the circumstances of each individual case[11]. See page 99 for further guidance.

It is worth noting that dyskinesia indistinguishable from TD was seen in psychiatric patients long before the introduction of antipsychotic drugs[12,13] (and indeed occurs independently of psychiatric illness in around 2% of the normal elderly population)[14]. There was a recorded prevalence of 5% in patients with schizophrenia before the introduction of antipsychotics, rising to up to 20% thereafter[14]. Recent studies of older patients with schizophrenia who have never been treated with antipsychotic drugs show a prevalence rate similar to populations treated with antipsychotics. All patients treated with antipsychotics are at risk of developing TD, although patients with affective illness, diabetes and learning disabilities; females; and the elderly seem to be more likely to be affected[14]. Those with mood disorders may also be more at risk of developing tardive dystonia. The presence of EPSEs during treatment with antipsychotics is associated with a threefold increase in risk of TD, and it is likely that the newer atypical antipsychotics (which produce less frequent EPSEs) will be associated with a lower incidence of TD[9].

Hyperprolactinaemia

This is an expected phenomenon as prolactin is under the inhibitory control of dopamine. Hyperprolactinaemia can lead to galactorrhoea, amenorrhoea, gynaecomastia, hypogonadism, sexual dysfunction and an increased risk of osteoporosis[15-17]. Long-stay psychiatric female inpatients have been noted to have a ninefold increase in the risk of breast cancer when compared to the normal population[18]. Although other risk factors are undoubtedly important in this group of patients, prolonged hyperprolactinaemia is likely to be a contributing factor.

A measurement of serum prolactin can be a useful indicator that the (older, first generation) antipsychotic drug is being taken and is reaching CNS dopamine receptors. Prolactin levels of several thousand micrograms/litre may be seen when very high doses of antipsychotics are prescribed.

Of the newer antipsychotics, sertindole, quetiapine, ziprasidone, aripiprazole and clozapine have no important effect on prolactin. Olanzapine has a transient minimal effect. Risperidone, amisulpride and zotepine have potent prolactin-elevating effects, similar to conventional drugs. For further guidance on hyperprolactinaemia, see page 95.

Reduced seizure threshold

Grand mal seizures are a recognised side-effect of antipsychotic therapy (the higher the dose, the greater the risk). As a very general rule of thumb, the more sedative and less potent drugs carry a higher risk than the more potent, less sedative drugs. Clozapine carries the greatest risk[19]. Some antipsychotics have little or no effect on seizure threshold. See page 353 for further information on treating patients with pre-existing epilepsy.

Postural hypotension

Postural hypotension is mediated through adrenergic α_1-blockade, and so can usually be predicted for any drug with significant antagonist activity at this receptor. It is a particular risk when phenothiazines are prescribed for the elderly, but can also occur with higher doses of other antipsychotics in much younger patients. The atypical antipsychotics clozapine, risperidone, quetiapine and sertindole all have important affinity for α_1-receptors, making dosage titration necessary.

Anticholinergic side-effects

Anticholinergic side-effects include dry mouth (which may contribute to dental decay, ill-fitting dentures), blurred vision (which can contribute to falls in the elderly) and constipation (impaction can occur). Clozapine in particular has been associated with severe constipation resulting in gastrointestinal obstruction[20]. Anticholinergic effects may also have a detrimental impact on cognitive functioning.

Antipsychotics with potent anticholinergic effects (notably chlorpromazine and clozapine) should never be given to patients who have closed-angle glaucoma. Drugs with less potent anticholinergic side-effects (e.g. haloperidol) can be used with caution in open-angle glaucoma that is being treated and monitored, as long as the dosage used does not produce mydriasis. Drugs such as haloperidol, trifluoperazine and sulpiride may be used in prostatic hypertrophy.

Neuroleptic malignant syndrome (NMS)[21-23]

NMS may occur in as many as 0.5% of patients treated with first-generation antipsychotics and is thought to be greatly under-diagnosed. It is a potentially life-threatening complication of neuroleptic treatment, with the mortality rate estimated as being up to 20%. The main symptoms of NMS are mild hyperthermia, fluctuating consciousness, muscular rigidity, autonomic instability and severe EPSEs (primarily rigidity). Serum CPK is always raised. Leucocytosis (with a left shift) and abnormal LFTs are common. The enormous load of muscle breakdown products can lead to severe renal damage. The syndrome is believed to be caused by the rapid blockade of hypothalamic and striatal dopamine receptors, leading to a 'resetting' of the thermoregulatory systems and severe skeletal muscle spasm, which contributes to a considerable heat load that cannot be dissipated. The risk is greater the higher the starting dose of the antipsychotic and the more rapidly it is increased. All antipsychotics and other psychotropics, lithium and SSRIs have been implicated in NMS, with the majority of cases attributable to haloperidol. It is difficult to know if this is an inherent characteristic of haloperidol or if it is better explained by the fact that haloperidol is very widely prescribed in situations where initial high-dose antipsychotic therapy may be indicated.

Although it is primarily associated with antipsychotics, other drugs that interfere with dopaminergic neurotransmission have also been implicated in NMS[21] (e.g. MAOIs, TCAs, metoclopramide and tetrabenazine). Levodopa withdrawal has also been implicated.

Weight gain

In comparison with the general population, people with schizophrenia are more likely to be overweight and have increased quantities of visceral fat[24,25]. They are also at greater risk of developing hypertension, cardiovascular disease, type 2 diabetes and dyslipidaemia. In addition, antipsychotic-induced weight gain, particularly with atypicals, can be significant.

A substantial proportion of patients will gain 7% of their baseline body weight, which increases the risk of obesity-related morbidity (type 2 diabetes, heart disease, some cancers, etc.). Relative weight gain is difficult to determine, as there is no standard way of measuring it (5% gain, 7% gain, BMI, etc.). In general, clozapine has the greatest potential to cause weight gain, followed by olanzapine, then quetiapine and risperidone, and then amisulpride. Ziprasidone[26,27] and aripiprazole may be relatively weight neutral[28]. See page 110 for further information. Several case reports/case series associate clozapine and olanzapine with the development of hyperglycaemia, diabetes mellitus and ketoacidosis. Being male, non-Caucasian and aged around 40 years, and possibly being obese/having recent weight gain, would appear to be risk factors. The maximum period of risk may be the first 6 months of treatment. The likely mechanism is insulin resistance and this does not seem to be clearly dose-related. In approximately one-third of cases, ongoing treatment with oral hypoglycaemics or insulin is required, despite treatment with clozapine or olanzapine being discontinued[29]. See page XX for further guidance on weight gain and diabetes.

Others

Some antipsychotic drugs are sedative, some are cardiotoxic and many are associated with idiosyncratic side-effects. Further information can be found under the individual drug headings. Antipsychotic treatment is a risk factor for venous thromboembolism[30]; and in elderly patients who have dementia, for stroke[31,32]. All-cause mortality is higher in elderly patients who take first-generation as opposed to second-generation antipsychotic drugs[33].

References

1. American Psychiatric Association. Practice guideline for the treatment of patients with schizophrenia. Am J Psychiatry 1997;154:1–63.
2. Bollini P et al. Antipsychotic drugs: is more worse? A meta-analysis of the published randomized control trials. Psychol Med 1994;24:307–16.
3. Halstead SM et al. Akathisia: prevalence and associated dysphoria in an in-patient population with chronic schizophrenia. Br J Psychiatry 1994;164:177–83.
4. Miller CH et al. Managing antipsychotic-induced acute and chronic akathisia. Drug Saf 2000;22:73–81.
5. Weiss D et al. Cyproheptadine treatment in neuroleptic-induced akathisia. Br J Psychiatry 1995;167: 483–6.
6. Poyurovsky M et al. Serotonin-based pharmacotherapy for acute neuroleptic-induced akathisia: a new approach to an old problem. Br J Psychiatry 2001;179:4–8.
7. Fischel T et al. Cyproheptadine versus propranolol for the treatment of acute neuroleptic-induced akathisia: a comparative double-blind study. J Clin Psychopharmacol 2001;21:612–15.
8. Van Putten T et al. Behavioral toxicity of antipsychotic drugs. J Clin Psychiatry 1987;48(Suppl):13–19.
9. Glazer WM. Expected incidence of tardive dyskinesia associated with atypical antipsychotics. J Clin Psychiatry 2000;61(Suppl 4):21–6.
10. Simpson GM. The treatment of tardive dyskinesia and tardive dystonia. J Clin Psychiatry 2000; 61(Suppl 4):39–44.
11. Duncan D et al. Tardive dyskinesia: how is it prevented and treated? Psychiatr Bull 1997;21:422–5.
12. Fenton WS. Prevalence of spontaneous dyskinesia in schizophrenia. J Clin Psychiatry 2000;61(Suppl 4): 10–14.
13. McCreadie RG et al. Spontaneous dyskinesia and parkinsonism in never-medicated, chronically ill patients with schizophrenia: 18-month follow-up. Br J Psychiatry 2002;181:135–7.
14. American Psychiatric Association. Tardive dyskinesia: A task force report of the American Psychiatric Association. Hosp Community Psychiatry 1993;44:190.
15. Dickson RA et al. Hormonal side effects in women: typical versus atypical antipsychotic treatment. J Clin Psychiatry 2000;61(Suppl 3):10–15.
16. Halbreich U et al. Accelerated osteoporosis in psychiatric patients: possible pathophysiological processes. Schizophr Bull 1996;22:447–54.
17. Smith SM et al. Sexual dysfunction in patients taking conventional antipsychotic medication. Br J Psychiatry 2002;181:49–55.
18. Halbreich U et al. Are chronic psychiatric patients at increased risk for developing breast cancer? Am J Psychiatry 1996;153:559–60.
19. Devinsky O et al. Clozapine-related seizures. Neurology 1991;41:369–71.
20. MHRA and Committee on Safety in Medicines. Clozapine (Clozaril) and gastrointestinal obstruction. Curr Probl Pharmacovig 1999;25:5–8.
21. Velamoor VR. Neuroleptic malignant syndrome. Recognition, prevention and management. Drug Saf 1998;19:73–82.
22. Pelonero AL et al. Neuroleptic malignant syndrome: a review. Psychiatr Serv 1998;49:1163–72.
23. Adityanjee A et al. Epidemiology of neuroleptic malignant syndrome. Clin Neuropharmacol 1999;22: 151–8.
24. Meyer JM. Effects of atypical antipsychotics on weight and serum lipid levels. J Clin Psychiatry 2001;62(Suppl 27):27–34.
25. Thakore JH et al. Increased visceral fat distribution in drug-naive and drug-free patients with schizophrenia. Int J Obes Relat Metab Disord 2002;26:137–41.
26. Taylor DM et al. Atypical antipsychotics and weight gain – a systematic review. Acta Psychiatr Scand 2000;101:416–32.
27. Allison D et al. Antipsychotic-induced weight gain: a comprehensive research synthesis. Am J Psychiatry 1999;156:1686–96.

28. Jody D et al. Meta-analysis of weight effects with aripiprazole. Int J Neuropsychopharmacol 2002; 5(Suppl 1):S186.
29. Mir S et al. Atypical antipsychotics and hyperglycaemia. Int Clin Psychopharmacol 2001;16:63–74.
30. Zornberg GL et al. Antipsychotic drug use and risk of first-time idiopathic venous thromboembolism: a case-control study. Lancet 2000;356:1219–23.
31. Schneider LS et al. Atypical antipsychotic drug treatment for dementia. Meta-analysis of randomized placebo-controlled trials. JAMA 2005;294:1934–43.
32. Gill SS et al. Atypical antipsychotic drugs and risk of ischaemic stroke: population based retrospective cohort study. BMJ 2005;330:445.
33. Wang PS et al. Risk of death in elderly users of conventional vs. atypical antipsychotic medications. N Engl J Med 2005;353:2335–41.

Antipsychotics – equivalent doses

Antipsychotic drugs vary greatly in potency (not the same as efficacy), and this is usually expressed as differences in 'neuroleptic' or 'chlorpromazine' 'equivalents'. Some of the estimates relating to neuroleptic equivalents are based on early dopamine-binding studies and some largely on clinical experience or even guesswork. *BNF* maximum doses for antipsychotic drugs bear little relationship to their 'neuroleptic equivalents'. The following table gives some approximate equivalent doses for conventional drugs[1,2]. Values given should be seen as a rough guide when transferring from one conventional drug to another. An early review of progress is essential.

Table Equivalent doses

Drug	Equivalent dose (consensus) (mg/day)	Range of values in literature (mg/day)
Chlorpromazine	100	–
Fluphenazine	2	2–5
Trifluoperazine	5	2.5–5
Flupentixol	3	2–3
Zuclopenthixol	25	25–60
Haloperidol	3	1.5–5
Sulpiride	200	200–270
Pimozide	2	2
Loxapine	10	10–25
Fluphenazine *depot*	5/week	1–12.5/week
Pipotiazine *depot*	10/week	10–12.5/week
Flupentixol *depot*	10/week	10–20/week
Zuclopenthixol *depot*	100/week	40–100/week
Haloperidol *depot*	15/week	5–25/week

It is inappropriate to convert second-generation antipsychotic doses into 'equivalents' since the dose–response relationship is usually well-defined for these drugs. Dosage guidelines are discussed under each individual drug. See page 15 for further discussion. Those readers desperate to find chlorpromazine equivalents for the newer drugs are directed to the only published paper listing such data[3].

References

1. Foster P. Neuroleptic equivalence. Pharm J 1989;243:431–2.
2. Atkins M et al. Chlorpromazine equivalents: a consensus of opinion for both clinical and research implications. Psychiatr Bull 1997;21:224–6.
3. Woods SW. Chlorpromazine equivalent doses for the newer atypical antipsychotics. J Clin Psychiatry 2003;64:663–7.

Antipsychotics – minimum effective doses

The table below suggests the minimum dose of antipsychotic likely to be effective in schizophrenia (first episode or relapse). At least some patients will respond to the dose suggested, although others may require higher doses. Given the variation in individual response, all doses should be considered approximate. Primary references are provided where available, but consensus opinion has also been used (as have standard texts such as the *BNF* and *Summaries of Product Characteristics*). Only oral treatment with commonly used drugs is covered.

Table   Minimum effective dose/day – antipsychotics

Drug	1st episode	Relapse	References
FGAs			
Chlorpromazine	200 mg*	300 mg	–
Haloperidol	2 mg	>4 mg	1–5
Sulpiride	400 mg*	800 mg	6
Trifluoperazine	10 mg*	15 mg	7
SGAs			
Amisulpride	400 mg*	800 mg	8–10
Aripiprazole	10 mg*	10 mg	11, 12
Olanzapine	5 mg	10 mg	5, 13, 14
Quetiapine	150 mg*	300 mg	15–18
Risperidone	2 mg	4 mg	4, 19–21
Sertindole	Not appropriate	12 mg	22
Ziprasidone	80 mg*	80 mg	23–25
Zotepine	75 mg*	150 mg	26, 27

*Estimate – too few data available.

References

1. Oosthuizen P et al. Determining the optimal dose of haloperidol in first-episode psychosis. J Psychopharmacol 2001;15:251–5.
2. McGorry PD. Recommended haloperidol and risperidone doses in first-episode psychosis. J Clin Psychiatry 1999;60:794–5.
3. Waraich PS et al. Haloperidol dose for the acute phase of schizophrenia. Cochrane Database Syst Rev 2002;CD001951.
4. Schooler N et al. Risperidone and haloperidol in first-episode psychosis: a long-term randomized trial. Am J Psychiatry 2005;162:947–53.
5. Keefe RS et al. Long-term neurocognitive effects of olanzapine or low-dose haloperidol in first-episode psychosis. Biol Psychiatry 2006;59:97–105.
6. Soares BG et al. Sulpiride for schizophrenia. Cochrane Database Syst Rev 2000;CD001162.
7. Armenteros JL et al. Antipsychotics in early onset schizophrenia: systematic review and meta-analysis. Eur Child Adolesc Psychiatry 2006;15:141–8.
8. Mota NE et al. Amisulpride for schizophrenia. Cochrane Database Syst Rev 2002;CD001357.
9. Puech A et al. Amisulpride, an atypical antipsychotic, in the treatment of acute episodes of schizophrenia: a dose-ranging study vs. haloperidol. The Amisulpride Study Group. Acta Psychiatr Scand 1998;98:65–72.
10. Moller HJ et al. Improvement of acute exacerbations of schizophrenia with amisulpride: a comparison with haloperidol. PROD-ASLP Study Group. Psychopharmacology 1997;132:396–401.
11. Taylor D. Aripiprazole: a review of its pharmacology and clinical utility. Int J Clin Pract 2003;57:49–54.
12. Cutler AJ et al. The efficacy and safety of lower doses of aripiprazole for the treatment of patients with acute exacerbation of schizophrenia. CNS Spectr 2006;11:691–702.
13. Sanger TM et al. Olanzapine versus haloperidol treatment in first-episode psychosis. Am J Psychiatry 1999;156:79–87.
14. Kasper S. Risperidone and olanzapine: optimal dosing for efficacy and tolerability in patients with schizophrenia. Int Clin Psychopharmacol 1998;13:253–62.
15. Small JG et al. Quetiapine in patients with schizophrenia. A high- and low-dose double-blind comparison with placebo. Seroquel Study Group. Arch Gen Psychiatry 1997;54:549–57.
16. Peuskens J et al. A comparison of quetiapine and chlorpromazine in the treatment of schizophrenia. Acta Psychiatr Scand 1997;96:265–73.
17. Arvanitis LA et al. Multiple fixed doses of "Seroquel" (quetiapine) in patients with acute exacerbation of schizophrenia: a comparison with haloperidol and placebo. Biol Psychiatry 1997;42:233–46.
18. Kopala LC et al. Treatment of a first episode of psychotic illness with quetiapine: an analysis of 2 year outcomes. Schizophr Res 2006;81:29–39.
19. Lane HY et al. Risperidone in acutely exacerbated schizophrenia: dosing strategies and plasma levels. J Clin Psychiatry 2000;61:209–14.
20. Williams R. Optimal dosing with risperidone: updated recommendations. J Clin Psychiatry 2001;62:282–9.
21. Ezewuzie N et al. Establishing a dose–response relationship for oral risperidone in relapsed schizophrenia. J Psychopharmacol 2006;20:86–90.
22. Lindstrom E et al. Sertindole: efficacy and safety in schizophrenia. Expert Opin Pharmacother 2006;7:1825–34.
23. Bagnall A et al. Ziprasidone for schizophrenia and severe mental illness. Cochrane Database Syst Rev 2000;CD001945.
24. Taylor D. Ziprasidone – an atypical antipsychotic. Pharm J 2001;266:396–401.
25. Joyce AT et al. Effect of initial ziprasidone dose on length of therapy in schizophrenia. Schizophr Res 2006;83:285–92.
26. Petit M et al. A comparison of an atypical and typical antipsychotic, zotepine versus haloperidol in patients with acute exacerbation of schizophrenia: a parallel-group double-blind trial. Psychopharmacol Bull 1996;32:81–7.
27. Palmgren K et al. The safety and efficacy of zotepine in the treatment of schizophrenia: results of a one-year naturalistic clinical trial. Int J Psychiatry Clin Pract 2000;4:299–306.

Further reading

Davis JM et al. Dose response and dose equivalence of antipsychotics. J Clin Psychopharmacol 2004;24:192–208.

Antipsychotics – licensed maximum doses

The table below lists the UK licensed maximum doses of antipsychotics.

Drug	Maximum dose (mg/day)
FGAs	
Chlorpromazine	1000
Flupentixol	18
Fluphenazine	20
Haloperidol	30 (see *BNF*)
Levomepromazine	1000
Loxapine	250
Pericyazine	300
Perphenazine	24
Pimozide	20
Trifluoperazine	None (suggest 30)
Zuclopenthixol	150
SGAs	
Amisulpride	1200
Aripiprazole	30
Clozapine	900
Olanzapine	20
Quetiapine	750/800 (see *BNF*)
Risperidone	16 (see *BNF*)
Sertindole	24
Sulpiride	2400
Ziprasidone*	160
Zotepine	300
Depots	
Flupentixol depot	400/week
Fluphenazine depot	50/week
Haloperidol depot	300 every 4 weeks (see *BNF*)
Pipotiazine depot	50/week
Risperidone	25/week
Zuclopenthixol depot	600/week

Note: Doses above these maxima should only be used in extreme circumstances: there is no evidence for improved efficacy.
*Not available in the UK at time of publication. US labelling used.

New antipsychotics – costs

Newer antipsychotics are relatively costly medicines, although their benefits may make them cost-effective in practice. Cost minimisation is a practical option that reduces drug expenditure without compromising patient care or patient quality of life. It involves using the right drug for the most appropriate condition (see Protocols) and using the minimum effective dose in each patient. The table below gives the cost (£/patient per 30 days) in January 2007 of atypicals at their estimated lowest effective dose, their approximate average clinical dose and their licensed maximum dose. The table allows comparison of different doses of the same drug and of different drugs at any of the three doses. It is hoped that the table will encourage the use of lower doses of less expensive drugs, given equality in other respects and allowing for clinical requirements.

Table Monthly costs of new antipsychotics

Drug dose	Minimum effective dose cost (see page XX)	Approximate average clinical dose cost	Maximum cost
Amisulpride*	400 mg/day (depends on indication – see *BNF*) £61.38	800 mg/day £122.76	1200 mg/day £184.14
Aripiprazole	10 mg/day £108.89	20 mg/day £217.78	30 mg/day £217.78
Olanzapine	10 mg/day £85.12	15 mg/day £127.69	20 mg/day £170.25
Quetiapine	300 mg/day £85.00	500 mg/day £141.55	750 mg/day £226.55
Risperidone *(injection)*	25 mg/2 weeks £165.84/28 days	37.5 mg/2 weeks £231.68/28 days	50 mg/2 weeks £297.10/28 days
Risperidone *(oral)*	4 mg/day £68.69	6 mg/day £101.01	16 mg/day £200.01
Sertindole	16 mg/day POA	20 mg/day POA	24 mg/day POA
Zotepine	150 mg/day £50.62	300 mg/day £94.55	300 mg/day £94.55

*Generic version expected – check latest price.

Notes:
- costs for UK adults (30 days), MIMS, January 2007
- average clinical doses for inpatients receiving maintenance therapy
- clozapine costs not included because it has different indications.

POA, price on application.

Choice of antipsychotic

The *BNF* states that 'the various antipsychotic drugs differ somewhat in predominant actions and side-effects. Selection is influenced by the degree of sedation required and the patient's susceptibility to EPSEs. However, the differences between antipsychotic drugs are less important than the greater variability in patient response.'

In general, second-generation antipsychotics (SGAs) are associated with fewer EPSEs than first-generation antipsychotics (FGAs), and some do not raise prolactin. With the exception of clozapine, efficacy advantages are minimal. Most SGAs have relatively narrow licensed indications compared with FGAs, and are considerably more expensive.

Phenothiazines

These are often divided into a further three subgroups, depending on their basic chemistry and, coincidentally, the degree of sedation they produce.

Chlorpromazine and **promazine** are the most sedative, and chlorpromazine the most widely prescribed phenothiazine. Chlorpromazine causes photosensitivity reactions (hence the need for liberal amounts of high-factor sunscreen in the summer), and occasionally a hypersensitivity reaction resembling obstructive jaundice (the block being biochemical and not mechanical). Chlorpromazine is epileptogenic in a dose-dependent fashion and can cause significant weight gain. Promazine has a relatively good side-effect profile and so is suitable for the elderly, if it is sufficient to control symptoms. It is not effective in schizophrenia.

Pericyazine and **pipotiazine** are relatively less likely to produce EPSEs. Pericyazine is particularly sedative and rarely prescribed. Pipotiazine is available only in depot form. Thioridazine has been withdrawn from the UK market because of its potential to cause QTc prolongation[1].

Fluphenazine and **trifluoperazine** are the least sedative phenothiazines but are more likely to cause EPSEs. Trifluoperazine is available as tablets, liquid and controlled-release capsules. There is little rationale in prescribing the more expensive controlled-release preparation, as, sedation aside, most antipsychotics can be administered once daily in their conventional form.

Butyrophenones

Haloperidol is the most widely prescribed drug in this group. It is a very potent D_2 blocker. It has been suggested that plasma levels of 5–12 µg/l are associated with optimal response and that such levels are achievable with daily doses of no more than 20 mg. Studies have shown that optimal response is achieved from daily doses of no more than 10 mg although much higher doses are commonly seen (and are associated with a high prevalence of EPSEs)[2]. Some studies suggest a non-linear relationship between dose and response, with a paradoxical response being possible when high doses are used. It has been suggested that the observed paradoxical response may be due to an increased incidence of EPSEs, akathisia and akinesia being interpreted as increased agitation and an increase in negative symptoms, respectively. The *BNF* maximum dose for oral haloperidol has decreased over the past few years from 120 to 15 mg/day (or 30 mg in treatment-resistant schizophrenia). **Droperidol** is no longer available in the UK (because of an association with QTc prolongation). Benperidol is rarely prescribed.

Thioxanthines

Flupentixol is the most widely prescribed member of this group and is used mostly in depot form. Low doses of flupentixol are claimed to have an antidepressant effect and, although there is a small hint (by no means proven) in some very old literature that this may be the case in psychosis, it is not a suitable treatment for depression.

Diphenylbutylpiperidines

Pimozide is a relatively specific D_2 antagonist and therefore has a side-effect profile consisting mainly of EPSEs and prolactin-related problems. The major disadvantage of pimozide is its potential to cause QTc prolongation and postulated association with sudden unexplained death[3]. A pre-treatment ECG is required, other drugs with the potential to prolong the QTc or cause electrolyte disturbances should not be co-prescribed and all patients should have an annual ECG. These restrictions mean that pimozide is rarely prescribed. Pimozide is claimed to be particularly useful in the treatment of monosymptomatic hypochondriacal psychoses (originating from a small open case series – a very poor evidence base).

Second-generation (atypical) antipsychotics

The term 'atypical' was originally associated with the inability of a compound to produce catalepsy in laboratory animals (a screening model thought to have good predictive validity in identifying potential antipsychotic agents). Atypical antipsychotics were also defined as having no effect on serum prolactin. More recently, the term has been used to describe antipsychotics that are highly selective D_2 blockers, those that are relatively selective for D_2 receptors in mesolimbic areas, those that have a high $5HT_2:D_2$ receptor blocking ratio and those that are claimed to have an effect on negative symptomatology. The definition of this term is likely to become even more confused in the future, should any of the more novel compounds presently being developed reach the market (dopamine autoreceptor agonists, NMDA agonists, $5HT_3$ antagonists, sigma antagonists, etc.). Atypical antipsychotics do cause fewer EPSEs than most of the older drugs, but are not devoid of other side-effects. These effects are discussed for individual drugs below.

Clozapine

Clozapine is the archetypal atypical antipsychotic. Clozapine has been around since the 1960s and was withdrawn from use after an association with neutropenia (incidence 3%) and agranulocytosis (0.8%) was made. The pivotal study by Kane et al.[4] in the late 1980s proved that clozapine was more effective than conventional antipsychotics, and it was reintroduced in the UK with compulsory haematological monitoring. Patients must be registered with an approved clozapine monitoring service (CPMS, ZTAS, etc.) and have a full blood count performed weekly for the first 18 weeks (when the risk of neutropenia/agranulocytosis is greatest)[5], fortnightly until 52 weeks of treatment, and then monthly thereafter if haematologically stable (the incidence of agranulocytosis after 1 year is similar to that associated with the phenothiazines[4]). Studies have shown that 30% of patients who have previously been refractory to treatment improve significantly after 6 weeks' treatment with clozapine, and up to 60% respond after 1 year. Although claims are made for the efficacy of clozapine in negative symptomatology, clinical gains in this area are much less marked[6,7]. Clozapine treatment reduces suicidality[8] and the data are sufficient[9] for specific labelling for this indication in the USA.

The pharmacology of clozapine is unusual compared with other antipsychotics in that it only binds weakly to D_1 and D_2 receptors, while having an affinity for D_4, $5HT_2$, $5HT_3$, α_1 and α_2 adrenergic, and ACh M_1 and H_1 receptors. Which one/combination of any of these effects is responsible for the superior clinical profile of clozapine is a subject of extensive speculation, but as of yet, no firm conclusion.

Clozapine also has a unique side-effect profile in that it has been associated with an extremely low incidence of EPSEs, and is thought not to cause/precipitate TD (it has even been suggested that clozapine can be an effective treatment for existing TD – see page 99). Clozapine does not raise prolactin levels and so is not associated with amenorrhoea. Menstruation will return and effective contraception is essential in sexually active females.

The side-effects commonly associated with clozapine and advice on their management can be found on page 70. Rare, serious side-effects are outlined on page 75.

Other SGAs[10]

The other SGAs, sulpiride, amisulpride, risperidone, sertindole, olanzapine, quetiapine, ziprasidone, aripiprazole and zotepine, have not been proven to be effective in treating resistant illness. They are advocated as better tolerated first-line treatments[11].

Sulpiride was arguably the first member of this group to be marketed and is often termed typical or at least grouped with them. FGAs are all effective in treating positive symptoms (i.e. formal thought disorder, passivity feelings, delusions and hallucinations) and, given prophylactically, they substantially reduce the relapse rate for many patients (see page 57). None of these compounds, however, directly or significantly, improves the manifestations of negative symptomatology (i.e. anergia, apathy, flattening of affect and poverty of speech), all of which are a major cause of long-term deterioration, withdrawal and isolation amongst patients with schizophrenia.

Sulpiride was the first antipsychotic for which claims were made regarding its effect upon negative symptomatology (although it must be noted that this effect is not striking). It has a dose-related selectivity for pre-synaptic D_4 and post-synaptic D_2 receptors. In low doses (less than 800 mg/day) the main affinity is for D_4 receptors, which are auto-inhibitory. The inhibitory control of dopamine release is therefore decreased and more dopamine is available in the synaptic cleft. Above 800 mg/day the affinity for D_2 receptors dominates, resulting in the post-synaptic blockade of D_2 receptors.

Sulpiride is associated with slightly less frequent EPSEs than the older drugs and, as such, may also be associated with less potential for causing TD. It can cause marked increases in serum prolactin.

Amisulpride is similar to sulpiride in that lower doses (300 mg/day or less) selectively block pre-synaptic dopamine receptors, leading to an increase in dopamine transmission in the prefrontal cortex (the site supposedly responsible for the genesis of negative symptoms). At higher doses, it blocks post-synaptic dopamine receptors and is relatively selective for limbic rather than striatal areas, which translates clinically into a low potential for EPSEs. Amisulpride is relatively free from sedation, anticholinergic side-effects and postural hypotension, but, like sulpiride, is a particularly potent elevator of serum prolactin. The difference clinically between amisulpride and sulpiride is unclear; there are no head-to-head studies. Amisulpride is significantly more expensive at the time of writing, but a cheaper generic form is expected.

Risperidone is a potent $5HT_2:D_2$ antagonist. It was developed in line with the observation that ritanserin (a potent $5HT_2$ receptor antagonist), when given in combination with conventional antipsychotics, was effective in treating the negative and affective symptoms of schizophrenia[12]. In doses of 6 mg or less per day, risperidone is associated with a low incidence of EPSEs and sedation. It is associated with hyperprolactinaemia. Risperidone has a first-dose hypotensive effect (due to α_1 blockade), and in order to minimise this, an increasing-dosage regimen is used over the first few days. There have been reports of nausea, dyspepsia, abdominal pain, dyspnoea and chest pain associated with its use.

Sertindole is also associated with significant α_1 blockade and therefore dosage titration is required. Its major advantages are that it produces virtually no EPSEs within the licensed dosage range and has no effect on prolactin. Its major disadvantage is that it is associated with QTc prolongation, and it is recommended that an ECG is obtained before initiating therapy. Sertindole has been tentatively linked with a number of cases of 'antipsychotic-associated sudden death'[13], and in November 1998 its licence was suspended by several European countries. Sertindole was subsequently voluntarily withdrawn from general use by the manufacturers, but has now been reintroduced, following studies demonstrating its apparent safety.

Olanzapine is also a $5HT_2:D_2$ blocker. It is sedative, produces some postural hypotension and has anticholinergic side-effects. Although chemically and pharmacologically very similar to clozapine, olanzapine has been licensed as a first-line antipsychotic, and there is currently no compelling evidence to support its efficacy in treatment-resistant illness. Olanzapine has minimal effects on serum prolactin and may be associated with a lower incidence of sexual dysfunction than other antipsychotics. Clinical trials have shown that 10–20 mg olanzapine/day is the most effective dose. Because it is well tolerated, with the exception of weight gain and associated adverse metabolic effects, prescribers may feel tempted to increase the dose above 20 mg (the licensed maximum) in partial or non-responders. Such patients would be more appropriately treated with clozapine. Olanzapine plasma levels can be measured and this may be useful when non-compliance is suspected. See page 4 for further guidance on plasma level monitoring.

Quetiapine has a low affinity for D_1, D_2 and $5HT_2$ receptors and moderate affinity for adrenergic α_1 and α_2 receptors. It is relatively mesolimbic-specific and does not raise serum prolactin; however, it does require dosage titration (like risperidone and sertindole). Quetiapine is considered to be a well-tolerated antipsychotic. There are very few data to suggest that it may be effective in treatment-resistant illness.

Zotepine is an antagonist at $5HT_{2a}$, $5HT_{2c}$, D_1, D_2, D_3 and D_4 receptors, a potent inhibitor of norepinephrine reuptake, and a potent H_1 antagonist (sedative), with some α_1 adrenergic blocking activity (postural hypotension) and possibly some activity at NMDA receptors. It raises serum prolactin and is associated with a high incidence of seizures. Doses above 300 mg/day (frequently used according to the available literature) and antipsychotic polypharmacy increase this risk. There are very few trial data comparing zotepine with other atypical antipsychotics. There is no study of any quality in refractory illness reported in the English language literature. Zotepine is rarely prescribed in the UK.

Ziprasidone has been available in the USA and some European countries for several years. It is a $5HT_2$:D_2 antagonist with significant agonist activity at $5HT_{1A}$ receptors and moderately potent inhibition of monoamine reuptake[14,15]. Efficacy is similar to haloperidol[16] and olanzapine[17] and tolerability is good; most adverse effects occur at the same frequency as placebo and EPSEs, hyperprolactinaemia and weight gain are uncommon[18,19]. Ziprasidone has a moderate effect on the QT interval, which may, at least in theory, make it relatively more likely than other antipsychotics to cause ventricular arrhythmia (see page 116)[20]. This potential problem should be set against the clear advantages of ziprasidone in relation to weight gain[21] and impaired glucose tolerance[22]. Switching to ziprasidone because of the adverse effects of other antipsychotics seems to be safe and effective[23].

Aripiprazole is a partial agonist at D_2 receptors: full binding to D_2 receptors reduces dopaminergic neuronal activity by about 30% (in the absence of dopamine, aripiprazole acts as a weak agonist)[24]. It is a potent antagonist at $5HT_{2A}$ receptors and a partial agonist at $5HT_{1A}$ receptors[25]. Aripiprazole appears to be at least as effective as haloperidol[26] and risperidone[27] and is well tolerated with a low incidence (placebo level) of extra-pyramidal symptoms[28]. It is not associated with symptomatic hyperprolactinaemia, QTc prolongation, impaired glucose tolerance or substantial weight gain[29–31]. Switching to aripiprazole from other antipsychotics seems safe and effective by any method[32]. Clinical experience suggests tolerability may be improved in some by starting at 10 mg daily.

References

1. Reilly JG et al. QTc-interval abnormalities and psychotropic drug therapy in psychiatric patients. Lancet 2000;355:1048–52.
2. Hilton T et al. Which dose of haloperidol? Psychiatr Bull 1996;20:359–62.
3. Committee on Safety of Medicines. Cardiotoxic effects of pimozide. Curr Probl Pharmacovig 1990;29:1.
4. Kane J et al. Clozapine for the treatment-resistant schizophrenic. A double-blind comparison with chlorpromazine. Arch Gen Psychiatry 1988;45:789–96.
5. Atkin K et al. Neutropenia and agranulocytosis in patients receiving clozapine in the UK and Ireland. Br J Psychiatry 1996;169:483–8.
6. Rosenheck R et al. Impact of clozapine on negative symptoms and on the deficit syndrome in refractory schizophrenia. Department of Veterans Affairs Cooperative Study Group on Clozapine in Refractory Schizophrenia. Am J Psychiatry 1999;156:88–93.
7. Breier AF et al. Clozapine and risperidone in chronic schizophrenia: effects on symptoms, parkinsonian side effects, and neuroendocrine response. Am J Psychiatry 1999;156:294–8.
8. Meltzer HY et al. Reduction of suicidality during clozapine treatment of neuroleptic-resistant schizophrenia: impact on risk–benefit assessment. Am J Psychiatry 1995;152:183–90.
9. Meltzer HY et al. Clozapine treatment for suicidality in schizophrenia: International Suicide Prevention Trial (InterSePT). Arch Gen Psychiatry 2003;60:82–91.
10. Gardner DM et al. Modern antipsychotic drugs: a critical overview. CMAJ 2005;172:1703–11.
11. Taylor DM et al. Refractory schizophrenia and atypical antipsychotics. J Psychopharmacol 2000;14: 409–18.
12. Duinkerke SJ et al. Ritanserin, a selective 5-HT2/1C antagonist, and negative symptoms in schizophrenia. A placebo-controlled double-blind trial. Br J Psychiatry 1993;163:451–5.
13. Fritze J et al. The QT interval and the atypical antipsychotic sertindole. Int J Psychiatry Clin Pract 1998; 2:265–73.
14. Taylor D. Ziprasidone – an atypical antipsychotic. Pharm J 2001;266:396–401.
15. Davis R et al. Ziprasidone. CNS Drugs 1997;8:153–9.
16. Goff DC et al. An exploratory haloperidol-controlled dose-finding study of ziprasidone in hospitalized patients with schizophrenia or schizoaffective disorder. J Clin Psychopharmacol 1998;18:296–304.
17. Simpson GM et al. Randomized, controlled, double-blind multicenter comparison of the efficacy and tolerability of ziprasidone and olanzapine in acutely ill inpatients with schizophrenia or schizoaffective disorder. Am J Psychiatry 2004;161:1837–47.
18. Keck P Jr. et al. Ziprasidone 40 and 120 mg/day in the acute exacerbation of schizophrenia and schizoaffective disorder: a 4-week placebo-controlled trial. Psychopharmacology 1998;140:173–84.
19. Keck PE Jr. et al. Ziprasidone in the short-term treatment of patients with schizoaffective disorder: results from two double-blind, placebo-controlled, multicenter studies. J Clin Psychopharmacol 2001;21:27–35.
20. Taylor D. Ziprasidone in the management of schizophrenia: the QT interval issue in context. CNS Drugs 2003;17:423–30.
21. Taylor DM et al. Atypical antipsychotics and weight gain – a systematic review. Acta Psychiatr Scand 2000;101:416–32.
22. Kingsbury SJ et al. The apparent effects of ziprasidone on plasma lipids and glucose. J Clin Psychiatry 2001;62:347–9.
23. Weiden PJ et al. Effectiveness of switching to ziprasidone for stable but symptomatic outpatients with schizophrenia. J Clin Psychiatry 2003;64:580–8.
24. Burris KD et al. Aripiprazole, a novel antipsychotic, is a high-affinity partial agonist at human dopamine D_2 receptors. J Pharmacol Exp Ther 2002;302:381–9.
25. Jordan S et al. The antipsychotic aripiprazole is a potent, partial agonist at the human 5-HT$_{1A}$ receptor. Eur J Pharmacol 2002;441:137–40.
26. Kane JM et al. Efficacy and safety of aripiprazole and haloperidol versus placebo in patients with schizophrenia and schizoaffective disorder. J Clin Psychiatry 2002;63:763–71.
27. Potkin SG et al. Aripiprazole, an antipsychotic with a novel mechanism of action, and risperidone vs placebo in patients with schizophrenia and schizoaffective disorder. Arch Gen Psychiatry 2003;60: 681–90.
28. Petrie JL et al. Aripiprazole, a new typical antipsychotic: Phase 2 clinical trial result. Eur Neuropsychopharmacol 1997;7:227.
29. Pigott TA et al. Aripiprazole for the prevention of relapse in stabilized patients with chronic schizophrenia: a placebo-controlled 26-week study. J Clin Psychiatry 2003;64:1048–56.
30. Marder SR et al. Aripiprazole in the treatment of schizophrenia: safety and tolerability in short-term, placebo-controlled trials. Schizophr Res 2003;61:123–36.
31. Jody D et al. Meta-analysis of weight effects with aripiprazole. Int J Neuropsychopharmacol 2002; 5(Suppl 1):S186.
32. Casey DE et al. Switching patients to aripiprazole from other antipsychotic agents: a multicenter randomized study. Psychopharmacology 2003;166:391–9.

New antipsychotics

Paliperidone

Paliperidone (9-OH risperidone) is the major active metabolite of risperidone; in-vitro data demonstrate rapid dissociation from D_2 receptors, predicting a low propensity to cause EPS[1]. It is a D_2 and $5HT_{2a}$ antagonist[2] currently in phase 3 clinical trials for schizophrenia formulated as an osmotic controlled-release oral delivery system (OROS) to reduce fluctuations in plasma levels and remove the need for dosage titration[3]. Paliperidone undergoes limited hepatic metabolism and this may reduce the potential for drug interactions[4].

A pooled analysis of three 6-week placebo controlled studies found paliperidone 3–15 mg to be more effective than placebo and relatively well tolerated[5]. In common with risperidone, paliperidone can cause headache. With respect to weight gain, 9% of paliperidone-treated patients gained >7% of their baseline bodyweight compared with 5% of patients treated with placebo[6]. Extra-pyramidal side effects are fairly common in people receiving 9 mg and 12 mg daily[7]. Doses of 6 mg and 12 mg have been shown to be more effective than placebo and to have equivalent efficacy to olanzapine 10 mg in a 6-week study in adults with schizophrenia[8]. Doses of 6–9 mg are effective and well tolerated in patients with schizophrenia who are >65 years old[9]. There are limited long-term data[10] suggesting efficacy in preventing relapse.

Bifeprunox

Bifeprunox is a D_2 partial agonist and $5HT_{1a}$ agonist with minimal propensity to increase serum prolactin[11].

Asenapine

Asenapine has affinity for D_2, $5HT_{2a}$, $5HT_{2c}$ and α_1 and α_2 adrenergic receptors along with relatively low affinity for H_1 and ACh receptors[12]. At a dose of 5 mg twice daily, asenapine has been demonstrated to be more effective than placebo in the acute treatment of schizophrenia and more effective than risperidone in the treatment of negative symptoms[13]; perhaps through selective affinity for different dopamine pathways, most notably in the pre-frontal cortex[14]. Asenapine has less potential to raise prolactin than risperidone and may also be associated with a lower risk of weight gain[15].

References

1. Seeman P. An update of fast-off dopamine D_2 atypical antipsychotics. Am J Psychiatry 2005;162:1984–5.
2. Karlsson P et al. Pharmacokinetics, dopamine D_2 and serotonin 5-HT_{2A} receptor occupancy and safety profile of paliperidone in healthy subjects: two open-label, single-dose studies. Poster presented at ASCPT 8–11 March, 2006, Baltimore.
3. Conley R et al. Review of the clinical spectrum of the osmotic-controlled release oral delivery system (OROS) and application in central nervous system disorders. Poster presented at CINP 9–13 July, 2006, Chicago, IL, USA.
4. Vermeir M et al. Absorption, metabolism and excretion of a single oral dose of 14C-paliperidone 1 mg in healthy subjects. Clin Pharmacol Ther 2006;79:80.
5. Meltzer H et al. Efficacy and tolerability of oral paliperidone extended-release tablets in the treatment of acute schizophrenia: pooled data from three 6-week placebo-controlled studies. Poster presented at CINP 9–13 July, 2006, Chicago, IL, USA.
6. Meyer J et al. Metabolic outcomes in patients with schizophrenia treated with oral paliperidone extended-release tablets: pooled analysis of three 6-week placebo-controlled studies. Poster presented at CINP 9–13 July, 2006, Chicago, IL, USA.
7. Aspiazu S et al. Insight and depressive symptoms in first episode psychosis. Eur Neuropsychopharmacol 2006;16(Suppl 4):S385.
8. Marder S et al. A 6-week, US based, placebo-controlled study on the efficacy and tolerability of two fixed dosages of oral paliperidone extended-release tablets in the treatment of acute schizophrenia. Poster presented at APA 20–25 May, 2006, Toronto, Canada.
9. Tzimos A et al. A 6-week placebo-controlled study on the safety and tolerability of flexible doses of oral paliperidone extended-release tablets in the treatment of schizophrenia in elderly patients. Poster presented at the CINP 9–13 July, 2006, Chicago, IL, USA.
10. Kramer M et al. Delaying symptom recurrence in patients with schizophrenia with paliperidone extended-release tablet: an international, randomised, double-blind, placebo-controlled study. Poster presented at CINP 9–13 July, 2006, Chicago, IL, USA.
11. Cosi C et al. Partial agonist properties of the antipsychotics SSR181507, aripiprazole and bifeprunox at dopamine D_2 receptors: G protein activation and prolactin release. Eur J Pharmacol 2006;535:135–44.
12. Shahid M et al. Asenapine: a novel psychopharmacologic agent with a unique human receptor binding signature. Schizophr Res 2006;81(Suppl 1):107.
13. Potkin G et al. Asenapine: a novel psychotherapeutic agent with efficacy in positive and negative symptoms during acute episodes of schizophrenia: a randomised, placebo and risperidone controlled trial. Schizophr Res 2006;81(Suppl 1):62.
14. Moran-Gates T. Long-term administration of asenapine causes differential regional and dose-related effects on dopamine receptor subtypes. Biol Psychiatry 2006;59(Suppl 1):1475.
15. Potkin SG. Asenapine efficacy, safety and tolerability in the treatment of acute schizophrenia: a randomised, placebo- and risperidone-controlled trial. Biol Psychiatry 2006;59(Suppl 1):1545.

Antipsychotics – general principles of prescribing

- The **lowest possible** dose should be used. For each patient, the dose should be titrated to the lowest known to be effective (see page 15); dose increases should then take place only after 2 weeks of assessment during which the patient is clearly showing poor or no response. With depot medication, plasma levels rise for 6–12 weeks after initiation, even without a change in dose. Dose increases during this time are therefore inappropriate (see page 42).

- For the large majority of patients, the use of a **single antipsychotic** (with or without additional mood stabiliser or sedatives) is recommended (see page 50). Apart from exceptional circumstances (e.g. clozapine augmentation) antipsychotic polypharmacy should be avoided because of the risks associated with QT prolongation.

- **Polypharmacy** of antipsychotics may be undertaken only where response to a single antipsychotic (including clozapine) has been clearly demonstrated to be inadequate. In such cases, the effect of polypharmacy should be carefully evaluated and documented. Where there is no clear benefit, treatment should revert to single antipsychotic therapy (see page 50).

- In general, **antipsychotics should not be used as 'PRN' sedatives**. Short courses of benzodiazepines or general sedatives (e.g. promethazine) are recommended.

- Responses to antipsychotic drug treatment should be **assessed by recognised rating scales** and be documented in patients' records.

- Those receiving antipsychotics should undergo close monitoring of physical health (see page 38).

Further reading

Pharmacovigilance Working Party. Public Assessment Report on Neuroleptics and Cardiac safety, in particular QT prolongation, cardiac arrhythmias, ventricular tachycardia and torsades de pointes. http://www.mhra.gov.uk. 2006.

Atypical antipsychotics – summary of NICE guidance[1]

NICE guidance on the use of SGAs remains extant in the UK despite being developed as long ago as 2001/2002. Although it predates full appreciation of the metabolic effects of many SGAs, the guidance does offer reasonable advice on the use of newer antipsychotics. This is summarised below.

- Choice of antipsychotic should be made jointly by the prescriber and the (properly informed) patient and/or carer.

- When consultation with the patient is not possible and where there is no advance directive, a second-generation drug should be used. The patient's carer or advocate should be consulted whenever possible.

- Second-generation antipsychotics (SGAs) should be considered in the choice of first-line treatments.

- SGAs should be considered for patients showing or reporting unacceptable adverse effects caused by typical agents (see page 33).

- Patients unresponsive to two different antipsychotics (one a SGA) should be given clozapine.

- Depot medication should be used where there are grounds to suspect that a patient may be unlikely to adhere to prescribed oral therapy.

- Where more than one SGA is appropriate, the drug with the lowest purchase cost should be prescribed.

- 'Advance directives' regarding patients' preference for treatment should be developed and documented.

- Drug treatment should be considered only part of a comprehensive package of care.

- SGAs and FGAs should not be prescribed together except during changeover of medication.

Reference

1. National Institute for Clinical Excellence. Guidance on the use of newer (atypical) antipsychotic drugs for the treatment of schizophrenia. Health Technology Appraisal No. 43. http://www.nice.org.uk. 2002.

1st episode schizophrenia

Treatment algorithm

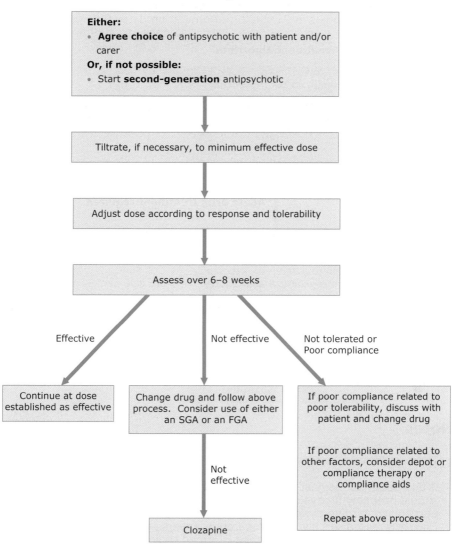

Either:
- **Agree choice** of antipsychotic with patient and/or carer

Or, if not possible:
- Start **second-generation** antipsychotic

↓

Tiltrate, if necessary, to minimum effective dose

↓

Adjust dose according to response and tolerability

↓

Assess over 6–8 weeks

Effective → Continue at dose established as effective

Not effective → Change drug and follow above process. Consider use of either an SGA or an FGA

Not effective → Clozapine

Not tolerated or Poor compliance → If poor compliance related to poor tolerability, discuss with patient and change drug

If poor compliance related to other factors, consider depot or compliance therapy or compliance aids

Repeat above process

Relapse or acute exacerbation of schizophrenia

(full adherence to medication confirmed)

Treatment algorithm

Investigate social or psychological precipitants

Provide appropriate support and/or therapy

Continue usual drug treatment

Acute drug treatment required

Add short-term sedative
or
Switch to a different, acceptable antipsychotic if appropriate

Assess over at least 6 weeks

Treatment ineffective

Switch to **clozapine**

Notes

- There is little to choose between antipsychotics in respect to efficacy or effectiveness (with the notable exception of clozapine). First-generation drugs seem to be just as effective as non-clozapine SGAs[1,2] but FGAs should probably be avoided because of the high risk of movement disorder, particularly tardive dyskinesia[3,4].
- Choice is based largely on comparative adverse-effect profile and relative toxicity. Patients seem able to make informed choices based on these factors[5] although in practice they may only very rarely be involved in drug choice[6].
- Where there is prior treatment failure (but not confirmed treatment refractoriness), olanzapine or risperidone may be better options than quetiapine[7].
- Where there is confirmed treatment resistance (failure to respond to at least two antipsychotics), evidence supporting the use of clozapine (and only clozapine) is now overwhelming[8,9].

Relapse or acute exacerbation of schizophrenia

(adherence doubtful or known to be poor)

Treatment algorithm

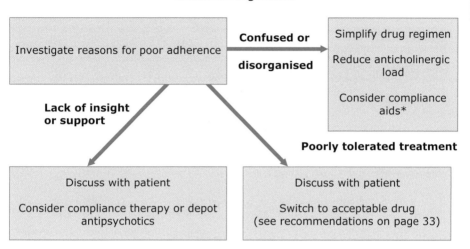

*Compliance aids (e.g. Medidose system) are not a substitute for patient education. The ultimate aim should be to promote independent living, perhaps with patients filling their own compliance aid, having first been given support and training. Note that such compliance aids are of little use unless the patient is clearly motivated to adhere to prescribed treatment. Note also that some medicines are not suitable for storage in compliance aids.

References

1. Jones PB et al. Randomized controlled trial of the effect on Quality of Life of second- vs first-generation antipsychotic drugs in schizophrenia: Cost Utility of the Latest Antipsychotic Drugs in Schizophrenia Study (CUtLASS 1). Arch Gen Psychiatry 2006;63:1079–87.
2. Lieberman JA et al. Effectiveness of antipsychotic drugs in patients with chronic schizophrenia. N Engl J Med 2005;353:1209–23.
3. Schooler N et al. Risperidone and haloperidol in first-episode psychosis: a long-term randomized trial. Am J Psychiatry 2005;162:947–53.
4. Oosthuizen PP et al. Incidence of tardive dyskinesia in first-episode psychosis patients treated with low-dose haloperidol. J Clin Psychiatry 2003;64:1075–80.
5. Whiskey E et al. Evaluation of an antipsychotic information sheet for patients. Int J Psychiatry Clin Pract 2005;9:264–70.
6. Olofinjana B et al. Antipsychotic drugs – information and choice: a patient survey. Psychiatr Bull 2005;29:369–71.
7. Stroup TS et al. Effectiveness of olanzapine, quetiapine, risperidone, and ziprasidone in patients with chronic schizophrenia following discontinuation of a previous atypical antipsychotic. Am J Psychiatry 2006;163:611–22.
8. McEvoy JP et al. Effectiveness of clozapine versus olanzapine, quetiapine, and risperidone in patients with chronic schizophrenia who did not respond to prior atypical antipsychotic treatment. Am J Psychiatry 2006;163:600–10.
9. Lewis SW et al. Randomized controlled trial of effect of prescription of clozapine versus other second-generation antipsychotic drugs in resistant schizophrenia. Schizophr Bull 2006;32:715–23.

Switching antipsychotics because of poor tolerability – recommendations

Adverse effect	Suggested drugs	Alternatives
Acute EPSEs[1-5]	Aripiprazole Olanzapine Quetiapine	Clozapine Risperidone (<6 mg/day) Ziprasidone
Dyslipidaemia[6-9]	Amisulpride Aripiprazole Ziprasidone	
Impaired glucose tolerance[10-13]	Amisulpride Aripiprazole Ziprasidone	Risperidone
Hyperprolactinaemia[14-16]	Aripiprazole Olanzapine *(small, transient rise in prolactin[17], although symptoms rarely observed[18])* Quetiapine	Clozapine Ziprasidone
Postural hypotension	Amisulpride Aripiprazole Haloperidol Sulpiride Trifluoperazine	
QT prolongation[19-21]	Aripiprazole	Olanzapine
Sedation	Amisulpride Aripiprazole Haloperidol Risperidone Sulpiride	
Sexual dysfunction[22-26]	Aripiprazole Quetiapine	
Tardive dyskinesia[27-30]	Clozapine	Aripiprazole Olanzapine Quetiapine Risperidone (<6 mg/day)
Weight gain[31-34]	Amisulpride Aripiprazole Haloperidol Trifluoperazine Ziprasidone	Quetiapine Risperidone

References

1. Stanniland C et al. Tolerability of atypical antipsychotics. Drug Saf 2000;22:195–214.
2. Tarsy D et al. Effects of newer antipsychotics on extrapyramidal function. CNS Drugs 2002;16:23–45.
3. Caroff SN et al. Movement disorders associated with atypical antipsychotic drugs. J Clin Psychiatry 2002;63(Suppl 4):12–19.
4. Lemmens P et al. A combined analysis of double-blind studies with risperidone vs. placebo and other antipsychotic agents: factors associated with extrapyramidal symptoms. Acta Psychiatr Scand 1999;99:160–70.
5. Taylor DM. Aripiprazole: a review of its pharmacology and clinical use. Int J Clin Pract 2003;57:49–54.
6. Rettenbacher MA et al. Early changes of plasma lipids during treatment with atypical antipsychotics. Int Clin Psychopharmacol 2006;21:369–72.
7. Ball MP et al. Clozapine-induced hyperlipidemia resolved after switch to aripiprazole therapy. Ann Pharmacother 2005;39:1570–2.
8. De Hert M et al. A case series: evaluation of the metabolic safety of aripiprazole. Schizophr Bull 2006;Epub ahead of print.
9. Chrzanowski WK et al. Effectiveness of long-term aripiprazole therapy in patients with acutely relapsing or chronic, stable schizophrenia: a 52-week, open-label comparison with olanzapine. Psychopharmacology 2006;189:259–66.
10. Haddad PM. Antipsychotics and diabetes: review of non-prospective data. Br J Psychiatry Suppl 2004; 47:S80–S86.
11. Berry S et al. Improvement of insulin indices after switch from olanzapine to risperidone. Eur Neuropsychopharmacol 2002;12:316.
12. Gianfrancesco FD et al. Differential effects of risperidone, olanzapine, clozapine, and conventional antipsychotics on type 2 diabetes: findings from a large health plan database. J Clin Psychiatry 2002; 63:920–30.
13. Mir S et al. Atypical antipsychotics and hyperglycaemia. Int Clin Psychopharmacol 2001;16:63–74.
14. Turrone P et al. Elevation of prolactin levels by atypical antipsychotics. Am J Psychiatry 2002;159: 133–5.
15. David SR et al. The effects of olanzapine, risperidone, and haloperidol on plasma prolactin levels in patients with schizophrenia. Clin Ther 2000;22:1085–96.
16. Hamner MB et al. Hyperprolactinaemia in antipsychotic-treated patients: guidelines for avoidance and management. CNS Drugs 1998;10:209–22.
17. Crawford AM et al. The acute and long-term effect of olanzapine compared with placebo and haloperidol on serum prolactin concentrations. Schizophr Res 1997;26:41–54.
18. Licht RW et al. Olanzapine-induced galactorrhea. Psychopharmacology 2002;162:94–5.
19. Glassman AH et al. Antipsychotic drugs: prolonged QTc interval, torsade de pointes, and sudden death. Am J Psychiatry 2001;158:1774–82.
20. Taylor D. Antipsychotics and QT prolongation. Acta Psychiatr Scand 2003;107:85–95.
21. Titier K et al. Atypical antipsychotics: from potassium channels to torsade de pointes and sudden death. Drug Saf 2005;28:35–51.
22. Byerly MJ et al. An open-label trial of quetiapine for antipsychotic-induced sexual dysfunction. J Sex Marital Ther 2004;30:325–32.
23. Montejo Gonzalez AL et al. A 6-month prospective observational study on the effects of quetiapine on sexual functioning. J Clin Psychopharmacol 2005;25:533–8.
24. Dossenbach M et al. Effects of atypical and typical antipsychotic treatments on sexual function in patients with schizophrenia: 12-month results from the Intercontinental Schizophrenia Outpatient Health Outcomes (IC-SOHO) study. Eur Psychiatry 2006;21:251–8.
25. Byerly MJ et al. Sexual dysfunction associated with second-generation antipsychotics in outpatients with schizophrenia or schizoaffective disorder: an empirical evaluation of olanzapine, risperidone, and quetiapine. Schizophr Res 2006;86:244–50.
26. Kerwin R et al. Effectiveness of aripiprazole versus standard of care: Schizophrenia Trial of Aripiprazole: STAR Trial. 2006. Poster presentation at the 159th annual meeting of the American Psychiatric Association, Abstract NR929, May 20–25, 2006.
27. Lieberman J et al. Clozapine pharmacology and tardive dyskinesia. Psychopharmacology 1989; 99(Suppl):S54–9.
28. O'Brien J et al. Marked improvement in tardive dyskinesia following treatment with olanzapine in an elderly subject. Br J Psychiatry 1998;172:186.
29. Sacchetti E et al. Quetiapine, clozapine, and olanzapine in the treatment of tardive dyskinesia induced by first-generation antipsychotics: a 124-week case report. Int Clin Psychopharmacol 2003;18:357–9.
30. Witschy JK et al. Improvement in tardive dyskinesia with aripiprazole use. Can J Psychiatry 2005; 50:188.
31. Taylor DM. Atypical antipsychotics and weight gain – a systematic review. Acta Psychiatr Scand 2000;101:416–32.
32. Allison D et al. Antipsychotic-induced weight gain: a comprehensive research synthesis. Am J Psychiatry 1999;156:1686–96.

33. Brecher M et al. The long term effect of quetiapine (Seroquel^{TM}) monotherapy on weight in patients with schizophrenia. Int J Psychiatry Clin Pract 2000;4:287–91.
34. Casey DE et al. Switching patients to aripiprazole from other antipsychotic agents: a multicenter randomized study. Psychopharmacology 2003;166:391–9.

Further reading

Devlin MJ et al. Obesity: what mental health professionals need to know. Am J Psychiatry 2000; 157:854–66.

National Institute of Clinical Excellence. Guidance on the use of newer (atypical) antipsychotic drugs for the treatment of schizophrenia. Health Technology Appraisal No. 43, NICE, London, 2002.

Slovenko R. Update of legal issues associated with tardive dyskinesia. J Clin Psychiatry 1999;61(Suppl 4): 45–57.

Van Harten PN et al. Acute dystonia induced by drug treatment. BMJ 1999;319:623–6.

First-generation antipsychotics – place in therapy

Typical and atypical antipsychotics are not categorically delineated. Typical (first-generation) drugs are those which can be expected to give rise to acute EPSEs, hyperprolactinaemia and, in the longer term, tardive dyskinesia. Atypicals (second-generation antipsychotics), by any sensible definition, might be expected not to be associated with these adverse effects. However, some atypicals show dose-related EPSEs, some induce hyperprolactinaemia and some may eventually give rise to tardive dyskinesia. To complicate matters further, it has been suggested that the therapeutic and adverse effects of typical drugs can be separated by careful dosing[1] – thus making typical drugs atypical (there is much evidence to the contrary, incidentally[2–4]).

Given these observations, it seems unwise to consider so-called typical and atypical drugs as distinct groups of drugs. The essential difference between the two is the therapeutic index in relation to acute EPSEs; for instance, haloperidol has an extremely narrow index (probably less than 0.5 mg/day); olanzapine a wide index (20–40 mg/day).

Typical drugs still play an important role in schizophrenia and offer a valid alternative to atypicals where atypicals are poorly tolerated. Typicals are probably no less effective than non-clozapine atypicals[5,6]. Their main drawbacks are, of course, acute EPSEs (see page 92), hyperprolactinaemia and tardive dyskinesia. Hyperprolactinaemia is probably unavoidable in practice and, even when not symptomatic, may grossly affect hypothalamic function[7]. It is also firmly associated with sexual dysfunction[8], but be aware that the autonomic effects of some atypicals may also cause sexual dysfunction[9].

Tardive dyskinesia probably occurs much more frequently with typicals than atypicals[10–13] (notwithstanding difficulties in defining what is atypical), although there remains some uncertainty[14]. Careful observation of patients and the prescribing of the lowest effective dose are essential to help reduce the risk of this serious adverse event[15,16]. Even with these precautions, the risk of tardive dyskinesia may be unacceptably high[17].

References

1. Oosthuizen P et al. Determining the optimal dose of haloperidol in first-episode psychosis. J Psychopharmacol 2001;15:251–5.
2. Zimbroff DL et al. Controlled, dose-response study of sertindole and haloperidol in the treatment of schizophrenia. Sertindole Study Group. Am J Psychiatry 1997;154:782–91.
3. Jeste DV et al. Incidence of tardive dyskinesia in early stages of low-dose treatment with typical neuroleptics in older patients. Am J Psychiatry 1999;156:309–11.
4. Meltzer HY et al. The effect of neuroleptics on serum prolactin in schizophrenic patients. Arch Gen Psychiatry 1976;33:279–86.
5. Lieberman JA et al. Effectiveness of antipsychotic drugs in patients with chronic schizophrenia. N Engl J Med 2005;353:1209–23.
6. Jones PB et al. Randomized controlled trial of the effect on Quality of Life of second- vs first-generation antipsychotic drugs in schizophrenia: Cost Utility of the Latest Antipsychotic Drugs in Schizophrenia Study (CUtLASS 1). Arch Gen Psychiatry 2006;63:1079–87.
7. Smith S et al. The effects of antipsychotic-induced hyperprolactinaemia on the hypothalamic–pituitary–gonadal axis. J Clin Psychopharmacol 2002;22:109–14.
8. Smith SM et al. Sexual dysfunction in patients taking conventional antipsychotic medication. Br J Psychiatry 2002;181:49–55.
9. Aizenberg D et al. Comparison of sexual dysfunction in male schizophrenia patients maintained on treatment with classical antipsychotics versus clozapine. J Clin Psychiatry 2001;62:541–4.
10. Tollefson GD et al. Blind, controlled, long-term study of the comparative incidence of treatment-emergent tardive dyskinesia with olanzapine or haloperidol. Am J Psychiatry 1997;154:1248–54.
11. Beasley C et al. Randomised double-blind comparison of the incidence of tardive dyskinesia in patients with schizophrenia during long-term treatment with olanzapine or haloperidol. Br J Psychiatry 1999; 174:23–30.
12. Correll CU et al. Lower risk for tardive dyskinesia associated with second-generation antipsychotics: a systematic review of 1-year studies. Am J Psychiatry 2004;161:414–25.
13. Tenback DE et al. Effects of antipsychotic treatment on tardive dyskinesia: a 6-month evaluation of patients from the European Schizophrenia Outpatient Health Outcomes (SOHO) Study. J Clin Psychiatry 2005;66:1130–3.
14. Halliday J et al. Nithsdale Schizophrenia Surveys 23: movement disorders. 20-year review. Br J Psychiatry 2002;181:422–7.
15. Jeste DV et al. Tardive dyskinesia. Schizophr Bull 1993;19:303–15.
16. Cavallaro R et al. Recognition, avoidance, and management of antipsychotic-induced tardive dyskinesia. CNS Drugs 1995;4:278–93.
17. Oosthuizen PP et al. Incidence of tardive dyskinesia in first-episode psychosis patients treated with low-dose haloperidol. J Clin Psychiatry 2003;64:1075–80.

Antipsychotics – monitoring

Parameter/test	Suggested frequency	Action to be taken if results outside reference range	Drugs with special precautions	Drugs for which monitoring is not required
Urea and electrolytes (including creatinine or estimated GFR)	Baseline and yearly	Investigate all abnormalities detected	Amisulpride and sulpiride renally excreted – consider reducing dose if GFR reduced	None
Full blood count (FBC)[1–6]	Baseline and yearly	Stop suspect drug if neutrophils fall below 1.5 x10^9/l. Refer to specialist medical care if neutrophils below 0.5 x 10^9/l. Note high frequency of benign ethnic neutropenia in certain ethnic groups (see page 77)	Clozapine – FBC weekly for 18 weeks, then fortnightly up to 1 year, then monthly	None
Blood lipids[7,8] (cholesterol; triglycerides) Fasting sample, if possible	Baseline, at 3 months, then yearly	Offer lifestyle advice. Consider changing antipsychotic and/or statin therapy (see page 128)	Clozapine, olanzapine, quetiapine, phenothiazines – 3 monthly for first year, then yearly	Some antipsychotics not clearly associated with dyslipidaemia (see page 128) but prevalence is high in this patient group[9–11]

Weight[7,8,11] (include waist size and BMI, if possible)	Baseline, frequently for 3 months, then yearly	Offer lifestyle advice. Consider changing antipsychotic and/or dietary/pharmacological intervention (see page 112)	Clozapine, olanzapine – frequently for 3 months then 3 monthly for first year, then yearly	Aripiprazole and ziprasidone not clearly associated with weight gain but monitoring recommended nonetheless – obesity prevalence high in this patient group
Plasma glucose (fasting sample, if possible)	Baseline, at 4–6 months, then yearly (see page XX)	Offer lifestyle advice. Obtain fasting sample and HbA_{1C}. Refer to GP or specialist	Clozapine, olanzapine – test at baseline, 1 month, then 4–6 monthly	Some antipsychotics not clearly associated with IFG (see page 123) but prevalence is high in this patient group[12,13]
ECG	Baseline and after dose changes (see page 116) (ECG changes rare in practice[14])	Refer to cardiologist if abnormality detected (see page 116)	Haloperidol, pimozide, sertindole – ECG mandatory. Ziprasidone, zotepine – ECG mandatory in some situations	Antipsychotics with no or low to moderate effect on QT_c (see page 116) where there are no other risk factors for arrhythmia
Blood pressure	Baseline; frequently during dose titration	If severe hypotension or hypertension (clozapine) observed, slow rate of titration	Clozapine, chlorpromazine and quetiapine most likely to be associated with postural hypotension	Amisulpride, aripiprazole, trifluoperazine, sulpiride

Table Antipsychotics–monitoring (Cont.)

Parameter/test	Suggested frequency	Action to be taken if results outside reference range	Drugs with special precautions	Drugs for which monitoring is not required
Prolactin	Baseline, then at 6 months, then yearly	Switch drugs if hyperprolactinaemia confirmed and symptomatic (see page 95)		Aripiprazole, clozapine, quetiapine, olanzapine (<20 mg), ziprasidone (see page 95)
Liver function tests (LFTs)[15–17]	Baseline, then yearly	Stop suspect drug if LFTs indicate hepatitis (transaminases x 3 normal) or functional damage (PT/albumin change)	Clozapine and chlorpromazine associated with hepatic failure	Amisulpride, sulpiride
Creatinine phosphokinase (CPK)	Baseline, then if NMS suspected	See page 103	NMS more likely with first-generation antipsychotics	None

Other tests:
Patients on clozapine may benefit from an **EEG**[18,19] as this may help determine the need for valproate. Those on quetiapine should have **thyroid** function tests yearly, although the risk of abnormality is very small[20,21].

Key:
BMI, body mass index; ECG, electrocardiograph; EEG, electroencephalogram; GFR, glomerula filtration rate; IFG, impaired fasting glucose.

References

1. Burckart GJ et al. Neutropenia following acute chlorpromazine ingestion. Clin Toxicol 1981;18:797–801.
2. Grohmann R et al. Agranulocytosis and significant leucopenia with neuroleptic drugs: results from the AMUP program. Psychopharmacology 1989;99(Suppl):S109–S112.
3. Esposito D et al. Risperidone-induced morning pseudoneutropenia. Am J Psychiatry 2005;162:397.
4. Montgomery J. Ziprasidone-related agranulocytosis following olanzapine-induced neutropenia. Gen Hosp Psychiatry 2006;28:83–5.
5. Cowan C et al. Leukopenia and neutropenia induced by quetiapine. Prog Neuropsychopharmacol Biol Psychiatry 2007;31:292–4.
6. Buchman N et al. Olanzapine-induced leukopenia with human leukocyte antigen profiling. Int Clin Psychopharmacol 2001;16:55–7.
7. Marder SR et al. Physical health monitoring of patients with schizophrenia. Am J Psychiatry 2004;161:1334–49.
8. Fenton WS et al. Medication-induced weight gain and dyslipidemia in patients with schizophrenia. Am J Psychiatry 2006;163:1697–704.
9. Weissman EM et al. Lipid monitoring in patients with schizophrenia prescribed second-generation antipsychotics. J Clin Psychiatry 2006;67:1323–6.
10. Cohn TA et al. Metabolic monitoring for patients treated with antipsychotic medications. Can J Psychiatry 2006;51:492–501.
11. Paton C et al. Obesity, dyslipidaemias and smoking in an inpatient population treated with antipsychotic drugs. Acta Psychiatr Scand 2004;110:299–305.
12. Taylor D et al. Undiagnosed impaired fasting glucose and diabetes mellitus amongst inpatients receiving antipsychotic drugs. J Psychopharmacol 2005;19:182–6.
13. Citrome L et al. Incidence, prevalence, and surveillance for diabetes in New York State psychiatric hospitals, 1997–2004. Psychiatr Serv 2006;57:1132–9.
14. Novotny T et al. Monitoring of QT interval in patients treated with psychotropic drugs. Int J Cardiol 2006; [Epub ahead of print].
15. Hummer M et al. Hepatotoxicity of clozapine. J Clin Psychopharmacol 1997;17:314–17.
16. Erdogan A et al. Management of marked liver enzyme increase during clozapine treatment: a case report and review of the literature. Int J Psychiatry Med 2004;34:83–9.
17. Regal RE et al. Phenothiazine-induced cholestatic jaundice. Clin Pharm 1987;6:787–94.
18. Centorrino F et al. EEG abnormalities during treatment with typical and atypical antipsychotics. Am J Psychiatry 2002;159:109–15.
19. Gross A et al. Clozapine-induced QEEG changes correlate with clinical response in schizophrenic patients: a prospective, longitudinal study. Pharmacopsychiatry 2004;37:119–22.
20. Twaites BR et al. The safety of quetiapine: results of a post-marketing surveillance study on 1728 patients in England. J Psychopharmacol 2006; [Epub ahead of print].
21. Kelly DL et al. Thyroid function in treatment-resistant schizophrenia patients treated with quetiapine, risperidone, or fluphenazine. J Clin Psychiatry 2005;66:80–4.

Depot antipsychotics

Advice on prescribing depot medication

- **Give a test dose.**
  Depots are long-acting. Any adverse effects that result from injection are likely to be long-lived. Thus a small test dose is essential to help avoid severe, prolonged adverse effects. See table below and manufacturer's information.

- **Begin with the lowest therapeutic dose.**
  There are few data showing clear dose–response effects for depot preparations. There is some information indicating that low doses are at least as effective as higher ones. Low doses are likely to be better tolerated and are certainly less expensive.

- **Administer at the longest possible licensed interval.**
  All depots can be safely administered at their licensed dosing intervals. There is no evidence to suggest that shortening the dose interval improves efficacy. Moreover, injections are painful, so less frequent administration is desirable. The 'observation' that some patients deteriorate in the days before the next depot is due is probably fallacious. For some hours (or even days with some preparations) plasma levels of antipsychotics continue to fall, albeit slowly, after the next injection. Thus patients are most at risk of deterioration immediately after a depot injection and not before it. Moreover, in trials, relapse seems only to occur 3–6 months after withdrawing depot therapy; roughly the time required to clear steady-state depot drug levels from the blood.

- **Adjust doses only after an adequate period of assessment.**
  Attainment of peak plasma levels, therapeutic effect and steady-state plasma levels are all delayed with depot injections. Doses may be *reduced* if adverse effects occur, but should only be increased after careful assessment over at least 1 month, and preferably longer. The use of adjunctive oral medication to assess depot requirements may be helpful, but it too is complicated by the slow emergence of antipsychotic effects. Note that at the start of therapy, plasma levels of antipsychotic released from a depot increase over several weeks without increasing the given dose. Dose increases during this time to steady-state plasma levels are thus illogical and impossible to evaluate properly.

Differences between depots

Zuclopenthixol is claimed to be more effective in aggressive patients, flupentixol decanoate in those who are depressed, haloperidol decanoate in the prophylaxis of manic illness and pipotiazine palmitate when EPSEs are problematic. Fluphenazine decanoate is said to be associated with depressed mood (which is common anyway in this patient group). Cochrane reviews have been completed for pipotiazine[1], flupentixol[2], zuclopenthixol[3], haloperdiol[4] and fluphenazine[5]. With the exception of zuclopenthixol[3], these depot preparations are equally effective, both with respect to oral antipsychotics and each other. Standard doses are as effective as high doses for flupentixol[2]. It has been argued that compliance with oral antipsychotics decreases over time and that relapse rates in patients prescribed depots decrease in comparison to oral antipsychotics in the longer term[6]. That is, depots reveal advantages over oral treatment only after several years.

Two differences that do exist between depot antipsychotics are (1) zuclopenthixol may be more effective in preventing relapses than other depots, although this may be at the expense of an increased burden of side-effects[3], and (2) flupentixol decanoate can be given in very much higher 'neuroleptic equivalent' doses than the other depot preparations and still remain 'within *BNF* limits'. It is doubtful that this confers any real therapeutic advantage.

Table Antipsychotic depot injections – suggested doses and frequencies[7]

Drug	Trade name	Test dose (mg)	Dose range (mg/week)	Dosing interval (weeks)	Comments
Flupentixol decanoate	Depixol	20	12.5–400	2–4	? Mood elevating; may worsen agitation
Fluphenazine decanoate	Modecate	12.5	6.25–50	2–5	? Avoid in depression High EPS
Haloperidol decanoate	Haldol	25*	12.5–75	4	High EPS, low incidence of sedation
Pipothiazine palmitate	Piportil	25	12.5–50	4	? Lower incidence of EPS (unproven)
Zuclopenthixol decanoate	Clopixol	100	100–600	2–4	? Useful in agitation and aggression

Notes:
- Give a quarter or half stated doses in elderly.
- After test dose, wait 4–10 days before starting titration to maintenance therapy (see product information for individual drugs).
- Dose range is given in mg/week for convenience only – avoid using shorter dose intervals than those recommended except in exceptional circumstances (e.g. long interval necessitates high volume (>3–4 ml) injection).

*Test dose not stated by manufacturer.

Intramuscular anticholinergics and depots

Depot antipsychotics do not produce acute movement disorder at the time of administration[8]: this may take hours to days. The administration of intramuscular procyclidine routinely with each depot is illogical, as the effects of the anticholinergic drug will have worn off before plasma antipsychotic levels peak.

References

1. Dinesh M et al. Depot pipotiazine palmitate and undecylenate for schizophrenia. Cochrane Database Syst Rev 2006;CD001720.
2. David A et al. Depot flupenthixol decanoate for schizophrenia or other similar psychotic disorders. Cochrane Database Syst Rev 2006;CD001470.
3. da Silva Freire Coutinho E et al. Zuclopenthixol decanoate for schizophrenia and other serious mental illnesses. Cochrane Database Syst Rev 2006;CD001164.
4. Quraishi S et al. Depot haloperidol decanoate for schizophrenia. Cochrane Database Syst Rev 2006; CD001361.
5. David A et al. Depot fluphenazine decanoate and enanthate for schizophrenia. Cochrane Database Syst Rev 2006;CD000307.
6. Schooler NR. Relapse and rehospitalization: comparing oral and depot antipsychotics. J Clin Psychiatry 2003;64(Suppl 16):14–17.
7. Taylor D et al. Antipsychotic depot injections – suggested doses and frequencies. Psychiatr Bull 1995; 19:357.
8. Kane JM et al. Guidelines for depot antipsychotic treatment in schizophrenia. European Neuropsychopharmacology Consensus Conference in Siena, Italy. Eur Neuropsychopharmacol 1998;8:55–66.

Further reading

Adams CE et al. Systematic meta-review of depot antipsychotic drugs for people with schizophrenia. Br J Psychiatry 2001;179:290–9.

Barnes TRE. Why indeed?: Invited commentary on . . . . why aren't depot antipsychotics prescribed more often and what can be done about it? Adv Psychiatr Treat 2005;11:211–13.

Patel MX et al. Why aren't depot antipsychotics prescribed more often and what can be done about it? Adv Psychiatr Treat 2005;11:203–11.

Taylor D. Depot antipsychotics revisited. Psychiatr Bull 1999;23:551–3.

Walburn J et al. Systematic review of patient and nurse attitudes to depot antipsychotic medication. Br J Psychiatry 2001;179:300–7.

Risperidone long-acting injection (RLAI)

Risperidone is the only second-generation drug available as a depot or long-acting, injectable formulation. Doses of 25–50 mg every 2 weeks appear to be as effective as oral doses of 2–6 mg/day[1]. The long-acting injection also seems to be well tolerated – less than 10% experience EPSEs and less than 6% withdrew from a long-term trial because of adverse effects[2]. Few data are available relating to effects on prolactin but, although problems might be predicted[3], prolactin levels appear to reduce somewhat following a switch from oral to injectable risperidone[4]. Rates of tardive dyskinesia are said to be low[5].

There is confusion over the dose–response relationship for RLAI. Studies randomising subjects to different doses of RLAI show no differences in response according to dose[6]. One randomised, fixed-dose year-long study suggested better outcome for 50 mg every 2 weeks than with 25 mg, although no observed difference reached statistical significance[7]. Naturalistic studies indicate doses higher than 25 mg/2 weeks are frequently used[8,9]. One study suggests higher doses are associated with better outcome[10].

Plasma levels afforded by 25 mg/2 weeks seem to be similar to, or even lower than, levels provided by 2 mg/day oral risperidone[11,12]. Striatal dopamine D_2 occupancies are similarly low in people receiving 25 mg/2 weeks[13,14]. So, although fixed dose studies have not revealed clear advantages for doses above 25 mg/2 weeks other indicators cast doubt on the assumption that 25 mg/2 weeks will be adequate for all or even most patients. While this conundrum remains unresolved, the need for careful dose titration becomes of great importance. This is perhaps most efficiently achieved by establishing the required dose of oral risperidone and converting this dose into the equivalent injection dose. Trials have clearly established that switching from 2 mg oral to 25 mg injection and 4 mg oral to 50 mg injection is usually successful[2,15,16]. There remains a question over the equivalent dose for 6 mg oral: in theory, patients should be switched to 75 mg injection, but this showed no advantage over lower doses in trials and is, in any case, above the licensed maximum dose.

Risperidone long-acting injection differs importantly from other depots and the following should be noted:

- Risperidone depot is not an esterified form of the parent drug. It contains risperidone coated in polymer to form microspheres. These microspheres have to be suspended in an aqueous base immediately before use.

- The injection must be stored in a fridge (consider the practicalities for CPNs).

- It is available as doses of 25, 37.5 and 50 mg. The whole vial must be used (because of the nature of the suspension). This means that there is limited flexibility in dosing.

- A test dose is not required or sensible. (Testing tolerability with oral risperidone is desirable but not always practical.)

- It takes 3–4 weeks for the first injection to produce therapeutic plasma levels. Patients must be maintained on a full dose of their previous antipsychotic for at least 3 weeks after the administration of the first risperidone injection. Oral antipsychotic cover is sometimes required for longer (6–8 weeks). If the patient is not already receiving an oral antipsychotic, oral risperidone should be prescribed. (See table for advice on switching from depots.) Patients who refuse oral treatment and are acutely ill should not be given RLAI because of the long delay in drug release.

- Risperidone depot must be administered every 2 weeks. The pharmacokinetic profile does not allow longer intervals between doses. There is no flexibility to negotiate with patients about the frequency of administration.

- The most effective way of predicting response to RLAI is to establish dose and response with oral risperidone.

- Risperidone injection is not suitable for patients with treatment refractory schizophrenia.

For guidance on switching to risperidone long-acting injection see below.

Switching to risperidone long-acting injection (RLAI)

Table		
Switching from	*Recommended method of switching*	*Comments*
No treatment (new patient or recently non-compliant)	Start risperidone oral at 2 mg/day and titrate to effective dose. If tolerated, prescribe equivalent dose of RLAI. Continue with oral risperidone for at least 3 weeks, then taper over 1–2 weeks. Be prepared to continue oral risperidone for longer	Use oral risperidone before giving injection to assure good tolerability. Those stabilised on 2 mg/day – start on 25 mg/2 weeks. Those on higher doses – start on 37.5 mg/2 weeks.
Oral risperidone	Prescribe equivalent dose of RLAI	See above
Oral antipsychotics (not risperidone)	*Either:* (a) Switch to oral risperidone and titrate to effective dose. If tolerated, prescribe equivalent dose of RLAI. Continue with oral risperidone for at least 3 weeks then taper over 1–2 weeks. Be prepared to continue oral risperidone for longer. or: (b) Give RLAI and then slowly discontinue oral antipsychotics after 3–4 weeks. Be prepared to continue oral antipsychotics for longer	Dose assessment is difficult in those switching from another antipsychotic. Broadly speaking, those on low oral doses should be switched to 25 mg/2 weeks. 'Low' in this context means towards the lower end of the licensed dose range or around the minimum dose known to be effective (see page 15). Those on higher oral doses should initially receive 37.5 mg every 2 weeks. The continued need for oral antipsychotics after 3–4 weeks usually indicates that higher doses of RLAI are required
Depot anti-psychotic	Give RLAI 1 week *before* the last depot is given	Dose of RLAI difficult to predict. For those on low doses (see above) start at 25 mg every 2 weeks and then adjust as necessary. Start RLAI at 37.5 mg/2 weeks in those previously maintained on doses in the middle or upper range of licensed doses
Antipsychotic polypharmacy with depot	Give RLAI 1 week before the last depot is given. Slowly taper oral antipsychotics 3–4 weeks later. Be prepared to continue oral antipsychotics for longer	Aim to treat patient with RLAI as the sole antipsy-chotic. As before, RLAI dose should be dictated as far as is possible by the total dose of oral and injectable antipsychotic

References

1. Chue P et al. Comparative efficacy and safety of long-acting risperidone and risperidone oral tablets. Eur Neuropsychopharmacol 2005;15:111–17.
2. Fleischhacker WW et al. Treatment of schizophrenia with long-acting injectable risperidone: a 12-month open-label trial of the first long-acting second-generation antipsychotic. J Clin Psychiatry 2003;64: 1250–7.
3. Kleinberg DL et al. Prolactin levels and adverse events in patients treated with risperidone. J Clin Psychopharmacol 1999;19:57–61.
4. Bai YM et al. A comparative efficacy and safety study of long-acting risperidone injection and risperidone oral tablets among hospitalized patients: 12-week randomized, single-blind study. Pharmacopsychiatry 2006;39:135–41.
5. Gharabawi GM et al. An assessment of emergent tardive dyskinesia and existing dyskinesia in patients receiving long-acting, injectable risperidone: results from a long-term study. Schizophr Res 2005;77: 129–39.
6. Kane JM et al. Long-acting injectable risperidone: efficacy and safety of the first long-acting atypical antipsychotic. Am J Psychiatry 2003;160:1125–32.
7. Simpson GM et al. A 1-year double-blind study of 2 doses of long-acting risperidone in stable patients with schizophrenia or schizoaffective disorder. J Clin Psychiatry 2006;67:1194–203.
8. Turner M et al. Long-acting injectable risperidone: safety and efficacy in stable patients switched from conventional depot antipsychotics. Int Clin Psychopharmacol 2004;19:241–9.
9. Taylor DM et al. Early clinical experience with risperidone long-acting injection: a prospective, 6-month follow-up of 100 patients. J Clin Psychiatry 2004;65:1076–83.
10. Taylor DM et al. Prospective 6-month follow-up of patients prescribed risperidone long-acting injection: factors predicting favourable outcome. Int J Neuropsychopharmacol 2006;9:685–94.
11. Nesvag R et al. Serum concentrations of risperidone and 9-OH risperidone following intramuscular injection of long-acting risperidone compared with oral risperidone medication. Acta Psychiatr Scand 2006; 114:21–6.
12. Castberg I et al. Serum concentrations of risperidone and 9-hydroxyrisperidone after administration of the long-acting injectable form of risperidone: evidence from a routine therapeutic drug monitoring service. Ther Drug Monit 2005;27:103–6.
13. Gefvert O et al. Pharmacokinetics and D_2 receptor occupancy of long-acting injectable risperidone (Risperdal Consta™) in patients with schizophrenia. Int J Neuropsychopharmacol 2005;8:27–36.
14. Remington G et al. A PET study evaluating dopamine D_2 receptor occupancy for long-acting injectable risperidone. Am J Psychiatry 2006;163:396–401.
15. Lasser RA et al. Clinical improvement in 336 stable chronically psychotic patients changed from oral to long-acting risperidone: a 12-month open trial. Int J Neuropsychopharmacol 2005;8:427–38.
16. Lauriello J et al. Long-acting risperidone vs. placebo in the treatment of hospital inpatients with schizophrenia. Schizophr Res 2005;72:249–58.

Management of patients on long-term depots

All patients receiving long-term treatment with antipsychotic medication should be seen by their consultant at least once a year (ideally more frequently) in order to review their progress and treatment. There is no simple formula for deciding when to reduce the dose of maintenance antipsychotic treatment; therefore, a risk/benefit analysis must be done for every patient. The following prompts may be helpful:

- Is the patient symptom-free and if so for how long? Long-standing, non-distressing symptoms which have not previously been responsive to medication may be excluded.
- What is the severity of the side-effects (EPSEs, TD, obesity, etc.)?
- What is the previous pattern of illness? Consider the speed of onset, duration and severity of episodes and any danger posed to self or others.
- Has dosage reduction been attempted before? If so, what was the outcome?
- What are the patient's current social circumstances? Is it a period of relative stability, or are stressful life events anticipated?
- What is the social cost of relapse (e.g. is the patient the sole breadwinner for a family)?
- Is the patient able to monitor his/her own symptoms? If so, will he/she seek help?

If after consideration of the above, the decision is taken to reduce medication, the patient's carers should be involved and a clear explanation given of what should be done if symptoms return/worsen. It would then be reasonable to proceed in the following manner:

- If it has not already been done, oral antipsychotic medication should be discontinued first.
- The interval between injections should be increased to up to 4 weeks before decreasing the dose given each time. Note: *not* with risperidone.
- The dose should be reduced by no more than a third at any one time. Note: special considerations apply to risperidone.
- Decrements should, if possible, be made no more frequently than every 3 months.
- Discontinuation should be seen as the end point of the above process.

If the patient becomes symptomatic, this should be seen not as a failure, but rather as an important step in determining the minimum effective dose that the patient requires.

Combined antipsychotics

There is no good objective evidence that combined antipsychotics offer any efficacy advantage over the use of a single antipsychotic. The evidence base supporting combinations that do not include clozapine consists entirely of small open studies and case series[1–3]. There are a number of published case reports of clinically significant side-effects such as severe EPSE[4], grand mal seizures[5] and prolonged QTc[6] associated with this strategy. Despite this, prescriptions for combined antipsychotics are commonly seen[7]. National surveys have repeatedly shown that up to 50% of patients prescribed atypical antipsychotics receive a typical drug as well[8,9]. Anticholinergic medication is then often required[9].

A UK audit of antipsychotic prescribing in hospitalised patients found that 20% of all patients prescribed antipsychotics were prescribed doses above the *BNF* maximum. Very few of these prescriptions were for single antipsychotics[7] (high doses were the result of combined antipsychotics). Monitoring of patients receiving high doses or combinations was very poor. Prescribers would seem not to be aware of the additive side-effects resulting from antipsychotic polypharmacy. Clinical factors such as age (young), gender (male) and diagnosis (schizophrenia) were associated with antipsychotic polypharmacy, albeit only a small proportion of the total[10]. One study has shown a past history of violence to be an important factor[11]. A recent national audit conducted through the Prescribing Observatory for Mental Health (POMH-UK) found that combined antipsychotics were prescribed to 43% of patients in acute adult wards in the UK. In the majority of cases, the second antipsychotic was prescribed PRN and the most common reason given for prescribing in this way was to manage behavioural disturbance[12]. A large proportion of such prescribing, however, remains unexplained.

A study which followed a cohort of patients with schizophrenia prospectively over a 10-year period found that receiving more than one antipsychotic concurrently was associated with increased mortality[13]. There was no association with the total number of antipsychotics given sequentially as monotherapy, the maximum daily antipsychotic dose, duration of exposure, lifetime intake, or any other measure of illness severity. Interestingly, the prescription of anticholinergics was associated with increased survival. Another study followed up 99 patients with schizophrenia over a 25-year period and found that those who were prescribed three antipsychotics simultaneously were twice as likely to die as those who were prescribed only one[14]. Although these data should be interpreted with some important caveats in mind, they should serve to remind us that antipsychotic monotherapy is desirable and should be the norm. This is emphasised by a recent study which demonstrated longer patient hospital stay and more frequent adverse effects in people receiving combined antipsychotics[15]. It follows that it should be standard practice to document the rationale for combined antipsychotics in individual cases in clinical notes along with a clear account of any benefits and side-effects. Medicolegally, that would seem to be wise although in practice it is rarely done[16].

Note that the NICE explicitly demands that first- and second-generation antipsychotics be not prescribed together except when switching[17]. On the basis of risk associated with QT prolongation (common to almost all antipsychotics), concomitant use of antipsychotics should be avoided. Note, however, that clozapine augmentation strategies often involve combining antipsychotics and this is perhaps the sole therapeutic area where such practice is supportable[18,19]. See page 63.

References

1. Bacher NM et al. Combining risperidone with standard neuroleptics for refractory schizophrenic patients. Am J Psychiatry 1996;153:137.
2. Waring EW et al. Treatment of schizophrenia with antipsychotics in combination. Can J Psychiatry 1999;44:189–90.
3. Zink M et al. Combination of amisulpride and olanzapine in treatment-resistant schizophrenic psychoses. Eur Psychiatry 2004;19:56–8.
4. Gomberg RF. Interaction between olanzapine and haloperidol. J Clin Psychopharmacol 1999;19:272–3.
5. Hedges DW et al. New-onset seizure associated with quetiapine and olanzapine. Ann Pharmacother 2002;36:437–9.
6. Beelen AP et al. Asymptomatic QTc prolongation associated with quetiapine fumarate overdose in a patient being treated with risperidone. Hum Exp Toxicol 2001;20:215–19.
7. Harrington M et al. The results of a multi-centre audit of the prescribing of antipsychotic drugs for in-patients in the UK. Psychiatr Bull 2002;26:414–18.
8. Taylor D et al. A prescription survey of the use of atypical antipsychotics for hospital patients in the UK. Int J Psychiatry Clin Pract 2000;4:41–6.
9. Paton C et al. Patterns of antipsychotic and anticholinergic prescribing for hospital inpatients. J Psychopharmacol 2003;17:223–9.
10. Lelliott P et al. The influence of patient variables on polypharmacy and combined high dose of antipsychotic drugs prescribed for in-patients. Psychiatr Bull 2002;26:411–14.
11. Wilkie A et al. High dose neuroleptics – who gives them and why? Psychiatr Bull 2001;25:179–83.
12. Paton C et al. Prescribing of high dose and combined antipsychotics on acute adult and psychiatric intensive care wards: results of the Prescribing Observatory for Mental Health (POMH-UK) baseline audit. J Psychopharmacol 2006; in press.
13. Waddington JL et al. Mortality in schizophrenia. Antipsychotic polypharmacy and absence of adjunctive anticholinergics over the course of a 10-year prospective study. Br J Psychiatry 1998;173:325–9.
14. Joukamaa M et al. Schizophrenia, neuroleptic medication and mortality. Br J Psychiatry 2006;188:122–7.
15. Centorrino F et al. Multiple versus single antipsychotic agents for hospitalized psychiatric patients: case-control study of risks versus benefits. Am J Psychiatry 2004;161:700–6.
16. Taylor D et al. Co-prescribing of atypical and typical antipsychotics – prescribing sequence and documented outcome. Psychiatr Bull 2002;26:170–2.
17. National Institute of Clinical Excellence. Guidance on the use of newer (atypical) antipsychotic drugs for the treatment of schizophrenia. Health Technology Appraisal No. 43. http://www.nice. org.uk. 2002.
18. Shiloh R et al. Sulpiride augmentation in people with schizophrenia partially responsive to clozapine. A double-blind, placebo-controlled study. Br J Psychiatry 1997;171:569–73.
19. Josiassen RC et al. Clozapine augmented with risperidone in the treatment of schizophrenia: a randomized, double-blind, placebo-controlled trial. Am J Psychiatry 2005;162:130–6.

High-dose antipsychotics: prescribing and monitoring

'High dose' can result from the prescription of either:

1. a single antipsychotic in a dose that is above the recommended maximum

or

2. two or more antipsychotics that, when expressed as a percentage of their respective maximum recommended doses and added together, result in a cumulative dose of >100%.

Efficacy

There is no firm evidence that high doses of antipsychotics are any more effective than standard doses. This holds true for the use of antipsychotics in rapid tranquillisation, the management of acute psychotic episodes, chronic aggression and relapse prevention. Approximately a quarter of hospitalised patients are prescribed high-dose antipsychotics, the vast majority through the cumulative effect of combinations[1].

There are a small number of RCTs that examine the efficacy of high versus standard doses in patients with treatment-resistant schizophrenia[2,3]. Some demonstrated benefit[4] but the majority of these studies are old, the number of patients randomised is small and study design is poor by current standards. Some studies used doses equivalent to more than 10 g chlorpromazine. A recent review of the dose–response effects of a variety of antipsychotics revealed no evidence whatever for increasing doses above accepted therapeutic ranges[5]. Effect appears to be optimal at low doses: 4 mg/day risperidone; 300 mg/day quetiapine, etc.

Adverse effects

The majority of side-effects associated with antipsychotic treatment are dose-related. These include EPSEs, sedation, postural hypotension, anticholinergic effects and QTc prolongation. High-dose antipsychotic treatment has insufficient support in the scientific literature and clearly worsens adverse effect incidence and severity[6,7]. Polypharmacy (with the exception of augmentation strategies for clozapine) also seems to be ineffective[8,9] and to produce more severe adverse effects[9,10].

Recommendations

The use of high-dose antipsychotics should be an exceptional clinical practice and only ever employed when standard treatments, including clozapine, have failed. Documentation of target symptoms, response and side-effects, ideally using validated rating scales, should be standard practice so that there is ongoing consideration of the risk–benefit ratio for the patient.

References

1. Royal College of Psychiatrists. Consensus statement on high-dose antipsychotic medication (Council Report 138). 2006.
2. Hirsch SR et al. Clinical use of high-dose neuroleptics. Br J Psychiatry 1994;164:94–6.
3. Thompson C. The use of high-dose antipsychotic medication. Br J Psychiatry 1994;164:448–58.
4. Aubree JC et al. High and very high dosage antipsychotics: a critical review. J Clin Psychiatry 1980;41:341–50.
5. Davis JM et al. Dose response and dose equivalence of antipsychotics. J Clin Psychopharmacol 2004;24:192–208.
6. Bollini P et al. Antipsychotic drugs: is more worse? A meta-analysis of the published randomized control trials. Psychol Med 1994;24:307–16.
7. Baldessarini RJ et al. Significance of neuroleptic dose and plasma level in the pharmacological treatment of psychoses. Arch Gen Psychiatry 1988;45:79–90.
8. Taylor D et al. Co-prescribing of atypical and typical antipsychotics – prescribing sequence and documented outcome. Psychiatr Bull 2002;26:170–2.
9. Centorrino F et al. Multiple versus single antipsychotic agents for hospitalized psychiatric patients: case-control study of risks versus benefits. Am J Psychiatry 2004;161:700–6.
10. Waddington JL et al. Mortality in schizophrenia. Antipsychotic polypharmacy and absence of adjunctive anticholinergics over the course of a 10-year prospective study. Br J Psychiatry 1998;173:325–9.

Schizophrenia

Prescribing high-dose antipsychotics

Before using high doses, ensure that:
- Sufficient time has been allowed for response (see page 29).
- At least two different antipsychotics have been tried (one atypical).
- Clozapine has failed or not been tolerated due to agranulocytosis. Most other side-effects can be managed: see page 70 et seq. A very small proportion of patients may also refuse clozapine outright.
- Compliance is not in doubt (use of blood tests, liquids/dispersible tablets, depot preparations, etc.).
- Adjunctive medications such as antidepressants or mood stabilisers are not indicated.
- Psychological approaches have failed or are not appropriate.

The decision to use high doses should:
- Be made by a consultant psychiatrist
- Involve the multidisciplinary team
- Be done if possible, with the patient's informed consent

Process
- Exclude contraindications (ECG abnormalities, hepatic impairment).
- Consider and minimise any risks posed by concomitant medication (e.g. potential to cause QTc prolongation, electrolyte disturbance or pharmacokinetic interactions via CYP inhibition).
- Document the decision to prescribe high doses in the clinical notes along with a description of target symptoms. The use of an appropriate rating scale is advised.
- Adequate time for response should be allowed after each dosage increment before a further increase is made.

Monitoring
- Physical monitoring should be carried out as outlined on page 38.
- All patients on high doses should have regular ECGs (baseline, when steady-state serum levels have been reached after each dosage increment, and then every 6–12 months). Additional monitoring is advised if drugs that are known to cause electrolyte disturbances or QTc prolongation are subsequently co-prescribed.
- Target symptoms should be assessed after 6 weeks and 3 months. If insufficient improvement in these symptoms has occurred, the dose should be decreased to the normal range.

Negative symptoms

The aetiology of negative symptoms is complex and it is important to determine the most likely cause in any individual case before embarking on a treatment regimen. Negative symptoms can be either primary (transient or enduring) or secondary to positive symptoms (e.g. asociality secondary to paranoia), EPSEs (e.g. bradykinesia, lack of facial expression), depression (e.g. social withdrawal) or institutionalisation[1]. Secondary negative symptoms are obviously best dealt with by treating the relevant cause (EPSEs, depression, etc.). In general:

- The earlier a psychotic illness is effectively treated, the less likely is the development of negative symptoms over time[2].

- Older antipsychotics have only a small effect against primary negative symptoms and can cause secondary negative symptoms (via EPSEs).

- Although second-generation antipsychotics have been shown to be superior to first-generation antipsychotics in the treatment of negative symptoms, the magnitude of the effect is not convincingly clinically significant[3]. The most robust data support the effectiveness of amisulpride in primary negative symptoms[4,5] but even this effect seems no better than haloperidol[6]. There are many small RCTs in the literature reporting equivalent efficacy for different SGAs, e.g. quetiapine and olanzapine[7]; ziprasidone and amisulpride[8]. A well-conducted study appeared to show superiority for olanzapine (only at 5 mg/day) over amisulpride[9].

- Low serum folate[10] and glycine[11] concentrations have been found in patients with predominantly negative symptoms.

A Cochrane review concluded that antidepressants may be effective in the treatment of affective flattening, alogia and avolition[12]. Small RCTs have demonstrated some benefit for selegiline[13] but no benefit for rTMS (repetitive transcranial magnetic stimulation)[14] or donepezil (in elderly patients)[15]. Patients who abuse psychoactive substances experience fewer negative symptoms than patients who do not[16]. It is not clear if this is cause or effect.

References

1. Carpenter WT. The treatment of negative symptoms: pharmacological and methodological issues. Br J Psychiatry 1996;168:17–22.
2. Waddington JL et al. Sequential cross-sectional and 10-year prospective study of severe negative symptoms in relation to duration of initially untreated psychosis in chronic schizophrenia. Psychol Med 1995;25:849–57.
3. Erhart SM et al. Treatment of schizophrenia negative symptoms: future prospects. Schizophr Bull 2006; 32:234–7.
4. Boyer P et al. Treatment of negative symptoms in schizophrenia with amisulpride. Br J Psychiatry 1995; 166:68–72.
5. Danion JM et al. Improvement of schizophrenic patients with primary negative symptoms treated with amisulpride. Amisulpride Study Group. Am J Psychiatry 1999;156:610–16.
6. Speller JC et al. One-year, low-dose neuroleptic study of in-patients with chronic schizophrenia characterised by persistent negative symptoms. Amisulpride v. haloperidol. Br J Psychiatry 1997;171:564–8.
7. Sirota P et al. Quetiapine versus olanzapine for the treatment of negative symptoms in patients with schizophrenia. Hum Psychopharmacol 2006;21:227–34.
8. Olie JP et al. Ziprasidone and amisulpride effectively treat negative symptoms of schizophrenia: results of a 12-week, double-blind study. Int Clin Psychopharmacol 2006;21:143–51.
9. Lecrubier Y et al. The treatment of negative symptoms and deficit states of chronic schizophrenia: olanzapine compared to amisulpride and placebo in a 6-month double-blind controlled clinical trial. Acta Psychiatr Scand 2006;114:319–27.
10. Goff DC et al. Folate, homocysteine, and negative symptoms in schizophrenia. Am J Psychiatry 2004; 161:1705–8.
11. Sumiyoshi T et al. Prediction of the ability of clozapine to treat negative symptoms from plasma glycine and serine levels in schizophrenia. Int J Neuropsychopharmacol 2005;8:451–5.
12. Rummel C et al. Antidepressants for the negative symptoms of schizophrenia. Cochrane Database Syst Rev 2006;3:CD005581.
13. Lin A et al. Selegiline in the treatment of negative symptoms of schizophrenia. Prog Neurother Neuropsychopharmacol 2006;1:121–31.
14. Novak T et al. The double-blind sham-controlled study of high-frequency rTMS (20Hz) for negative symptoms in schizophrenia: negative results. Neuro Endocrinol Lett 2006;27:209–13.
15. Mazeh D et al. Donepezil for negative signs in elderly patients with schizophrenia: an add-on, double-blind, crossover, placebo-controlled study. Int Psychogeriatr 2006;18:429–36.
16. Potvin S et al. A meta-analysis of negative symptoms in dual diagnosis schizophrenia. Psychol Med 2006;36:431–40.

Antipsychotic prophylaxis

First episode of psychosis

A placebo-controlled study has shown that when no prophylactic treatment is given, 57% of first-episode patients have relapsed at 1 year[1]. After 1–2 years of being well on antipsychotic medication, the risk of relapse remains high (figures of 10–15% per month have been quoted), but this area is less well researched[2,3]. Although the current consensus is that antipsychotics should be prescribed for 1–2 years after a first episode of schizophrenia[4,5], Gitlin et al[6] found that withdrawing antipsychotic treatment in line with this consensus led to a relapse rate of almost 80% after 1 year medication-free and 98% after 2 years. Another study in first-episode patients found that discontinuing antipsychotics increased the risk of relapse fivefold[7].

In practice, a firm diagnosis of schizophrenia is rarely made after a first episode and the majority of prescribers and/or patients will have at least attempted to stop antipsychotic treatment within 1 year[8]. It is vital that patients, carers and keyworkers are aware of the early signs of relapse and how to access help. Antipsychotics should not be considered the only intervention. Psychosocial and psychological interventions are clearly also important[9,10].

Multi-episode schizophrenia

The majority of those who have one episode of schizophrenia will go on to have further episodes. With each subsequent episode, the baseline level of functioning deteriorates[11] and the majority of this decline is seen in the first decade of illness. Suicide risk (10%) is also concentrated in the first decade of illness. Those who receive targeted antipsychotics (i.e. only when symptoms re-emerge) have a worse outcome than those who receive prophylactic antipsychotics[12,13] and the risk of TD may also be higher. The figure below depicts the relapse rate in a large cohort of patients with psychotic illness, the majority of whom had already experienced multiple episodes[14]. All had originally received or were still receiving treatment with typical antipsychotics. Note that many of the studies included in this data set were old, and unstandardised diagnostic criteria were used. Variable definitions of relapse and short follow-up periods were the norm and other psychotropic drugs were not controlled for.

Figure Effect of prophylactic antipsychotics

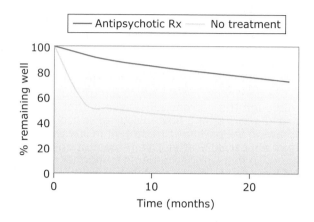

There are some data to support reduced relapse rates with depot antipsy-chotics compared with oral treatment, although differences may not be apparent until the second year of treatment[9].

There is some evidence to support improved long-term outcomes with SGAs; a meta-analysis that contained data for 2032 patients concluded that the risk of relapse with SGAs is less than that associated with FGAs[15]. Note that lack of relapse is not the same as good functioning[9].

Adherence to antipsychotic treatment

Amongst people with schizophrenia, non-adherence with antipsychotic treat-ment is high; only 10 days after discharge from hospital up to 25% are partially or non-adherent, rising to 50% at 1 year and 75% at 2 years[16]. Not only does non-adherence increase the risk of relapse, it may also increase the severity of relapse and the duration of hospitalisation[16]. The risk of suicide attempts also increases fourfold[16].

Dose for prophylaxis

Many patients probably receive higher doses than necessary (particularly of the older drugs) when acutely psychotic[17,18]. In the longer term a balance needs to be made between effectiveness and side-effects. Lower doses of the older drugs (8 mg haloperidol/day or equivalent) are, when compared with higher doses, associated with less severe side-effects[19], better subjective state and better community adjustment[20]. Very low doses increase the risk of psychotic relapse[17,21]. There are no data to support the use of lower than standard doses of the newer drugs as prophylaxis: doses that are acutely effective should generally be continued as prophylaxis.

How and when to stop[22]

The decision to stop antipsychotic drugs requires a thorough risk–benefit analysis for each patient. Withdrawal of antipsychotic drugs after long-term treatment should be gradual and closely monitored. The relapse rate in the first 6 months after abrupt withdrawal is double that seen after gradual withdrawal (defined as slow taper down over at least 3 weeks for oral antipsychotics or abrupt withdrawal of depot preparations)[23]. Abrupt withdrawal may also lead to discontinuation symptoms (e.g. headache, nausea, insomnia) in some patients[24].

The following factors should be considered[22]:

- Is the patient symptom-free, and if so, for how long? Long-standing, non-distressing symptoms which have not previously been responsive to medication may be excluded.
- What is the severity of side-effects (EPSEs, TD, obesity, etc.)?
- What was the previous pattern of illness? Consider the speed of onset, duration and severity of episodes and any danger posed to self and others.
- Has dosage reduction been attempted before, and, if so, what was the outcome?
- What are the patient's current social circumstances? Is it a period of relative stability, or are stressful life events anticipated?
- What is the social cost of relapse (e.g. is the patient the sole breadwinner for a family)?
- Is the patient/carer able to monitor symptoms, and, if so, will they seek help?

As with first-episode patients, patients, carers and keyworkers should be aware of the early signs of relapse and how to access help. Those with a history of aggressive behaviour or serious suicide attempts and those with residual psychotic symptoms should be considered for life-long treatment.

Key points that patients should know

- Antipsychotics do not 'cure' schizophrenia. They treat symptoms in the same way that insulin treats diabetes.
- Long-term treatment is required to prevent relapses.
- Psychoeducation[10], social skills training[9] and CBT[9] increase the chance of staying well.
- Many antipsychotic drugs are available. Different drugs suit different patients. Perceived side-effects should always be discussed, so that the best tolerated drug can be found.
- Antipsychotics should not be stopped suddenly.

References

1. Crow TJ et al. The Northwick Park study of first episodes of schizophrenia 11. A randomised controlled trial of prophylactic neuroleptic treatment. Br J Psychiatry 1986;148:120–7.
2. Nuechterlein KH et al. The early course of schizophrenia and long-term maintenance neuroleptic therapy. Arch Gen Psychiatry 1995;52:203–5.
3. Davis JM et al. Depot antipsychotic drugs. Place in therapy. Drugs 1994;47:741–73.
4. Sheitman BB et al. The evaluation and treatment of first-episode psychosis. Schizophr Bull 1997;23:653–61.
5. American Psychiatric Association. Practice guideline for the treatment of patients with schizophrenia. Am J Psychiatry 1997;154:1–63.
6. Gitlin M et al. Clinical outcome following neuroleptic discontinuation in patients with remitted recent-onset schizophrenia. Am J Psychiatry 2001;158:1835–42.
7. Robinson D et al. Predictors of relapse following response from a first episode of schizophrenia or schizoaffective disorder. Arch Gen Psychiatry 1999;56:241–7.
8. Johnson DAW et al. Professional attitudes in the UK towards neuroleptic maintenance therapy in schizophrenia. Psychiatr Bull 1997;21:394–7.
9. Schooler NR. Relapse prevention and recovery in the treatment of schizophrenia. J Clin Psychiatry 2006;67(Suppl 5):19–23.
10. Motlova L et al. Relapse prevention in schizophrenia: does group family psychoeducation matter? One-year prospective follow-up field study. Int J Psychiatry Clin Pract 2006;10:38–44.
11. Wyatt RJ. Neuroleptics and the natural course of schizophrenia. Schizophr Bull 1991;17:325–51.
12. Jolley AG et al. Trial of brief intermittent neuroleptic prophylaxis for selected schizophrenic outpatients: clinical and social outcome at two years. Br Med J 1990;301:837–42.
13. Herz MI et al. Intermittent vs maintenance medication in schizophrenia. Two-year results. Arch Gen Psychiatry 1991;48:333–9.
14. Gilbert PL et al. Neuroleptic withdrawal in schizophrenic patients. A review of the literature. Arch Gen Psychiatry 1995;52:173–88.
15. Leucht S et al. Relapse prevention in schizophrenia with new-generation antipsychotics: a systematic review and exploratory meta-analysis of randomized, controlled trials. Am J Psychiatry 2003;160:1209–22.
16. Leucht S et al. Epidemiology, clinical consequences, and psychosocial treatment of nonadherence in schizophrenia. J Clin Psychiatry 2006;67(Suppl 5):3–8.
17. Baldessarini RJ et al. Significance of neuroleptic dose and plasma level in the pharmacological treatment of psychoses. Arch Gen Psychiatry 1988;45:79–90.
18. Harrington M et al. The results of a multi-centre audit of the prescribing of antipsychotic drugs for in-patients in the UK. Psychiatr Bull 2002;26:414–18.
19. Geddes J et al. Atypical antipsychotics in the treatment of schizophrenia: systematic overview and meta-regression analysis. Br Med J 2000;321:1371–6.
20. Hogarty GE et al. Dose of fluphenazine, familial expressed emotion, and outcome in schizophrenia. Results of a two-year controlled study. Arch Gen Psychiatry 1988;45:797–805.
21. Marder SR et al. Low- and conventional-dose maintenance therapy with fluphenazine decanoate. Two-year outcome. Arch Gen Psychiatry 1987;44:518–21.
22. Wyatt RJ. Risks of withdrawing antipsychotic medications. Arch Gen Psychiatry 1995;52:205–8.
23. Viguera AC et al. Clinical risk following abrupt and gradual withdrawal of maintenance neuroleptic treatment. Arch Gen Psychiatry 1997;54:49–55.
24. Chouinard G et al. Withdrawal symptoms after long-term treatment with low-potency neuroleptics. J Clin Psychiatry 1984;45:500–2.

Further reading

Bosveld-van Haandel LJM et al. Reasoning about the optimal duration of prophylactic antipsychotic medication in schizophrenia: evidence arguments. Acta Psychiatr Scand 2001;103:335–46.
Csernansky JG et al. Relapse and rehospitalisation rates in patients with schizophrenia: effects of second generation antipsychotics. CNS Drugs 2002;16:473–84.

Schizophrenia

Refractory schizophrenia

Clozapine – dosing regimen

Many of the adverse effects of clozapine are dose-dependent and associated with speed of titration. Adverse effects also tend to be more common at the beginning of therapy. To minimise these problems it is important to start treatment at a low dose and to increase dosage slowly.

Clozapine should normally be started at a dose of 12.5 mg once a day, at night. Blood pressure should be monitored hourly for 6 hours because of the hypotensive effect of clozapine. This monitoring is not usually necessary if the first dose is given at night. On day 2, the dose can be increased to 12.5 mg twice daily. If the patient is tolerating clozapine, the dose can be increased by 25–50 mg a day, until a dose of 300 mg a day is reached. This can usually be achieved in 2–3 weeks. Further dosage increases should be made slowly in increments of 50–100 mg each week. A plasma level of 350 μg/l should be aimed for to ensure an adequate trial, but response may occur at a lower plasma level. The *average* (there is substantial variation) dose at which this plasma level is reached varies according to gender and smoking status. The range is approximately 250 mg/day (female non-smoker) to 550 mg/day (male smoker)[1]. The total clozapine dose should be divided and, if sedation is a problem, the larger portion of the dose can be given at night.

The following table is a suggested starting regimen for clozapine. This is a cautious regimen – more rapid increases have been used in exceptional circumstances. Slower titration may be necessary where sedation is severe. If the patient is not tolerating a particular dose, decrease to one that was previously tolerated. If the adverse effect resolves, increase the dose again but at a slower rate. If for any reason a patient misses less than 2 days' clozapine, restart at the dose prescribed before the event. Do not administer extra tablets to catch up. If more than 2 days are missed, restart at 12.5 mg once daily and increase slowly (but at a faster rate than in drug-naïve patients).

Table Suggested starting regimen for clozapine (inpatients)

Day	Morning dose (mg)	Evening dose (mg)
1	–	12.5
2	12.5	12.5
3	25	25
4	25	25
5	25	50
6	25	50
7	50	50
8	50	75
9	75	75
10	75	100
11	100	100
12	100	125
13	125	125[a]
14	125	150
15	150	150
18	150	200[b]
21	200	200
28	200	250[c]

[a]Target dose for female non-smokers.
[b]Target dose for male non-smokers.
[c]Target dose for female smokers.

Reference

1. Rostami-Hodjegan A et al. Influence of dose, cigarette smoking, age, sex, and metabolic activity on plasma clozapine concentrations: a predictive model and nomograms to aid clozapine dose adjustment and to assess compliance in individual patients. J Clin Psychopharmacol 2004;24:70–8.

Refractory schizophrenia – optimising clozapine treatment

Using clozapine alone

Target dose (*Note that dose is best adjusted according to patient tolerability*)	• Average dose in UK is around 450 mg/day[1] • Response usually seen in the range 150–900 mg/day[2] • Lower doses required in the elderly, females and non-smokers, and in those prescribed certain enzyme inhibitors[3,4]
Plasma levels	• Most studies indicate that threshold for response is in the range 350–420 µg/l[5,6]. Threshold may be as high as 500 µg//l[7] (see page 4) • Importance of norclozapine levels not established but clozapine/norclozapine ratio may aid assessment of recent compliance

Clozapine augmentation

Clozapine 'augmentation' has become common practice because inadequate response to clozapine alone is a frequent clinical event. The evidence base supporting augmentation strategies is weak and not nearly sufficient to allow the development of any algorithm or schedule of treatment options. In practice, the result of clozapine augmentation is often disappointing and substantial changes in symptom severity are rarely observed. This clinical impression is supported by the equivocal results of many studies, which suggest a small effect size at best.

It is recommended that all augmentation attempts are carefully monitored and, if no clear benefit is forthcoming, abandoned after 3–6 months. The addition of another drug to clozapine treatment might be expected to worsen overall adverse effect burden and so continued ineffective treatment is not appropriate. In some cases, the addition of an augmenting agent may reduce the severity of some adverse effects (e.g. weight gain, dyslipidaemia – see below) or allow a reduction in clozapine dose. This aspect of clozapine therapy is poorly researched.

The table below shows other suggested options (in alphabetical order) where 3–6 months of clozapine alone has provided unsatisfactory benefit.

Table Suggested options for augmenting clozapine

Option	Comment
Add amisulpride[8-12] (400–800 mg/day)	• Developing evidence and experience suggest amisulpride augmentation is worthwhile. No RCT evidence. May allow clozapine dose reduction[13]
Add aripiprazole[14-17] (15–30 mg/day)	• Limited evidence of therapeutic benefit. May improve metabolic parameters
Add haloperidol (2 mg/day)	• Modest evidence of benefit[18]
Add lamotrigine[19-21] (25–300 mg/day)	• May be useful in partial or non-responders. May reduce alcohol consumption[22]. One negative report[23]
Add omega-3 triglycerides[24,25] (2–3 g EPA daily)	• Modest, and contested, evidence to support efficacy in non- or partial responders to antipsychotics, including clozapine (see page 89)
Add risperidone[26,27] (2–6 mg/day)	• Increases clozapine plasma levels. May have additive antipsychotic effects. Supported by an RCT but there are two negative RCTs, each with minuscule response rates[28,29]
Add sulpiride[30] (400 mg/day)	• May be useful in partial or non-responders. Supported by a randomised trial

Notes:
- Always consider the use of mood stabilisers and/or antidepressants, especially where mood disturbance is thought to contribute to symptoms[31,32].
- Topiramate has also been suggested, either to augment clozapine or to induce weight loss. It may be effective as augmentation[33] but can worsen psychosis[20,34].
- Other options include adding pimozide[35] and olanzapine[36]. Neither is recommended: pimozide has important cardiac toxicity and the addition of olanzapine is expensive and poorly supported. There is developing evidence supporting ziprasidone augmentation of clozapine[37-39].

References

1. Taylor D et al. A prescription survey of the use of atypical antipsychotics for hospital patients in the UK. Int J Psychiatry Clin Pract 2000;4:41–6.
2. Murphy B et al. Maintenance doses for clozapine. Psychiatr Bull 1998;22:12–14.
3. Taylor D. Pharmacokinetic interactions involving clozapine. Br J Psychiatry 1997;171:109–12.
4. Lane HY et al. Effects of gender and age on plasma levels of clozapine and its metabolites: analyzed by critical statistics. J Clin Psychiatry 1999;60:36–40.
5. Taylor D et al. The use of clozapine plasma levels in optimising therapy. Psychiatr Bull 1995;19:753–5.
6. Spina E et al. Relationship between plasma concentrations of clozapine and norclozapine and therapeutic response in patients with schizophrenia resistant to conventional neuroleptics. Psychopharmacology 2000;148:83–9.
7. Perry PJ. Therapeutic drug monitoring of antipsychotics. Psychopharmacol Bull 2001;35:19–29.
8. Matthiasson P et al. Relationship between dopamine D_2 receptor occupancy and clinical response in amisulpride augmentation of clozapine non-response. J Psychopharmacol 2001;15:S41.
9. Munro J et al. Amisulpride augmentation of clozapine: an open non-randomized study in patients with schizophrenia partially responsive to clozapine. Acta Psychiatr Scand 2004;110:292–8.
10. Zink M et al. Combination of clozapine and amisulpride in treatment-resistant schizophrenia – case reports and review of the literature. Pharmacopsychiatry 2004;37:26–31.
11. Ziegenbein M et al. Augmentation of clozapine with amisulpride in patients with treatment-resistant schizophrenia. An open clinical study. German J Psychiatry 2006;9:17–21.
12. Kampf P et al. Augmentation of clozapine with amisulpride: a promising therapeutic approach to refractory schizophrenic symptoms. Pharmacopsychiatry 2005;38:39–40.

13. Croissant B et al. Reduction of side effects by combining clozapine with amisulpride: case report and short review of clozapine-induced hypersalivation – a case report. Pharmacopsychiatry 2005;38:38–9.
14. Lim S et al. Possible increased efficacy of low-dose clozapine when combined with aripiprazole. J Clin Psychiatry 2004;65:1284–5.
15. Clarke LA et al. Clozapine augmentation with aripiprazole for negative symptoms. J Clin Psychiatry 2006; 67:675–6.
16. Ziegenbein M et al. Combination of clozapine and aripiprazole: a promising approach in treatment-resistant schizophrenia. Aust N Z J Psychiatry 2005;39:840–1.
17. Henderson DC et al. An exploratory open-label trial of aripiprazole as an adjuvant to clozapine therapy in chronic schizophrenia. Acta Psychiatr Scand 2006;113:142–7.
18. Rajarethinam R et al. Augmentation of clozapine partial responders with conventional antipsychotics. Schizophr Res 2003;60:97–8.
19. Dursun SM et al. Clozapine plus lamotrigine in treatment-resistant schizophrenia. Arch Gen Psychiatry 1999;56:950.
20. Dursun SM et al. Augmenting antipsychotic treatment with lamotrigine or topiramate in patients with treatment-resistant schizophrenia: a naturalistic case-series outcome study. J Psychopharmacol 2001; 15:297–301.
21. Tiihonen J et al. Lamotrigine in treatment-resistant schizophrenia: a randomized placebo-controlled crossover trial. Biol Psychiatry 2003;54:1241–8.
22. Kalyoncu A et al. Use of lamotrigine to augment clozapine in patients with resistant schizophrenia and comorbid alcohol dependence: a potent anti-craving effect? J Psychopharmacol 2005;19:301–5.
23. Heck AH et al. Addition of lamotrigine to clozapine in inpatients with chronic psychosis. J Clin Psychiatry 2005;66:1333.
24. Peet M et al. Double-blind placebo controlled trial of N-3 polyunsaturated fatty acids as an adjunct to neuroleptics. Schizophr Res 1998;29:160–1.
25. Puri BK et al. Sustained remission of positive and negative symptoms of schizophrenia following treatment with eicosapentaenoic acid. Arch Gen Psychiatry 1998;55:188–9.
26. Josiassen RC et al. Clozapine augmented with risperidone in the treatment of schizophrenia: a randomized, double-blind, placebo-controlled trial. Am J Psychiatry 2005;162:130–6.
27. Raskin S et al. Clozapine and risperidone: combination/augmentation treatment of refractory schizophrenia: a preliminary observation. Acta Psychiatr Scand 2000;101:334–6.
28. Anil Yagcioglu AE et al. A double-blind controlled study of adjunctive treatment with risperidone in schizophrenic patients partially responsive to clozapine: efficacy and safety. J Clin Psychiatry 2005;66: 63–72.
29. Honer WG et al. Clozapine alone versus clozapine and risperidone with refractory schizophrenia. N Engl J Med 2006;354:472–82.
30. Shiloh R et al. Sulpiride augmentation in people with schizophrenia partially responsive to clozapine. A double-blind, placebo-controlled study. Br J Psychiatry 1997;171:569–73.
31. Citrome L. Schizophrenia and valproate. Psychopharmacol Bull 2003;37(Suppl 2):74–88.
32. Tranulis C et al. Somatic augmentation strategies in clozapine resistance – what facts? Clin Neuropharmacol 2006;29:34–44.
33. Tiihonen J et al. Topiramate add-on in treatment-resistant schizophrenia: a randomized, double-blind, placebo-controlled, crossover trial. J Clin Psychiatry 2005;66:1012–15.
34. Millson RC et al. Topiramate for refractory schizophrenia. Am J Psychiatry 2002;159:675.
35. Friedman J et al. Pimozide augmentation for the treatment of schizophrenic patients who are partial responders to clozapine. Biol Psychiatry 1997;42:522–3.
36. Gupta S et al. Olanzapine augmentation of clozapine. Ann Clin Psychiatry 1998;10:113–15.
37. Zink M et al. Combination of ziprasidone and clozapine in treatment-resistant schizophrenia. Hum Psychopharmacol 2004;19:271–3.
38. Ziegenbein M et al. Clozapine and ziprasidone: a useful combination in patients with treatment-resistant schizophrenia. J Neuropsychiatry Clin Neurosci 2006;18:246–7.
39. Ziegenbein M et al. Combination of clozapine and ziprasidone in treatment-resistant schizophrenia: an open clinical study. Clin Neuropharmacol 2005;28:220–4.

Further reading

Kontaxakis VP et al. Randomized controlled augmentation trials in clozapine-resistant schizophrenic patients: a critical review. Eur Psychiatry 2005;20:409–15.
Kontaxakis VP et al. Case studies of adjunctive agents in clozapine-resistant schizophrenic patients. Clin Neuropharmacol 2005;28:50–3.
Mouaffak F et al. Augmentation strategies of clozapine with antipsychotics in the treatment of ultra-resistant schizophrenia. Clin Neuropharmacol 2006;29:28–33.
Remington G et al. Augmenting strategies in clozapine-resistant schizophrenia. CNS Drugs 2006;20:171.

Refractory schizophrenia – alternatives to clozapine

Clozapine is the established treatment of choice in refractory schizophrenia. Where treatment resistance is established, clozapine treatment should not normally be delayed or withheld. The practice of using successive antipsychotics (or the latest) instead of clozapine is widespread but not supported by any cogent research. Where clozapine cannot be used (toxicity, patient refusal) other drugs or drug combinations may be tried (see below) but outcome is usually disappointing. Available data do not allow the drawing of any distinction between treatment regimens but it seems wise to use single drugs before trying multiple drug regimens. Many of the treatments listed below are somewhat experimental and some of the compounds difficult to obtain (e.g. glycine, D-serine).

Table Alternatives to clozapine
(Treatments in alphabetical order: no preference is implied by position in table)

Treatment	Comments
Allopurinol 300–600 mg/day **(+ antipsychotic)**[1-3]	Increases adenosinergic transmission, which may reduce effects of dopamine. Two positive RCTs[1,2]
Amisulpride[4] (up to 1200 mg/day)	Single, small open study
Aripiprazole[5] (15–30 mg/day)	Single RCT indicating moderate effect in patients resistant to risperidone or olanzapine (+ others). Higher doses (60 mg/day) have been used[6]
CBT[7]	Non-drug therapies should always be considered
D-Alanine 100 mg/kg/day (+ antipsychotic)[8]	Glycine (NMDA) agonist. One positive RCT
D-Serine 30 mg/kg/day (+ olanzapine)[9]	Glycine (NMDA) agonist. One positive RCT
ECT[10-13]	Open studies suggest moderate effect. Often reserved for last-line treatment in practice
Ginkgo biloba **(+ antipsychotic)**[14,15]	Possibly effective in combination with haloperidol. Unlikely to give rise to additional adverse effects but clinical experience limited
Mianserin + FGA 30 mg/day[16]	$5HT_2$ antagonist. One, small positive RCT
Olanzapine[17-22] 5–25 mg/day	Supported by some well-conducted trials but clinical experience disappointing. Some patients show moderate response

Table Alternatives to clozapine (Cont.)

Olanzapine[23-26] 30–60 mg/day	Contradictory findings in the literature but possibly effective. Expensive and unlicenced. High-dose olanzapine is not atypical[27] and can be poorly tolerated[28]
Olanzapine + amisulpride[29] (up to 800 mg/day)	Small open study suggests benefit
Olanzapine + aripiprazole[30]	Single case report suggests benefit
Olanzapine + glycine[31] (0.8 g/kg/day)	Small, double-blind crossover trial suggests clinically relevant improvement in negative symptoms
Olanzapine + lamotrigine[32,33] (up to 400 mg/day)	Reports contradictory and rather unconvincing. Reasonable theoretical basis for adding lamotrigine, which is usually well tolerated
Olanzapine + sulpiride[34] (600 mg/day)	Some evidence that this combination improves mood symptoms
Omega-3-triglycerides[35,36]	Suggested efficacy but data very limited (see page 89)
Quetiapine[37-39]	Very limited evidence and clinical experience not encouraging
Quetiapine + haloperidol[40]	Two case reports
Risperidone[41-43] 4–8 mg/day	Doubtful efficacy in true treatment-refractory schizophrenia but some supporting evidence. May also be tried in combination with glycine[31] or lamotrigine[32] or indeed with other atypicals[44]
Sarcosine (2 g/day) **(+ antipsychotic)**	Enhances glycine action. Supported by two RCTs
Topiramate (30 mg/day) **(+ antipsychotic)**[45]	Small effect shown in single RCT
Transcranial magnetic stimulation[46,47]	Probably not effective
Valproate[48]	Doubtful effect but may be useful where there is a clear affective component

References

1. Akhondzadeh S et al. Beneficial antipsychotic effects of allopurinol as add-on therapy for schizophrenia: a double blind, randomized and placebo controlled trial. Prog Neuropsychopharmacol Biol Psychiatry 2005;29:253–9.
2. Brunstein MG et al. A clinical trial of adjuvant allopurinol therapy for moderately refractory schizophrenia. J Clin Psychiatry 2005;66:213–19.
3. Buie LW et al. Allopurinol as adjuvant therapy in poorly responsive or treatment refractory schizophrenia. Ann Pharmacother 2006;40:2200–4.
4. Kontaxakis VP et al. Switching to amisulpride monotherapy for treatment-resistant schizophrenia. Eur Psychiatry 2006;21:214–17.
5. Kungel M et al. Efficacy and tolerability of aripiprazole compared to perphenazine in treatment-resistant schizophrenia. Pharmacopsychiatry 36, DOI: 10.1055/s-2003-825416. 2003.
6. Crossman AM et al. Tolerability of high-dose aripiprazole in treatment-refractory schizophrenic patients. J Clin Psychiatry 2006;67:1158–9.
7. Valmaggia LR et al. Cognitive-behavioural therapy for refractory psychotic symptoms of schizophrenia resistant to atypical antipsychotic medication. Randomised controlled trial. Br J Psychiatry 2005;186: 324–30.
8. Tsai GE et al. D-alanine added to antipsychotics for the treatment of schizophrenia. Biol Psychiatry 2006;59:230–4.
9. Heresco-Levy U et al. D-serine efficacy as add-on pharmacotherapy to risperidone and olanzapine for treatment-refractory schizophrenia. Biol Psychiatry 2005;57:577–85.
10. Chanpattana W et al. Combined ECT and neuroleptic therapy in treatment-refractory schizophrenia: prediction of outcome. Psychiatry Res 2001;105:107–15.
11. Tang WK et al. Efficacy of electroconvulsive therapy in treatment-resistant schizophrenia: a prospective open trial. Prog Neuropsychopharmacol Biol Psychiatry 2003;27:373–9.
12. Chanpattana W et al. Acute and maintenance ECT with flupenthixol in refractory schizophrenia: sustained improvements in psychopathology, quality of life, and social outcomes. Schizophr Res 2003;63: 189–93.
13. Chanpattana W et al. ECT for treatment-resistant schizophrenia: a response from the Far East to the UK. NICE report. J ECT 2006;22:4–12.
14. Zhou D et al. The effects of classic antipsychotic haloperidol plus the extract of Ginkgo biloba on superoxide dismutase in patients with chronic refractory schizophrenia. Chin Med J 1999; 112:1093–6.
15. Zhang XY et al. A double-blind, placebo-controlled trial of extract of Ginkgo biloba added to haloperidol in treatment-resistant patients with schizophrenia. J Clin Psychiatry 2001;62:878–83.
16. Shiloh R et al. Mianserin or placebo as adjuncts to typical antipsychotics in resistant schizophrenia. Int Clin Psychopharmacol 2002;17:59–64.
17. Breier A et al. Comparative efficacy of olanzapine and haloperidol for patients with treatment-resistant schizophrenia. Biol Psychiatry 1999;45:403–11.
18. Conley RR et al. Olanzapine compared with chlorpromazine in treatment-resistant schizophrenia. Am J Psychiatry 1998;155:914–20.
19. Sanders RD et al. An open trial of olanzapine in patients with treatment-refractory psychoses. J Clin Psychopharmacol 1999;19:62–6.
20. Taylor D et al. Olanzapine in practice: a prospective naturalistic study. Psychiatr Bull 1999;23:178–80.
21. Bitter I et al. Olanzapine versus clozapine in treatment-resistant or treatment-intolerant schizophrenia. Prog Neuropsychopharmacol Biol Psychiatry 2004;28:173–80.
22. Tollefson GD et al. Double-blind comparison of olanzapine versus clozapine in schizophrenic patients clinically eligible for treatment with clozapine. Biol Psychiatry 2001;49:52–63.
23. Sheitman BB et al. High-dose olanzapine for treatment-refractory schizophrenia. Am J Psychiatry 1997; 154:1626.
24. Fanous A et al. Schizophrenia and schizoaffective disorder treated with high doses of olanzapine. J Clin Psychopharmacol 1999;19:275–6.
25. Dursun SM et al. Olanzapine for patients with treatment-resistant schizophrenia: a naturalistic case-series outcome study. Can J Psychiatry 1999;44:701–4.
26. Conley RR et al. The efficacy of high-dose olanzapine versus clozapine in treatment-resistant schizophrenia: a double-blind crossover study. J Clin Psychopharmacol 2003;23:668–71.
27. Bronson BD et al. Adverse effects of high-dose olanzapine in treatment-refractory schizophrenia. J Clin Psychopharmacol 2000;20:382–4.
28. Kelly DL et al. Adverse effects and laboratory parameters of high-dose olanzapine vs. clozapine in treatment-resistant schizophrenia. Ann Clin Psychiatry 2003;15:181–6.
29. Zink M et al. Combination of amisulpride and olanzapine in treatment-resistant schizophrenic psychoses. Eur Psychiatry 2004;19:56–8.
30. Duggal HS. Aripiprazole–olanzapine combination for treatment of schizophrenia. Can J Psychiatry 2004; 49:151.
31. Heresco-Levy U et al. High-dose glycine added to olanzapine and risperidone for the treatment of schizophrenia. Biol Psychiatry 2004;55:165–71.
32. Kremer I et al. Placebo-controlled trial of lamotrigine added to conventional and atypical antipsychotics in schizophrenia. Biol Psychiatry 2004;56:441–6.

33. Dursun SM et al. Augmenting antipsychotic treatment with lamotrigine or topiramate in patients with treatment-resistant schizophrenia: a naturalistic case-series outcome study. J Psychopharmacol 2001; 15:297–301.
34. Kotler M et al. Sulpiride augmentation of olanzapine in the management of treatment-resistant chronic schizophrenia: evidence for improvement of mood symptomatology. Int Clin Psychopharmacol 2004;19:23–6.
35. Mellor JE et al. Omega-3 fatty acid supplementation in schizophrenic patients. Hum Psychopharmacol 1996;11:39–46.
36. Puri BK et al. Sustained remission of positive and negative symptoms of schizophrenia following treatment with eicosapentaenoic acid. Arch Gen Psychiatry 1998;55:188–9.
37. Reznik I et al. Long-term efficacy and safety of quetiapine in treatment-refractory schizophrenia: A case report. Int J Psychiatry Clin Pract 2000;4:77–80.
38. De Nayer A et al. Efficacy and tolerability of quetiapine in patients with schizophrenia switched from other antipsychotics. Int J Psychiatry Clin Pract 2003;7:66.
39. Larmo I et al. Efficacy and tolerability of quetiapine in patients with schizophrenia who switched from haloperidol, olanzapine or risperidone. Hum Psychopharmacol 2005;20:573–81.
40. Aziz MA et al. Remission of positive and negative symptoms in refractory schizophrenia with a combination of haloperidol and quetiapine: two case studies. J Psychiatr Pract 2006;12:332–6.
41. Breier AF et al. Clozapine and risperidone in chronic schizophrenia: effects on symptoms, parkinsonian side effects, and neuroendocrine response. Am J Psychiatry 1999;156:294–8.
42. Bondolfi G et al. Risperidone versus clozapine in treatment-resistant chronic schizophrenia: a randomized double-blind study. The Risperidone Study Group. Am J Psychiatry 1998;155:499–504.
43. Conley RR et al. Risperidone, quetiapine, and fluphenazine in the treatment of patients with therapy-refractory schizophrenia. Clin Neuropharmacol 2005;28:163–8.
44. Lerner V et al. Combination of "atypical" antipsychotic medication in the management of treatment-resistant schizophrenia and schizoaffective disorder. Prog Neuropsychopharmacol Biol Psychiatry 2004;28:89–98.
45. Tiihonen J et al. Topiramate add-on in treatment-resistant schizophrenia: a randomized, double-blind, placebo-controlled, crossover trial. J Clin Psychiatry 2005;66:1012–15.
46. Franck N et al. Left temporoparietal transcranial magnetic stimulation in treatment-resistant schizophrenia with verbal hallucinations. Psychiatry Res 2003;120:107–9.
47. Fitzgerald PB et al. A double-blind sham-controlled trial of repetitive transcranial magnetic stimulation in the treatment of refractory auditory hallucinations. J Clin Psychopharmacol 2005;25:358–62.
48. Basan A et al. Valproate as an adjunct to antipsychotics for schizophrenia: a systematic review of randomized trials. Schizophr Res 2004;70:33–7.

Further reading

Henderson DC et al. Switching from clozapine to olanzapine in treatment-refractory schizophrenia: safety, clinical efficacy, and predictors of response. J Clin Psychiatry 1998;59:585–8.
Lindenmayer JP et al. Olanzapine in refractory schizophrenia after failure of typical or atypical antipsychotic treatment: an open-label switch study. J Clin Psychiatry 2002;63:931–5.
Still DJ et al. Effects of switching inpatients with treatment-resistant schizophrenia from clozapine to risperidone. Psychiatr Serv 1996;47:1382–4.

Clozapine – management of common adverse effects

Clozapine has a wide range of adverse effects, many of which are serious or potentially life-threatening. The table below describes some more common adverse effects; tables on the following pages deal with rare or serious events.

Table

Adverse effect	Time course	Action
Sedation	First few months. May persist, but usually wears off	Give smaller dose in the morning. Reduce dose if necessary
Hypersalivation	First few months. May persist, but usually wears off. Often very troublesome at night	Give hyoscine 300 µg (Kwells) sucked and swallowed at night. Pirenzepine[1] (not licensed in the UK) up to 50 mg tds should be tried (see page 81)
Constipation	Usually persists	Recommend high-fibre diet. Bulk-forming and stimulant laxatives should be used. Effective treatment or prevention of constipation is essential as death may result[2]
Hypotension	First 4 weeks	Advise patient to take time when standing up. Reduce dose or slow down rate of increase. If severe, consider moclobemide and Bovril[3], or fludrocortisone
Hypertension	First 4 weeks, sometimes longer	Monitor closely and increase dose as slowly as is necessary. Hypotensive therapy (e.g. atenolol 25 mg/day) is sometimes necessary[4]
Tachycardia	First 4 weeks, but sometimes persists	Very common in early stages of treatment but usually benign. Tachycardia, if persistent at rest and associated with fever, hypotension or chest pain, may indicate myocarditis[5,6] (see page 75). Referral to a cardiologist is advised. Clozapine should be stopped if tachycardia occurs in the context of chest pain or heart failure. Benign tachycardia can be treated with atenolol

Table (Cont.)

Weight gain	Usually during the first year of treatment	Dietary counselling is essential. Advice may be more effective if given before weight gain occurs. Weight gain is common and often profound (>10 lbs) (see page 110)
Fever	First 3 weeks	Give antipyretic but check FBC. This fever is not usually related to blood dyscrasias[7,8] but beware myocarditis (see page 75)
Seizures	May occur at any time[9]	Dose-/dose increase-related. Consider prophylactic valproate* if on high dose or with high plasma level (>500 μg/l). After a seizure: withhold clozapine for 1 day; restart at reduced dose; give sodium valproate. EEG abnormalities are common in those on clozapine[10]
Nausea	First 6 weeks	May give antiemetic. Avoid prochlorperazine and metoclopramide if previous EPSEs
Nocturnal enuresis	May occur at any time	Try manipulating dose schedule. Avoid fluids before bedtime. May resolve spontaneously[11]. In severe cases, desmopressin is usually effective[12] but is not without risk: hyponatraemia may result[13]. Anticholinergic agents may be effective[14] but support for this is weak
Neutropenia/ agranulocytosis	First 18 weeks (but may occur at any time)	Stop clozapine; admit to hospital

* Usual dose is 1000–2000 mg/day. Plasma levels may be useful as a rough guide to dosing – aim for 50–100 mg/l. Use of modified-release preparation (Epilim Chrono) may aid compliance: can be given once daily and may be better tolerated.

References

1. Fritze J et al. Pirenzepine for clozapine-induced hypersalivation. Lancet 1995;346:1034.
2. Townsend G et al. Case report: rapidly fatal bowel ischaemia on clozapine treatment. BMC Psychiatry 2006;6:43.
3. Taylor D et al. Clozapine-induced hypotension treated with moclobemide and Bovril. Br J Psychiatry 1995; 167:409–10.
4. Henderson DC et al. Clozapine and hypertension: a chart review of 82 patients. J Clin Psychiatry 2004; 65:686–9.
5. Committee on Safety of Medicines. Clozapine and cardiac safety: updated advice for prescribers. Curr Probl Pharmacovig 2002;28:8.
6. Hagg S et al. Myocarditis related to clozapine treatment. J Clin Psychopharmacol 2001;21:382–8.
7. Tham JC et al. Clozapine-induced fevers and 1-year clozapine discontinuation rate. J Clin Psychiatry 2002; 63:880–4.
8. Tremeau F et al. Spiking fevers with clozapine treatment. Clin Neuropharmacol 1997;20:168–70.
9. Pacia SV et al. Clozapine-related seizures: experience with 5,629 patients. Neurology 1994;44:2247–9.
10. Centorrino F et al. EEG abnormalities during treatment with typical and atypical antipsychotics. Am J Psychiatry 2002;159:109–15.
11. Warner JP et al. Clozapine and urinary incontinence. Int Clin Psychopharmacol 1994;9:207–9.
12. Steingard S. Use of desmopressin to treat clozapine-induced nocturnal enuresis. J Clin Psychiatry 1994; 55:315–16.
13. Sarma S et al. Severe hyponatraemia associated with desmopressin nasal spray to treat clozapine-induced nocturnal enuresis. Aust N Z J Psychiatry 2005;39:949.
14. Praharaj SK et al. Amitriptyline for clozapine-induced nocturnal enuresis and sialorrhoea. Br J Clin Pharmacol 2006 Aug 30; [Epub ahead of print].

Further reading

Iqbal MM et al. Clozapine: a clinical review of adverse effects and management. Ann Clin Psychiatry 2003;15:33–48.
Lieberman JA. Maximizing clozapine therapy: managing side effects. J Clin Psychiatry 1998; 59(Suppl 3):38–43.

Clozapine – uncommon or unusual adverse effects

Pharmacoepidemiological monitoring of clozapine is more extensive than with any other drug. Our awareness of adverse effects related to clozapine treatment is therefore enhanced. The table below gives brief details of unusual or uncommon adverse effects of clozapine reported since its relaunch in 1990.

Table

Adverse effect	Comment
Agranulocytosis/neutropenia (delayed)[1–3]	Occasional reports of apparent clozapine-related blood dyscrasia even after 1 year of treatment
Delirium[4]	Reported to be fairly common, but rarely seen in practice if dose is titrated slowly and plasma level determinations are used
Eosinophilia[5,6]	Reasonably common but significance unclear. Some suggestion that eosinophilia predicts neutropenia but this is disputed. May be associated with colitis and related symptoms[7]
Heat stroke[8]	Occasional case reported. May be mistaken for NMS
Hepatic failure/enzyme abnormalities[9,10]	Benign changes in LFTs are common (up to 50% of patients) but worth monitoring because of the very small risk of fulminant hepatic failure. Rash may be associated with clozapine-related hepatitis[11]
Pancreatitis[12]	Rare reports of asymptomatic and symptomatic pancreatitis sometimes associated with eosinophilia. Some authors recommend monitoring serum amylase
Pneumonia[13]	Very rarely results from saliva aspiration. Infections in general may be more common in those on clozapine[14]. Note that respiratory infections may give rise to elevated clozapine levels[15,16]. (Possibly an artefact: smoking usually ceases during an infection)
Thrombocytopenia[17]	Few data but apparently fairly common. Probably transient and clinically unimportant
Vasculitis[18]	One report in the literature in which patient developed confluent erythematous rash on lower limbs

References

1. Thompson A et al. Late onset neutropenia with clozapine. Can J Psychiatry 2004;49:647–8.
2. Bhanji NH et al. Late-onset agranulocytosis in a patient with schizophrenia after 17 months of clozapine treatment. J Clin Psychopharmacol 2003;23:522–3.
3. Sedky K et al. Clozapine-induced agranulocytosis after 11 years of treatment (Letter). Am J Psychiatry 2005;162:814.
4. Centorrino F et al. Delirium during clozapine treatment: incidence and associated risk factors. Pharmacopsychiatry 2003;36:156–60.
5. Hummer M et al. Does eosinophilia predict clozapine induced neutropenia? Psychopharmacology 1996;124:201–4.
6. Ames D et al. Predictive value of eosinophilia for neutropenia during clozapine treatment. J Clin Psychiatry 1996;57:579–81.
7. Karmachatya R et al. Clozapine-induced eosinophilic colitis (Letter). Am J Psychiatry 2005;162:1386a.
8. Kerwin RW et al. Heat stroke in schizophrenia during clozapine treatment: rapid recognition and management. J Psychopharmacol 2004;18:121–3.
9. Erdogan A et al. Management of marked liver enzyme increase during clozapine treatment: a case report and review of the literature. Int J Psychiatry Med 2004;34:83–9.
10. Macfarlane B et al. Fatal acute fulminant liver failure due to clozapine: a case report and review of clozapine-induced hepatotoxicity. Gastroenterology 1997;112:1707–9.
11. Fong SY et al. Clozapine-induced toxic hepatitis with skin rash. J Psychopharmacol 2005;19:107.
12. Bergemann N et al. Asymptomatic pancreatitis associated with clozapine. Pharmacopsychiatry 1999;32:78–80.
13. Hinkes R et al. Aspiration pneumonia possibly secondary to clozapine-induced sialorrhea. J Clin Psychopharmacol 1996;16:462–3.
14. Landry P et al. Increased use of antibiotics in clozapine-treated patients. Int Clin Psychopharmacol 2003;18:297–8.
15. Raaska K et al. Bacterial pneumonia can increase serum concentration of clozapine. Eur J Clin Pharmacol 2002;58:321–2.
16. de Leon J et al. Serious respiratory infections can increase clozapine levels and contribute to side effects: a case report. Prog Neuropsychopharmacol Biol Psychiatry 2003;27:1059–63.
17. Jagadheesan K et al. Clozapine-induced thrombocytopenia: a pilot study. Hong Kong J Psychiatry 2003;13:12–15.
18. Penaskovic KM et al. Clozapine-induced allergic vasculitis (Letter). Am J Psychiatry 2005;162:1543.

Clozapine – serious haematological and cardiovascular adverse effects

Agranulocytosis, thromboembolism, cardiomyopathy and myocarditis

Clozapine clearly and substantially reduces overall mortality in schizophrenia, largely because of a reduction in the rate of suicide[1,2]. Nevertheless, clozapine can cause serious, life-threatening adverse effects, of which **agranulocytosis** is the best known. In the UK, the risk if death from agranulocytosis is probably less than 1 in 10,000 patients exposed (Novartis report 4 deaths from 47,000 exposed)[3]. Risk is well managed by the approved clozapine-monitoring systems.

A possible association between clozapine and **pulmonary embolism** has been suggested. Initially, Walker et al[1] uncovered a risk of fatal pulmonary embolism of 1 in 4500 – about 20 times the risk in the population as a whole. Following a case report of non-fatal pulmonary embolism possibly related to clozapine[4], data from the Swedish authorities were published[5]. Twelve cases of venous thromboembolism were described, of which five were fatal. The risk of thromboembolism was estimated to be 1 in 2000–6000 patients treated. Thromboembolism may be related to clozapine's observed effect on antiphospholipid antibodies[6]. It seems most likely to occur in the first 3 months of treatment. Other SGAs may also be linked to thromboembolism, at least in the elderly[7].

It has also been suggested that clozapine is associated with **myocarditis** and **cardiomyopathy**. Australian data identified 23 cases (15 myocarditis, 8 cardiomyopathy), of which 6 were fatal[8]. Risk of death from either cause is estimated from these data to be 1 in 1300. Myocarditis seems to occur within 6–8 weeks of starting clozapine (median 3 weeks[9]); cardiomyopathy may occur later in treatment (median 9 months[9]). It is notable that other data sources give rather different risk estimates: in Canada the risk of fatal myocarditis was estimated to be 1 in 12,500; in the USA, 1 in 67,000[10]. Conversely, an Australian study identified nine cases of possible (non-fatal) myocarditis in 94 patients treated[11]. Despite this uncertainty over incidence, patients should be closely monitored for signs of myocarditis especially in the first few months of treatment[12]. Symptoms include tachycardia, fever, flu-like symptoms, fatigue, dyspnoea and chest pain. Signs include ECG changes (ST depression), enlarged heart on radiography and eosinophilia. Many of these symptoms occur in patients on clozapine not developing myocarditis[13]. Nonetheless, signs of heart failure should provoke immediate cessation of clozapine. Rechallenge has been successfully completed[11] but recurrence is possible[14]. Cardiomyopathy should be suspected in any patient showing signs of heart failure, which should provoke immediate referral.

Note also that, despite an overall reduction in mortality, younger patients may have an increased risk of sudden death[15], perhaps because of clozapine-induced ECG changes[16]. The overall picture remains very unclear but caution is required. There may, of course, be similar problems with other antipsychotics[17–19].

Summary

- Overall mortality appears to be lower for those on clozapine than in schizophrenia as a whole.
- Risk of fatal agranulocytosis is less than 1 in 10 000 patients treated in the UK.
- Risk of fatal pulmonary embolism is estimated to be around 1 in 4500 patients treated.
- Risk of fatal myocarditis or cardiomyopathy may be as high as 1 in 1300 patients.
- Careful monitoring is essential especially during the first 3 months of treatment.

References

1. Walker AM et al. Mortality in current and former users of clozapine. Epidemiology 1997;8:671–7.
2. Munro J et al. Active monitoring of 12,760 clozapine recipients in the UK and Ireland. Beyond pharma-covigilance. Br J Psychiatry 1999;175:576–80.
3. Thuillier S. Clozapine and agranulocytosis. Personal communication 2006.
4. Lacika S et al. Pulmonary embolus possibly associated with clozapine treatment (Letter). Can J Psychiatry 1999;44:396–7.
5. Hagg S et al. Association of venous thromboembolism and clozapine. Lancet 2000;355:1155–6.
6. Davis S et al. Antiphospholipid antibodies associated with clozapine treatment. Am J Hematol 1994; 46:166–7.
7. Liperoti R et al. Venous thromboembolism among elderly patients treated with atypical and conventional antipsychotic agents. Arch Intern Med 2005;165:2677–82.
8. Killian JG et al. Myocarditis and cardiomyopathy associated with clozapine. Lancet 1999;354:1841–5.
9. La Grenade L et al. Myocarditis and cardiomyopathy associated with clozapine use in the United States (Letter). N Engl J Med 2001;345:224–5.
10. Warner B et al. Clozapine and sudden death. Lancet 2000;355:842.
11. Reinders J et al. Clozapine-related myocarditis and cardiomyopathy in an Australian metropolitan psychiatric service. Aust N Z J Psychiatry 2004;38:915–22.
12. Marder SR et al. Physical health monitoring of patients with schizophrenia. Am J Psychiatry 2004;161:1334–49.
13. Wehmeier PM et al. Chart review for potential features of myocarditis, pericarditis, and cardiomyopathy in children and adolescents treated with clozapine. J Child Adolesc Psychopharmacol 2004;14:267–71.
14. Roh S et al. Cardiomyopathy associated with clozapine. Exp Clin Psychopharmacol 2006;14:94–8.
15. Modai I et al. Sudden death in patients receiving clozapine treatment: a preliminary investigation. J Clin Psychopharmacol 2000;20:325–7.
16. Kang UG et al. Electrocardiographic abnormalities in patients treated with clozapine. J Clin Psychiatry 2000;61:441–6.
17. Thomassen R et al. Antipsychotic drugs and venous thromboembolism (Letter). Lancet 2000;356:252.
18. Hagg S et al. Antipsychotic-induced venous thromboembolism: a review of the evidence. CNS Drugs 2002;16:765–76.
19. Coulter DM et al. Antipsychotic drugs and heart muscle disorder in international pharmacovigilance: data mining study. BMJ 2001;322:1207–9.

Further reading

Razminia M et al. Clozapine induced myopericarditis: early recognition improves clinical outcome. Am J Ther 2006;13:274–6.

Wehmeier PM et al. Myocarditis, pericarditis and cardiomyopathy in patients treated with clozapine. J Clin Pharm Ther 2005;30:91–6.

Clozapine, neutropenia and lithium

Risk of clozapine-induced neutropenia

Around 2.7% of patients treated with clozapine develop neutropenia. Of these, half do so within the first 18 weeks of treatment and three-quarters by the end of the first year[1]. Risk factors[1] include being Afro-Caribbean (77% increase in risk) and young (17% decrease in risk per decade increase in age), and having a low baseline white cell count (WCC) (31% increase in risk for each 1×10^9/l drop). Risk is not dose-related.

After being released from the bone marrow, neutrophils can either circulate freely in the bloodstream or be deposited next to vessel walls (margination)[2]. All of these neutrophils are available to fight infection. The proportion of marginated neutrophils is greater in people of Afro-Caribbean or African origin than in Caucasians, leading to lower apparent WCCs in the former. This is benign ethnic neutropenia.

Many patients develop neutropenia on clozapine but not all are clozapine-related or even pathological. Benign ethnic neutropenia very probably accounts for a proportion of observed or apparent clozapine-associated neutropenias (hence higher rates among Afro-Caribbeans). Distinguishing between true clozapine toxicity and neutropenia unrelated to clozapine is not possible with certainty but some factors are important. True clozapine-induced neutropenia generally occurs early in treatment. White cell counts are normal to begin with but then fall precipitantly (over 1–2 weeks or less) and recover slowly once clozapine is withdrawn. In benign ethnic neutropenia, WCCs are generally low and may frequently fall below the lower limit of normal. This pattern may be observed before, during and after the use of clozapine. Of course, true clozapine-induced neutropenia can occur in the context of benign ethnic neutropenia. Partly because of this, **any iatrogenic manipulation of WCCs in benign ethnic neutropenia carries significant risk.**

Effect of lithium on the WCC

Lithium increases the neutrophil count and total WCC both acutely[3] and chronically[4]. The magnitude of this effect is poorly quantified, but a mean neutrophil count of 11.9×10^9/l has been reported in lithium-treated patients[3] and a mean rise in neutrophil count of 2×10^9/l was seen in clozapine-treated patients after the addition of lithium[5]. This effect does not seem to be clearly dose-related[3,4], although a minimum lithium serum level of 0.4 mmol/l may be required[6]. The mechanism is not completely understood: both stimulation of granulocyte–macrophage colony-stimulating factor (GM-CSF)[7] and demargination[5] have been suggested. Lithium has been successfully used to raise the WCC during cancer chemotherapy[8–10]. White cells are fully formed and function normally – there is no 'left shift'.

Case reports

Lithium has been used to increase the WCC in patients who have developed neutropenia with clozapine, thus allowing clozapine treatment to continue.

Several case reports in adults[6,11-14] and in children[15] have been published. All patients had serum lithium levels of >0.6 mmol/l. Lithium has also been reported to speed the recovery of the WCC when prescribed after the development of clozapine-induced agranulocytosis[6].

Other potential benefits of lithium–clozapine combinations

Combinations of clozapine and lithium may improve symptoms in schizoaffective patients[5] and refractory bipolar illness[16,17]. There are no data pertaining to schizophrenia.

Potential risks

At least 0.7% of clozapine-treated patients develop agranulocytosis, which is potentially fatal. Over 80% of cases develop within the first 18 weeks of treatment[1]. Risk factors include increasing age and Asian race[1]. Some patients may be genetically predisposed[18]. Although the timescale and individual risk factors for the development of agranulocytosis are different from those associated with neutropenia, it is impossible to be certain in any given patient that neutropenia is not a precursor to agranulocytosis. Lithium does not seem to protect against true clozapine-induced agranulocytosis: one case of fatal agranulocytosis has occurred with this combination[19] and a second case of agranulocytosis has been reported where the bone marrow was resistant to treatment with GCSF[20]. Note also that up to 20% of patients who receive clozapine–lithium combinations develop neurological symptoms typical of lithium toxicity despite lithium levels being maintained well within the therapeutic range[5,21].

The use of lithium to elevate WCC in patients with clear prior clozapine-induced neutropenia is not recommended. Lithium should only be used to elevate WCC where it is strongly felt that prior neutropenic episodes were unrelated to clozapine. One-third of patients who stop clozapine because they have developed neutropenia or agranulocytosis will develop a blood dyscrasia on rechallenge. In almost all cases, the second reaction will occur more rapidly, be more severe and last longer than the first[22].

Lithium for the management of patients with:

1. low initial WCC ($<4 \times 10^9$/l) or neutrophils ($<2.5 \times 10^9$/l)
or
2. clozapine-associated leucopenia (WCC $<3 \times 10^9$/l) or neutropenia (neutrophils $<1.5 \times 10^9$/l) thought to be linked to benign ethnic neutropenia.

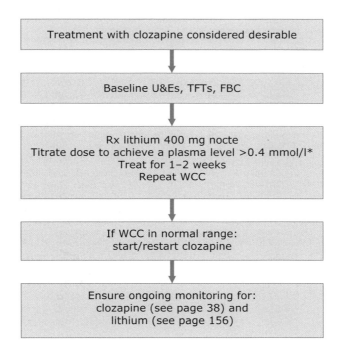

NB: Lithium does not protect against agranulocytosis: if the WCC continues to fall despite lithium treatment, consideration should be given to discontinuing clozapine. Particular vigilance is required in high-risk patients during the first 18 weeks of treatment.

*Higher plasma levels may be appropriate for patients who have an affective component to their illness.

References

1. Munro J et al. Active monitoring of 12,760 clozapine recipients in the UK and Ireland. Beyond pharma-covigilance. Br J Psychiatry 1999;175:576–80.
2. Abramson N et al. Leukocytosis: basics of clinical assessment. Am Fam Physician 2000;62:2053–60.
3. Lapierre G et al. Lithium carbonate and leukocytosis. Am J Hosp Pharm 1980;37:1525–8.
4. Carmen J et al. The effects of lithium therapy on leukocytes: a 1-year follow-up study. J Natl Med Assoc 1993;85:301–3.
5. Small JG et al. Tolerability and efficacy of clozapine combined with lithium in schizophrenia and schizoaffective disorder. J Clin Psychopharmacol 2003;23:223–8.
6. Blier P et al. Lithium and clozapine-induced neutropenia/agranulocytosis. Int Clin Psychopharmacol 1998; 13:137–40.
7. Ozdemir MA et al. Lithium-induced hematologic changes in patients with bipolar affective disorder. Biol Psychiatry 1994;35:210–13.
8. Johnke RM et al. Accelerated marrow recovery following total-body irradiation after treatment with vin-cristine, lithium or combined vincristine–lithium. Int J Cell Cloning 1991;9:78–88.
9. Greco FA et al. Effect of lithium carbonate on the neutropenia caused by chemotherapy: a preliminary clinical trial. Oncology 1977;34:153–5.
10. Ridgway D et al. Enhanced lymphocyte response to PHA among leukopenia patients taking oral lithium carbonate. Cancer Invest 1986;4:513–17.
11. Adityanjee A. Modification of clozapine-induced leukopenia and neutropenia with lithium carbonate. Am J Psychiatry 1995;152:648–9.
12. Silverstone PH. Prevention of clozapine-induced neutropenia by pretreatment with lithium. J Clin Psychopharmacol 1998;18:86–8.
13. Boshes RA et al. Initiation of clozapine therapy in a patient with preexisting leukopenia: a discussion of the rationale of current treatment options. Ann Clin Psychiatry 2001;13:233–7.
14. Papetti F et al. Treatment of clozapine-induced granulocytopenia with lithium (two observations). Encephale 2004;30:578–82.
15. Sporn A et al. Clozapine-induced neutropenia in children: management with lithium carbonate. J Child Adolesc Psychopharmacol 2003;13:401–4.
16. Suppes T et al. Clozapine treatment of nonpsychotic rapid cycling bipolar disorder: a report of three cases. Biol Psychiatry 1994;36:338–40.
17. Puri BK et al. Low-dose maintenance clozapine treatment in the prophylaxis of bipolar affective disorder. Br J Clin Pract 1995;49:333–4.
18. Dettling M et al. Further evidence of human leukocyte antigen-encoded susceptibility to clozapine-induced agranulocytosis independent of ancestry. Pharmacogenetics 2001;11:135–41.
19. Gerson SL et al. Polypharmacy in fatal clozapine-associated agranulocytosis. Lancet 1991;338:262–3.
20. Valevski A et al. Clozapine–lithium combined treatment and agranulocytosis. Int Clin Psychopharmacol 1993;8:63–5.
21. Blake LM et al. Reversible neurologic symptoms with clozapine and lithium. J Clin Psychopharmacol 1992;12:297–9.
22. Dunk LR et al. Rechallenge with clozapine following leucopenia or neutropenia during previous therapy. Br J Psychiatry 2006;188:255–63.

Further reading

Paton C et al. Managing clozapine-induced neutropenia with lithium. Psychiatr Bull 2005; 29:186–8.
Whiskey E et al. Restarting clozapine after neutropenia: evaluating the possibilities and practicalities. CNS Drugs 2007;21:25–5.

Clozapine-related hypersalivation

Clozapine is well known to be causally associated with apparent hypersalivation (drooling, particularly at night). This seems to be chiefly problematic in the early stages of treatment and is probably dose-related. Clinical observation suggests that hypersalivation reduces in severity over time (usually several months) but may persist. Clozapine-induced hypersalivation is socially embarrassing and potentially life-threatening[1], so treatment is a matter of some urgency.

The pharmacological basis of clozapine-related hypersalivation remains unclear[2]. Suggested mechanisms include muscarinic M_4 agonism, adrenergic α_2 antagonism and inhibition of the swallowing reflex[3,4]. The last of these is supported by trials which suggest that saliva production is not increased in clozapine-treated patients[5,6].

Whatever the mechanism, drugs which reduce saliva production are likely to diminish the severity of this adverse effect. The table below describes drug treatments so far examined.

Table Clozapine–related hypersalivation Summary

Treatment	Comments
Amisulpride 400 mg/day[7]	Supported by one, small positive RCT
Amitriptyline 75–100 mg/day[8]	Limited literature support. Adverse effects may be troublesome
Atropine eye drops (1%) – given sublingually[9]	Limited literature support. Rarely used
Benzhexol (trihexyphenidyl) 5–15 mg/day[10]	Small, open study suggests useful activity Widely used in some centres but may impair cognitive function
Benzatropine 2 mg/day + terazosin 2 mg/day[11]	Combination shown to be better than either drug alone Not widely used
Botulinum toxin[12] (Botox)	Effective in treating sialorrhoea associated with neurological disorders. Single case report of success in clozapine-treated patient
Clonidine (0.1 mg patch weekly or 0.1 mg orally at night)[13,14]	α_2 partial agonist. Limited literature support. May exacerbate psychosis and depression
Hyoscine 0.3 mg sucked and swallowed up to 3 times daily	Peripheral and central anticholinergic Very widely used but no published data available Patches also used[15] May cause cognitive impairment, drowsiness and constipation
Ipratropium nasal spray (0.03%) – given sublingually[16,17] or intranasally[17]	Limited literature support. Rarely used
Lofexidine 0.2 mg twice daily[18]	α_2 agonist. Very few data. May exacerbate psychosis and depression
Pirenzepine 25–100 mg/day[19–21]	Selective M_1, M_4 antagonist Does not affect clozapine metabolism Extensive clinical experience suggests efficacy in some but randomised trial suggests no effect. Still widely used
Propantheline 7.5 mg at night	Peripheral anticholinergic. No central effects. No published data
Quetiapine[22]	May reduce hypersalivation by allowing lower doses of clozapine to be used
Sulpiride 150–300 mg/day[23]	Supported by one, small positive RCT

References

1. Hinkes R et al. Aspiration pneumonia possibly secondary to clozapine-induced sialorrhea. J Clin Psychopharmacol 1996;16:462–3.
2. Praharaj SK et al. Clozapine-induced sialorrhea: pathophysiology and management strategies. Psychopharmacology 2006;185:265–73.
3. Davydov L et al. Clozapine-induced hypersalivation. Ann Pharmacother 2000;34:662–5.
4. Rogers DP et al. Therapeutic options in the treatment of clozapine-induced sialorrhea. Pharmacotherapy 2000;20:1092–5.
5. Rabinowitz T et al. The effect of clozapine on saliva flow rate: a pilot study. Biol Psychiatry 1996;40:1132–4.
6. Ben Aryeh H et al. Salivary flow-rate and composition in schizophrenic patients on clozapine: subjective reports and laboratory data. Biol Psychiatry 1996;39:946–9.
7. Kreinin A et al. Amisulpride treatment of clozapine-induced hypersalivation in schizophrenia patients: a randomized, double-blind, placebo-controlled cross-over study. Int Clin Psychopharmacol 2006;21:99–103.
8. Copp P et al. Amitriptyline in clozapine-induced sialorrhoea. Br J Psychiatry 1991;159:166.
9. Antonello C et al. Clozapine and sialorrhea: a new intervention for this bothersome and potentially dangerous side effect. J Psychiatry Neurosci 1999;24:250.
10. Spivak B et al. Trihexyphenidyl treatment of clozapine-induced hypersalivation. Int Clin Psychopharmacol 1997;12:213–15.
11. Reinstein M et al. Comparative efficacy and tolerability of benzatropine and terazosin in the treatment of hypersalivation secondary to clozapine. Clin Drug Invest 1999;17:97–102.
12. Kahl KG et al. Botulinum toxin as an effective treatment of clozapine-induced hypersalivation. Psychopharmacology 2004;173:229–30.
13. Grabowski J. Clonidine treatment of clozapine-induced hypersalivation. J Clin Psychopharmacol 1992;12:69–70.
14. Praharaj SK et al. Is clonidine useful for treatment of clozapine-induced sialorrhea? J Psychopharmacol 2005;19:426–8.
15. McKane JP et al. Hyoscine patches in clozapine-induced hypersalivation. Psychiatr Bull 2001;25:277c.
16. Calderon J et al. Potential use of ipatropium bromide for the treatment of clozapine-induced hypersalivation: a preliminary report. Int Clin Psychopharmacol 2000;15:49–52.
17. Freudenreich O et al. Clozapine-induced sialorrhea treated with sublingual ipratropium spray: a case series. J Clin Psychopharmacol 2004;24:98–100.
18. Corrigan FM et al. Clozapine-induced hypersalivation and the alpha 2 adrenoceptor. Br J Psychiatry 1995;167:412.
19. Fritze J et al. Pirenzepine for clozapine-induced hypersalivation. Lancet 1995;346:1034.
20. Bai YM et al. Therapeutic effect of pirenzepine for clozapine-induced hypersalivation: a randomized, double-blind, placebo-controlled, cross-over study. J Clin Psychopharmacol 2001;21:608–11.
21. Schneider B et al. Reduction of clozapine-induced hypersalivation by pirenzepine is safe. Pharmacopsychiatry 2004;37:43–5.
22. Reinstein MJ et al. Use of quetiapine to manage patients who experienced adverse effects with clozapine. Clin Drug Invest 2003;23:63–7.
23. Kreinin A et al. Sulpiride addition for the treatment of clozapine-induced hypersalivation: preliminary study. Isr J Psychiatry Relat Sci 2005;42:61–3.

Clozapine and cancer chemotherapy

The use of clozapine with agents which are known to cause neutropenia is contraindicated. Most chemotherapy treatments cause significant bone marrow suppression. When WCCs fall $<3.0 \times 10^9/l$, clozapine is usually discontinued. Chemotherapy is likely to reduce white blood cells below this level irrespective of the use of clozapine.

If possible, clozapine should be discontinued before chemotherapy. However, many patients will be at high risk of relapse or deterioration if clozapine is discontinued and other antipsychotics are unlikely to be as beneficial. The deteriorating patient may refuse or remove consent for chemotherapy, which poses a therapeutic dilemma in the patient prescribed clozapine and requiring chemotherapy.

There are several case reports in the literature supporting continuing clozapine during chemotherapy treatment[1-8]. Successful outcome probably depends on a collaborative approach between the oncologist, psychiatrist, pharmacy, patient and clozapine monitoring service.

The clozapine monitoring service will ask for the psychiatrist to sign an unlicensed use form and will request additional blood monitoring. There is one case report of neutropenia persisting for 6 months after doxorubicin, radiotherapy and clozapine[7]. Granulocyte-colony stimulating factor (G-CSF) has also been used to treat agranulocytosis associated with chemotherapy and clozapine in combination[8].

Summary

- If possible, clozapine should be discontinued before starting chemotherapy.
- The risk of relapse or deterioration must be considered before discontinuing clozapine.
- The relapsing patient may refuse or withdraw consent for chemotherapy.
- When clozapine is continued during chemotherapy, a collaborative approach is strongly recommended.

References

1. Wesson ML et al. Continuing clozapine despite neutropenia. Br J Psychiatry 1996;168:217–20.
2. Bareggi C et al. Clozapine and full-dose concomitant chemoradiation therapy in a schizophrenic patient with nasopharyngeal cancer. Tumori 2002;88:59–60.
3. Avnon M et al. Clozapine, cancer, and schizophrenia. Am J Psychiatry 1993;150:1562–3.
4. Hundertmark J et al. Reintroduction of clozapine after diagnosis of lymphoma. Br J Psychiatry 2001;178:576.
5. McKenna RC et al. Clozapine and chemotherapy. Hosp Community Psychiatry 1994;45:831.
6. Haut FA. Clozapine and chemotherapy. J Drug Dev Clin Pract 1995;7:237–9.
7. Rosenstock J. Clozapine therapy during cancer treatment. Am J Psychiatry 2004;161:175.
8. Lee SY et al. Combined antitumor chemotherapy in a refractory schizophrenic receiving clozapine. J Korean Neuropsychiatr Assoc 2000;39:234–9.

Schizophrenia

Guidelines for the initiation of clozapine for patients based in the community

Note: this section provides general guidance – refer to manufacturer's and local policies (where available) for detailed guidance.

Some points to check before starting:

- Is the patient likely to be adherent with oral medication?
- Has the patient understood the need for regular blood tests?
- Is it possible for the patient to be seen every day during the early titration phase?
- Is the patient able to attend the team base or pharmacy to collect medication every week or does medication need to be delivered?
- Does the patient live with other people?

Mandatory blood monitoring and registration with an approved clozapine monitoring service:

- Register with the relevant monitoring service.
- Perform baseline blood tests (WCC and differential count) before starting clozapine.
- Further blood testing continues weekly for the first 18 weeks and then every 2 weeks for the remainder of the year. After that, the blood monitoring is usually done monthly.

Dosing

Note: other schedules than that described below are possible (e.g. 12-week titration with twice-weekly monitoring).

Starting clozapine in the community requires a slow and flexible titration schedule. Prior antipsychotics should be slowly discontinued.

There are two basic methods for starting clozapine in the community. The first method is to give the first dose in the morning in clinic and then monitor as usual for 6 hours. The patient is then allowed home and the process repeated the next day. On the second day the patient takes home a night-time dose. The second method involves giving the first dose before retiring, so avoiding the need for close physical monitoring immediately after administration. This is described below. All initiations should take place on a Monday and Tuesday so that adequate staffing and monitoring are assured.

Table Suggested initial titration regimen – clozapine in the community

Day	Day of the week	Morning dose (mg)	Evening dose (mg)	Percentage dose of previous antipsychotic
1	Monday	–	6.25	100
2	Tuesday	6.25	6.25	
3	Wednesday	6.25	6.25	
4	Thursday	6.25	12.5	
5	Friday	12.5	12.5	
6	Saturday	12.5	12.5	
7	Sunday	12.5	12.5	
8	Monday	12.5	25	
9	Tuesday	12.5	25	
10	Wednesday	25	25	
11	Thursday	25	37.5	
12	Friday	25	37.5	
13	Saturday	25	37.5	
14	Sunday	25	37.5	
15	Monday	37.5	37.5	75
16	Tuesday	37.5	37.5	
17	Wednesday	37.5	50	
18	Thursday	37.5	50	
19	Friday	50	50	
20	Saturday	50	50	
21	Sunday	50	50	
22	Monday	50	75	
23	Tuesday	50	75	
24	Wednesday	75	75	
25	Thursday	75	75	
26	Friday	75	100	50
27	Saturday	75	100	
28	Sunday	75	100	

Further increments should be 25 mg/day until target dose is reached.

Switching from other antipsychotics

- The switching regimen will be largely dependent on the patient's mental state.
- Consider additive side-effects of the antipsychotics (e.g. effect on QTc interval) (see page 116).
- Consider drug interactions (e.g. risperidone may increase clozapine levels).
- All depots, sertindole, pimozide and ziprasidone should be stopped before clozapine is started.
- Other antipsychotics and clozapine may be cross-tapered with varying degrees of caution. ECG monitoring is prudent when clozapine is co-prescribed with other drugs known to affect QT interval.

Clozapine in the community – acute monitoring requirements

- *Blood pressure (BP), temperature and pulse*. After the first dose, monitor BP, temperature and pulse hourly for at least 3 (preferably 6) hours afterwards. (This may not be necessary if the first dose is given at bedtime.) Thereafter, the patient should be seen at least once a day (twice a day if faster titration is used), and all three parameters should be monitored before and after the morning dose.
- Continue daily monitoring for at least 2 weeks or until there are no unacceptable adverse effects. Twice-weekly monitoring may then be undertaken until a stable dose is reached. Thereafter, monitor at time of blood testing.
- If the patient is attending a day hospital they should be accompanied to and from the unit for the first week.
- A full physical examination should be undertaken each week during titration.
- The formal carer (usually the Community Psychiatric Nurse) should inform the prescriber if:
  - **temperature** rises above **38°C** (this is very common and is not a good reason, on its own, for stopping clozapine); see page 70
  - **pulse** is >**100 bpm** (also common but may rarely be linked to myocarditis)
  - **postural drop** of >**30 mmHg**
  - patient is clearly oversedated
  - any other **adverse effect is intolerable**.

Additional monitoring requirements (see page 38)

Baseline	1 month	3 months	4–6 months	12 months
Weight, lipids	Weight	Weight, lipids	Weight, lipids	Weight, lipids
Plasma glucose	Plasma glucose		Plasma glucose	Plasma glucose
LFTs			LFTs	

Where available, consider also use of ECG (benefit not established, but see above). Oral glucose tolerance test is preferred to plasma glucose.

Adverse effects

- Sedation and hypotension are common at the start of treatment. These effects can usually be managed by reducing the dose or slowing down the rate of titration.
- Many other adverse effects associated with clozapine can also be managed by dose reduction.

Management of adverse effects

See page 70 et seq.

Serious cardiac adverse effects (see page 75)

Patients who have *persistent* tachycardia at rest, especially during the first 2 months of treatment, should be closely observed for other signs or symptoms of myocarditis. These include palpitations, arrhythmia, symptoms mimicking myocardial infarction, chest pain and other unexplained symptoms of heart failure.

In patients with suspected clozapine-induced myocarditis or cardiomyopathy, the drug must be stopped and the patient referred to a cardiologist. If clozapine-induced myocarditis or cardiomyopathy is confirmed, the patient must not be re-exposed to clozapine.

Further reading

O'Brien A. Starting clozapine in the community: a UK perspective. CNS Drugs 2004;18:845–52.

Lovett L et al. Initiation of clozapine treatment at home. Progress in Neurology and Psychiatry. 2004; 8:19–21.

Fish oils in schizophrenia

Fish oils contain the omega-3 fatty acids, eicosapentaenoic acid (EPA) and docosahexaenoic acid (DHA). These compounds are thought to be involved in maintaining neuronal membrane structure, in the modulation of membrane proteins and in the production of prostaglandins and leukotrienes[1]. They have been suggested as treatments for a variety of psychiatric illnesses[2] but most research relates to their use in schizophrenia, where case reports[3–5] and prospective trials suggest useful efficacy (see the following table).

Table A summary of the evidence – fish oils in schizophrenia

References	n	Design	Outcome
Mellor et al 1995[6]	20	Open-label evaluation of fish oil (EPA+DHA) added to usual medication	Significant improvement in symptoms
Peet et al 2001[7]	45	Double-blind, randomised comparison of EPA (2 g daily), DHA and placebo (12 weeks)	EPA significantly more effective than DHA or placebo
Peet et al 2001[7]	26	Double-blind, randomised comparison of EPA (2 g daily) or placebo as sole drug treatment (12 weeks)	All 12 patients given placebo required conventional antipsychotic treatment; 8 of 14 given EPA required antipsychotics. EPA more effective
Peet et al 2002[8]	115	Double-blind randomised comparison of ethyl-EPA (1, 2 or 4 g/day) and placebo added to antipsychotic treatment (conventional, atypical or clozapine) (12 weeks)	Ethyl-EPA significantly improved response in patients receiving clozapine. 2 g/day most effective dose
Fenton et al 2001[9]	87	Double-blind, randomised comparison of EPA (3 g daily) and placebo added to standard drug treatment (16 weeks)	No differences between EPA and placebo

Table A summary of the evidence – fish oils in schizophrenia (Cont.)

References	n	Design	Outcome
Emsley et al 2002[10]	40	Double-blind, randomised comparison of EPA (3 g daily) and placebo added to standard drug treatment (12 weeks)	EPA associated with significantly greater reduction in symptoms and tardive dyskinesia (9 patients in each group received clozapine)

On balance, evidence suggests that EPA (2–3 g daily) is a worthwhile option in schizophrenia when added to standard treatment, particularly clozapine[11,12]. However, doubt still remains over the true extent of the beneficial effect derived from fish oils, and research in this area has dwindled in the last few years[12]. Set against doubts over efficacy are the observations that fish oils are relatively cheap, well tolerated (mild GI symptoms may occur) and may benefit physical health[1].

Fish oils are therefore very tentatively recommended for the treatment of residual symptoms of schizophrenia but particularly in patients responding poorly to clozapine. Careful assessment of response is essential and fish oils should be withdrawn if no effect is observed after 3 months' treatment.

The recommended dose is

Omacor (414 mg EPA) 5 capsules daily

or

Maxepa (170 mg EPA) 10 capsules daily

References

1. Fenton WS et al. Essential fatty acids, lipid membrane abnormalities, and the diagnosis and treatment of schizophrenia. Biol Psychiatry 2000;47:8–21.
2. Freeman MP. Omega-3 fatty acids in psychiatry: a review. Ann Clin Psychiatry 2000;12:159–65.
3. Richardson AJ et al. Red cell and plasma fatty acid changes accompanying symptom remission in a patient with schizophrenia treated with eicosapentaenoic acid. Eur Neuropsychopharmacol 2000; 10:189–93.
4. Puri BK et al. Eicosapentaenoic acid treatment in schizophrenia associated with symptom remission, normalisation of blood fatty acids, reduced neuronal membrane phospholipid turnover and structural brain changes. Int J Clin Pract 2000;54:57–63.
5. Su KP et al. Omega-3 fatty acids as a psychotherapeutic agent for a pregnant schizophrenic patient. Eur Neuropsychopharmacol 2001;11:295–9.
6. Mellor JE et al. Schizophrenic symptoms and dietary intake of n-3 fatty acids. Schizophr Res 1995; 18:85–6.
7. Peet M et al. Two double-blind placebo-controlled pilot studies of eicosapentaenoic acid in the treatment of schizophrenia. Schizophr Res 2001;49:243–51.
8. Peet M et al. A dose-ranging exploratory study of the effects of ethyl-eicosapentaenoate in patients with persistent schizophrenic symptoms. J Psychiatr Res 2002;36:7–18.
9. Fenton WS et al. A placebo-controlled trial of omega-3 fatty acid (ethyl eicosapentaenoic acid) supplementation for residual symptoms and cognitive impairment in schizophrenia. Am J Psychiatry 2001; 158:2071–4.
10. Emsley R et al. Randomized, placebo-controlled study of ethyl-eicosapentaenoic acid as supplemental treatment in schizophrenia. Am J Psychiatry 2002;159:1596–8.
11. Emsley R et al. Clinical potential of omega-3 fatty acids in the treatment of schizophrenia. CNS Drugs 2003;17:1081–91.
12. Joy CB et al. Polyunsaturated fatty acid supplementation for schizophrenia. Cochrane Database Syst Rev 2006;3:CD001257.

Schizophrenia

Extrapyramidal side-effects

Table Most common extrapyramidal side-effects

	Dystonia (uncontrolled muscular spasm)	Pseudo-parkinsonism (tremor, etc.)	Akathisia (rest-lessness)[1]	Tardive dyskinesia (abnormal movements)
Signs and symptoms[2]	Muscle spasm in any part of the body, e.g. • Eyes rolling upwards (oculogyric crisis) • Head and neck twisted to the side (torticollis) *The patient may be unable to swallow or speak clearly. In extreme cases, the back may arch or the jaw dislocate* Acute dystonia can be both painful and very frightening	• Tremor and/or rigidity • Bradykinesia (decreased facial expression, flat monotone voice, slow body movements, inability to initiate movement) • Bradyphrenia (slowed thinking) • Salivation Pseudoparkinsonism can be mistaken for depression or the negative symptoms of schizophrenia	A subjectively unpleasant state of inner restlessness where there is a strong desire or compulsion to move • Foot stamping when seated • Constantly crossing/ uncrossing legs • Rocking from foot to foot • Constantly pacing up and down Akathisia can be mistaken for psychotic agitation and has been (weakly) linked with suicide and aggression towards others[3]	A wide variety of movements can occur such as: • Lip smacking or chewing • Tongue protrusion (fly catching) • Choreiform hand movements (pill-rolling or piano-playing) • Pelvic thrusting Severe orofacial movements can lead to difficulty speaking, eating or breathing. Movements are worse when under stress
Rating scales	No specific scale Small component of general EPSE scales	Simpson–Angus EPSE Rating Scale[4]	Barnes Akathisia Scale[5]	Abnormal Involuntary Movement Scale[6] (AIMS)
Prevalence (with FGA drugs)	Approximately 10%[7], but more common[8]: • In young males • In the neuroleptic-naive • With high potency	Approximately 20%[9], but more common in: • Elderly females • Those with pre-existing neurological damage	Approximately 25%[10]. Less with SGAs. In decreasing order: risperidone, olanzapine, quetiapine and	5% of patients per year of antipsychotic exposure[12]. More common in: • Elderly women

	drugs (e.g. haloperidol) Dystonic reactions are rare in the elderly	(head injury, stroke, etc.)	clozapine[11]	• Those with affective illness • Those who have had acute EPSEs early on in treatment
Time taken to develop	Acute dystonia can occur within hours of starting antipsychotics (minutes if the IM or IV route is used) Tardive dystonia occurs after months to years of antipsychotic treatment	Days to weeks after antipsychotic drugs are started or the dose is increased	Acute akathisia occurs within hours to weeks of starting antipsychotics or increasing the dose. Tardive akathisia takes longer to develop and can persist after antipsychotics have been withdrawn	Months to years Approximately 50% of cases are reversible[12]
Treatment	Anticholinergic drugs given orally, IM or IV depending on the severity of symptoms[8] • Remember the patient may be unable to swallow • Response to IV administration will be seen within 5 minutes • Response to IM administration takes around 20 minutes • Tardive dystonia may respond to ECT[13]	Several options are available depending on the clinical circumstances: • Reduce the antipsychotic dose • Change to an atypical drug (as antipsychotic monotherapy!) • Prescribe an anticholinergic. The majority of patients do not require long-term anticholinergics. Use should be reviewed at least every 3 months	• Reduce the antipsychotic dose • Change to a SGA drug • A reduction in symptoms may be seen with[14]: propranolol 30–80 mg/day, clonazepam (low dose) $5HT_2$ antagonists such as cyproheptadine[13], mirtazapine[14], trazodone[15], mianserin[16], and cyproheptadine[13] may help, as may diphenhydramine[17] All are unlicensed for this indication Anticholinergics are generally unhelpful[18]	• Stop anticholinergic if prescribed • Reduce dose of antipsychotic • Change to an atypical drug[19–22] • Clozapine is the antipsychotic most likely to be associated with resolution of symptoms[23] • For other treatment options see page 99[24]

EPSEs are:

- dose-related
- more likely with high-potency FGAs
- uncommon with most SGAs.

Patients who experience one type of EPSE may be more vulnerable to developing others[25].

References

1. Barnes TRE. The Barnes akathisia scale – revisited. J Psychopharmacol 2003;17:365–70.
2. Gervin M et al. Assessment of drug-related movement disorders in schizophrenia. Adv Psychiatr Treat 2000;6:332–41.
3. Leong GB et al. Neuroleptic-induced akathisia and violence: a review. J Forensic Sci 2003;48:187–9.
4. Simpson GM et al. A rating scale for extrapyramidal side effects. Acta Psychiatr Scand 1970; 212:11–19.
5. Barnes TRE. A rating scale for drug-induced akathisia. Br J Psychiatry 1989;154:672–6.
6. Guy W. ECDEU Assessment Manual for Psychopharmacology. Washington, DC: US Department of Health, Education, and Welfare 1976;534–7.
7. American Psychiatric Association. Practice guideline for the treatment of patients with schizophrenia. Am J Psychiatry 1997;154:1–63.
8. van Harten PN et al. Acute dystonia induced by drug treatment. Br Med J 1999;319:623–6.
9. Bollini P et al. Antipsychotic drugs: is more worse? A meta-analysis of the published randomized control trials. Psychol Med 1994;24:307–16.
10. Halstead SM et al. Akathisia: prevalence and associated dysphoria in an in-patient population with chronic schizophrenia. Br J Psychiatry 1994;164:177–83.
11. Hirose S. The causes of underdiagnosing akathisia. Schizophr Bull 2003;29:547–58.
12. American Psychiatric Association. Tardive Dyskinesia: A task force report of the American Psychiatric Association. Hosp Community Psychiatry 1993;44:190.
13. Miller CH et al. Managing antipsychotic-induced acute and chronic akathisia. Drug Saf 2000;22:73–81.
14. Poyurovsky M et al. Efficacy of low-dose mirtazapine in neuroleptic-induced akathisia: a double-blind randomized placebo-controlled pilot study. J Clin Psychopharmacol 2003;23:305–8.
15. Stryjer R et al. Treatment of neuroleptic-induced akathisia with the 5-HT$_{2A}$ antagonist trazodone. Clin Neuropharmacol 2003;26:137–41.
16. Stryjer R et al. Mianserin for the rapid improvement of chronic akathisia in a schizophrenia patient. Eur Psychiatry 2004;19:237–8.
17. Vinson DR. Diphenhydramine in the treatment of akathisia induced by prochlorperazine. J Emerg Med 2004;26:265–70.
18. Lima AR et al. Anticholinergics for neuroleptic-induced acute akathisia. Cochrane Database Syst Rev 2004;CD003727.
19. Glazer WM. Expected incidence of tardive dyskinesia associated with atypical antipsychotics. J Clin Psychiatry 2000;61(Suppl 4):21–6.
20. Kinon BJ et al. Olanzapine treatment for tardive dyskinesia in schizophrenia patients: a prospective clinical trial with patients randomized to blinded dose reduction periods. Prog Neuropsychopharmacol Biol Psychiatry 2004;28:985–96.
21. Bai YM et al. Risperidone for severe tardive dyskinesia: a 12-week randomized, double-blind, placebo-controlled study. J Clin Psychiatry 2003;64:1342–8.
22. Tenback DE et al. Effects of antipsychotic treatment on tardive dyskinesia: a 6-month evaluation of patients from the European Schizophrenia Outpatient Health Outcomes (SOHO) Study. J Clin Psychiatry 2005;66:1130–3.
23. Simpson GM. The treatment of tardive dyskinesia and tardive dystonia. J Clin Psychiatry 2000; 61(Suppl 4):39–44.
24. Duncan D et al. Tardive dyskinesia: how is it prevented and treated? Psychiatr Bull 1997;21:422–5.
25. Kim JH et al. Prevalence and characteristics of subjective akathisia, objective akathisia, and mixed akathisia in chronic schizophrenic subjects. Clin Neuropharmacol 2003;26:312–16.

Further reading

El Sayeh HG et al. Non-neuroleptic catecholaminergic drugs for neuroleptic-induced tardive dyskinesia. Cochrane Database Syst Rev 2006;CD000458.
McGrath JJ et al. Neuroleptic reduction and/or cessation and neuroleptics as specific treatments for tardive dyskinesia. Cochrane Database Syst Rev 2000;CD000459.
Margolese HC et al. Tardive dyskinesia in the era of typical and atypical antipsychotics. Part 2: Incidence and management strategies in patients with schizophrenia. Can J Psychiatry 2005;50:703–14.

Hyperprolactinaemia

Because dopamine inhibits prolactin release, dopamine antagonists can be expected to increase prolactin plasma levels. All antipsychotics cause measurable changes in prolactin but some do not increase prolactin above the normal range at standard doses. These drugs are clozapine, olanzapine, quetiapine, aripiprazole and ziprasidone[1-3]. Even with these drugs, raised prolactin and prolactin-related symptoms are occasionally reported[4-6]. With all drugs, the degree of prolactin elevation is probably dose-related[7].

Hyperprolactinaemia is often superficially asymptomatic (i.e. the patient does not spontaneously report problems) and there is evidence that hyperprolactinaemia does not affect subjective quality of life[8]. Nonetheless, persistent elevation of plasma prolactin is associated with a number of adverse consequences. These include sexual dysfunction[9-12] (but note that other pharmacological activities also give rise to sexual dysfunction), reductions in bone mineral density[13-16], menstrual disturbances[2,17], breast growth and galactorrhoea[17], suppression of the hypothalamic–pituitary–gonadal axis[18] and a possible increase in the risk of breast cancer[2,19,20].

Treatment

For most patients with symptomatic hyperprolactinaemia, a switch to a non-prolactin-elevating drug is the first choice[2,12,21,22]. Symptoms resolve slowly and symptom severity does not always reflect prolactin changes[21]. Genetic differences may play a part[23].

For patients who need to remain on a prolactin-elevating antipsychotic, dopamine agonists may be effective[3,21,24]. Amantadine, cabergoline and bromocriptine have all been used, but each has the potential to worsen psychosis (although this has not been reported in trials).

References

1. David SR et al. The effects of olanzapine, risperidone, and haloperidol on plasma prolactin levels in patients with schizophrenia. Clin Ther 2000;22:1085–96.
2. Haddad PM et al. Antipsychotic-induced hyperprolactinaemia: mechanisms, clinical features and management. Drugs 2004;64:2291–314.
3. Hamner MB et al. Hyperprolactinaemia in antipsychotic-treated patients: guidelines for avoidance and management. CNS Drugs 1998;10:209–22.
4. Melkersson K. Differences in prolactin elevation and related symptoms of atypical antipsychotics in schizophrenic patients. J Clin Psychiatry 2005;66:761–7.
5. Kopecek M et al. Ziprasidone-induced galactorrhea: a case report. Neuro Endocrinol Lett 2005;26:69–70.
6. Buhagiar K et al. Quetiapine-induced hyperprolactinemic galactorrhea in an adolescent male. German J Psychiatry 2006;9:118–20.
7. Staller J. The effect of long-term antipsychotic treatment on prolactin. J Child Adolesc Psychopharmacol 2006;16:317–26.
8. Kaneda Y. The impact of prolactin elevation with antipsychotic medications on subjective quality of life in patients with schizophrenia. Clin Neuropharmacol 2003;26:182–4.
9. Bobes J et al. Frequency of sexual dysfunction and other reproductive side-effects in patients with schizophrenia treated with risperidone, olanzapine, quetiapine, or haloperidol: the results of the EIRE study. J Sex Marital Ther 2003;29:125–47.
10. Smith S. Effects of antipsychotics on sexual and endocrine function in women: implications for clinical practice. J Clin Psychopharmacol 2003;23:S27–S32.
11. Spollen JJ III et al. Prolactin levels and erectile function in patients treated with risperidone. J Clin Psychopharmacol 2004;24:161–6.
12. Knegtering R et al. A randomized open-label study of the impact of quetiapine versus risperidone on sexual functioning. J Clin Psychopharmacol 2004;24:56–61.
13. Halbreich U et al. Accelerated osteoporosis in psychiatric patients: possible pathophysiological processes. Schizophr Bull 1996;22:447–54.
14. Becker D et al. Risperidone, but not olanzapine, decreases bone mineral density in female premenopausal schizophrenia patients. J Clin Psychiatry 2003;64:761–6.
15. Meaney AM et al. Reduced bone mineral density in patients with schizophrenia receiving prolactin raising antipsychotic medication. J Psychopharmacol 2003;17:455–8.
16. Meaney AM et al. Effects of long-term prolactin-raising antipsychotic medication on bone mineral density in patients with schizophrenia. Br J Psychiatry 2004;184:503–8.
17. Wieck A et al. Antipsychotic-induced hyperprolactinaemia in women: pathophysiology, severity and consequences. Selective literature review. Br J Psychiatry 2003;182:199–204.
18. Smith S et al. The effects of antipsychotic-induced hyperprolactinaemia on the hypothalamic–pituitary–gonadal axis. J Clin Psychopharmacol 2002;22:109–14.
19. Halbreich U et al. Are chronic psychiatric patients at increased risk for developing breast cancer? Am J Psychiatry 1996;153:559–60.
20. Wang PS et al. Dopamine antagonists and the development of breast cancer. Arch Gen Psychiatry 2002;59:1147–54.
21. Duncan D et al. Treatment of psychotropic-induced hyperprolactinaemia. Psychiatr Bull 1995;19:755–7.
22. Anghelescu I et al. Successful switch to aripiprazole after induction of hyperprolactinemia by ziprasidone: a case report. J Clin Psychiatry 2004;65:1286–7.
23. Young RM et al. Prolactin levels in antipsychotic treatment of patients with schizophrenia carrying the DRD2*A1 allele. Br J Psychiatry 2004;185:147–51.
24. Cavallaro R et al. Cabergoline treatment of risperidone-induced hyperprolactinemia: a pilot study. J Clin Psychiatry 2004;65:187–90.

Algorithm for the treatment of antipsychotic-induced akathisia

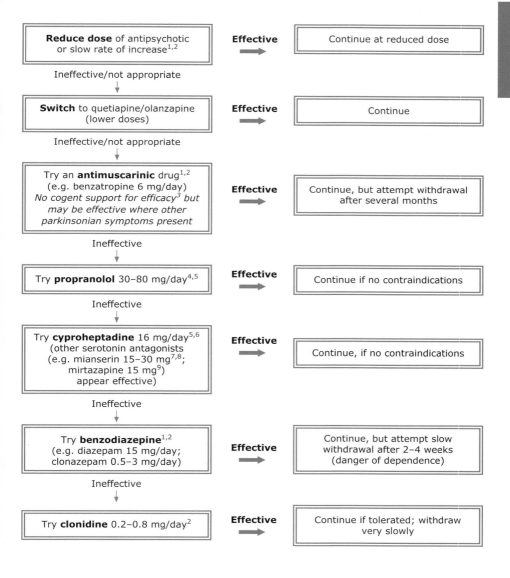

Reduce dose of antipsychotic or slow rate of increase[1,2] → **Effective** → Continue at reduced dose

Ineffective/not appropriate ↓

Switch to quetiapine/olanzapine (lower doses) → **Effective** → Continue

Ineffective/not appropriate ↓

Try an **antimuscarinic** drug[1,2] (e.g. benzatropine 6 mg/day) *No cogent support for efficacy[3] but may be effective where other parkinsonian symptoms present* → **Effective** → Continue, but attempt withdrawal after several months

Ineffective ↓

Try **propranolol** 30–80 mg/day[4,5] → **Effective** → Continue if no contraindications

Ineffective ↓

Try **cyproheptadine** 16 mg/day[5,6] (other serotonin antagonists (e.g. mianserin 15–30 mg[7,8]; mirtazapine 15 mg[9]) appear effective) → **Effective** → Continue, if no contraindications

Ineffective ↓

Try **benzodiazepine**[1,2] (e.g. diazepam 15 mg/day; clonazepam 0.5–3 mg/day) → **Effective** → Continue, but attempt slow withdrawal after 2–4 weeks (danger of dependence)

Ineffective ↓

Try **clonidine** 0.2–0.8 mg/day[2] → **Effective** → Continue if tolerated; withdraw very slowly

Notes:

- Akathisia is sometimes difficult to diagnose with certainty. A careful history of symptoms, medication and illicit substance use is essential. Note that severe akathisia may be linked to violent or suicidal behaviour[10-12].
- Evaluate efficacy of each treatment option over at least 1 month. Some effect may be seen after a few days but it may take much longer to become apparent in those with chronic akathisia.
- Withdraw previously ineffective treatments before starting the next option in the algorithm.
- Combinations of treatment may be used in refractory cases if carefully monitored.
- Consider tardive akathisia in patients on long-term therapy.
- Other possible treatments include vitamin B_6[8,13] and zolmitriptan[14].

References

1. Fleischhacker WW et al. The pharmacologic treatment of neuroleptic-induced akathisia. J Clin Psychopharmacol 1990;10:12–21.
2. Sachdev P. The identification and management of drug-induced akathisia. CNS Drugs 1995;4:28–46.
3. Rathbone J et al. Anticholinergics for neuroleptic-induced acute akathisia. Cochrane Database Syst Rev 2006;CD003727.
4. Adler L et al. A controlled assessment of propranolol in the treatment of neuroleptic-induced akathisia. Br J Psychiatry 1986;149:42–5.
5. Fischel T et al. Cyproheptadine versus propranolol for the treatment of acute neuroleptic-induced akathisia: a comparative double-blind study. J Clin Psychopharmacol 2001;21:612–15.
6. Weiss D et al. Cyproheptadine treatment in neuroleptic-induced akathisia. Br J Psychiatry 1995; 167:483–6.
7. Poyurovsky M et al. Treatment of neuroleptic-induced akathisia with the 5-HT$_2$ antagonist mianserin. Double-blind, placebo-controlled study. Br J Psychiatry 1999;174:238–42.
8. Miodownik C et al. Vitamin B_6 versus mianserin and placebo in acute neuroleptic-induced akathisia: a randomized, double-blind, controlled study. Clin Neuropharmacol 2006;29:68–72.
9. Poyurovsky M et al. Low-dose mirtazapine: a new option in the treatment of antipsychotic-induced akathisia. A randomized, double-blind, placebo- and propranolol-controlled trial. Biol Psychiatry 2006;59:1071–7.
10. Drake RE et al. Suicide attempts associated with akathisia. Am J Psychiatry 1985;142:499–501.
11. Azhar MZ et al. Akathisia-induced suicidal behaviour. Eur Psychiatry 1992;7:239–41.
12. Hansen L. A critical review of akathisia, and its possible association with suicidal behaviour. Hum Psychopharmacol 2001;16:495–505.
13. Lerner V et al. Vitamin B_6 treatment in acute neuroleptic-induced akathisia: a randomized, double-blind, placebo-controlled study. J Clin Psychiatry 2004;65:1550–4.
14. Gross-Isseroff R et al. The 5-HT$_{1D}$ receptor agonist zolmitriptan for neuroleptic-induced akathisia: an open label preliminary study. Int Clin Psychopharmacol 2005;20:23–5.

Further reading

Maidment I. Use of serotonin antagonists in the treatment of neuroleptic-induced akathisia. Psychiatr Bull 2000;24:348–51.

Treatment of tardive dyskinesia (TD)

TD is now a somewhat less commonly encountered problem probably because of the introduction and widespread use of second-generation antipsychotics (SGAs)[1-4]. Treatment of established TD is often unsuccessful, so prevention and early detection are essential. There is now fairly good evidence that some newer 'atypical' antipsychotics are less likely to cause TD[5-8] although TD certainly does occur with these drugs[9-14]. The observation that SGAs produce less TD than typical drugs is consistent with the long-held belief that early acute movement disorders and akathisia predict later TD[15-17]. Note, also, that TD can occur after minuscule doses of conventional drugs and in the absence of portentous acute movement disorder[18].

Treatment – first steps

Most authorities recommend the withdrawal of anticholinergic drugs and a reduction in the dose of antipsychotic as initial steps in those with early signs of TD[19,20] (dose reduction may initially worsen TD). A Cochrane review, however, found little support for this approach[21]. It has now become common practice to withdraw the antipsychotic prescribed when TD was first observed and to substitute another drug. The use of clozapine[19] is probably best supported in this regard, but quetiapine, another weak striatal dopamine antagonist, is also effective[22-28]. Olanzapine is also an option[29,30] while there are a few supporting data for risperidone[31] and aripiprazole[32,33].

Treatment – additional agents

Switching or withdrawing antipsychotics is not always effective and so additional agents are often used. The table below describes the most frequently prescribed add-on drugs for TD.

Drug	Comments
Tetrabenazine[34]	Only licensed treatment for TD in UK. Has antipsychotic properties but reported to be depressogenic. Drowsiness and akathisia also occur[35]. Dose is 25–200 mg/day
Benzodiazepines[19,20]	Widely used and considered effective but Cochrane review suggests benzodiazepines are 'experimental'[36]. Intermittent use may be necessary to avoid tolerance to effects. Most used are clonazepam 1–4 mg/day and diazepam 6–25 mg/day
Vitamin E[37,38]	Numerous studies but efficacy remains to be conclusively established. Dose is in the range 400–1600 IU/day

Treatment – other possible options

The large number of proposed treatments for TD undoubtedly reflects the somewhat limited effectiveness of standard remedies. The following table lists some of these putative treatments in alphabetical order. Supporting evidence is slim in each case.

Drug	Comments
Amino acids[39]	Use is supported by a small randomised, placebo-controlled trial. Low risk of toxicity
Calcium antagonists[40]	A few published studies but not widely used. Cochrane is dismissive
Donepezil[41,42]	Supported by a single study and case series. Dose is 10 mg/day
Fish oils[43,44]	Very limited support for use of EPA at dose of 2 g/day
Gabapentin[45]	Data derived almost entirely from a single research group. Adds weight to theory that GABAergic mechansims improve TD. Dose is 900–1200 mg/day
Levetiracetam[46,47]	Two published reports. No RCT. Dose up to 3000 mg
Melatonin[48]	Use is supported by a well-conducted trial. Usually well tolerated. Dose is 10 mg/day
Naltrexone[49]	May be effective when added to benzodiazepines. Well tolerated. Dose is 200 mg/day
Ondansetron[50,51]	Limited evidence but low toxicity. Dose – up to 12 mg/day
Pyridoxine[52]	Supported by a well-conducted trial. Dose – up to 400 mg/day
Quercetin[53]	Plant compound which is thought to be an antioxidant. No human studies in TD but widely used in other conditions
Transcranial magnetic stimulation[54] (rTMS)	Single case report
Note: Botulinum toxin may have a role in tardive dyskinesia.[55,56]	

References

1. Halliday J et al. Nithsdale Schizophrenia Surveys 23: movement disorders. 20-year review. Br J Psychiatry 2002;181:422–7.
2. Kane JM. Tardive dyskinesia circa 2006. Am J Psychiatry 2006;163:1316–18.
3. de Leon J. The effect of atypical versus typical antipsychotics on tardive dyskinesia: a naturalistic study. Eur Arch Psychiatry Clin Neurosci 2006; [Epub ahead of print].
4. Eberhard J et al. Tardive dyskinesia and antipsychotics: a 5-year longitudinal study of frequency, correlates and course. Int Clin Psychopharmacol 2006;21:35–42.
5. Beasley C et al. Randomised double-blind comparison of the incidence of tardive dyskinesia in patients with schizophrenia during long-term treatment with olanzapine or haloperidol. Br J Psychiatry 1999; 174:23–30.
6. Glazer WM. Expected incidence of tardive dyskinesia associated with atypical antipsychotics. J Clin Psychiatry 2000;61(Suppl 4):21–6.
7. Correll CU et al. Lower risk for tardive dyskinesia associated with second-generation antipsychotics: a systematic review of 1-year studies. Am J Psychiatry 2004;161:414–25.
8. Dolder CR et al. Incidence of tardive dyskinesia with typical versus atypical antipsychotics in very high risk patients. Biol Psychiatry 2003;53:1142–5.
9. Karama S et al. Tardive dyskinesia following brief exposure to risperidone – a case study (Letter). Eur Psychiatry 2004;19:391–2.
10. Gafoor R et al. Three case reports of emergent dyskinesia with clozapine. Eur Psychiatry 2003;18: 260–1.
11. Bhanji NH et al. Tardive dyskinesia associated with olanzapine in a neuroleptic-naive patient with schizophrenia (Letter). Can J Psychiatry 2004;49:343.
12. Keck ME et al. Ziprasidone-related tardive dyskinesia. Am J Psychiatry 2004;161:175–6.
13. Maytal G et al. Aripiprazole-related tardive dyskinesia. CNS Spectr 2006;11:435–9.
14. Fountoulakis KN et al. Amisulpride-induced tardive dyskinesia. Schizophr Res 2006;88:232–4.
15. Sachdev P. Early extrapyramidal side-effects as risk factors for later tardive dyskinesia: a prospective study. Aust N Z J Psychiatry 2004;38:445–9.
16. Miller DD et al. Clinical correlates of tardive dyskinesia in schizophrenia: baseline data from the CATIE schizophrenia trial. Schizophr Res 2005;80:33–43.
17. Tenback DE et al. Evidence that early extrapyramidal symptoms predict later tardive dyskinesia: a prospective analysis of 10,000 patients in the European Schizophrenia Outpatient Health Outcomes (SOHO) Study. Am J Psychiatry 2006;163:1438–40.
18. Oosthuizen PP et al. Incidence of tardive dyskinesia in first-episode psychosis patients treated with low-dose haloperidol. J Clin Psychiatry 2003;64:1075–80.
19. Duncan D et al. Tardive dyskinesia: how is it prevented and treated? Psychiatr Bull 1997;21:422–5.
20. Simpson GM. The treatment of tardive dyskinesia and tardive dystonia. J Clin Psychiatry 2000; 61(Suppl 4):39–44.
21. Soares-Weiser K et al. Neuroleptic reduction and/or cessation and neuroleptics as specific treatments for tardive dyskinesia. Cochrane Database Syst Rev 2006;CD000459.
22. Vesely C et al. Remission of severe tardive dyskinesia in a schizophrenic patient treated with the atypical antipsychotic substance quetiapine. Int Clin Psychopharmacol 2000;15:57–60.
23. Alptekin K et al. Quetiapine-induced improvement of tardive dyskinesia in three patients with schizophrenia. Int Clin Psychopharmacol 2002;17:263–4.
24. Nelson MW et al. Adjunctive quetiapine decreases symptoms of tardive dyskinesia in a patient taking risperidone. Clin Neuropharmacol 2003;26:297–8.
25. Emsley R et al. A single-blind, randomized trial comparing quetiapine and haloperidol in the treatment of tardive dyskinesia. J Clin Psychiatry 2004;65:696–701.
26. Bressan RA et al. Atypical antipsychotic drugs and tardive dyskinesia: relevance of D_2 receptor affinity. J Psychopharmacol 2004;18:124–7.
27. Sacchetti E et al. Quetiapine, clozapine, and olanzapine in the treatment of tardive dyskinesia induced by first-generation antipsychotics: a 124-week case report. Int Clin Psychopharmacol 2003;18:357–9.
28. Gourzis P et al. Quetiapine in the treatment of focal tardive dystonia induced by other atypical antipsychotics: a report of 2 cases. Clin Neuropharmacol 2005;28:195–6.
29. Soutullo CA et al. Olanzapine in the treatment of tardive dyskinesia: a report of two cases. J Clin Psychopharmacol 1999;19:100–1.
30. Kinon BJ et al. Olanzapine treatment for tardive dyskinesia in schizophrenia patients: a prospective clinical trial with patients randomized to blinded dose reduction periods. Prog Neuropsychopharmacol Biol Psychiatry 2004;28:985–96.
31. Bai YM et al. Risperidone for severe tardive dyskinesia: a 12-week randomized, double-blind, placebo-controlled study. J Clin Psychiatry 2003;64:1342–8.
32. Duggal HS. Aripiprazole-induced improvement in tardive dyskinesia. Can J Psychiatry 2003;48:771–2.
33. Grant MJ et al. Possible improvement of neuroleptic-associated tardive dyskinesia during treatment with aripiprazole. Ann Pharmacother 2005;39:1953.
34. Jankovic J et al. Long-term effects of tetrabenazine in hyperkinetic movement disorders. Neurology 1997;48:358–62.
35. Kenney C et al. Long-term tolerability of tetrabenazine in the treatment of hyperkinetic movement disorders. Mov Disord 2006; [Epub ahead of print].

36. Bhoopathi PS et al. Benzodiazepines for neuroleptic-induced tardive dyskinesia. Cochrane Database Syst Rev 2006;3:CD000205.
37. Adler LA et al. Vitamin E treatment for tardive dyskinesia. Br J Psychiatry 1995;167:412.
38. Zhang XY et al. The effect of vitamin E treatment on tardive dyskinesia and blood superoxide dismu-tase: a double-blind placebo-controlled trial. J Clin Psychopharmacol 2004;24:83–6.
39. Richardson MA et al. Efficacy of the branched-chain amino acids in the treatment of tardive dyskinesia in men. Am J Psychiatry 2003;160:1117–24.
40. Soares-Weiser K et al. Calcium channel blockers for neuroleptic-induced tardive dyskinesia. Cochrane Database Syst Rev 2004;CD000206.
41. Caroff SN et al. Treatment of tardive dyskinesia with donepezil. J Clin Psychiatry 2001;62:128–9.
42. Bergman J et al. Beneficial effect of donepezil in the treatment of elderly patients with tardive movement disorders. J Clin Psychiatry 2005;66:107–10.
43. Emsley R et al. The effects of eicosapentaenoic acid in tardive dyskinesia: a randomized, placebo-controlled trial. Schizophr Res 2006;84:112–20.
44. Vaddadi K et al. Tardive dyskinesia and essential fatty acids. Int Rev Psychiatry 2006;18:133–43.
45. Hardoy MC et al. Gabapentin in antipsychotic-induced tardive dyskinesia: results of 1-year follow-up. J Affect Disord 2003;75:125–30.
46. McGavin CL et al. Levetiracetam as a treatment for tardive dyskinesia: a case report. Neurology 2003;61:419.
47. Meco G et al. Levetiracetam in tardive dyskinesia. Clin Neuropharmacol 2006;29:265–8.
48. Shamir E et al. Melatonin treatment for tardive dyskinesia: a double-blind, placebo-controlled, crossover study. Arch Gen Psychiatry 2001;58:1049–52.
49. Wonodi I et al. Naltrexone treatment of tardive dyskinesia in patients with schizophrenia. J Clin Psychopharmacol 2004;24:441–5.
50. Sirota P et al. Use of the selective serotonin 3 receptor antagonist ondansetron in the treatment of neu-roleptic-induced tardive dyskinesia. Am J Psychiatry 2000;157:287–9.
51. Naidu PS et al. Reversal of neuroleptic-induced orofacial dyskinesia by 5-HT$_3$ receptor antagonists. Eur J Pharmacol 2001;420:113–17.
52. Lerner V et al. Vitamin B$_6$ in the treatment of tardive dyskinesia: a double-blind, placebo-controlled, crossover study. Am J Psychiatry 2001;158:1511–14.
53. Naidu PS et al. Reversal of haloperidol-induced orofacial dyskinesia by quercetin, a bioflavonoid. Psychopharmacology 2003;167:418–23.
54. Brambilla P et al. Transient improvement of tardive dyskinesia induced with rTMS. Neurology 2003;61:1155.
55. Tarsy D et al. An open-label study of botulinum toxin A for treatment of tardive dystonia. Clin Neuro-pharmacol 1997;20:90–3.
56. Brashear A et al. Comparison of treatment of tardive dystonia and idiopathic cervical dystonia with botulinum toxin type A. Mov Disord 1998;13:158–61.

Further reading

Paleacu D et al. Tetrabenazine treatment in movement disorders. Clin Neuropharmacol 2004;27:230–3.

Neuroleptic malignant syndrome (NMS)

NMS is a rare but potentially serious even fatal adverse effect of all antipsychotics. NMS is a syndrome largely of sympathetic hyperactivity occurring as a result of dopaminergic antagonism in the context of psychological stressors (cont.)

Table Neuroleptic malignant syndrome	
Signs and symptoms[1,4,24,25]	Fever, diaphoresis, rigidity, confusion, fluctuating consciousness
	Fluctuating blood pressure, tachycardia
	Elevated creatine kinase, leukocytosis, altered liver function tests
Risk factors[24–28]	High-potency typical drugs, recent or rapid dose increase, rapid dose reduction, abrupt withdrawal of anticholinergics
	Psychosis, organic brain disease, alcoholism, Parkinson's disease, hyperthyroidism, psychomotor agitation, mental retardation
	Agitation, dehydration
Treatments[4,24,29–32]	In the psychiatric unit:
	Withdraw antipsychotics, monitor temperature, pulse, BP
	In the medical/A&E unit:
	Rehydration, bromocriptine + dantrolene, sedation with benzodiazepines, artificial ventilation if required
	L-dopa, apomorphine and carbamazepine have also been used, among many other drugs. Consider ECT for treatment of psychosis
Restarting antipsychotics[24,29,33]	Antipsychotic treatment will be required in most instances and rechallenge is associated with acceptable risk
	Stop antipsychotics for at least 5 days, preferably longer. Allow time for symptoms and signs to resolve completely
	Begin with very small dose and increase very slowly with close monitoring of temperature, pulse and blood pressure. CK monitoring may be used, but is controversial[25,34]. Close monitoring of physical and biochemical parameters is effective in reducing progression to full-blown NMS[35,36]
	Consider using an antipsychotic structurally unrelated to that associated with NMS or a drug with low dopamine affinity (quetiapine or clozapine)
	Avoid depots and high-potency conventional antipsychotics

and genetic predisposition[1]. Although widely seen as an acute, severe syndrome, NMS may, in many cases, have few signs and symptoms; 'full-blown' NMS may thus represent the extreme of a range of non-malignant related symptoms[2]. Certainly, asymptomatic rises in plasma creatine kinase (CK) are fairly common[3].

The incidence and mortality of NMS are difficult to establish and probably vary as drug use changes and recognition increases. It has been estimated that less than 1% of all patients treated with conventional antipsychotics will experience NMS[4]. Incidence figures for SGA drugs are not available, but all have been reported to be associated with the syndrome[5-11], even newer drugs like ziprasidone[12,13] and aripiprazole[14,15-17]. Mortality may be lower with SGAs[18]. NMS is also very rarely seen with other drugs such as antidepressants[19-22] and lithium[23].

References

1. Gurrera RJ. Sympathoadrenal hyperactivity and the etiology of neuroleptic malignant syndrome. Am J Psychiatry 1999;156:169–80.
2. Bristow MF et al. How "malignant" is the neuroleptic malignant syndrome? BMJ 1993;307:1223–4.
3. Meltzer HY et al. Marked elevations of serum creatine kinase activity associated with antipsychotic drug treatment. Neuropsychopharmacology 1996;15:395–405.
4. Guze BH et al. Current concepts. Neuroleptic malignant syndrome. N Engl J Med 1985;313:163–6.
5. Sing KJ et al. Neuroleptic malignant syndrome and quetiapine (Letter). Am J Psychiatry 2002;159: 149–50.
6. Suh H et al. Neuroleptic malignant syndrome and low-dose olanzapine (Letter). Am J Psychiatry 2003; 160:796.
7. Gallarda T et al. Neuroleptic malignant syndrome in a 72-year-old-man with Alzheimer's disease: a case report and review of the literature. Eur Neuropsychopharmacol 2000;10(Suppl 3):357.
8. Stanley AK et al. Possible neuroleptic malignant syndrome with quetiapine. Br J Psychiatry 2000; 176:497.
9. Sierra-Biddle D et al. Neuroleptic malignant syndrome and olanzapine. J Clin Psychopharmacol 2000;20: 704–5.
10. Hasan S et al. Novel antipsychotics and the neuroleptic malignant syndrome: a review and critique. Am J Psychiatry 1998;155:1113–16.
11. Tsai JH et al. Zotepine-induced catatonia as a precursor in the progression to neuroleptic malignant syndrome. Pharmacotherapy 2005;25:1156–9.
12. Leibold J et al. Neuroleptic malignant syndrome associated with ziprasidone in an adolescent. Clin Ther 2004;26:1105–8.
13. Borovicka MC et al. Ziprasidone- and lithium-induced neuroleptic malignant syndrome. Ann Pharmacother 2006;40:139–42.
14. Spalding S et al. Aripiprazole and atypical neuroleptic malignant syndrome. J Am Acad Child Adolesc Psychiatry 2004;43:1457–8.
15. Chakraborty N et al. Aripiprazole and neuroleptic malignant syndrome. Int Clin Psychopharmacol 2004;19:351–3.
16. Rodriguez OP et al. A case report of neuroleptic malignant syndrome without fever in a patient given aripiprazole. J Okla State Med Assoc 2006;99:435–8.
17. Srephichit S et al. Neuroleptic malignant syndrome and aripiprazole in an antipsychotic-naive patient. J Clin Psychopharmacol 2006;26:94–5.
18. Ananth J et al. Neuroleptic malignant syndrome and atypical antipsychotic drugs. J Clin Psychiatry 2004;65:464–70.
19. Kontaxakis VP et al. Neuroleptic malignant syndrome after addition of paroxetine to olanzapine. J Clin Psychopharmacol 2003;23:671–2.
20. Young C. A case of neuroleptic malignant syndrome and serotonin disturbance. J Clin Psychopharmacol 1997;17:65–6.
21. June R et al. Neuroleptic malignant syndrome associated with nortriptyline. Am J Emerg Med 1999; 17:736–7.
22. Lu TC et al. Neuroleptic malignant syndrome after the use of venlafaxine in a patient with generalized anxiety disorder. J Formos Med Assoc 2006;105:90–3.
23. Gill J et al. Acute lithium intoxication and neuroleptic malignant syndrome. Pharmacotherapy 2003;23: 811–15.
24. Levenson JL. Neuroleptic malignant syndrome. Am J Psychiatry 1985;142:1137–45.
25. Hermesh H et al. High serum creatinine kinase level: possible risk factor for neuroleptic malignant syndrome. J Clin Psychopharmacol 2002;22:252–6.

26. Viejo LF et al. Risk factors in neuroleptic malignant syndrome. A case-control study. Acta Psychiatr Scand 2003;107:45–9.
27. Spivak B et al. Neuroleptic malignant syndrome during abrupt reduction of neuroleptic treatment. Acta Psychiatr Scand 1990;81:168–9.
28. Spivak B et al. Neuroleptic malignant syndrome associated with abrupt withdrawal of anticholinergic agents. Int Clin Psychopharmacol 1996;11:207–9.
29. Olmsted TR. Neuroleptic malignant syndrome: guidelines for treatment and reinstitution of neuroleptics. South Med J 1988;81:888–91.
30. Shoop SA et al. Carbidopa/levodopa in the treatment of neuroleptic malignant syndrome (Letter). Ann Pharmacother 1997;31:119.
31. Terao T. Carbamazepine in the treatment of neuroleptic malignant syndrome (Letter). Biol Psychiatry 1999;45:381–2.
32. Lattanzi L et al. Subcutaneous apomorphine for neuroleptic malignant syndrome. Am J Psychiatry 2006;163:1450–1.
33. Wells AJ et al. Neuroleptic rechallenge after neuroleptic malignant syndrome: case report and literature review. Drug Intell Clin Pharm 1988;22:475–80.
34. Klein JP et al. Massive creatine kinase elevations with quetiapine: report of two cases. Pharmacopsychiatry 2006;39:39–40.
35. Shiloh R et al. Precautionary measures reduce risk of definite neuroleptic malignant syndrome in newly typical neuroleptic-treated schizophrenia inpatients. Int Clin Psychopharmacol 2003;18:147–9.
36. Hatch CD et al. Failed challenge with quetiapine after neuroleptic malignant syndrome with conventional antipsychotics. Pharmacotherapy 2001;21:1003–6.

Catatonia

Catatonia is a disorder characterised by movement abnormalities usually associated with schizophrenia, mood disorders and less frequently in general medical conditions. A number of neurological disorders, endocrine and metabolic disorders, infections and toxic drug states can precipitate catatonic symptoms. The clinical picture is characterised by marked psychomotor disturbance that may involve motoric immobility or excessive motor activity, extreme negativism, mutism, peculiarities of voluntary movement, echolalia or echopraxia.

The term lethal catatonia has now been replaced by malignant catatonia, which is used when motor symptoms of catatonia are accompanied by autonomic instability or hyperthermia. This potentially fatal condition cannot be distinguished either clinically or by laboratory testing from neuroleptic malignant syndrome (NMS), leading to the conclusion that NMS is a variant form of malignant catatonia[1]. In addition, both catatonia and antipsychotic treatment are recognised as risk factors for the development of NMS[2].

Prompt treatment of catatonia is crucial and may prevent complications, which include death, dehydration, venous thrombosis, pulmonary embolism and pneumonia[3]. Numerous studies and case reports indicate that benzodiazepines are rapidly effective, safe and easily administered and therefore are regarded as first-line treatment[4]. There is most experience with lorazepam. Many patients will respond to standard doses (up to 4 mg daily), but repeated and higher doses (between 8 and 24 mg/day of lorazepam) may be needed[5]. Approximately 80% of catatonic patients will respond to benzodiazepine treatment and response is usually seen within 3–7 days.

Patients with schizophrenia are somewhat less likely to respond to benzodiazepines, with response in the range of 40–50%[4]. A double-blind, placebo-controlled, cross-over trial with lorazepam up to 6 mg/day demonstrated no effect on catatonic symptoms in patients with chronic schizophrenia[6]. If catatonic symptoms do not resolve rapidly with lorazepam, ECT treatment is indicated[7]. The response of catatonic symptoms to ECT is about 85%. This rate is probably greater than that seen with benzodiazepines[8]. As with benzodiazepines, response to ECT may be lower in patients with schizophrenia than in patients with mood disorders.

The use of antipsychotics in patients with catatonic symptoms is controversial. Some authors recommend that antipsychotics should be avoided altogether in catatonic patients, although there are case reports of successful treatment with risperidone, olanzapine, ziprasidone and clozapine[9,10]. During the acute phase of catatonia, the use of an antipsychotic should be avoided, more so in cases of malignant catatonia where their use may be harmful. In patients with chronic persistent catatonic symptoms, treatment of the underlying cause is necessary. SGAs, because of their reduced potential for inducing movement disorders, may be used in those patients with schizophrenia who have a predisposition to catatonia, although clinicians should be vigilant to the signs of NMS and be ready for prompt discontinuation of any antipsychotic. Quetiapine is therefore cautiously recommended (short half-life, weak dopamine antagonist).

Treatment of catatonia

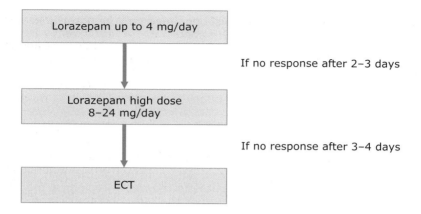

Lorazepam up to 4 mg/day

If no response after 2–3 days

Lorazepam high dose
8–24 mg/day

If no response after 3–4 days

ECT

References

1. Taylor MA et al. Catatonia in psychiatric classification: a home of its own. Am J Psychiatry 2003;160: 1233–41.
2. White DA et al. Catatonia: harbinger of the neuroleptic malignant syndrome. Br J Psychiatry 1991; 158:419–21.
3. Petrides G et al. Synergism of lorazepam and electroconvulsive therapy in the treatment of catatonia. Biol Psychiatry 1997;42:375–81.
4. Rosebush PI et al. Catatonia: re-awakening to a forgotten disorder. Mov Disord 1999;14:395–7.
5. Fink M et al. Neuroleptic malignant syndrome is malignant catatonia, warranting treatments efficacious for catatonia. Prog Neuropsychopharmacol Biol Psychiatry 2006;30:1182–3.
6. Ungvari GS et al. Lorazepam for chronic catatonia: a randomized, double-blind, placebo-controlled cross-over study. Psychopharmacology 1999;142:393–8.
7. Bush G et al. Catatonia. II. Treatment with lorazepam and electroconvulsive therapy. Acta Psychiatr Scand 1996;93:137–43.
8. Hawkins JM et al. Somatic treatment of catatonia. Int J Psychiatry Med 1995;25:345–69.
9. Van Den EF et al. The use of atypical antipsychotics in the treatment of catatonia. Eur Psychiatry 2005;20:422–9.
10. Caroff SN et al. Movement disorders associated with atypical antipsychotic drugs. J Clin Psychiatry 2002;63(Suppl 4):12–19.

Antipsychotics and hypertension

There are two ways in which antipsychotic drugs may be associated with the development or worsening of hypertension:

1. **Slow steady rise in blood pressure over time**. This may be associated with weight gain. Being overweight increases the risk of developing hypertension. The magnitude of the effect has been modelled using the Framingham data; for every 30 people who gain 4 kg, one will develop hypertension over the next 10 years[1]. Note that this is a very modest weight gain; the majority of patients treated with some antipsychotics gain more than this, increasing further the risk of developing hypertension.

2. **Unpredictable rapid sharp increase in blood pressure on starting a new drug or increasing the dose**. Increases in blood pressure occur shortly after starting, ranging from within hours of the first dose to a month. The information below relates to the pharmacological mechanism behind this and the antipsychotic drugs that are most implicated.

Postural hypotension is commonly associated with antipsychotic drugs that are antagonists at postsynaptic adrenergic α_1 receptors. Examples include clozapine, chlorpromazine, quetiapine and risperidone. Some antipsychotics are also antagonists at pre-synaptic α_2 adrenergic receptors; this can lead to increased plasma levels of norepinephrine, increased vagal activity and vasoconstriction. As all antipsychotics that are antagonists at α_2 receptors are also antagonists at α_1 receptors, the end result for any given patient can be difficult to predict, but for a very small number it can be hypertension. Some antipsychotics are more commonly implicated than others, but individual patient factors are undoubtedly also important.

Receptor binding studies have demonstrated that clozapine, olanzapine and risperidone have the highest affinity for α_2 adrenergic receptors[2] so it could be predicted that these drugs would be most likely to cause hypertension. Most case reports implicate clozapine[3–9] with some clearly describing normal blood pressure before clozapine was introduced, a sharp rise during treatment and return to normal when clozapine was discontinued. Blood pressure has also been reported to rise again on rechallenge and increased plasma catecholamines have been noted in some cases. Single case reports also implicate aripiprazole[10], sulpiride[11], risperdone[8] and quetiapine[8].

Data available through the CSM yellow card system indicate that clozapine is the antipsychotic drug most associated with hypertension. There are a small number of reports with aripiprazole, olanzapine, quetiapine and risperidone[12].

No antipsychotic is contraindicated in essential hypertension but extreme care is needed when clozapine is prescribed. Concomitant treatment with SSRIs may increase risk of hypertension, possibly via inhibition of the metabolism of the antipsychotic[8]. It is also (theoretically) possible that α_2 antagonism may be at least partially responsible for clozapine-induced tachycardia and nausea[13].

References

1. Fontaine KR et al. Estimating the consequences of anti-psychotic induced weight gain on health and mortality rate. Psychiatry Res 2001;101:277–88.
2. Abi-Dargham A et al. Mechanisms of action of second generation antipsychotic drugs in schizophrenia: insights from brain imaging studies. Eur Psychiatry 2005;20:15–27.
3. Gupta S et al. Paradoxical hypertension associated with clozapine. Am J Psychiatry 1994;151:148.
4. Krentz AJ et al. Drug points: pseudophaeochromocytoma syndrome associated with clozapine. BMJ 2001;322:1213.
5. George TP et al. Hypertension after initiation of clozapine. Am J Psychiatry 1996;153:1368–9.
6. Prasad SE et al. Pseudophaeochromocytoma associated with clozapine treatment. Ir J Psychol Med 2003;20:132–4.
7. Shiwach RS. Treatment of clozapine induced hypertension and possible mechanisms. Clin Neuropharmacol 1998;21:139–40.
8. Coulter D. Atypical antipsychotics may cause hypertension. http://www.medsafe.govt.nz/Profs/PUarticles/aahyp.htm. 2003. Accessed 22-8-2006.
9. Li JK et al. Clozapine: a mimicry of phaeochromocytoma. Aust N Z J Psychiatry 1997;31:889–91.
10. Borras L et al. Hypertension and aripiprazole. Am J Psychiatry 2005;162:2392.
11. Mayer RD et al. Acute hypertensive episode induced by sulpiride – a case report. Hum Psychopharmacol 1989;4:149–50.
12. Medicines and Healthcare Products Regulatory Agency. Reporting suspected adverse drug reactions. http://www.mhra.gov.uk/home. 2006. Accessed 22-8-2006.
13. Pandharipande P et al. Alpha-2 agonists: can they modify the outcomes in the Postanesthesia Care Unit? Curr Drug Targets 2005;6:749–54.

Antipsychotic-induced weight gain

Antipsychotics have long been recognised as weight-inducing agents. Suggested mechanisms include $5HT_{2C}$ antagonism, H_1 antagonism, hyperprolactinaemia and increased serum leptin (leading to leptin desensitisation)[1–3]. There is no evidence that drugs exert any direct metabolic effect: weight gain seems to result from increased food intake and, in some cases, reduced energy expenditure[4]. Risk of weight gain appears to be related to clinical response[5] and may also have a genetic basis[6,7].

All available antipsychotics have been associated with weight gain, although mean weight gained varies substantially between drugs. With all drugs, some patients gain no weight. Assessment of relative risk is made difficult by the poor quality of available data and the scarcity of long-term data. The following table suggests approximate relative risk of weight gain (based on two systematic reviews[8,9]).

(See also page 112 for advice on treating drug-induced weight gain and page 33 for switching strategies.)

Table   Antipsychotic-induced weight gain

Drug	*Risk/extent of weight gain*
Clozapine Olanzapine	**High**
Zotepine	**Moderate/high**
Chlorpromazine Quetiapine Risperidone	**Moderate**
Amisulpride Aripiprazole Haloperidol Trifluoperazine Ziprasidone	**Low**

References

1. Monteleone P et al. Pronounced early increase in circulating leptin predicts a lower weight gain during clozapine treatment. J Clin Psychopharmacol 2002;22:424–6.
2. Herran A et al. Effects of long-term treatment with antipsychotics on serum leptin levels. Br J Psychiatry 2001;179:59–62.
3. McIntyre RS et al. Mechanisms of antipsychotic-induced weight gain. J Clin Psychiatry 2001;62(Suppl 23): 23–9.
4. Virkkunen M et al. Decrease of energy expenditure causes weight increase in olanzapine treatment – a case study. Pharmacopsychiatry 2002;35:124–6.
5. Czobor P et al. Antipsychotic-induced weight gain and therapeutic response: a differential association. J Clin Psychopharmacol 2002;22:244–51.
6. Basile VS et al. Genetic dissection of atypical antipsychotic-induced weight gain: novel preliminary data on the pharmacogenetic puzzle. J Clin Psychiatry 2001;62(Suppl 23):45–66.
7. Reynolds GP et al. Polymorphism of the promoter region of the serotonin 5-HT$_{2C}$ receptor gene and clozapine-induced weight gain. Am J Psychiatry 2003;160:677–9.
8. Allison D et al. Antipsychotic-induced weight gain: a comprehensive research synthesis. Am J Psychiatry 1999;156:1686–96.
9. Taylor DM et al. Atypical antipsychotics and weight gain – a systematic review. Acta Psychiatr Scand 2000;101:416–32.

Schizophrenia

Further reading

Consensus Development Conference on Antipsychotic Drugs and Obesity and Diabetes. Diabetes Care 2004;27:596–601.

Treatment of drug-induced weight gain

Weight gain is an important adverse effect of nearly all antipsychotics with obvious consequences for self-image, morbidity and mortality. Prevention and treatment are therefore matters of clinical urgency.

Patients starting antipsychotic treatment or changing drugs should, as an absolute minimum, be weighed and their weight clearly recorded. Estimates of body mass index and waist circumference should, ideally, also be made at baseline and later at least every 6 months[1]. Frequent (weekly) monitoring of weight is recommended early in treatment – for the first 3 months at least. There is evidence that very few UK patients have anywhere near adequate monitoring of weight[2]. Clearly, monitoring of weight parameters is essential to assess the value of preventative and remedial measures.

Drug	Comments
Amantadine[3–6] (100–300 mg/day)	May attenuate olanzapine-related weight gain. Seems to be well tolerated
Bupropion[7,8] (amfebutamone)	Seems to be effective in obesity when combined with calorie-restricted diets. Few data of its effects on drug-induced weight gain. Note that pharmacology is essentially that of a dual-acting antidepressant. Caution in patients with bipolar illness
Fluoxetine[9,10] (and other SSRIs)	Probably not effective
H_2 antagonists[11–14] (e.g. nizatidine 300 mg bd or famotidine 40 mg/day)	Some positive studies but most negative. Effect, if any, is small. Few data supporting a reversal of weight gain
Metformin[15–18] (500 mg tds)	Limited data in drug-related weight gain: one positive, one negative RCT. Ideal for those with weight gain and diabetes
Methylcellulose (1500 mg ac)	Old-fashioned and rather unpalatable preparation. No data in drug-induced weight gain but fairly widely used. Also acts as a laxative so may be suitable for clozapine-related weight gain
Orlistat[19–21] (120 mg tds ac/pc)	Reliable effect in obesity, especially when combined with calorie restriction. Few published data in drug-induced weight gain but fairly widely used with some success. Failure to adhere to a low-fat diet will result in fatty diarrhoea and possible malabsorption of orally administered medication
Phenylpropanolamine[22]	Probably not effective
Reboxetine[23] (4 mg daily)	Attenuates olanzapine-induced weight gain. No data on weight reduction

Continued

Table   (Cont.)

Rimonabant[24,25]	Undoubted effect on weight and metabolic parameters in 'medical' populations. Few data in psychiatric population except to suggest that rimonabant is not antipsychotic[25]. Animal data suggest useful effect on antidepressant-induced weight gain[24]. Note that SPC lists depressive disorders occurring in 3.2%[26]
Sibutramine[21,27] (10–15 mg daily)	Effective, with one positive RCT[28]. Tachycardia, insomnia and hypertension may be problematic. Note that the SPC lists 'psychiatric illness' as a contraindication. Panic[29] and psychosis[30] have been reported
Topiramate[31–36] (up to 150 mg daily)	Reliably reduces weight even when drug-induced, but data are mainly observational. Problems may arise because of topiramate's propensity for causing sedation, confusion and cognitive impairment
Zonisamide[37] (400–600 mg/day)	Newer antiepileptic drug with weight-reducing properties. No data on drug-induced weight gain

Most of the relevant literature in this area relates to attempts at reversing antipsychotic-related weight gain[38]. There are relatively few data suggesting that early interventions can prevent weight gain[39–41] although this seems a more sensible approach.

When weight gain occurs, initial options involve switching drugs or instituting behavioural programmes (or both). Switching always presents a risk of relapse but there is fairly strong support for switching to aripiprazole[42–44] or ziprasidone[45,46] as a method for reversing weight gain. It is possible that switching to other drugs with a low propensity for weight gain is also beneficial[47,48].

A variety of behavioural methods have been proposed and evaluated with fairly good results[49]. Methods include calorie restriction[50], low glycaemic index diet[51], Weight Watchers[52] and diet/exercise programmes[38,40,41,53–55].

Pharmacological methods should be considered only where behavioural methods have failed or where obesity presents a clear, immediate physical risk to the patient. Some options are described in the table above (alphabetical order – no preference implied by position in table).

References

1. Marder SR et al. Physical health monitoring of patients with schizophrenia. Am J Psychiatry 2004;161: 1334–49.
2. Paton C et al. Obesity, dyslipidaemias and smoking in an inpatient population treated with antipsychotic drugs. Acta Psychiatr Scand 2004;110:299–305.
3. Floris M et al. Effect of amantadine on weight gain during olanzapine treatment. Eur Neuropsychopharmacol 2001;11:181–2.
4. Gracious BL et al. Amantadine treatment of psychotropic-induced weight gain in children and adolescents: case series. J Child Adolesc Psychopharmacol 2002;12:249–57.
5. Bahk WM et al. Open label study of the effect of amantadine on weight gain induced by olanzapine. Psychiatry Clin Neurosci 2004;58:163–7.
6. Deberdt W et al. Amantadine for weight gain associated with olanzapine treatment. Eur Neuropsychopharmacol 2005;15:13–21.
7. Gadde KM et al. Bupropion for weight loss: an investigation of efficacy and tolerability in overweight and obese women. Obes Res 2001;9:544–51.
8. Jain AK et al. Bupropion SR vs. placebo for weight loss in obese patients with depressive symptoms. Obes Res 2002;10:1049–56.
9. Poyurovsky M et al. Olanzapine-induced weight gain in patients with first-episode schizophrenia: a double-blind, placebo-controlled study of fluoxetine addition. Am J Psychiatry 2002;159:1058–60.
10. Bustillo JR et al. Treatment of weight gain with fluoxetine in olanzapine-treated schizophrenic outpatients. Neuropsychopharmacology 2003;28:527–9.
11. Cavazzoni P et al. Nizatidine for prevention of weight gain with olanzapine: a double-blind placebo-controlled trial. Eur Neuropsychopharmacol 2003;13:81–5.
12. Pae CU et al. Effect of nizatidine on olanzapine-associated weight gain in schizophrenic patients in Korea: a pilot study. Hum Psychopharmacol 2003;18:453–6.
13. Poyurovsky M et al. The effect of famotidine addition on olanzapine-induced weight gain in first-episode schizophrenia patients: a double-blind placebo-controlled pilot study. Eur Neuropsychopharmacol 2004;14:332–6.
14. Atmaca M et al. Nizatidine for the treatment of patients with quetiapine-induced weight gain. Hum Psychopharmacol 2004;19:37–40.
15. Morrison JA et al. Metformin for weight loss in pediatric patients taking psychotropic drugs. Am J Psychiatry 2002;159:655–7.
16. Mogul HR et al. Long-term (2–4 year) weight reduction with metformin plus carbohydrate-modified diet in euglycemic, hyperinsulinemic, midlife women (Syndrome W). Heart Dis 2003;5:384–92.
17. Baptista T et al. Metformin for prevention of weight gain and insulin resistance with olanzapine: a double-blind placebo-controlled trial. Can J Psychiatry 2006;51:192–6.
18. Klein DJ et al. A randomized, double-blind, placebo-controlled trial of metformin treatment of weight gain associated with initiation of atypical antipsychotic therapy in children and adolescents. Am J Psychiatry 2006;163:2072–9.
19. Sjostrom L et al. Randomised placebo-controlled trial of orlistat for weight loss and prevention of weight regain in obese patients. European Multicentre Orlistat Study Group. Lancet 1998;352:167–72.
20. Hilger E et al. The effect of orlistat on plasma levels of psychotropic drugs in patients with long-term psychopharmacotherapy. J Clin Psychopharmacol 2002;22:68–70.
21. Werneke U et al. Options for pharmacological management of obesity in patients treated with atypical antipsychotics. Int Clin Psychopharmacol 2002;17:145–60.
22. Borovicka MC et al. Phenylpropanolamine appears not to promote weight loss in patients with schizophrenia who have gained weight during clozapine treatment. J Clin Psychiatry 2002;63:345–8.
23. Poyurovsky M et al. Attenuation of olanzapine-induced weight gain with reboxetine in patients with schizophrenia: a double-blind, placebo-controlled study. Am J Psychiatry 2003;160:297–302.
24. Gobshtis N et al. Antidepressant-induced undesirable weight gain: prevention with rimonabant without interference with behavioral effectiveness. Eur J Pharmacol 2007;554:155–63.
25. Meltzer HY et al. Placebo-controlled evaluation of four novel compounds for the treatment of schizophrenia and schizoaffective disorder. Am J Psychiatry 2004;161:975–84.
26. Sanofi-Aventis. Acomplia 20 mg film-coated tablets. http://emc.medicines.org.uk/. 2006.
27. Arterburn DE et al. The efficacy and safety of sibutramine for weight loss: a systematic review. Arch Intern Med 2004;164:994–1003.
28. Henderson DC et al. A double-blind, placebo-controlled trial of sibutramine for olanzapine-associated weight gain. Am J Psychiatry 2005;162:954–62.
29. Binkley K et al. Sibutramine and panic attacks. Am J Psychiatry 2002;159:1793–4.
30. Taflinski T et al. Sibutramine-associated psychotic episode. Am J Psychiatry 2000;157:2057–8.
31. Dursun SM et al. Clozapine weight gain, plus topiramate weight loss. Can J Psychiatry 2000; 45:198.
32. Levy E et al. Topiramate produced weight loss following olanzapine-induced weight gain in schizophrenia. J Clin Psychiatry 2002;63:1045.
33. Van Ameringen M et al. Topiramate treatment for SSRI-induced weight gain in anxiety disorders. J Clin Psychiatry 2002;63:981–4.
34. Appolinario JC et al. Topiramate use in obese patients with binge eating disorder: an open study. Can J Psychiatry 2002;47:271–3.

35. Chengappa KN et al. Changes in body weight and body mass index among psychiatric patients receiving lithium, valproate, or topiramate: an open-label, nonrandomized chart review. Clin Ther 2002;24: 1576–84.
36. Pavuluri MN et al. Topiramate plus risperidone for controlling weight gain and symptoms in preschool mania. J Child Adolesc Psychopharmacol 2002;12:271–3.
37. Gadde KM et al. Zonisamide for weight loss in obese adults: a randomized controlled trial. JAMA 2003;289:1820–5.
38. Kwon JS et al. Weight management program for treatment-emergent weight gain in olanzapine-treated patients with schizophrenia or schizoaffective disorder: a 12-week randomized controlled clinical trial. J Clin Psychiatry 2006;67:547–53.
39. Littrell KH et al. The effects of an educational intervention on antipsychotic-induced weight gain. J Nurs Scholarsh 2003;35:237–41.
40. Mauri M et al. Effects of an educational intervention on weight gain in patients treated with antipsychotics. J Clin Psychopharmacol 2006;26:462–6.
41. Alvarez-Jimenez M et al. Attenuation of antipsychotic-induced weight gain with early behavioral intervention in drug-naive first-episode psychosis patients: a randomized controlled trial. J Clin Psychiatry 2006;67:1253–60.
42. Casey DE et al. Switching patients to aripiprazole from other antipsychotic agents: a multicenter randomized study. Psychopharmacology 2003;166:391–9.
43. De Hert M et al. A case series: evaluation of the metabolic safety of aripiprazole. Schizophr Bull 2006; [Epub ahead of print].
44. Lin SK et al. Reversal of antipsychotic-induced hyperprolactinemia, weight gain, and dyslipidemia by aripiprazole: a case report. J Clin Psychiatry 2006;67:1307.
45. Weiden PJ et al. Improvement in indices of health status in outpatients with schizophrenia switched to ziprasidone. J Clin Psychopharmacol 2003;23:595–600.
46. Montes JM et al. Improvement in antipsychotic-related metabolic disturbances in patients with schizophrenia switched to ziprasidone. Prog Neuropsychopharmacol Biol Psychiatry 2006; [Epub ahead of print].
47. Gupta S et al. Weight decline in patients switching from olanzapine to quetiapine. Schizophr Res 2004;70:57–62.
48. Ried LD et al. Weight change after an atypical antipsychotic switch. Ann Pharmacother 2003;37:1381–6.
49. Werneke U et al. Behavioural management of antipsychotic-induced weight gain: a review. Acta Psychiatr Scand 2003;108:252–9.
50. Cohen S et al. Weight gain with risperidone among patients with mental retardation: effect of calorie restriction. J Clin Psychiatry 2001;62:114–16.
51. Smith H et al. Low glycaemic index diet in patients prescribed clozapine: pilot study. Psychiatr Bull 2004;28:292–4.
52. Ball MP et al. A program for treating olanzapine-related weight gain. Psychiatr Serv 2001;52:967–9.
53. Pendlebury J et al. Evaluation of a behavioural weight management programme for patients with severe mental illness: 3 year results. Hum Psychopharmacol 2005;20:447–8.
54. Vreeland B et al. A program for managing weight gain associated with atypical antipsychotics. Psychiatr Serv 2003;54:1155–7.
55. Ohlsen RI et al. A dedicated nurse-led service for antipsychotic-induced weight gain: an evaluation. Psychiatr Bull 2004;28:164–6.

Further reading

Appolinario JC et al. Psychotropic drugs in the treatment of obesity. What promise? CNS Drugs 2004; 18:629–51.

Psychotropic-related QT prolongation

Introduction

Many psychotropic drugs are associated with ECG changes and it is probable that certain drugs are causally linked to serious ventricular arrhythmia and sudden cardiac death. Specifically, some antipsychotics block cardiac potassium channels and are linked to prolongation of the cardiac QT interval, a risk factor for the ventricular arrhythmia torsade de pointes, which is occasionally fatal. Recent case-control studies have suggested that the use of some antipsychotics (mainly haloperidol) is associated with an increase in the rate of sudden cardiac death[1-5]. Overall risk, however, remains extremely low. Tricyclic antidepressants are sodium channel antagonists which prolong QRS interval and QT interval, but this is usually evident only following overdose[6,7].

ECG monitoring of drug-induced changes in a mental health trust is complicated by a number of factors. Psychiatrists may have limited expertise in ECG interpretation, for example. (Self-reading, computerised ECG devices are available and to some extent compensate for some lack of expertise.) In addition, ECG machines may not be as readily available in all clinical areas as they are in general medicine. Also, time for ECG determination may not be available in many areas (e.g. outpatients). Lastly, ECG determination may be difficult to perform in acutely disturbed, physically uncooperative patients.

ECG monitoring of all patients is therefore impractical and, given that risks are probably very small, of dubious benefit. This section sets out a pragmatic strategy for risk reduction and should be seen as general guidance on minimising the possible risk associated with some drugs.

QT prolongation

- The cardiac QT interval (usually cited as QTc – QT corrected for heart rate) is a useful, but imprecise indicator of risk of torsade de pointes and of increased cardiac mortality[8]. Different correction factors and methods may give markedly different values[9].
- There is some controversy over the exact association between QTc and risk of arrhythmia. Very limited evidence suggests that risk is exponentially related to the extent of prolongation beyond normal limits (440 ms for men; 470 ms for women), although there are well-known exceptions which appear to disprove this theory[10]. Rather stronger evidence links QTc values over 500 ms to a clearly increased risk of arrhythmia[11]. Despite these uncertainties, QTc determination remains an important measure in estimating risk of arrhythmia and sudden death.
- QTc measurements and evaluation are complicated by:
  - difficulty in determining the end of the T wave, particularly where U waves are present (this applies both to manual and self-reading ECG machines)[11]
  - normal physiological variation in QTc interval: QT varies with gender, time of day, food intake, alcohol intake, menstrual cycle, ECG lead, etc.[9,10]

– variation in the extent of drug-induced prolongation of QTc because of changes in plasma levels. QTc prolongation is most prominent at peak drug plasma levels and least obvious at trough levels[9,10].

Other ECG changes

Tricyclics and other antidepressants may prolong the QRS interval, particularly in overdose. Other reported antipsychotic-induced changes include atrial fibrillation, giant P waves, T-wave changes and heart block[10].

Quantifying risk

Drugs are categorised here according to data available on their effects on the cardiac QTc interval (as calculated by Bazett's correction formula). 'No-effect' drugs are those with which QTc prolongation has not been reported

(Continued)

Table   Psychotropics – effect on QTc[9,10,13–28]

No effect	Moderate effect
Aripiprazole	Chlorpromazine
	Melperone
SSRIs (except citalopram)	Quetiapine
Reboxetine	Ziprasidone
Mirtazapine	Zotepine
MAOIs	
	TCAs
Carbamazepine	
Gabapentin	**High effect**
Lamotrigine	Any intravenous antipsychotic
Valproate	Haloperidol
	Methadone (see page 318)
Benzodiazepines	Pimozide
	Sertindole
Low effect	
Amisulpride	Any drug or combination of drugs
Clozapine	used in doses exceeding
Flupentixol	recommended maximum
Fluphenazine	
Perphenazine	**Unknown effect**
Olanzapine*	Loxapine
Risperidone	Pipothiazine
Sulpiride	Trifluoperazine
	Zuclopenthixol
Bupropion	
Citalopram	Anticholinergic drugs (procyclidine,
Moclobemide	benzhexol, etc.)
Venlafaxine	
Trazodone	
Lithium	

*Isolated cases of QTc prolongation[17,29], all other data suggest no effect[10,15,16].

either at therapeutic doses or in overdose. 'Low-effect' drugs are those for which severe QTc prolongation has been reported only following overdose or where only small average increases (<10 ms) have been observed at clinical doses. 'Moderate-effect' drugs are those which have been observed to prolong QTc by >10 ms on average when given at normal clinical doses or where ECG monitoring is officially recommended in some circumstances. 'High-effect' drugs are those for which extensive average QTc prolongation (usually >20 ms at normal clinical doses) has been noted or where ECG monitoring is mandated by the manufacturer's data sheet.

Note that effect on QTc may not necessarily equate directly to risk of torsade de pointes or sudden death[12], although this is often assumed. Note also that categorisation is inevitably approximate given the problems associated with QTc measurements.

Other risk factors

A number of physiological/pathological factors are associated with an increased risk of QT changes and of arrhythmia (Table 1) and many non-psychotropic drugs are linked to QT prolongation (Table 2)[11].

Table 1 Physiological risk factors for QTc prolongation and arrhythmia
Cardiac
Long QT syndrome
Bradycardia
Ischaemic heart disease
Myocarditis
Myocardial infarction
Left ventricular hypertrophy
Metabolic
Hypokalaemia
Hypomagnesaemia
Hypocalcaemia
Others
Extreme physical exertion
Stress or shock
Anorexia nervosa
Extremes of age – children and elderly may be more susceptible to QT changes
Female gender
Note: Hypokalaemia-related QTc prolongation is more commonly observed in acute psychotic admissions[30]. Also, be aware that there are a number of physical and genetic factors which may not be discovered on routine examination but which probably predispose patients to arrhythmia[31,32].

Table 2 Non-psychotropics associated with QT prolongation

Antibiotics	**Antiarrhythmics**
Erythromycin	Quinidine
Clarithromycin	Disopyramide
Ampicillin	Procainamide
Co-trimoxazole	Sotalol
Pentamidine	Amiodarone
(Some 4-quinolones affect QTc – see	Bretylium
manufacturers' literature)	
Antimalarials	**Others**
Chloroquine	Amantadine
Mefloquine	Ciclosporin
Quinine	Diphenhydramine
	Hydroxyzine
	Nicardipine
	Tamoxifen

Note: β_2 agonists and sympathomimetics may provoke torsade de pointes in patients with prolonged QTc.

ECG monitoring recommendations

Generally, prescribing should be such that the need for ECG monitoring is minimised. This can be achieved by prescribing drugs with the lowest effect on QT at their minimum effective dose and by avoiding polypharmacy of other QT-prolonging drugs and hepatic enzyme inhibitors. (see table overleaf.)

Table ECG monitoring recommendations

	No other risk factors	Physiological/ pathological risk factors*	When co-administered with other QT-prolonging drugs**
'No-effect' drugs	None	None	None
'Low-effect' drugs	None	None	Baseline ECG, then after dose change, consider referral to cardiologist
'Moderate-effect' drugs	None	Correct risk factors if possible, if not baseline ECG, then after dose change, consider referral to cardiologist	Avoid or refer to cardiologist
'High-effect' drugs	Baseline ECG, then after dose change, consider referral to cardiologist	Correct risk factors if possible, if not – avoid	Avoid
'Unknown-effect' drugs	None	Correct risk factors if possible if not – baseline ECG, then after dose change, consider referral to cardiologist	Avoid or refer to cardiologist

Notes
* Many conditions necessitate close cardiac monitoring, regardless of drugs prescribed. Recommendations in this column therefore represent additional requirements to those already mandated by the patient's condition.
** Defined as any drug in Table 2 on page 119 or psychotropics of moderate or high effect. The use of some of these drugs may necessitate cardiac monitoring. Recommendations in this column therefore represent *additional* requirements to those already mandated by the use of these drugs alone.

Actions to be taken

- **QTc   <440 ms (men) or <470 ms (women)**
  No action required unless abnormal T-wave morphology – consider referral to cardiologist if in doubt.
- **QTc   >440 ms (men) or >470 ms (women) but <500 ms**
  Consider switch to drug of lower effect; reperform ECG and consider referral to cardiologist.
- **QTc   >500 ms**
  Stop suspected causative drug(s) and switch to drug of lower effect; refer to cardiologist immediately.
- **Abnormal T-wave morphology**
  Review treatment. Consider switch to drug of lower effect. Refer to cardiologist immediately.

Metabolic inhibition

The effect of drugs on the QTc interval is plasma level-dependent. Drug interactions are therefore important, especially when metabolic inhibition results in increased plasma levels of the drug affecting QTc. Commonly used metabolic inhibitors include fluvoxamine, fluoxetine, paroxetine and valproate. This is a complex area with an expanding database.

Other cardiovascular risk factors

The risk of drug-induced arrhythmia and sudden cardiac death with psychotropics is very small with a few drugs and probably non-existent with many others. Of much greater concern are other patient-related risk factors for cardiovascular disease. These include smoking, obesity and impaired glucose tolerance, and present a much greater risk to patient mortality than the uncertain outcome of QT changes. See relevant sections for discussion of these problems.

References

1. Reilly JG et al. Thioridazine and sudden unexplained death in psychiatric in-patients. Br J Psychiatry 2002;180:515–22.
2. Ray WA et al. Antipsychotics and the risk of sudden cardiac death. Arch Gen Psychiatry 2001;58:1161–7.
3. Hennessy S et al. Cardiac arrest and ventricular arrhythmia in patients taking antipsychotic drugs: cohort study using administrative data. BMJ 2002;325:1070.
4. Straus SM et al. Antipsychotics and the risk of sudden cardiac death. Arch Intern Med 2004;164:1293–7.
5. Liperoti R et al. Conventional and atypical antipsychotics and the risk of hospitalization for ventricular arrhythmias or cardiac arrest. Arch Intern Med 2005;165:696–701.
6. Cohen H et al. Antidepressant poisoning and treatment: a review and case illustration. J Pharm Pract 1997;10:249–70.
7. Whyte IM et al. Relative toxicity of venlafaxine and selective serotonin reuptake inhibitors in overdose compared to tricyclic antidepressants. QJM 2003;96:369–74.
8. Malik M et al. Evaluation of drug-induced QT interval prolongation: implications for drug approval and labelling. Drug Saf 2001;24:323–51.
9. Haddad PM et al. Antipsychotic-related QTc prolongation, torsade de pointes and sudden death. Drugs 2002;62:1649–71.
10. Taylor DM. Antipsychotics and QT prolongation. Acta Psychiatr Scand 2003;107:85–95.

11. Botstein P. Is QT interval prolongation harmful? A regulatory perspective. Am J Cardiol 1993;72: 50B–2B.
12. Witchel HJ et al. Psychotropic drugs, cardiac arrhythmia, and sudden death. J Clin Psychopharmacol 2003; 23:58–77.
13. Glassman AH et al. Antipsychotic drugs: prolonged QTc interval, torsade de pointes, and sudden death. Am J Psychiatry 2001;158:1774–82.
14. Warner B et al. Investigation of the potential of clozapine to cause torsade de pointes. Adverse Drug React Toxicol Rev 2002;21:189–203.
15. Harrigan EP et al. A randomized evaluation of the effects of six antipsychotic agents on QTc, in the absence and presence of metabolic inhibition. J Clin Psychopharmacol 2004;24:62–9.
16. Lindborg SR et al. Effects of intramuscular olanzapine vs. haloperidol and placebo on QTc intervals in acutely agitated patients. Psychiatry Res 2003;119:113–23.
17. Dineen S et al. QTc prolongation and high-dose olanzapine (Letter). Psychosomatics 2003;44:174–5.
18. Gupta S et al. Quetiapine and QTc issues: a case report (Letter). J Clin Psychiatry 2003;64:612–13.
19. Su KP et al. A pilot cross-over design study on QTc interval prolongation associated with sulpiride and haloperidol. Schizophr Res 2003;59:93–4.
20. Lin CH et al. Predictive factors for QTc prolongation in schizophrenic patients taking antipsychotics. J Formos Med Assoc 2004;103:437–41.
21. Chong SA et al. Prolonged QTc intervals in medicated patients with schizophrenia. Hum Psychopharmacol 2003;18:647–9.
22. Krantz MJ et al. Dose-related effects of methadone on QT prolongation in a series of patients with torsade de pointes. Pharmacotherapy 2003;23:802–5.
23. Gil M et al. QT prolongation and torsades de pointes in patients infected with human immunodeficiency virus and treated with methadone. Am J Cardiol 2003;92:995–7.
24. Piguet V et al. QT interval prolongation in patients on methadone with concomitant drugs (Letter). J Clin Psychopharmacol 2004;24:446–8.
25. Stollberger C et al. Antipsychotic drugs and QT prolongation. Int Clin Psychopharmacol 2005; 20:243–51.
26. Isbister GK et al. Amisulpride deliberate self-poisoning causing severe cardiac toxicity including QT prolongation and torsade de pointes. Med J Aust 2006;184:354–6.
27. Ward DI. Two cases of amisulpride overdose: a cause for prolonged QT syndrome. Emerg Med Australas 2005;17:274–6.
28. Vieweg WV et al. Torsade de pointes in a patient with complex medical and psychiatric conditions receiving low-dose quetiapine. Acta Psychiatr Scand 2005;112:318–22.
29. Su KP et al. Olanzapine-induced QTc prolongation in a patient with Wolff–Parkinson–White syndrome. Schizophr Res 2004;66:191–2.
30. Hatta K et al. Prolonged QT interval in acute psychotic patients. Psychiatry Res 2000;94:279–85.
31. Priori SG et al. Low penetrance in the long-QT syndrome: clinical impact. Circulation 1999;99:529–33.
32. Frassati D et al. Hidden cardiac lesions and psychotropic drugs as a possible cause of sudden death in psychiatric patients: a report of 14 cases and review of the literature. Can J Psychiatry 2004;49:100–5.

Further reading

Abdelmawla N et al. Sudden cardiac death and antipsychotics. Part 1: Risk factors and mechanisms. Adv Psychiatr Treat 2006;12:35–44.
Titier K et al. Atypical antipsychotics – from potassium channels to torsade de pointes and sudden death. Drug Saf 2005;28:35–51.

Antipsychotics, diabetes and impaired glucose tolerance

Schizophrenia

Schizophrenia seems to be associated with relatively high rates of insulin resistance and diabetes[1,2] – an observation that predates the discovery of effective antipsychotics[3–5].

Antipsychotics

Data relating to diabetes and antipsychotic use are numerous but less than perfect[6–9]. The main problem is that incidence and prevalence studies assume full or uniform screening for diabetes. Neither is likely to be correct[6]. Many studies do not account for other factors affecting risk of diabetes[9]. Small differences between drugs are therefore difficult to substantiate but may in any case be ultimately unimportant: risk is increased for all those with schizophrenia receiving any antipsychotic.

First-generation antipsychotics

Phenothiazine derivatives have long been associated with impaired glucose tolerance and diabetes[10]. Diabetes prevalence rates were reported to have substantially increased following the introduction and widespread use of conventional drugs[11]. Prevalence of impaired glucose tolerance seems to be higher with aliphatic phenothiazines than with fluphenazine or haloperidol[12]. Hyperglycaemia has also been reported with other conventional drugs, such as loxapine[13], and other data confirm an association with haloperidol[14]. Some data suggest that FGAs are no different from SGAs in their propensity to cause diabetes[15,16].

Second-generation antipsychotics

Clozapine
Clozapine has been strongly linked to hyperglycaemia, impaired glucose tolerance and diabetic ketoacidosis[17]. The risk of diabetes appears to be higher with clozapine than with other SGAs and conventional drugs, especially in younger patients[18–21], although this is not a consistent finding[22,23].

As many as a third of patients may develop diabetes after 5 years of treatment[24]. Many cases of diabetes are noted in the first 6 months of treatment and some occur within 1 month[25], some after many years[23]. Death from ketoacidosis has also been reported[25]. Diabetes associated with clozapine is not necessarily linked to obesity or to family history of diabetes[17,26].

Clozapine appears to increase plasma levels of insulin in a clozapine level-dependent fashion[27,28]. It has been shown to be more likely than typical drugs to increase plasma glucose and insulin following oral glucose challenge[29].

Much clozapine-related diabetes may go unnoticed[30]. Testing for diabetes is essential given the high prevalence of diabetes in people receiving clozapine[31].

Olanzapine
Like clozapine, olanzapine has been strongly linked to impaired glucose tolerance, diabetes and diabetic ketoacidosis[32]. Olanzapine and clozapine appear to directly induce insulin resistance[33,34]. Risk of diabetes has also been reported to be higher than with FGA drugs[35], again with a particular risk in younger patients[19]. The time course of development of diabetes has not been established but impaired glucose tolerance seems to occur even in the absence of obesity and family history of diabetes[17,26]. Olanzapine may be more diabetogenic than risperidone[36–39].

Olanzapine is associated with plasma levels of glucose and insulin higher than those seen with conventional drugs (after oral glucose load)[29,40].

Risperidone
Risperidone has been linked mainly in case reports to impaired glucose tolerance[41], diabetes[42] and ketoacidosis[43]. The number of reports of such adverse effects is substantially smaller than with either clozapine or olanzapine[44]. At least one study has suggested that changes in fasting glucose are significantly less common with risperidone than with olanzapine[36] but other studies have detected no difference[45].

Risperidone seems no more likely than FGA drugs to be associated with diabetes[19,35,37], although there may be an increased risk in patients under 40 years of age[19]. Risperidone has, however, been observed to adversely affect fasting glucose and plasma glucose (following glucose challenge) compared with levels seen in healthy volunteers (but not compared with patients taking typical drugs)[29].

Quetiapine
Like risperidone, quetiapine has been linked to cases of new-onset diabetes and ketoacidosis[46,47]. Again, the number of reports is much fewer than with olanzapine or clozapine. Quetiapine appears to be more likely than conventional drugs to be associated with diabetes[19,48]. One study showed quetiapine to be equal to olanzapine in incidence of diabetes[45]. Inexplicably, quetiapine may ameliorate clozapine-related diabetes when given in conjunction with clozapine[49].

Other SGAs

There are relatively few data relating to other atypical drugs. Amisulpride appears not to elevate plasma glucose[50] and seems not to be associated with diabetes[51]. Data for aripiprazole[52,53] and ziprasidone[54] suggest that neither drug alters glucose homeostasis. Aripiprazole may even reverse diabetes caused by other drugs[55] (although ketoacidosis has been reported with aripiprazole[56,57]). These three drugs are cautiously recommended for those with a history of or predisposition to diabetes mellitus.

Monitoring

Diabetes is a growing problem in Western society and has a strong association with obesity, (older) age, (lower) educational achievement and certain racial groups[58,59]. Diabetes markedly increases cardiovascular mortality, largely as a consequence of atherosclerosis[60]. Likewise, the use of antipsychotics also increases cardiovascular mortality[61-63]. Intervention to reduce plasma glucose levels and minimise other risk factors (obesity, hypercholesterolaemia) is therefore essential[64].

There is no clear consensus on diabetes-monitoring practice for those receiving antipsychotics[65]. Given the known parlous state of testing for diabetes in the UK[6], arguments over precisely which tests are done and when seem redundant. There is an overwhelming need to improve monitoring by any means and so any tests for diabetes are supported – urine glucose (UG) and random plasma glucose (RPG) included.

Ideally, though, all patients should have an oral glucose tolerance test (OGTT) performed, as this is the most sensitive method[66]. A fasting plasma glucose (FPG) test is less sensitive but recommended[67]. Fasting tests are often difficult to achieve in acutely ill, disorganised patients so measurement of RPG or glycosylated haemoglobin (HbA_{1c}) may also be used (fasting not required). Frequency of monitoring should then be determined by physical factors (e.g. weight gain) and known risk factors (e.g. family history of diabetes). The absolute minimum is yearly testing for diabetes for all patients.

Recommended monitoring		
	Ideally	**Minimum**
Baseline	OGTT or FPG	Urine glucose (UG) Random plasma glucose (RPG)
Continuation	All drugs: OGTT or FPG every 12 months For clozapine and olanzapine or if other risk factors present: OGTT or FPG after 1 month, then every 4–6 months	UG or RPG every 12 months

References

1. Schimmelbusch WH et al. The positive correlation between insulin resistance and duration of hospitalization in untreated schizophrenia. Br J Psychiatry 1971;118:429–36.
2. Waitzkin L. A survey for unknown diabetics in a mental hospital. I. Men under age fifty. Diabetes 1966; 15:97–104.
3. Kasanin J. The blood sugar curve in mental disease. II. The schizophrenia (dementia praecox) groups. Arch Neurol Psychiatry 1926;16:414–19.
4. Braceland FJ et al. Delayed action of insulin in schizophrenia. Am J Psychiatry 1945;102:108–10.
5. Kohen D. Diabetes mellitus and schizophrenia: historical perspective. Br J Psychiatry Suppl 2004; 47:S64–6.
6. Taylor D et al. Testing for diabetes in hospitalised patients prescribed antipsychotic drugs. Br J Psychiatry 2004;185:152–6.
7. Haddad PM. Antipsychotics and diabetes: review of non-prospective data. Br J Psychiatry Suppl 2004; 47:S80–S86.
8. Bushe C et al. Association between atypical antipsychotic agents and type 2 diabetes: review of prospective clinical data. Br J Psychiatry 2004;184:S87–S93.
9. Gianfrancesco F et al. The influence of study design on the results of pharmacoepidemiologic studies of diabetes risk with antipsychotic therapy. Ann Clin Psychiatry 2006;18:9–17.
10. Arneson GA. Phenothiazine derivatives and glucose metabolism. J Neuropsychiatr 1964;5:181.
11. Lindenmayer JP et al. Hyperglycemia associated with the use of atypical antipsychotics. J Clin Psychiatry 2001;62(Suppl 23):30–8.
12. Keskiner A et al. Psychotropic drugs, diabetes and chronic mental patients. Psychosomatics 1973;14: 176–81.
13. Tollefson G et al. Nonketotic hyperglycemia associated with loxapine and amoxapine: case report. J Clin Psychiatry 1983;44:347–8.
14. Lindenmayer JP et al. Changes in glucose and cholesterol levels in patients with schizophrenia treated with typical or atypical antipsychotics. Am J Psychiatry 2003;160:290–6.
15. Carlson C et al. Diabetes mellitus and antipsychotic treatment in the United Kingdom. Eur Neuropsychopharmacol 2006;16:366–75.
16. Ostbye T et al. Atypical antipsychotic drugs and diabetes mellitus in a large outpatient population: a retrospective cohort study. Pharmacoepidemiol Drug Saf 2005;14:407–15.
17. Mir S et al. Atypical antipsychotics and hyperglycaemia. Int Clin Psychopharmacol 2001;16:63–74.
18. Lund BC et al. Clozapine use in patients with schizophrenia and the risk of diabetes, hyperlipidemia, and hypertension: a claims-based approach. Arch Gen Psychiatry 2001;58:1172–6.
19. Sernyak MJ et al. Association of diabetes mellitus with use of atypical neuroleptics in the treatment of schizophrenia. Am J Psychiatry 2002;159:561–6.
20. Gianfrancesco FD et al. Differential effects of risperidone, olanzapine, clozapine, and conventional antipsychotics on type 2 diabetes: findings from a large health plan database. J Clin Psychiatry 2002;63: 920–30.
21. Guo JJ et al. Risk of diabetes mellitus associated with atypical antipsychotic use among patients with bipolar disorder: a retrospective, population-based, case-control study. J Clin Psychiatry 2006;67: 1055–61.
22. Wang PS et al. Clozapine use and risk of diabetes mellitus. J Clin Psychopharmacol 2002;22:236–43.
23. Sumiyoshi T et al. A comparison of incidence of diabetes mellitus between atypical antipsychotic drugs: a survey for clozapine, risperidone, olanzapine, and quetiapine (Letter). J Clin Psychopharmacol 2004; 24:345–8.
24. Henderson DC et al. Clozapine, diabetes mellitus, weight gain, and lipid abnormalities: A five-year naturalistic study. Am J Psychiatry 2000;157:975–81.
25. Koller E et al. Clozapine-associated diabetes. Am J Med 2001;111:716–23.
26. Sumiyoshi T et al. The effect of hypertension and obesity on the development of diabetes mellitus in patients treated with atypical antipsychotic drugs (Letter). J Clin Psychopharmacol 2004;24:452–4.
27. Melkersson KI et al. Different influences of classical antipsychotics and clozapine on glucose–insulin homeostasis in patients with schizophrenia or related psychoses. J Clin Psychiatry 1999;60:783–91.
28. Melkersson K. Clozapine and olanzapine, but not conventional antipsychotics, increase insulin release in vitro. Eur Neuropsychopharmacol 2004;14:115–19.
29. Newcomer JW et al. Abnormalities in glucose regulation during antipsychotic treatment of schizophrenia. Arch Gen Psychiatry 2002;59:337–45.
30. Sernyak MJ et al. Undiagnosed hyperglycemia in clozapine-treated patients with schizophrenia. J Clin Psychiatry 2003;64:605–8.
31. Lamberti JS et al. Diabetes mellitus among outpatients receiving clozapine: prevalence and clinical-demographic correlates. J Clin Psychiatry 2005;66:900–6.
32. Wirshing DA et al. Novel antipsychotics and new onset diabetes. Biol Psychiatry 1998;44:778–83.
33. Engl J et al. Olanzapine impairs glycogen synthesis and insulin signaling in L6 skeletal muscle cells. Mol Psychiatry 2005;10:1089–96.
34. Vestri HS et al. Atypical antipsychotic drugs directly impair insulin action in adipocytes: effects on glucose transport, lipogenesis, and antilipolysis. Neuropsychopharmacology 2006; [Epub ahead of print].
35. Koro CE et al. Assessment of independent effect of olanzapine and risperidone on risk of diabetes among patients with schizophrenia: population based nested case-control study. BMJ 2002;325:243.

36. Meyer JM. A retrospective comparison of weight, lipid, and glucose changes between risperidone- and olanzapine-treated inpatients: metabolic outcomes after 1 year. J Clin Psychiatry 2002;63:425–33.
37. Gianfrancesco F et al. Antipsychotic-induced type 2 diabetes: evidence from a large health plan database. J Clin Psychopharmacol 2003;23:328–35.
38. Leslie DL et al. Incidence of newly diagnosed diabetes attributable to atypical antipsychotic medications. Am J Psychiatry 2004;161:1709–11.
39. Duncan E et al. Relative risk of glucose elevation during antipsychotic exposure in a Veterans Administration population. Int Clin Psychopharmacol 2007;22:1–11.
40. Ebenbichler CF et al. Olanzapine induces insulin resistance: results from a prospective study. J Clin Psychiatry 2003;64:1436–9.
41. Mallya A et al. Resolution of hyperglycemia on risperidone discontinuation: a case report. J Clin Psychiatry 2002;63:453–4.
42. Wirshing DA et al. Risperidone-associated new-onset diabetes. Biol Psychiatry 2001;50:148–9.
43. Croarkin PE et al. Diabetic ketoacidosis associated with risperidone treatment? Psychosomatics 2000; 41:369–70.
44. Koller EA et al. Risperidone-associated diabetes mellitus: a pharmacovigilance study. Pharmacotherapy 2003;23:735–44.
45. Lambert BL et al. Diabetes risk associated with use of olanzapine, quetiapine, and risperidone in veterans health administration patients with schizophrenia. Am J Epidemiol 2006;164:672–81.
46. Henderson DC. Atypical antipsychotic-induced diabetes mellitus: how strong is the evidence? CNS Drugs 2002;16:77–89.
47. Koller EA et al. A survey of reports of quetiapine-associated hyperglycemia and diabetes mellitus. J Clin Psychiatry 2004;65:857–63.
48. Citrome L et al. Relationship between antipsychotic medication treatment and new cases of diabetes among psychiatric inpatients. Psychiatr Serv 2004;55:1006–13.
49. Reinstein MJ et al. Effect of clozapine–quetiapine combination therapy on weight and glycaemic control. Clin Drug Invest 1999;18:99–104.
50. Vanelle JM et al. Metabolic control in patients with comorbid schizophrenia and depression treated with amisulpride. 2004. Poster presented at: 17th Congress of the European College of Neuropsychopharmacology; June 20–21, Stockholm, Sweden.
51. De Hert MA et al. Prevalence of the metabolic syndrome in patients with schizophrenia treated with antipsychotic medication. Schizophr Res 2006;83:87–93.
52. Keck PE Jr et al. Aripiprazole: a partial dopamine D_2 receptor agonist antipsychotic. Expert Opin Investig Drugs 2003;12:655–62.
53. Pigott TA et al. Aripiprazole for the prevention of relapse in stabilized patients with chronic schizophrenia: a placebo-controlled 26-week study. J Clin Psychiatry 2003;64:1048–56.
54. Simpson GM et al. Randomized, controlled, double-blind multicenter comparison of the efficacy and tolerability of ziprasidone and olanzapine in acutely ill inpatients with schizophrenia or schizoaffective disorder. Am J Psychiatry 2004;161:1837–47.
55. De Hert M et al. A case series: evaluation of the metabolic safety of aripiprazole. Schizophr Bull 2006; [Epub ahead of print].
56. Church CO et al. Diabetic ketoacidosis associated with aripiprazole. Diabet Med 2005;22:1440–3.
57. Reddymasu S et al. Elevated lipase and diabetic ketoacidosis associated with aripiprazole. JOP 2006; 7:303–5.
58. Mokdad AH et al. The continuing increase of diabetes in the US. Diabetes Care 2001;24:412.
59. Mokdad AH et al. Diabetes trends in the U.S.: 1990–1998. Diabetes Care 2000;23:1278–83.
60. Beckman JA et al. Diabetes and atherosclerosis: epidemiology, pathophysiology, and management. JAMA 2002;287:2570–81.
61. Henderson DC et al. Clozapine, diabetes mellitus, hyperlipidemia, and cardiovascular risks and mortality: results of a 10-year naturalistic study. J Clin Psychiatry 2005;66:1116–21.
62. Lamberti J et al. Prevalence of the metabolic syndrome among patients receiving clozapine. Am J Psychiatry 2006;163:1273–6.
63. Goff DC et al. A comparison of ten-year cardiac risk estimates in schizophrenia patients from the CATIE study and matched controls. Schizophr Res 2005;80:45–53.
64. Haupt DW et al. Hyperglycemia and antipsychotic medications. J Clin Psychiatry 2001;62(Suppl 27): 15–26.
65. Cohn TA et al. Metabolic monitoring for patients treated with antipsychotic medications. Can J Psychiatry 2006;51:492–501.
66. De Hert M et al. Oral glucose tolerance tests in treated patients with schizophrenia. Data to support an adaptation of the proposed guidelines for monitoring of patients on second generation antipsychotics? Eur Psychiatry 2006;21:224–6.
67. Marder SR et al. Physical health monitoring of patients with schizophrenia. Am J Psychiatry 2004; 161:1334–49.

Antipsychotics and dyslipidaemia

Morbidity and mortality from cardiovascular disease are higher in people with schizophrenia than in the general population[1]. Dyslipidaemia is an established risk factor for cardiovascular disease along with obesity, hypertension, smoking, diabetes and sedentary lifestyle. The majority of patients with schizophrenia have several of these risk factors and can be considered at 'high risk' of developing cardiovascular disease. Dyslipidaemia is treatable and intervention is known to reduce morbidity and mortality[2]. Aggressive treatment is particularly important in people with diabetes, the prevalence of which is increased two- to threefold over population norms in people with schizophrenia (see page 123).

Effect of antipsychotic drugs on lipids

First-generation antipsychotics
Phenothiazines are known to be associated with increases in triglycerides and low-density lipoprotein (LDL) cholesterol and decreases in high-density lipoprotein (HDL)[3] cholesterol, but the magnitude of these effects is poorly quantified[4]. Haloperidol seems to have minimal effect on lipid profiles[3].

Second-generation antipsychotics
Although there are relatively more data pertaining to some atypicals, they are derived from a variety of sources and are reported in different ways, making it difficult to compare drugs directly. While cholesterol levels can rise, the most profound effect of these drugs seems to be on triglycerides. Raised triglycerides are, in general, associated with obesity and diabetes. From the available data, olanzapine would seem to have the greatest propensity to increase lipids; quetiapine, moderate propensity; and risperidone, moderate or minimal propensity. Data for other atypicals are scarce, but recent data suggest that aripiprazole may be unique in having no adverse effect on blood lipids[5] and may even reverse dyslipidaemias associated with previous antipsychotics[6].

Olanzapine has been shown to increase triglyceride levels by 40% over the short (12 weeks) and medium (16 months) term[7,8]. Levels may continue to rise for up to a year[9]. Up to two-thirds of olanzapine-treated patients have raised triglycerides[10] and just under 10% may develop severe hypertriglyceridaemia[11]. While weight gain with olanzapine is generally associated with both increases in cholesterol[8,12] and triglycerides[11], severe hypertriglyceridaemia can occur independently of weight gain[11]. In one study, patients treated with olanzapine and risperidone gained a similar amount of weight, but in olanzapine patients serum triglyceride levels increased by four times as much (80 mg/dl) as in risperidone patients (20 mg/dl)[11]. Quetiapine[13] seems to have more modest effects than olanzapine.

A case-control study conducted in the UK found that patients with schizophrenia who were treated with olanzapine were five times more likely to develop hyperlipidaemia than controls and three times more likely to develop hyperlipidaemia than patients receiving typical antipsychotics[14]. Risperidone-treated patients could not be distinguished from controls.

Clozapine
Mean triglyceride levels have been shown to double and cholesterol levels to increase by at least 10% after 5 years' treatment with clozapine[15]. Patients treated with clozapine have triglyceride levels that are almost double those of patients who are treated with typical antipsychotics[16,17]. Cholesterol levels do not seem to be significantly different.

Particular care should be taken before prescribing clozapine, olanzapine, quetiapine and possibly phenothiazines for patients who are obese, diabetic or known to have pre-existing hyperlipidaemia[18].

Screening

All patients should have their lipids measured at baseline. Those prescribed clozapine, olanzapine, quetiapine or phenothiazines should have their serum lipids measured every 3 months for the first year of treatment[9]. Those prescribed other antipsychotics should have their lipids measured after 3 months then annually. Clinically significant changes in cholesterol are unlikely over the short term but triglycerides can increase dramatically[19]. In practice, dyslipidaemia is widespread in patients taking long-term antipsychotics irrespective of drug prescribed or diagnosis[20]. Severe hypertriglyceridaemia (fasting level of >5 mmol/l) is a risk factor for pancreatitis.

Treatment of dyslipidaemia

If moderate to severe hyperlipidaemia develops during antipsychotic treatment, a switch to another antipsychotic less likely to cause this problem should be considered in the first instance. Although not recommended as a strategy in patients with treatment-resistant illness, clozapine-induced hypertriglyceridaemia has been shown to reverse after a switch to risperidone[21]. This may hold true with other switching regimens but data are scarce.

Patients with raised cholesterol may benefit from dietary advice and/or treatment with statins. Risk tables and treatment guidelines can be found in the *British National Formulary* (*BNF*). Evidence supports the treatment of cholesterol concentrations as low as 4 mmol/l in high-risk patients[22]. Coronary heart disease and stroke risk can be reduced by a third by reducing cholesterol to as low as 3.5 mmol/l[2]. When triglycerides alone are raised, diets low in saturated fats and the taking of fish oil and fibrates are effective treatments[9]. Such patients should be screened for IGT and diabetes (see page 123). Note the suggested effective use of fish oils in some psychiatric conditions.

Summary

Monitoring	
Drug	**Suggested monitoring**
Clozapine Olanzapine Quetiapine Phenothiazines	Fasting lipids at baseline, then every 3 months for a year, then annually
Other antipsychotics	Fasting lipids at baseline and at 3 months, and then annually

References

1. Brown S et al. Causes of the excess mortality of schizophrenia. Br J Psychiatry 2000;177:212–17.
2. Durrington P. Dyslipidaemia. Lancet 2003;362:717–31.
3. Sasaki J et al. Lipids and apolipoproteins in patients treated with major tranquilizers. Clin Pharmacol Ther 1985;37:684–7.
4. Henkin Y et al. Secondary dyslipidemia. Inadvertent effects of drugs in clinical practice. JAMA 1992; 267:961–8.
5. Olfson M et al. Hyperlipidemia following treatment with antipsychotic medications. Am J Psychiatry 2006;163:1821–5.
6. De Hert M et al. A case series: evaluation of the metabolic safety of aripiprazole. Schizophr Bull 2006; [Epub ahead of print].
7. Sheitman BB et al. Olanzapine-induced elevation of plasma triglyceride levels. Am J Psychiatry 1999; 156:1471–2.
8. Osser DN et al. Olanzapine increases weight and serum triglyceride levels. J Clin Psychiatry 1999; 60:767–70.
9. Meyer JM. Effects of atypical antipsychotics on weight and serum lipid levels. J Clin Psychiatry 2001; 62(Suppl 27):27–34.
10. Melkersson KI et al. Elevated levels of insulin, leptin, and blood lipids in olanzapine-treated patients with schizophrenia or related psychoses. J Clin Psychiatry 2000;61:742–9.
11. Meyer JM. Novel antipsychotics and severe hyperlipidemia. J Clin Psychopharmacol 2001;21:369–74.
12. Kinon BJ et al. Long-term olanzapine treatment: weight change and weight-related health factors in schizophrenia. J Clin Psychiatry 2001;62:92–100.
13. Atmaca M et al. Serum leptin and triglyceride levels in patients on treatment with atypical antipsychotics. J Clin Psychiatry 2003;64:598–604.
14. Koro CE et al. An assessment of the independent effects of olanzapine and risperidone exposure on the risk of hyperlipidemia in schizophrenic patients. Arch Gen Psychiatry 2002;59:1021–6.
15. Henderson DC et al. Clozapine, diabetes mellitus, weight gain, and lipid abnormalities: a five-year naturalistic study. Am J Psychiatry 2000;157:975–81.
16. Ghaeli P et al. Serum triglyceride levels in patients treated with clozapine. Am J Health Syst Pharm 1996;53:2079–81.
17. Spivak B et al. Diminished suicidal and aggressive behavior, high plasma norepinephrine levels, and serum triglyceride levels in chronic neuroleptic-resistant schizophrenic patients maintained on clozapine. Clin Neuropharmacol 1998;21:245–50.
18. Baptista T et al. Novel antipsychotics and severe hyperlipidemia: comments on the Meyer paper. J Clin Psychopharmacol 2002;22:536–7.
19. Meyer JM et al. The effects of antipsychotic therapy on serum lipids: a comprehensive review. Schizophr Res 2004;70:1–17.
20. Paton C et al. Obesity, dyslipidaemias and smoking in an inpatient population treated with antipsychotic drugs. Acta Psychiatr Scand 2004;110:299–305.
21. Ghaeli P et al. Elevated serum triglycerides in clozapine resolve with risperidone. Pharmacotherapy 1995;15:382–5.
22. Heart Protection Study Collaborative Group. MRC/BHF Heart Protection Study of cholesterol lowering with simvastatin in 20,536 high-risk individuals: a randomised placebo-controlled trial. Lancet 2002; 360:7–22.

Further reading

American Diabetes Association, American Psychiatric Association, American Association of Clinical Endocrinologists et al. Consensus development conference on antipsychotic drugs and obesity and diabetes. J Clin Psychiatry 2004;65:267–72.

Bushe C et al. The potential impact of antipsychotics on lipids in schizophrenia: is there enough evidence to confirm a link? J Psychopharmacol 2005;19:76–83.

Young IS. Lipids for Psychiatrists – an overview. J Psychopharmacol 2005;19:66–75.

Antipsychotics and sexual dysfunction

Primary sexual disorders are common, although reliable normative data are lacking[1]. Reported prevalence rates vary depending on the method of data collection (low numbers with spontaneous reports, increasing with confidential questionnaires and further still with direct questioning[2]). Physical illness, psychiatric illness, substance misuse and prescribed drug treatment can all cause sexual dysfunction[2].

Baseline sexual functioning should be determined if possible (questionnaires may be useful) because sexual function can affect quality of life[3] and affect compliance with medication (sexual dysfunction is one of the major causes of treatment dropout)[4]. Complaints of sexual dysfunction may also indicate progression or inadequate treatment of underlying medical or psychiatric conditions. It may also be due to drug treatment, and intervention may greatly improve quality of life[5].

The human sexual response

There are four phases of the human sexual response, as detailed in the table below[2,6–8].

Table	The human sexual response
Desire	• Related to testosterone levels in men • Possibly increased by dopamine and decreased by prolactin • Psychosocial context and conditioning significantly affect desire
Arousal	• Influenced by testosterone in men and oestrogen in women • Other potential mechanisms include: central dopamine stimulation, modulation of the cholinergic/adrenergic balance, peripheral α_1 agonism and nitric oxide • Physical pathology such as hypertension or diabetes can have a significant effect
Orgasm	• May be related to oxytocin • Inhibition of orgasm may be caused by an increase in serotonin activity, as well as α_1 blockade
Resolution	• Occurs passively after orgasm
Note: Many other hormones and neurotransmitters may interact in a complex way at each phase.	

Effects of psychosis

Sexual dysfunction is a problem in first-episode schizophrenia[9] and up to 82% of men and 96% of women with established illness report problems with associated reductions in quality of life[3]. Men[10] complain of reduced desire, inability to achieve an erection and premature ejaculation, whereas women

132

complain more generally about reduced enjoyment[10,11]. Women with psychosis are known to have reduced fertility[12]. People with psychosis are less able to develop good psychosexual relationships and, for some, treatment with an antipsychotic can improve sexual functioning[13]. Assessment of sexual functioning can clearly be difficult in someone who is psychotic. The Arizona Sexual Experiences Scale (ASEX) may be useful in this respect[14].

Effects of antipsychotic drugs

Sexual dysfunction has been reported as a side-effect of all antipsychotics[5], and up to 45% of people taking conventional antipsychotics experience sexual dysfunction[15]. Individual susceptibility varies and all effects are reversible. Antipsychotics decrease dopaminergic transmission, which in itself can decrease libido but may also increase prolactin levels via negative feedback. This can cause amenorrhoea in women and a lack of libido, breast enlargement and galactorrhoea in both men and women[16]. Anticholinergic effects can cause disorders of arousal[17] and drugs that block peripheral α_1 receptors cause particular problems with erection and ejaculation in men[5]. Drugs that are antagonists at both peripheral α_1 receptors and cholinergic receptors can cause priapism[18]. Antipsychotic-induced sedation and weight gain may reduce sexual desire[18]. These principles can be used to predict the sexual side-effects of different antipsychotic drugs (see table below).

Table Sexual adverse effects of antipsychotics

Drug	Type of problem
Phenothiazines	• Hyperprolactinaemia and anticholinergic effects. Reports of delayed orgasm at lower doses followed by normal orgasm but without ejaculation at higher doses[11] • Most problems occur with thioridazine (which can also reduce testosterone levels)[19] • Priapism has been reported with thioridazine, risperidone and chlorpromazine (probably due to α_1 blockade)[20-22]
Thioxanthenes	• Arousal problems and anorgasmia[13]
Haloperidol	• Similar problems to the phenothiazines[23] but anticholinergic effects reduced[20]
Olanzapine	• Possibly less sexual dysfunction due to relative lack of prolactin-related effects[23] • Priapism reported rarely[24,25]
Risperidone	• Potent elevator of serum prolactin • Less anticholinergic • Specific peripheral α_1 adrenergic blockade leads to a moderately high reported incidence of ejaculatory problems such as retrograde ejaculation[26,27] • Priapism reported rarely[18]
Sulpiride/amisulpride	• Potent elevators of serum prolactin[15]

Table Sexual adverse effects of antipsychotics (Cont.)

Drug	Type of problem
Quetiapine	• No effect on serum prolactin[28] • Possibly associated with low risk of sexual dysfunction[29–32], but studies are conflicting[33,34]
Clozapine	• Significant α_1 adrenergic blockade and anticholinergic effects[35]. No effect on prolactin[36] • Probably fewer problems than with typical antipsychotics[37]
Aripiprazole	• Few data but problems not expected. No effect on prolactin or α_1 receptors

Treatment

Before attempting to treat sexual dysfunction, a thorough assessment is essential to determine the most likely cause. Assuming that physical pathology has been excluded, the following principles apply.

Spontaneous remission may occasionally occur[18]. The most obvious first step is to decrease the dose or discontinue the offending drug where appropriate. The next step is to switch to a different drug that is less likely to cause the specific sexual problem experienced (see table above). If this fails or is not practicable, 'antidote' drugs can be tried: for example, cyproheptadine (a $5HT_2$ antagonist at doses of 4–16 mg/day) has been used to treat SSRI-induced sexual dysfunction but sedation is a common side-effect. Amantadine, buproprion, buspirone, bethanechol and yohimbine have all been used with varying degrees of success but have a number of unwanted side-effects and interactions with other drugs (see opposite). Given that hyperprolactinaemia may contribute to sexual dysfunction, selegiline (enhances dopamine activity) has been tested in an RCT. This was negative[38].

The evidence base supporting the use of 'antidotes' is poor[18].

Drugs such as sildenafil (Viagra) or alprostadil (Caverject) are effective only in the treatment of erectile dysfunction. In the UK they are available for prescription by GPs for a limited number of medical indications, not including psychosis or antipsychotic-induced impotence[51]. The psychological approaches used by sexual dysfunction clinics may be difficult for clients with mental health problems to engage in[5].

Table Remedial treatments for psychotropic-induced sexual dysfunction (alphabetical order)

Drug	Pharmacology	Potential treatment for	Side-effects
Alprostadil[1,7]	Prostaglandin	Erectile dysfunction	Pain, fibrosis, hypotension, priapism
Amantadine[1,39]	Dopamine agonist	Prolactin-induced reduction in desire and arousal (dopamine increases libido and facilitates ejaculation)	Return of psychotic symptoms, GI effects, nervousness, insomnia
Bethanechol[40]	Cholinergic or cholinergic potentiation of adrenergic neurotransmission	Anticholinergic-induced arousal problems and anorgasmia (from TCAs, antipsychotics, etc.)	Nausea and vomiting, colic, bradycardia, blurred vision, sweating
Bromocriptine[5]	Dopamine agonist	Prolactin-induced reduction in desire and arousal	Return of psychotic symptoms, GI effects
Bupropion[41]	Norepinephrine and dopamine reuptake inhibitor	SSRI-induced sexual dysfunction (evidence poor)	Concentration problems, reduced sleep, tremor
Buspirone[42]	$5HT_{1a}$ partial agonist	SSRI-induced sexual dysfunction, particularly decreased libido and anorgasmia	Nausea, dizziness, headache
Cyproheptadine[1,42,43]	$5HT_2$ antagonist	Sexual dysfunction caused by increased serotonin transmission (e.g. SSRIs), particularly anorgasmia	Sedation and fatigue. Reversal of the therapeutic effect of antidepressants
Sildenafil[7,44-47]	Phosphodiesterase inhibitor	Erectile dysfunction of any aetiology. Anorgasmia in women. Effective when prolactin raised	Mild headaches, dizziness, nasal congestion
Yohimbine[1,7,48-50]	Central and peripheral α_2 adrenoceptor antagonist	SSRI-induced sexual dysfunction, particularly erectile dysfunction, decreased libido and anorgasmia (evidence poor)	Anxiety, nausea, fine tremor, increased BP, sweating, fatigue

Note: The use of the drugs listed above should ideally be under the care or supervision of a specialist in sexual dysfunction.

References

1. Baldwin DS et al. Effects of antidepressant drugs on sexual function. Int J Psychiatry Clin Pract 1997; 1:47–58.
2. Pollack MH et al. Genitourinary and sexual adverse effects of psychotropic medication. Int J Psychiatry Med 1992;22:305–27.
3. Olfson M et al. Male sexual dysfunction and quality of life in schizophrenia. J Clin Psychiatry 2005;66: 331–8.
4. Montejo AL et al. Incidence of sexual dysfunction associated with antidepressant agents: a prospective multicenter study of 1022 outpatients. Spanish Working Group for the Study of Psychotropic-Related Sexual Dysfunction. J Clin Psychiatry 2001;62(Suppl 3):10–21.
5. Segraves RT. Effects of psychotropic drugs on human erection and ejaculation. Arch Gen Psychiatry 1989;46:275–84.
6. Stahl SM. The psychopharmacology of sex, Part 1: Neurotransmitters and the 3 phases of the human sexual response. J Clin Psychiatry 2001;62:80–1.
7. Garcia-Reboll L et al. Drugs for the treatment of impotence. Drugs Aging 1997;11:140–51.
8. deGroat WC et al. Physiology of male sexual function. Ann Intern Med 1980;92:329–31.
9. Bitter I et al. Antipsychotic treatment and sexual functioning in first-time neuroleptic-treated schizo- phrenic patients. Int Clin Psychopharmacol 2005;20:19–21.
10. Macdonald S et al. Nithsdale Schizophrenia Surveys 24: sexual dysfunction. Case-control study. Br J Psychiatry 2003;182:50–6.
11. Smith S. Effects of antipsychotics on sexual and endocrine function in women: implications for clinical practice. J Clin Psychopharmacol 2003;23:S27–S32.
12. Howard LM et al. The general fertility rate in women with psychotic disorders. Am J Psychiatry 2002;159:991–7.
13. Aizenberg D et al. Sexual dysfunction in male schizophrenic patients. J Clin Psychiatry 1995;56:137–41.
14. Byerly MJ et al. An empirical evaluation of the Arizona sexual experience scale and a simple one-item screening test for assessing antipsychotic-related sexual dysfunction in outpatients with schizophrenia and schizoaffective disorder. Schizophr Res 2006;81:311–16.
15. Smith SM et al. Sexual dysfunction in patients taking conventional antipsychotic medication. Br J Psychiatry 2002;181:49–55.
16. Anon. Adverse effects of the atypical antipsychotics. Collaborative Working Group on Clinical Trial Evaluations. J Clin Psychiatry 1998;59(Suppl 12):17–22.
17. Aldridge SA. Drug-induced sexual dysfunction. Clin Pharm 1982;1:141–7.
18. Baldwin D et al. Sexual side-effects of antidepressant and antipsychotic drugs. Adv Psychiatr Treat 2003;9:202–10.
19. Kotin J et al. Thioridazine and sexual dysfunction. Am J Psychiatry 1976;133:82–5.
20. Mitchell JE et al. Antipsychotic drug therapy and sexual dysfunction in men. Am J Psychiatry 1982;139: 633–7.
21. Loh C et al. Risperidone-induced retrograde ejaculation: case report and review of the literature. Int Clin Psychopharmacol 2004;19:111–12.
22. Thompson JW Jr et al. Psychotropic medication and priapism: a comprehensive review. J Clin Psychiatry 1990;51:430–3.
23. Crawford AM et al. The acute and long-term effect of olanzapine compared with placebo and haloperidol on serum prolactin concentrations. Schizophr Res 1997;26:41–54.
24. Eli Lilly and Company Limited. Zyprexa. Summary of Product Characteristics. www.medicines.org.uk. 2005.
25. Dossenbach M et al. Effects of atypical and typical antipsychotic treatments on sexual function in patients with schizophrenia: 12-month results from the Intercontinental Schizophrenia Outpatient Health Outcomes (IC-SOHO) study. Eur Psychiatry 2006;21:251–8.
26. Tran PV et al. Double-blind comparison of olanzapine versus risperidone in the treatment of schizophre- nia and other psychotic disorders. J Clin Psychopharmacol 1997;17:407–18.
27. Raja M. Risperidone-induced absence of ejaculation. Int Clin Psychopharmacol 1999;14:317–19.
28. Peuskens J et al. A comparison of quetiapine and chlorpromazine in the treatment of schizophrenia. Acta Psychiatr Scand 1997;96:265–73.
29. Bobes J et al. Frequency of sexual dysfunction and other reproductive side-effects in patients with schizophrenia treated with risperidone, olanzapine, quetiapine, or haloperidol: the results of the EIRE study. J Sex Marital Ther 2003;29:125–47.
30. Byerly MJ et al. An open-label trial of quetiapine for antipsychotic-induced sexual dysfunction. J Sex Marital Ther 2004;30:325–32.
31. Knegtering R et al. A randomized open-label study of the impact of quetiapine versus risperidone on sexual functioning. J Clin Psychopharmacol 2004;24:56–61.
32. Montejo Gonzalez AL et al. A 6-month prospective observational study on the effects of quetiapine on sexual functioning. J Clin Psychopharmacol 2005;25:533–8.
33. Atmaca M et al. A new atypical antipsychotic: quetiapine-induced sexual dysfunctions. Int J Impot Res 2005;17:201–3.
34. Kelly DL et al. A randomized double-blind 12-week study of quetiapine, risperidone or fluphenazine on sexual functioning in people with schizophrenia. Psychoneuroendocrinology 2006;31:340–6.
35. Coward DM. General pharmacology of clozapine. Br J Psychiatry 1992;160:5–11.

36. Meltzer HY et al. Effect of clozapine on human serum prolactin levels. Am J Psychiatry 1979;136: 1550–5.
37. Aizenberg D et al. Comparison of sexual dysfunction in male schizophrenic patients maintained on treatment with classical antipsychotics versus clozapine. J Clin Psychiatry 2001;62:541–4.
38. Kodesh A et al. Selegiline in the treatment of sexual dysfunction in schizophrenic patients maintained on neuroleptics: a pilot study. Clin Neuropharmacol 2003;26:193–5.
39. Valevski A et al. Effect of amantadine on sexual dysfunction in neuroleptic-treated male schizophrenic patients. Clin Neuropharmacol 1998;21:355–7.
40. Gross MD. Reversal by bethanechol of sexual dysfunction caused by anticholinergic antidepressants. Am J Psychiatry 1982;139:1193–4.
41. Masand PS et al. Sustained-release bupropion for selective serotonin reuptake inhibitor-induced sexual dysfunction: a randomized, double-blind, placebo-controlled, parallel-group study. Am J Psychiatry 2001;158:805–7.
42. Rothschild AJ. Sexual side effects of antidepressants. J Clin Psychiatry 2000;61(Suppl 11):28–36.
43. Lauerma H. Successful treatment of citalopram-induced anorgasmia by cyproheptadine. Acta Psychiatr Scand 1996;93:69–70.
44. Nurnberg HG et al. Sildenafil for women patients with antidepressant-induced sexual dysfunction. Psychiatr Serv 1999;50:1076–8.
45. Salerian AJ et al. Sildenafil for psychotropic-induced sexual dysfunction in 31 women and 61 men. J Sex Marital Ther 2000;26:133–40.
46. Nurnberg HG et al. Treatment of antidepressant-associated sexual dysfunction with sildenafil: a randomized controlled trial. JAMA 2003;289:56–64.
47. Gopalakrishnan R et al. Sildenafil in the treatment of antipsychotic-induced erectile dysfunction: a randomized, double-blind, placebo-controlled, flexible-dose, two-way crossover trial. Am J Psychiatry 2006;163:494–9.
48. Jacobsen FM. Fluoxetine-induced sexual dysfunction and an open trial of yohimbine. J Clin Psychiatry 1992;53:119–22.
49. Michelson D et al. Mirtazapine, yohimbine or olanzapine augmentation therapy for serotonin reuptake-associated female sexual dysfunction: a randomized, placebo controlled trial. J Psychiatr Res 2002;36: 147–52.
50. Woodrum ST et al. Management of SSRI-induced sexual dysfunction. Ann Pharmacother 1998;32: 1209–15.
51. Department of Health. HSC 1999/117: The new NHS guidance on out of area treatments. http://www.dh.gov.uk/. 1999.

Schizophrenia

Antipsychotic-induced hyponatraemia

Hyponatraemia can occur in the context of:

1. **Water intoxication** where water consumption exceeds the maximal renal clearance capacity. Serum and urine osmolality are low. Cross-sectional studies of chronically ill, hospitalised, psychiatric patients have found the prevalence of water intoxication to be approximately 5%[1,2]. A longitudinal study found that 10% of severely ill patients with a diagnosis of schizophrenia had episodic hyponatraemia secondary to fluid overload[3]. The primary aetiology is poorly understood. It has been postulated that it may be driven, at least in part, by an extreme compensatory response to the anticholinergic side-effects of antipsychotic drugs[4].
2. Drug-induced **syndrome of inappropriate antidiuretic hormone (SIADH)** where the kidney retains an excessive quantity of solute-free water, serum osmolality is low and urine osmolality relatively high. The prevalence of SIADH is estimated to be as high as 11% in acutely ill psychiatric patients[5]. Risk factors for antidepressant-induced SIADH (increasing age, female gender, medical co-morbidity and polypharmacy) seem to be less relevant in the population of patients treated with antipsychotic drugs[6]. SIADH usually develops in the first few weeks of treatment with the offending drug. Phenothiazines, haloperidol, pimozide, risperidone, quetiapine, olanzapine, aripiprazole and clozapine have all been implicated[6,7]. Note, however, that the literature consists entirely of case reports and case series. Desmopressin use (for clozapine-induced enuresis) can also result in hyponatraemia[8].
3. Severe **hyperlipidaemia** and/or **hyperglycaemia** lead to secondary increases in plasma volume and 'pseudohyponatraemia'[4]. Both are more common in people treated with antipsychotic drugs than in the general population and should be excluded as causes.

Mild to moderate hyponatraemia presents as confusion, nausea, headache and lethargy. As the plasma sodium falls, these symptoms become increasingly severe and seizures and coma can develop.

Monitoring of plasma sodium is probably not strictly necessary for all those receiving antipsychotics, but is desirable. Signs of confusion or lethargy should provoke thorough diagnostic analysis, including plasma sodium determination.

Table Treatment[4,5]

Cause of hyponatraemia	Antipsychotic drugs implicated	Treatment
Water intoxication (serum and urine osmolality low)	Only very speculative evidence to support drugs as a cause. Core part of illness in a minority of patients (e.g. psychotic polydipsia)	• **Fluid restriction** with careful monitoring of serum sodium, particularly diurnal variation (Na drops as the day progresses). Refer to specialist medical care if Na <125 mmol/l. Note that the use of IV saline to correct hyponatraemia has been reported to precipitate rhabdomyolysis[9] • Consider treatment with **clozapine**: shown to increase plasma osmolality into the normal range and increase urine osmolality (not usually reaching the normal range)[10]. These effects are consistent with reduced fluid intake. This effect is not clearly related to improvements in mental state[11] • There are both[6] positive and negative reports for olanzapine[12] and risperidone[13] and one positive case report for quetiapine[14]. Compared with clozapine, the evidence base is weak • There is no evidence that either reducing or increasing the dose of an antipsychotic results in improvements in serum sodium in water-intoxicated patients[15] • Demeclocycline should not be used (exerts its effect by interfering with ADH and increasing water excretion, already at capacity in these patients)
SIADH (serum osmolality low; urine osmolality relatively high)	All antipsychotic drugs	• If mild, **fluid restriction** with careful monitoring of serum sodium. Refer to specialist medical care if Na <125 mmol/l • **Switching to a different antipsychotic drug**. There are insufficient data available to guide choice. Be aware that cross-sensitivity may occur (the individual may be predisposed and the choice of drug is unimportant) • Consider **demeclocycline** (see *BNF* for details) • Lithium may be effective[6] but is a potentially toxic drug. Remember that hyponatraemia predisposes to lithium toxicity

References

1. de Leon J et al. Polydipsia and water intoxication in psychiatric patients: a review of the epidemiological literature. Biol Psychiatry 1994;35:408–19.
2. Patel JK. Polydipsia, hyponatremia, and water intoxication among psychiatric patients. Hosp Community Psychiatry 1994;45:1073–4.
3. de Leon J. Polydipsia – a study in a long-term psychiatric unit. Eur Arch Psychiatry Clin Neurosci 2003; 253:37–9.
4. Siegel AJ et al. Primary and drug-induced disorders of water homeostasis in psychiatric patients: principles of diagnosis and management. Harv Rev Psychiatry 1998;6:190–200.
5. Siegler EL et al. Risk factors for the development of hyponatremia in psychiatric inpatients. Arch Intern Med 1995;155:953–7.
6. Madhusoodanan S et al. Hyponatraemia associated with psychotropic medications. A review of the literature and spontaneous reports. Adverse Drug React Toxicol Rev 2002;21:17–29.
7. Bachu K et al. Aripiprazole-induced syndrome of inappropriate antidiuretic hormone secretion (SIADH). Am J Ther 2006;13:370–2.
8. Sarma S et al. Severe hyponatraemia associated with desmopressin nasal spray to treat clozapine-induced nocturnal enuresis. Aust N Z J Psychiatry 2005;39:949.
9. Zaidi AN. Rhabdomyolysis after correction of hyponatremia in psychogenic polydipsia possibly complicated by ziprasidone. Ann Pharmacother 2005;39:1726–31.
10. Canuso CM et al. Clozapine restores water balance in schizophrenic patients with polydipsia-hyponatremia syndrome. J Neuropsychiatry Clin Neurosci 1999;11:86–90.
11. Spears NM et al. Clozapine treatment in polydipsia and intermittent hyponatremia. J Clin Psychiatry 1996;57:123–8.
12. Littrell KH et al. Effects of olanzapine on polydipsia and intermittent hyponatremia. J Clin Psychiatry 1997;58:549.
13. Kawai N et al. Risperidone failed to improve polydipsia-hyponatremia of the schizophrenic patients. Psychiatry Clin Neurosci 2002;56:107–10.
14. Montgomery JH et al. Adjunctive quetiapine treatment of the polydipsia, intermittent hyponatremia, and psychosis syndrome: a case report. J Clin Psychiatry 2003;64:339–41.
15. Canuso CM et al. Does minimizing neuroleptic dosage influence hyponatremia? Psychiatry Res 1996;63:227–9.

Antipsychotics: relative adverse effects – a rough guide

Drug	Sedation	Weight gain	Extra-pyramidal	Anti-cholinergic	Hypotension	Prolactin elevation
Amisulpride	−	+	+	−	−	+++
Aripiprazole	−	+/−	+/−	−	−	−
Benperidol	+	+	+++	+	+	+++
Chlorpromazine	+++	++	++	++	+++	+++
Clozapine	+++	+++	−	+++	+++	−
Flupentixol	+	++	++	++	+	+++
Fluphenazine	+	+	+++	++	+	+++
Haloperidol	+	+	+++	+	+	+++
Loxapine	++	+	+++	+	++	+++
Olanzapine	++	+++	+/−	+	+	+
Perphenazine	+	+	+++	+	+	+++
Pimozide	+	+	+	+	+	+++
Pipothiazine	++	++	++	++	++	+++
Promazine	+++	++	+	++	++	++
Quetiapine	++	++	−	+	++	−
Risperidone	+	++	+	+	++	+++
Sertindole	−	+	−	−	+++	+/−
Sulpiride	−	+	+	−	−	+++
Trifluoperazine	+	+	+++	+/−	+	+++
Ziprasidone	+	+/−	+/−	−	+	+/−
Zotepine	+++	++	+	+	++	+++
Zuclopenthixol	++	++	++	++	+	+++

Key: +++ High incidence/severity
++ Moderate
+ Low
− Very low

Note: the table above is made up of approximate estimates of relative incidence and/or severity, based on clinical experience, manufacturers' literature and published research. This is a rough guide – see individual sections for more precise information.

Other side effects not mentioned in this table do occur. Please see dedicated sections on other side effects included in this book for more information.

chapter 3

Bipolar disorder

Valproate

Valproate is available in the UK in three forms: sodium valproate (Epilim) and valproic acid (Convulex), licensed for the treatment of epilepsy, and semi-sodium valproate (Depakote), licensed for the acute treatment of mania. Both semisodium and sodium valproate are metabolised to valproic acid, which is apparently responsible for the pharmacological activity of all three preparations[1]. Clinical studies of the treatment of affective disorders variably use sodium valproate, semisodium valproate, 'valproate' or valproic acid. The great majority have used valproate semisodium.

Randomised, controlled trials (RCTs) have shown valproate to be effective in the treatment of mania[2,3]. Approximately 50% of patients respond during the acute phase[1]. One study[3] found lithium to be more effective overall than valproate, while another[4] found that patients who had depressive symptoms at baseline were more likely to respond to valproate than lithium. Patients who have experienced 10 or more episodes of mania may also respond better to valproate (as semisodium) than lithium[5]. In a further double-blind, placebo-controlled study of valproate in 36 patients who had failed to respond to or could not tolerate lithium, the median decrease in Young Mania Rating Scale scores was 54% in the valproate group and 5% in the placebo group[6]. Open studies and one small randomised placebo controlled study[7] suggest that valproate may have some efficacy in bipolar depression. The attrition rate in all of these studies was high (a feature of all bipolar studies).

Although open-label studies suggest that valproate is effective in the prophylaxis of bipolar affective disorder[8,9], only two RCTs have been published to date[10,11]. In the first[8], no difference was found between lithium, valproate semisodium and placebo in the primary outcome measure, time to any mood episode, although valproate was superior to lithium and placebo on some secondary outcome measures. This study can be criticised for including patients who were 'not ill enough' and for not lasting 'long enough' (1 year). In the second RCT[11], which lasted for 47 weeks, there was no difference in relapse rates between divalproex (valproate semisodium) and olanzapine. This study had no placebo arm and the attrition rate was high, so is difficult to interpret. A post-hoc analysis of data from this study found that patients with rapid cycling illness had a better very early response to valproate than to olanzapine but that this advantage was not maintained[12]. Outcomes with respect to manic symptoms for those who did not have a rapid cycling illness were better at 1 year with olanzapine than valproate[12]. NICE recommends valproate as a first-line option for the treatment of acute episodes of mania, in combination with an antidepressant for the treatment of acute episodes of depression and for prophylaxis[13]. See page XX for recommendations in women of childbearing age.

Valproate is sometimes used to treat aggressive behaviour of variable aetiology[14].

Plasma levels

Valproate has a complex pharmacokinetic profile, following a three-compartment model and showing protein-binding saturation. Plasma level monitoring is supposedly, therefore, of more limited use than with carbamazepine or lithium. There may be a linear association between valproate serum level and response in acute mania, with serum levels <55 mg/l being no more effective than placebo and levels >94 mg/l being associated with the most robust response[15]. Note that this is the top of the reference range (for epilepsy) that is quoted on laboratory request forms. Optimal serum levels during the maintenance phase are unknown, but are likely to be at least 50 mg/l[16]. Achieving therapeutic plasma levels rapidly using a loading dose regimen is generally well tolerated. Plasma levels can also be useful to detect non-compliance or predict or confirm toxicity.

Adverse effects[17]

Sodium valproate causes both hyperammonaemia and gastric irritation, which can sometimes lead to intense nausea. Lethargy and confusion can occasionally occur with starting doses of above 750 mg a day. Weight gain can be significant[18], particularly when valproate is used in conjunction with clozapine. Hair loss with curly regrowth, and peripheral oedema can also occur. Sodium valproate may very rarely cause fulminant hepatic failure[19]. All cases reported to date have occurred in children, often receiving multiple anticonvulsants and with family histories of hepatic problems. It would seem wise to evaluate clinically any patient with raised LFTs and to also monitor other markers of hepatic function such as albumin and prothrombin time. Valproate can cause hyperandrogenism in women and has been linked with the development of polycystic ovaries; the evidence supporting this association is conflicting. It is also associated with thrombocytopenia, leucopenia, red cell hypoplasia and pancreatitis. Many side-effects of valproate are dose-related (peak plasma level-related) and increase in frequency and severity when the plasma level is >100 mg/l. The once-daily 'chrono' form of sodium valproate does not produce as high peaks as the conventional forms of valproate and may be better tolerated. There is also a suggestion that valproate semisodium may be better tolerated in some.

Use of valproate in women of childbearing age

Valproate is an established teratogen. The risk of fetal malformations is 7.2%[20], much of which is due to neural tube defects. NICE recommends that alternative anticonvulsants are to be preferred in women with epilepsy[20] and that valproate should not be routinely used to treat bipolar illness in women of childbearing age[13].

The SPCs[21] for sodium and semisodium valproate state that:

- These drugs should not be initiated in women of childbearing potential without specialist advice (from a neurologist or psychiatrist).
- Women who are trying to conceive and require valproate, should be prescribed prophylactic folate.

Women who have mania are likely to be sexually disinhibited. The risk of unplanned pregnancy is likely to be above population norms (where 50% of pregnancies are unplanned). If valproate cannot be avoided, adequate contraception should be ensured and prophylactic folate prescribed.

The teratogenic potential of valproate is not widely understood[22] and many women of childbearing age who are prescribed valproate are not advised of the need for contraception or prophylactic folate[23].

Interactions with other drugs[24,25]

Valproate is highly protein-bound (up to 94%): other drugs that are highly protein-bound can displace valproate from albumin and precipitate toxicity (e.g. *aspirin*[26]). Other, less strongly protein-bound drugs, can be displaced by valproate, leading to higher free levels and increased therapeutic effect or toxicity (e.g. *warfarin*). Valproate is hepatically metabolised: drugs that inhibit CYP enzymes can increase valproate levels (e.g. *erythromycin*, *fluoxetine* and *cimetidine*). Valproate can increase the plasma levels of some drugs, possibly by inhibition/competitive inhibition of their metabolism. Examples include *TCAs* (particularly clomipramine[27]), *lamotrigine*[28] and *phenobarbital*.

Pharmacodynamic interactions also occur. The anticonvulsant effect of valproate is antagonised by drugs that lower the seizure threshold (e.g. antipsychotics and antidepressants). Weight gain can be exacerbated by other drugs that have this effect (e.g. antipsychotics, particularly clozapine and olanzapine).

Bipolar disorder

References

1. Fisher C et al. Sodium valproate or valproate semisodium: is there a difference in the treatment of bipolar disorder? Psychiatr Bull 2003;27:446–8.
2. Bowden CL et al. Efficacy of divalproex vs lithium and placebo in the treatment of mania. The Depakote Mania Study Group. JAMA 1994;271:918–24.
3. Freeman TW et al. A double-blind comparison of valproate and lithium in the treatment of acute mania. Am J Psychiatry 1992;149:108–11.
4. Swann AC et al. Depression during mania. Treatment response to lithium or divalproex. Arch Gen Psychiatry 1997;54:37–42.
5. Swann AC et al. Differential effect of number of previous episodes of affective disorder on response to lithium or divalproex in acute mania. Am J Psychiatry 1999;156:1264–6.
6. Pope HG Jr et al. Valproate in the treatment of acute mania. A placebo-controlled study. Arch Gen Psychiatry 1991;48:62–8.
7. Davis LL et al. Divalproex in the treatment of bipolar depression: a placebo-controlled study. J Affect Disord 2005;85:259–66.
8. Calabrese JR et al. Spectrum of efficacy of valproate in 55 patients with rapid-cycling bipolar disorder. Am J Psychiatry 1990;147:431–4.
9. McElroy SL et al. Sodium valproate: its use in primary psychiatric disorders. J Clin Psychopharmacol 1987;7:16–24.
10. Bowden CL et al. A randomized, placebo-controlled 12-month trial of divalproex and lithium in treatment of outpatients with bipolar I disorder. Divalproex Maintenance Study Group. Arch Gen Psychiatry 2000;57:481–9.
11. Tohen M et al. Olanzapine versus divalproex sodium for the treatment of acute mania and maintenance of remission: a 47-week study. Am J Psychiatry 2003;160:1263–71.
12. Suppes T et al. Rapid versus non-rapid cycling as a predictor of response to olanzapine and divalproex sodium for bipolar mania and maintenance of remission: post hoc analyses of 47-week data. J Affect Disord 2005;89:69–77.
13. National Institute for Clinical Excellence. Bipolar disorder. The management of bipolar disorder in adults, children and adolescents, in primary and secondary care. Clinical Guidance 38. http://www.nice.org.uk. 2006.
14. Lindenmayer JP et al. Use of sodium valproate in violent and aggressive behaviors: a critical review. J Clin Psychiatry 2000;61:123–8.
15. Allen MH et al. Linear relationship of valproate serum concentration to response and optimal serum levels for acute mania. Am J Psychiatry 2006;163:272–5.
16. Taylor D et al. Doses of carbamazepine and valproate in bipolar affective disorder. Psychiatr Bull 1997;21:221–3.
17. Sanofi-Aventis. Depakote tablets. Summary of Product Characteristics. www.medicines.org.uk. 2004.
18. Vanina Y et al. Body weight changes associated with psychopharmacology. Psychiatr Serv 2002;53: 842–7.
19. Rimmer EM et al. An update on sodium valproate. Pharmacotherapy 1985;5:171–84.
20. National Institute for Clinical Excellence. The clinical effectiveness and cost effectiveness of newer drugs for epilepsy in adults. Technology Appraisal 76. http://www.nice.org.uk. 2004.
21. Sanofi-Aventis. Epilim Chrono. Summary of Product Characteristics. www.medicines.org.uk. 2006.
22. James L et al. Mood stabilisers and teratogenicity – prescribing practice and awareness amongst practising psychiatrists. J Ment Health 2007; Submitted.

23. James L et al. Informing patients of the teratogenic potential of mood stabilising drugs; a case notes review of the practice of psychiatrists. J Psychopharmacol 2007; in press.
24. Spina E et al. Clinical significance of pharmacokinetic interactions between antiepileptic and psychotropic drugs. Epilepsia 2002;43(Suppl 2):37–44.
25. Patsalos PN et al. The importance of drug interactions in epilepsy therapy. Epilepsia 2002;43:365–85.
26. Goulden KJ et al. Clinical valproate toxicity induced by acetylsalicylic acid. Neurology 1987;37:1392–4.
27. Fehr C et al. Increase in serum clomipramine concentrations caused by valproate. J Clin Psychopharmacol 2000;20:493–4.
28. Morris RG et al. Clinical study of lamotrigine and valproic acid in patients with epilepsy: using a drug interaction to advantage? Ther Drug Monit 2000;22:656–60.

Lithium

Lithium is widely used for the prophylaxis and treatment of mania and hypo-mania, recurrent depression and bipolar affective disorder. Its use in the treatment of acute mania[1] is limited by the fact that it usually takes at least a week to achieve a response[2] and that the co-administration of high doses of potent antipsychotics may increase the risk of neurological side-effects. It can also be difficult to achieve therapeutic serum levels rapidly and monitor-ing can be problematic if the patient is uncooperative.

Lithium augmentation of an antidepressant is recommended by NICE in patients with unipolar depression who have failed to respond to sequential trials of two or more antidepressants in adequate doses for adequate periods of time[3]. There is some evidence that lithium is underutilised for this purpose, at least in the USA[4].

Lithium is used in the prophylaxis of bipolar affective disorder where it reduces both the number and the severity of relapses[1,5]. Lithium is more effective in preventing manic than depressive relapse[6,7]; the NNT to prevent relapse into mania or depression has been calculated to be 10 and 14, respectively[6]. Lithium also offers some protection against antidepressant-induced hypoma-nia. It is recommended by NICE that a mood stabiliser should be prescribed prophylactically (1) after a single manic episode that was associated with sig-nificant risk and adverse consequences or (2) in the case of bipolar I illness, two or more acute episodes or (3) in the case of bipolar II illness, significant functional impairment, frequent episodes or significant risk of suicide[8]. NICE support the use of lithium as a first-line mood stabiliser. Although numerous factors have been studied in an attempt to identify patients who are likely to respond to lithium, an empirical trial is still the best predictor of long-term out-come. Relapse within 1 year of starting lithium prophylaxis is highly suggestive of a poor long-term response. Some evidence points to the previous pattern of illness as a predictor of response to lithium[9]: patients whose illness shows a pattern of mania followed by depression followed by a euthymic interval, or those whose illness shows an irregular pattern, are more likely to respond to lithium prophylaxis than those who show a pattern of depression – mania – euthymia or have a rapidly cycling illness (four or more episodes/year)[10].

Intermittent treatment with lithium may worsen the natural course of bipolar illness (a much greater than expected incidence of manic relapse is seen in the first few months after discontinuing lithium[11-13], even in patients who have been symptom-free for as long as 5 years[14]). There is a suggestion that depressive relapses may also increase[13]. This has led to recommendations that lithium treatment should not be started unless there is a clear intention to continue it for at least 3 years[15]. This advice has obvious implications for initiating lithium treatment against a patient's will (or in someone known to be non-compliant) during a period of acute illness. The risk of relapse may be reduced by decreasing the dose of lithium gradually over a period of 1 month[16]. Intermittent treatment with lithium does not seem to have the same detrimental effect on the course of unipolar depressive illness.

It is estimated that 15% of those with bipolar illness take their own life[17]. Mortality from physical illness is also increased. Chronic treatment with lithium reduces mortality from suicide to the same level as that seen in the general population[10,18,19]. Incidents of self-harm are also reduced and there is no convincing evidence that mortality from other causes is increased[20].

Bipolar disorder

Lithium is used in combination with antipsychotics in the treatment of schizo-affective illness[21], and is also used to treat aggressive[22] and self-mutilating behaviour and in steroid-induced psychosis[23]. The neuropharmacology of lithium[24] is not clearly understood but its therapeutic effect is thought to be related, among other things, to its ability to block neuronal calcium channels, and its effects on GABA pathways. The efficacy of lithium does not go unchallenged. For a review, see Moncrieff[25].

Plasma levels

Lithium is rapidly absorbed from the gastrointestinal tract, but has a long distribution phase. Blood should ideally be taken 12 hours after the last dose was administered. Pharmacokinetic data show that the level, for any given individual, is reproducible if blood is taken 10–14 hours post-dose (for once-daily dosing with modified-release preparations)[26]. On average, the plasma level can be expected to fall by 0.2 mmol/l between 12 and 24 hours post-dose[27].

Lithium should be started at a dose of 400 mg at night: lower in the elderly or in renal impairment. The serum level should be measured after 7 days, and then 1 week after each dose change until the desired level has been achieved. Once the serum level is stable, it should be checked 3 monthly: more often if problems are suspected or the patient is elderly or is co-prescribed interacting drugs. Full guidance on monitoring can be found on pages XX–XX. Plasma levels of 0.6–1.0 mmol/l are usually aimed for; 0.6–0.8 mmol/l initially, increased to 0.8–1.0 mmol/l if response is suboptimal[8]. A re-analysis of the original lithium clinical data concluded that the absolute level used for maintenance may be less important than the rapid reduction in serum lithium level that occurred in these trials when patients were switched from one treatment group to another[28]. Children and adolescents may require higher serum levels than adults to ensure that an adequate brain concentration is achieved[29].

Formulations of lithium

There is no significant difference in the pharmacokinetics of the two most widely prescribed brands of lithium in the UK: Priadel and Camcolit[2]. Not all preparations are bioequivalent, however, and care must be taken to make sure that the patient receives the same preparation each time a new prescription is supplied.

- Lithium carbonate 400 mg tablets each contain 10.8 mmol lithium.
- Lithium citrate liquid is available in two strengths and should be administered twice daily:
  - 5.4 mmol/5 ml equivalent to 200 mg lithium carbonate
  - 10.8 mmol/5 ml equivalent to 400 mg lithium carbonate.

Lack of clarity over which preparation is intended when prescribing can lead to the patient receiving a subtherapeutic or toxic dose.

Adverse effects

Side-effects tend to be directly related to plasma levels and their frequency increases dramatically at levels above 1 mmol/l. Mild gastrointestinal symptoms can occur when therapy is initiated and are usually transient. Fine hand tremor may occur, as may mild thirst and polyuria. Polyuria may occur more frequently with twice-daily dosing[30]. Propranolol can be useful in the treatment of lithium-induced tremor. Certain skin conditions such as psoriasis and acne can be aggravated by lithium therapy.

In the longer term, hypothyroidism may occur, although this should not be a reason for stopping lithium treatment: thyroxine replacement therapy is indicated. TFTs usually return to normal when lithium is discontinued. The risk of developing hypothyroidism is probably very much higher than is commonly believed, particularly in middle-aged women (prevalence up to 20%[31]). There is a strong case for testing for thyroid autoantibodies in this group before starting lithium (to better estimate risk) and for measuring TFTs more frequently in the first year of treatment[31]. Lithium treatment also increases the risk of hyperparathyroidism, and patients receiving long-term lithium should have their serum calcium level monitored[32].

Some patients complain that lithium 'curbs creativity' or produces 'mental dulling'. A study of artists and writers found that, for the majority, creativity actually increased with lithium treatment, because of thoughts and actions being more organised. A small minority reported diminished creativity (those who felt inspired by high mood)[33].

The long-term complication that has received the most attention is nephrotoxicity. A small reduction in glomerular filtration rate is seen in 20% of patients[26]. In the vast majority of patients this effect is benign[34]. A very small number of lithium-treated patients may develop interstitial nephritis. Lithium can also cause a reduction in urinary concentrating capacity (nephrogenic diabetes insipidus – hence occurrence of thirst and polyuria), which is reversible in the short-to-medium term but may be irreversible after long-term treatment (>15 years)[26,34].

Lithium toxicity

Toxic effects reliably occur at levels >1.5 mmol/l and usually consist of gastrointestinal effects (increasing anorexia, nausea and diarrhoea) and CNS effects (muscle weakness, drowsiness, ataxia, coarse tremor and muscle twitching). Above 2 mmol/l, increased disorientation and seizures are seen, which can progress to coma and death. In the presence of more severe symptoms, osmotic diuresis or forced alkaline diuresis should be initiated.[35] (*Note:* not thiazide or loop diuretics under any circumstances.) Above 3 mmol/l, peritoneal or haemodialysis is often used[35]. These plasma levels are only a guide and individuals can vary in their susceptibility to symptoms of toxicity.

Before prescribing lithium

Before prescribing lithium, renal, cardiac and thyroid function should be checked[26]. Women of childbearing age should be advised to use reliable contraception. Patients should be informed about symptoms of toxicity: why they might occur and what to do. Bouts of vomiting/diarrhoea or any form of dehydration will lead to sodium depletion and therefore to increased plasma lithium levels. Similarly, a salt-free diet is contraindicated. It is also wise to ensure that the patient is aware of the importance of maintaining an adequate fluid balance and of the need not to double today's dose because yesterday's was forgotten.

Basic information about lithium and how to minimise the risk of toxicity is contained in the *Patient Information Leaflet* found inside each box of lithium tablets.

Interactions with other drugs

Because of lithium's relatively narrow therapeutic index, interactions with other drugs can be very important. The most commonly encountered interactions are as follows.

Diuretics can increase serum lithium levels markedly by reducing its clearance. Thiazides are the worst culprits, while loop diuretics are somewhat safer. Initial thiazide diuresis is accompanied by the loss of sodium. This loss is compensated for within a few days by an increase in sodium reabsorption in the proximal tubule. As the kidney cannot distinguish between sodium and lithium at this site, it follows that there is also an increase in lithium reabsorption, leading to decreased renal clearance.

Non-steroidal anti-inflammatory drugs (NSAIDs) can increase serum lithium levels by up to 40%[36]. The mechanism of this interaction is not clearly understood, although it is thought to be related to the effects of NSAIDs on fluid balance, and is particularly important if PRN NSAIDs are added to a long-standing regular prescription of lithium. Lithium toxicity secondary to NSAID co-prescription has led to legal cases where substantial damages have been awarded against psychiatrists. One case in 1999 was settled for £600,000[37]. Some NSAIDs can be obtained without a prescription. Patients should be aware of the potential interaction. Lithium toxicity has also been reported with the COX 2 inhibitors rofecoxib (now withdrawn) and celecoxib[38]. There is one case report of lithium toxicity in a patient stabilised on lithium and ibuprofen when celecoxib was added[39]. Caution is required with all COX 2 inhibitors.

Haloperidol: Although, Cohen and Cohen[40] have reported severe neurotoxicity with this combination, if lithium levels are maintained in the therapeutic range (0.6–1.0 mmol/l) and the haloperidol dose is not increased rapidly above the recommended maximum, the chance of inducing a toxic state is very low.

Carbamazepine, in combination with lithium, has been reported to cause neurotoxic reactions. Again, higher (>1 mmol/l) plasma lithium levels were involved than are now thought acceptable, and most of the references state that a previous neurotoxic reaction to lithium alone is a risk factor; carbamazepine and lithium may be usefully co-prescribed[41].

SSRIs have been linked to an increased incidence of CNS toxicity when used with lithium. Although the mechanism of this interaction is not completely understood, it is likely to be mediated through serotonin pathways. It is prudent to be aware and to check lithium levels soon after starting treatment with an SSRI (although it must be noted that some reports claim neurotoxic reactions in the absence of raised lithium levels). Clinical experience has shown any interaction to be rare[42].

ACE inhibitors decrease the excretion of lithium. They can also precipitate renal failure, so extra care is needed in monitoring both serum creatinine and lithium, if these drugs are prescribed together. Care is also required with **angiotensin 2 antagonists**[43] (losartan, valsartan, candesartan, eprosartan, irbesartan and telmisartan).

Summary table – lithium

Indications	Mania, hypomania; prophyaxis in bipolar disorder and recurrent depression. Also effective in schizo-affective disorder and aggression
Pre-lithium work-up	ECG, thyroid function tests, renal function tests (serum creatinine and urea), U&Es
Monitoring	Start at 400 mg once daily (200 mg in the elderly). Plasma level after 7 days, then every 7 days until the required level is reached (0.6–1.0 mmol/l). Blood should be taken 12 hours after the last dose. Once stable, check level every 3 months. Check U&Es and TFTs every 6 months
Stopping	Slowly reduce over at least 1 month

References

1. Cookson J. Lithium: balancing risks and benefits. Br J Psychiatry 1997;171:120–4.
2. Ferrier IN et al. Lithium therapy. Adv Psychiatr Treat 1995;1:102–10.
3. National Institute for Clinical Excellence. Depression: management of depression in primary and secondary care – clinical guidance. http://www.nice.org.uk. 2004.
4. Valenstein M et al. What happened to lithium? Antidepressant augmentation in clinical settings. Am J Psychiatry 2006;163:1219–25.
5. Tondo L et al. Long-term clinical effectiveness of lithium maintenance treatment in types I and II bipolar disorders. Br J Psychiatry Suppl 2001;41:s184–s190.
6. Geddes JR et al. Long-term lithium therapy for bipolar disorder: systematic review and meta-analysis of randomized controlled trials. Am J Psychiatry 2004;161:217–22.
7. Muzina DJ et al. Maintenance therapies in bipolar disorder: focus on randomized controlled trials. Aust N Z J Psychiatry 2005;39:652–61.
8. National Institute for Clinical Excellence. Bipolar disorder. The management of bipolar disorder in adults, children and adolescents, in primary and secondary care. Clinical Guidance 38. http://www.nice.org.uk. 2006.
9. Faedda GL et al. Episode sequence in bipolar disorder and response to lithium treatment. Am J Psychiatry 1991;148:1237–9.
10. Tondo L et al. Lower suicide risk with long-term lithium treatment in major affective illness: a meta-analysis. Acta Psychiatr Scand 2001;104:163–72.
11. Mander AJ et al. Rapid recurrence of mania following abrupt discontinuation of lithium. Lancet 1988;2:15–17.
12. Suppes T et al. Risk of recurrence following discontinuation of lithium treatment in bipolar disorder. Arch Gen Psychiatry 1991;48:1082–8.
13. Cavanagh J et al. Relapse into mania or depression following lithium discontinuation: a 7-year follow-up. Acta Psychiatr Scand 2004;109:91–5.
14. Yazici O et al. Controlled lithium discontinuation in bipolar patients with good response to long-term lithium prophylaxis. J Affect Disord 2004;80:269–71.
15. Goodwin GM. Recurrence of mania after lithium withdrawal. Implications for the use of lithium in the treatment of bipolar affective disorder. Br J Psychiatry 1994;164:149–52.
16. Baldessarini RJ et al. Effects of the rate of discontinuing lithium maintenance treatment in bipolar disorders. J Clin Psychiatry 1996;57:441–8.
17. Harris EC et al. Excess mortality of mental disorder. Br J Psychiatry 1998;173:11–53.
18. Schou M. Forty years of lithium treatment. Arch Gen Psychiatry 1997;54:9–13.
19. Rucci P et al. Suicide attempts in patients with bipolar I disorder during acute and maintenance phases of intensive treatment with pharmacotherapy and adjunctive psychotherapy. Am J Psychiatry 2002;159:1160–4.
20. Cipriani A et al. Lithium in the prevention of suicidal behavior and all-cause mortality in patients with mood disorders: a systematic review of randomized trials. Am J Psychiatry 2005;162:1805–19.
21. Baethge C et al. Prophylaxis of schizoaffective disorder with lithium or carbamazepine: outcome after long-term follow-up. J Affect Disord 2004;79:43–50.
22. Tyrer SP. Lithium and treatment of aggressive behaviour. Eur Neuropsychopharmacol 1994;4:234–6.
23. Falk WE et al. Lithium prophylaxis of corticotropin-induced psychosis. JAMA 1979;241:1011–12.
24. Peet M et al. Lithium. Current status in psychiatric disorders. Drugs 1993;46:7–17.
25. Moncrieff J. Lithium: evidence reconsidered. Br J Psychiatry 1997;171:113–19.

Bipolar disorder

26. Anon. Using lithium safely. Drug Ther Bull 1999;37:22–4.
27. Anon. Priadel: Psychiatrist's Handbook. Canterbury, Kent, UK: Delandale Laboratories, 1986.
28. Perlis RH et al. Effect of abrupt change from standard to low serum levels of lithium: a reanalysis of double-blind lithium maintenance data. Am J Psychiatry 2002;159:1155–9.
29. Moore CM et al. Brain-to-serum lithium ratio and age: an in vivo magnetic resonance spectroscopy study. Am J Psychiatry 2002;159:1240–2.
30. Bowen RC et al. Less frequent lithium administration and lower urine volume. Am J Psychiatry 1991; 148:189–92.
31. Johnston AM et al. Lithium-associated clinical hypothyroidism. Prevalence and risk factors. Br J Psychiatry 1999;175:336–9.
32. Bendz H et al. Hyperparathyroidism and long-term lithium therapy – a cross-sectional study and the effect of lithium withdrawal. J Intern Med 1996;240:357–65.
33. Muller-Oerlinghausen B. Mental functioning. In: Johnson FN, ed. Depression and Mania: Modern Lithium Therapy, Oxford: IRL Press, 1987: 246–52.
34. Gitlin M. Lithium and the kidney: an updated review. Drug Saf 1999;20:231–43.
35. Tyrer SP. Lithium intoxication: appropriate treatment. CNS Drugs 1996;6:426–39.
36. Reimann IW et al. Indomethacin but not aspirin increases plasma lithium ion levels. Arch Gen Psychiatry 1983;40:283–6.
37. Nicholson J et al. Monitoring patients on lithium – a good practice guideline. Psychiatr Bull 2002;26: 348–51.
38. Phelan KM et al. Lithium interaction with the cyclooxygenase 2 inhibitors rofecoxib and celecoxib and other nonsteroidal anti-inflammatory drugs. J Clin Psychiatry 2003;64:1328–34.
39. Slordal L et al. A life-threatening interaction between lithium and celecoxib. Br J Clin Pharmacol 2003;55: 413–14.
40. Cohen WJ et al. Lithium carbonate, haloperidol, and irreversible brain damage. JAMA 1974;230: 1283–7.
41. Freeman MP et al. Mood stabilizer combinations: a review of safety and efficacy. Am J Psychiatry 1998;155:12–21.
42. Hawley CJ et al. Efficacy, safety and tolerability of combined administration of lithium and selective serotonin reuptake inhibitors: a review of the current evidence. Hertfordshire Neuroscience Research Group. Int Clin Psychopharmacol 2000;15:197–206.
43. Zwanzger P et al. Lithium intoxication after administration of AT_1 blockers. J Clin Psychiatry 2001; 62:208–9.

Further reading

Kleindienst N et al. Which clinical factors predict response to prophylactic lithium? A systematic review for bipolar disorders. Bipolar Disord 2005;7:404–17.
Wilting I et al. Drug–drug interactions as a determinant of elevated lithium serum levels in daily clinical practice. Bipolar Disord 2005;7:274–80.
Young AH. Treatment of bipolar affective disorder. BMJ 2000;321:1302–1303.

Carbamazepine

Carbamazepine is primarily used as an anticonvulsant in the treatment of grand mal and focal seizures. It is also used in the management of trigeminal neuralgia and, in the UK, is licensed for the prophylaxis of bipolar illness in patients who do not respond to lithium. Two recent placebo-controlled randomised studies have found the extended-release formulation of carbamazepine to be effective in the treatment of mania; in both studies, the response rate in the carbamazepine arm was twice that of the placebo arm[1,2]. Carbamazepine was not particularly well tolerated in these studies; the incidence of dizziness, somnolence and nausea was high. NICE does not recommend carbamazepine as a first-line treatment for mania[3].

Open studies also suggest that monotherapy has some efficacy in bipolar depression[4]: carbamazepine has a similar molecular structure to TCAs, but without possessing their ability to induce mania in bipolar depression; note that the evidence base supporting other strategies is stronger (see page XX). Carbamazepine may also usefully augment antidepressants or other mood stabilisers in refractory unipolar depression[5,6], although its enzyme-inducing properties complicate treatment. Carbamazepine is generally considered to be less effective than lithium in the prophylaxis of bipolar illness[7]; several published studies report a very low response rate and high drop-out rate[8,9]. A recent blinded, randomised trial of lithium versus carbamazepine found lithium to be the superior prophylactic agent[10]. Most of the lithium treatment failures occurred in the first 3 months of treatment, whereas relapses on carbamazepine occurred at a rate of 40% per year. Lithium is superior to carbamazepine in reducing suicidal behaviour[11]. NICE consider carbamazepine to be a third-line prophylactic agent[3].

It is 'perceived wisdom' that carbamazepine is more effective than lithium in rapid-cycling illness (four or more episodes/year). Although some evidence supports this view[12], negative studies have also been published[13].

There are also reports of carbamazepine being successful in treating aggressive behaviour in patients with schizophrenia[14]. This is apparently not a result of its anticonvulsant effect, as patients with normal EEGs may respond. A trial of carbamazepine is often thought worthwhile, as a last resort, in various psychiatric illnesses (such as panic disorder, borderline personality disorder and episodic dyscontrol syndrome) where no other drug is specifically indicated. The literature consists primarily of case reports and open case series. Carbamazepine is also used in the management of alcohol withdrawal symptoms[15], although the high doses required initially are often poorly tolerated.

Plasma levels

When carbamazepine is used as an anticonvulsant the therapeutic range is stated as being 4–12 mg/l, although the supporting evidence is not strong. A dose of at least 600 mg/day and a plasma level of at least 7 mg/l seem to be required in affective illness[16], although some studies do not support this view[17].

Carbamazepine serum levels vary significantly within a dosage interval. It is important to sample at a point in time where levels are likely to be reproducible for any given individual. The most appropriate way of monitoring is to take a trough level before the first dose of the day. Carbamazepine is an hepatic-enzyme inducer that induces its own metabolism as well as that of other drugs. An initial plasma half-life of around 30 hours is reduced to around 12 hours on chronic dosing. For this reason, plasma levels should be checked 2–4 weeks after an increase in dose to ensure that the desired level is still being obtained.

The published clinical trials that demonstrate the efficacy of carbamazepine as a mood stabiliser used doses that are significantly higher (usually in the order of 800–1200 mg/day) than those prescribed in everyday UK clinical practice[18].

Adverse effects

The main problems encountered with carbamazepine therapy are dizziness, drowsiness, ataxia and nausea. They can be largely avoided by starting with a low dose and increasing it slowly. Around 3% of patients treated with carba-mazepine develop a generalised erythematous rash. Serious dermatological reactions can rarely occur (e.g. toxic epidermal necrolysis). Hyponatraemia can also be a problem. Carbamazepine is a known human teratogen (see page XX).

Carbamazepine can induce a chronic low white blood cell (WBC) count. Many patients treated with carbamazepine have a WBC count at the lower end of the normal range, which rises on discontinuing treatment. One patient in 20,000 develops agranulocytosis and/or aplastic anaemia[19]. Raised ALP and GGT are, potentially, a sign of a hypersensitivity reaction to carbamazepine (a GGT of up to twice normal is common and should not cause concern). Normally, it would be recommended that therapy should be withdrawn, as this can progress to a multi-system hypersensitivity reaction (mainly manifesting itself as various skin reactions and a low WBC count, along with raised ALP and GGT), which can in turn lead to hepatitis. Fatalities have been reported. There is no clear timescale for these events, so it must not be assumed that raised LFTs for 6 months with no other clinical complications will not produce problems in the future. FBC and LFTs should be monitored in patients on long-term therapy.

Interactions with other drugs[20–22]

Carbamazepine is a potent inducer of hepatic cytochrome P450 enzymes and is metabolised by CYP3A4. Plasma levels of most **antidepressants**, most **antipsychotics**, **benzodiazepines**, some **cholinesterase inhibitors**, **methadone**, **thyroxine**, **theophylline**, **oestrogens**[23] and other steroids may be reduced by carbamazepine, resulting in treatment failure. Drugs that inhibit CYP3A4 will increase carbamazepine plasma levels and may precipitate toxicity. Examples include cimetidine, diltiazem, verapamil, erythromycin and SSRIs.

Pharmacodynamic interactions also occur. The anticonvulsant activity of carbamazepine is reduced by drugs that lower the seizure threshold (e.g. antipsychotics and antidepressants), the potential for carbamazepine to cause neutropenia may be increased by other drugs that have the potential to depress the bone marrow (e.g. clozapine), and the risk of hyponatraemia may be increased by other drugs that can deplete sodium (e.g. diuretics). Neurotoxicity has been reported with lithium and carbamazepine combinations[24]. This is rare. There are many complex interactions with other anticonvulsant drugs.

The latest edition of the *BNF* should be checked before prescribing anticonvulsant polypharmacy (see also page 159).

As carbamazepine is structurally similar to the TCAs, in theory it should not be given within 14 days of discontinuing a MAOI. Most side-effects of carbamazepine are dose-related (peak plasma level-related), and increase in frequency and severity when the plasma level is >12 mg/l (this varies substantially from patient to patient). Side-effects can be minimised by using the slow-release preparation.

References

1. Weisler RH et al. A multicenter, randomized, double-blind, placebo-controlled trial of extended-release carbamazepine capsules as monotherapy for bipolar disorder patients with manic or mixed episodes. J Clin Psychiatry 2004;65:478–84.
2. Weisler RH et al. Extended-release carbamazepine capsules as monotherapy for acute mania in bipolar disorder: a multicenter, randomized, double-blind, placebo-controlled trial. J Clin Psychiatry 2005; 66:323–30.
3. National Institute for Clinical Excellence. Bipolar disorder. The management of bipolar disorder in adults, children and adolescents, in primary and secondary care. Clinical Guidance 38. http://www.nice.org.uk. 2006.
4. Dilsaver SC et al. Treatment of bipolar depression with carbamazepine: results of an open study. Biol Psychiatry 1996;40:935–7.
5. Cullen M et al. Carbamazepine for treatment-resistant melancholia. J Clin Psychiatry 1991;52:472–6.
6. Kramlinger KG et al. The addition of lithium to carbamazepine. Antidepressant efficacy in treatment-resistant depression. Arch Gen Psychiatry 1989;46:794–800.
7. Muzina DJ et al. Maintenance therapies in bipolar disorder: focus on randomized controlled trials. Aust N Z J Psychiatry 2005;39:652–61.
8. Keck PE Jr et al. Anticonvulsants and antipsychotics in the treatment of bipolar disorder. J Clin Psychiatry 1998;59(Suppl 6):74–81.
9. Post RM et al. Carbamazepine prophylaxis in refractory affective disorders: a focus on long-term follow-up. J Clin Psychopharmacol 1990;10:318–27.
10. Hartong EG et al. Prophylactic efficacy of lithium versus carbamazepine in treatment-naive bipolar patients. J Clin Psychiatry 2003;64:144–51.
11. Kleindienst N et al. Differential efficacy of lithium and carbamazepine in the prophylaxis of bipolar disorder: results of the MAP study. Neuropsychobiology 2000;42(Suppl 1):2–10.
12. Joyce PR. Carbamazepine in rapid cycling bipolar affective disorder. Int Clin Psychopharmacol 1988;3: 123–9.
13. Okuma T. Effects of carbamazepine and lithium on affective disorders. Neuropsychobiology 1993;27: 138–45.
14. Brieden T et al. Psychopharmacological treatment of aggression in schizophrenic patients. Pharmacopsychiatry 2002;35:83–9.
15. Malcolm R et al. The effects of carbamazepine and lorazepam on single versus multiple previous alcohol withdrawals in an outpatient randomized trial. J Gen Intern Med 2002;17:349–55.
16. Taylor D et al. Doses of carbamazepine and valproate in bipolar affective disorder. Psychiatr Bull 1997;21:221–3.
17. Simhandl C et al. The comparative efficacy of carbamazepine low and high serum level and lithium carbonate in the prophylaxis of affective disorders. J Affect Disord 1993;28:221–31.
18. Taylor DM et al. Prescribing and monitoring of carbamazepine and valproate – a case note review. Psychiatr Bull 2000;24:174–7.
19. Kaufman DW et al. Drugs in the aetiology of agranulocytosis and aplastic anaemia. Eur J Haematol Suppl 1996;60:23–30.
20. Spina E et al. Clinical significance of pharmacokinetic interactions between antiepileptic and psychotropic drugs. Epilepsia 2002;43(Suppl 2):37–44.
21. Patsalos PN et al. The importance of drug interactions in epilepsy therapy. Epilepsia 2002;43:365–85.
22. Ketter TA et al. Principles of clinically important drug interactions with carbamazepine. Part I. J Clin Psychopharmacol 1991;11:198–203.
23. Crawford P. Interactions between antiepileptic drugs and hormonal contraception. CNS Drugs 2002;16: 263–72.
24. Shukla S et al. Lithium-carbamazepine neurotoxicity and risk factors. Am J Psychiatry 1984; 141: 1604–6.

Table Physical monitoring for people with bipolar disorder (Based on NICE Guidelines[1])

Test or measurement	Monitoring for all patients		Additional monitoring for specific drugs			
	Initial health check	Annual check up	Antipsychotics	Lithium	Valproate	Carbamazepine
Thyroid function	Yes	Yes		At start and every 6 months; more often if evidence of deterioration		
Liver function	Yes	Yes			At start and at 6 months	At start and at 6 months
Renal function	Yes	Yes		At start and every 6 months; more often if there is evidence of deterioration or the patient starts taking interacting drugs		Urea and electrolytes every 6 months
Full blood count	Yes	Yes		Only if clinically indicated	At start and 6 months	At start and at 6 months
Blood (plasma) glucose	Yes	Yes	At start and then every 4–6 months (and at 1 month if taking olanzapine); more often if evidence of elevated levels			

Lipid profile	Yes	Over 40s only	At start and at 3 months; more often initially if evidence of elevated levels		
Blood pressure	Yes	Yes			
Prolactin	Children and adolescents only		At start and if symptoms of raised prolactin develop. Raised prolactin unlikely with olanzapine, quetiapine, aripiprazole (see page 95)		
ECG	If indicated by history or clinical picture		At start if there are risk factors for or existing cardiovascular disease (or haloperidol is prescribed)	At start if risk factors for or existing cardiovascular disease	
Weight and height	Yes	Yes	At start, then frequently for 3 months, then 3 monthly for first year	At start and when needed if the patient gains weight rapidly	At start and at 3 and 6 months	At start and at 6 months
Plasma levels of drug			One week after initiation and 1 week after every dose; change until levels stable, then every 3 months	Titrate by effect and tolerability. Use plasma levels to assure adequate dosing and/or compliance	Two weeks after initiation and 2 weeks after dose change. Then every 6 months

For patients on **lamotrigine**, do an annual health check, but no special monitoring tests are needed.

Reference

1. National Institute for Clinical Excellence. Bipolar disorder. The management of bipolar disorder in adults, children and adolescents, in primary and secondary care. Clinical Guidance 38. http://www.nice.org.uk. 2006.

Treatment of acute mania or hypomania

Drug treatment is the mainstay of therapy for mania and hypomania. Both antipsychotics and so-called mood stabilisers are effective. Sedative and anxiolytic drugs (e.g. benzodiazepines) may add to the effects of these drugs. Drug choice is made difficult by the dearth of useful comparative data – no one drug can be recommended over another on efficacy grounds. The value of antipsychotic–mood stabiliser combinations is established for those relapsing while on mood stabilisers but unclear for those presenting on no treatment[1-5].

Treatment strategy

The diagram below outlines a treatment strategy for mania and hypomania. These recommendations are based on UK NICE guidelines[6], BAP guidelines[2], APA guidelines[3], UK NICE guidance on olanzapine and valproate[4], and individual references cited.

Treatment of acute mania or hypomania[1-16]

Stop antidepressant treatment

Is the patient taking antimanic medication?

No

Consider:
An antipsychotic (if symptoms severe or behaviour disturbed)

Or

Valproate (avoid in women of childbearing potential)

Or

Lithium (if future adherence likely)

If response is inadequate
Combine antipsychotic and valproate or lithium

Consider adding short-term benzodiazepine[17-19]
(lorazepam or clonazepam)

Yes

If taking an antipsychotic
Check compliance and dose
Increase if necessary
Consider adding lithium or valproate

If taking lithium
Check plasma levels
Increase dose to give levels
1.0–1.2 mmol/l
Consider adding antipsychotic

If taking valproate
Check plasma levels[2,3,20,21]
Increase dose to give levels
up to 125 mg/l if tolerated
Consider adding antipsychotic

If taking lithium or valproate and mania is severe
Check level
Add an antipsychotic[1]

If taking carbamazepine
Consider adding antipsychotic
(higher doses may be needed)

All patients – consider adding short-term benzodiazepine[17-19]
(lorazepam or clonazepam)

Note that lithium may be less effective in mixed states[22] or substance misuse[23].

Suggested doses – mania

Drug	Dose
Lithium	400 mg/day, increasing every 5–7 days according to plasma levels
Valproate	As semisodium – 250 mg three times daily, increasing according to tolerability and plasma levels
	As sodium valproate slow release – 500 mg/day, increasing as above
	Higher, so-called loading doses, have been used, both oral[24–26] and intravenous[27] Dose is 20–30 mg/kg/day
Olanzapine	10 mg/day, increasing to 15 mg or 20 mg as required
Risperidone	2 mg or 3 mg/day, increased to 6 mg/day as required
Quetiapine	100 mg/day, increasing to 800 mg as required. Higher starting doses have been used[28]
Haloperidol	5–10 mg, increasing to 15 mg if required
Lorazepam[18,19]	Up to 4 mg/day (some centres use higher doses)
Clonzapam[17,19]	Up to 8 mg/day

Other treatments – mania

Treatment	Comments
Aripiprazole[29-31] 15–30 mg/day	Strong support for antimanic effect from several placebo-controlled trials. May be considered as first-line treatment
Clozapine[32,33]	Established treatment option for refractory mania
Donepezil[34] (5–10 mg)	Probably not effective
Gabapentin[35-37] (up to 2.4 g/day)	Probably only effective by virtue of an anxiolytic effect. Rarely used. May be useful as prophylaxis[38]
Lamotrigine[39,40] (up to 200 mg/day)	Possibly effective but better efficacy in bipolar depression
Levetiracetam[41,42] (up to 4000 mg/day)	Possibly effective but controlled studies required
Oxcarbazepine[43-46] (around 300–3000 mg/day)	Possibly effective. One controlled study conducted (in youths) was negative[47]
Phenytoin[48] (300–400 mg/day)	Rarely used. Limited data
Ritanserin[49] (10 mg/day)	Supported by a single randomised, controlled trial. Well tolerated. May protect against EPSEs
Topiramate[50-53] (up to 300 mg/day)	Possibly effective, even in refractory mania. Causes weight loss
Ziprasidone[54]	Supported by a randomised, placebo-controlled study

Alphabetical order – no preference implied by order in the table.
Consult specialist and primary literature before using any treatment listed.

References

1. Smith LA et al. Acute bipolar mania: a systematic review and meta-analysis of co-therapy vs. monotherapy. Acta Psychiatr Scand 2007;115:12–20.
2. Goodwin GM et al. The British Association for Psychopharmacology guidelines for treatment of bipolar disorder: a summary. J Psychopharmacol 2003;17:3–6.
3. American Psychiatric Association. Practice guideline for the treatment of patients with bipolar disorder. Am J Psychiatry 2002;159:1–50.
4. National Institute for Clinical Excellence. The clinical effectiveness and cost effectiveness of new drugs for bipolar disorder. Technical Appraisal 66. http://www.nice.org.uk. 2003.
5. Sachs GS. Decision tree for the treatment of bipolar disorder. J Clin Psychiatry 2003;64(Suppl 8):35–40.
6. National Institute for Clinical Excellence. Bipolar disorder. The management of bipolar disorder in adults, children and adolescents, in primary and secondary care. Clinical Guidance 38. http:// www.nice.org.uk. 2006.
7. Tohen M et al. A 12-week, double-blind comparison of olanzapine vs haloperidol in the treatment of acute mania. Arch Gen Psychiatry 2003;60:1218–26.
8. Baldessarini RJ et al. Olanzapine versus placebo in acute mania treatment responses in subgroups. J Clin Psychopharmacol 2003;23:370–6.
9. Applebaum J et al. Intravenous fosphenytoin in acute mania. J Clin Psychiatry 2003;64:408–9.
10. Sachs G et al. Quetiapine with lithium or divalproex for the treatment of bipolar mania: a randomized, double-blind, placebo-controlled study. Bipolar Disord 2004;6:213–23.
11. Yatham LN et al. Quetiapine versus placebo in combination with lithium or divalproex for the treatment of bipolar mania. J Clin Psychopharmacol 2004;24:599–606.
12. Yatham LN et al. Risperidone plus lithium versus risperidone plus valproate in acute and continuation treatment of mania. Int Clin Psychopharmacol 2004;19:103–9.
13. Bowden CL et al. Risperidone in combination with mood stabilizers: a 10-week continuation phase study in bipolar I disorder. J Clin Psychiatry 2004;65:707–14.
14. Hirschfeld RM et al. Rapid antimanic effect of risperidone monotherapy: a 3-week multicenter, double-blind, placebo-controlled trial. Am J Psychiatry 2004;161:1057–65.
15. Bowden CL et al. A randomized, double-blind, placebo-controlled efficacy and safety study of quetiapine or lithium as monotherapy for mania in bipolar disorder. J Clin Psychiatry 2005;66:111–21.
16. Khanna S et al. Risperidone in the treatment of acute mania: double-blind, placebo-controlled study. Br J Psychiatry 2005;187:229–34.
17. Sachs GS et al. Adjunctive clonazepam for maintenance treatment of bipolar affective disorder. J Clin Psychopharmacol 1990;10:42–7.
18. Modell JG et al. Inpatient clinical trial of lorazepam for the management of manic agitation. J Clin Psychopharmacol 1985;5:109–13.
19. Curtin F et al. Clonazepam and lorazepam in acute mania: a Bayesian meta-analysis. J Affect Disord 2004;78:201–8.
20. Taylor D et al. Doses of carbamazepine and valproate in bipolar affective disorder. Psychiatr Bull 1997; 21:221–3.
21. Allen MH et al. Linear relationship of valproate serum concentration to response and optimal serum levels for acute mania. Am J Psychiatry 2006;163:272–5.
22. Swann AC et al. Lithium treatment of mania: clinical characteristics, specificity of symptom change, and outcome. Psychiatry Res 1986;18:127–41.
23. Goldberg JF et al. A history of substance abuse complicates remission from acute mania in bipolar disorder. J Clin Psychiatry 1999;60:733–40.
24. McElroy SL et al. A randomized comparison of divalproex oral loading versus haloperidol in the initial treatment of acute psychotic mania. J Clin Psychiatry 1996;57:142–6.
25. Hirschfeld RM et al. Safety and tolerability of oral loading divalproex sodium in acutely manic bipolar patients. J Clin Psychiatry 1999;60:815–18.
26. Hirschfeld RM et al. The safety and early efficacy of oral-loaded divalproex versus standard-titration divalproex, lithium, olanzapine, and placebo in the treatment of acute mania associated with bipolar disorder. J Clin Psychiatry 2003;64:841–6.
27. Jagadheesan K et al. Acute antimanic efficacy and safety of intravenous valproate loading therapy: an open-label study. Neuropsychobiology 2003;47:90–3.
28. Pajonk FG et al. Rapid dose titration of quetiapine for the treatment of acute schizophrenia and acute mania: a case series. J Psychopharmacol 2006;20:119–24.
29. Lyseng-Williamson KA et al. Aripiprazole: in acute mania associated with bipolar I disorder. CNS Drugs 2004;18:367–76.
30. Keck PE Jr et al. A placebo-controlled, double-blind study of the efficacy and safety of aripiprazole in patients with acute bipolar mania. Am J Psychiatry 2003;160:1651–8.
31. Sachs G et al. Aripiprazole in the treatment of acute manic or mixed episodes in patients with bipolar I disorder: a 3-week placebo-controlled study. J Psychopharmacol 2006;20:536–46.
32. Mahmood T et al. Clozapine in the management of bipolar and schizoaffective manic episodes resistant to standard treatment. Aust N Z J Psychiatry 1997;31:424–6.
33. Green AI et al. Clozapine in the treatment of refractory psychotic mania. Am J Psychiatry 2000; 157:982–6.

34. Eden EA et al. A double-blind, placebo-controlled trial of adjunctive donepezil in treatment-resistant mania. Bipolar Disord 2006;8:75–80.
35. Macdonald KJ et al. Newer antiepileptic drugs in bipolar disorder: rationale for use and role in therapy. CNS Drugs 2002;16:549–62.
36. Cabras PL et al. Clinical experience with gabapentin in patients with bipolar or schizoaffective disorder: results of an open-label study. J Clin Psychiatry 1999;60:245–8.
37. Pande AC et al. Gabapentin in bipolar disorder: a placebo-controlled trial of adjunctive therapy. Gabapentin Bipolar Disorder Study Group. Bipolar Disord 2000;2(3 Pt 2):249–55.
38. Vieta E et al. A double-blind, randomized, placebo-controlled, prophylaxis study of adjunctive gabapentin for bipolar disorder. J Clin Psychiatry 2006;67:473–7.
39. Calabrese JR et al. Spectrum of activity of lamotrigine in treatment-refractory bipolar disorder. Am J Psychiatry 1999;156:1019–23.
40. Bowden CL et al. A placebo-controlled 18-month trial of lamotrigine and lithium maintenance treatment in recently manic or hypomanic patients with bipolar I disorder. Arch Gen Psychiatry 2003;60:392–400.
41. Grunze H et al. Levetiracetam in the treatment of acute mania: an open add-on study with an on-off-on design. J Clin Psychiatry 2003;64:781–4.
42. Goldberg JF et al. Levetiracetam for acute mania (Letter). Am J Psychiatry 2002;159:148.
43. Benedetti A et al. Oxcarbazepine as add-on treatment in patients with bipolar manic, mixed or depressive episode. J Affect Disord 2004;79:273–7.
44. Lande RG. Oxcarbazepine: efficacy, safety, and tolerability in the treatment of mania. Int J Psychiatry Clin Pract 2004;8:37–40.
45. Ghaemi SN et al. Oxcarbazepine treatment of bipolar disorder. J Clin Psychiatry 2003;64:943–5.
46. Pratoomsri W et al. Oxcarbazepine in the treatment of bipolar disorder: a review. Can J Psychiatry 2006;51:540–5.
47. Wagner KD et al. A double-blind, randomized, placebo-controlled trial of oxcarbazepine in the treatment of bipolar disorder in children and adolescents. Am J Psychiatry 2006;163:1179–86.
48. Mishory A et al. Phenytoin as an antimanic anticonvulsant: a controlled study. Am J Psychiatry 2000;157:463–5.
49. Akhondzadeh S et al. Ritanserin as an adjunct to lithium and haloperidol for the treatment of medication-naive patients with acute mania: a double blind and placebo controlled trial. BMC Psychiatry 2003;3:7.
50. Grunze HC et al. Antimanic efficacy of topiramate in 11 patients in an open trial with an on-off-on design. J Clin Psychiatry 2001;62:464–8.
51. Yatham LN et al. Third generation anticonvulsants in bipolar disorder: a review of efficacy and summary of clinical recommendations. J Clin Psychiatry 2002;63:275–83.
52. Vieta E et al. 1-year follow-up of patients treated with risperidone and topiramate for a manic episode. J Clin Psychiatry 2003;64:834–9.
53. Vieta E et al. Use of topiramate in treatment-resistant bipolar spectrum disorders. J Clin Psychopharmacol 2002;22:431–5.
54. Keck PE Jr et al. Ziprasidone in the treatment of acute bipolar mania: a three-week, placebo-controlled, double-blind, randomized trial. Am J Psychiatry 2003;160:741–8.

Bipolar disorder

Table Drugs for acute mania – relative costs (January 2007)

Drug	Costs for 30 days' treatment	Comments
Lithium (Priadel) 800 mg/day	£2.95	Add cost of plasma level monitoring
Carbamazepine (Tegretol Retard) 800 mg/day	£11.08	Self-induction complicates acute treatment
Sodium valproate (Epilim Chrono) 1500 mg/day	£18.19	Not licensed for mania, but may be given once daily
Valproate semisodium (Depakote) 1500 mg/day	£24.29	Licensed for mania, but given two or three times daily
Haloperidol (Serenace) 10 mg/day	£8.81	Most widely used FGA
Olanzapine (Zyprexa) 15 mg/day	£127.69	Most widely used SGA
Quetiapine (Seroquel) 600 mg/day	£170.00	
Risperidone (Risperdal) 4 mg/day	£66.67	Non-sedative but effective

Antipsychotics in bipolar disorder

First-generation antipsychotics have long been used in mania and several studies support their use in a variety of hypomanic and manic presentations[1-3]. Their effectiveness seems to be enhanced by the addition of a mood stabiliser[4,5]. In the longer-term treatment of bipolar disorder, typicals are widely used (presumably as prophylaxis)[6] but robust supporting data are absent[7]. The observation that typical antipsychotics can induce depression and tardive dyskinesia in bipolar patients militates against their long-term use[7-9].

Among atypical antipsychotics, olanzapine, risperidone and quetiapine have been most robustly evaluated and are licensed in the UK for the treatment of mania. Olanzapine is probably most widely used. It is more effective than placebo in mania[10,11], and at least as effective as valproate semisodium[12] and lithium[13]. As with typical drugs, olanzapine may be most effective when used in combination with a mood stabiliser[14,15]. Data suggest olanzapine may offer benefits in longer-term treatment[16,17]; it may be more effective than lithium[18], and it is formally licensed as prophylaxis.

Clozapine seems to be effective in refractory bipolar conditions, including refractory mania[19-22]. Risperidone has shown efficacy in mania[23], particularly in combination with a mood stabiliser[2,24]. Data relating to quetiapine[25-27] are compelling but those relating to amisulpride[28] and zotepine[29] are scarce. Aripiprazole is effective in mania[30], perhaps to a greater extent than haloperidol[31,32]. It is licensed for mania in a number of countries.

References

1. Prien RF et al. Comparison of lithium carbonate and chlorpromazine in the treatment of mania. Report of the Veterans Administration and National Institute of Mental Health Collaborative Study Group. Arch Gen Psychiatry 1972;26:146–53.
2. Sachs GS et al. Combination of a mood stabilizer with risperidone or haloperidol for treatment of acute mania: a double-blind, placebo-controlled comparison of efficacy and safety. Am J Psychiatry 2002; 159:1146–54.
3. McElroy SL et al. A randomized comparison of divalproex oral loading versus haloperidol in the initial treatment of acute psychotic mania. J Clin Psychiatry 1996;57:142–6.
4. Chou JC et al. Acute mania: haloperidol dose and augmentation with lithium or lorazepam. J Clin Psychopharmacol 1999;19:500–5.
5. Small JG et al. A placebo-controlled study of lithium combined with neuroleptics in chronic schizophrenic patients. Am J Psychiatry 1975;132:1315–17.
6. Soares JC et al. Adjunctive antipsychotic use in bipolar patients: an open 6-month prospective study following an acute episode. J Affect Disord 1999;56:1–8.
7. Keck PE Jr et al. Anticonvulsants and antipsychotics in the treatment of bipolar disorder. J Clin Psychiatry 1998;59(Suppl 6):74–81.
8. Tohen M et al. Antipsychotic agents and bipolar disorder. J Clin Psychiatry 1998;59(Suppl 1):38–48.
9. Zarate CA Jr et al. Double-blind comparison of the continued use of antipsychotic treatment versus its discontinuation in remitted manic patients. Am J Psychiatry 2004;161:169–71.
10. Tohen M et al. Olanzapine versus placebo in the treatment of acute mania. Olanzapine HGEH Study Group. Am J Psychiatry 1999;156:702–9.
11. Tohen M et al. Efficacy of olanzapine in acute bipolar mania: a double-blind, placebo-controlled study. The Olanzapine HGGW Study Group. Arch Gen Psychiatry 2000;57:841–9.
12. Tohen M et al. Olanzapine versus divalproex in the treatment of acute mania. Am J Psychiatry 2002;159:1011–17.
13. Berk M et al. Olanzapine compared to lithium in mania: a double-blind randomized controlled trial. Int Clin Psychopharmacol 1999;14:339–43.
14. Tohen M et al. Efficacy of olanzapine in combination with valproate or lithium in the treatment of mania in patients partially nonresponsive to valproate or lithium monotherapy. Arch Gen Psychiatry 2002;59:62–9.
15. Tohen M et al. Relapse prevention in bipolar I disorder: 18-month comparison of olanzapine plus mood stabiliser v. mood stabiliser alone. Br J Psychiatry 2004;184:337–45.
16. Sanger TM et al. Long-term olanzapine therapy in the treatment of bipolar I disorder: an open-label continuation phase study. J Clin Psychiatry 2001;62:273–81.
17. Vieta E et al. Olanzapine as long-term adjunctive therapy in treatment-resistant bipolar disorder. J Clin Psychopharmacol 2001;21:469–73.
18. Tohen M et al. Olanzapine versus lithium in the maintenance treatment of bipolar disorder: a 12-month, randomized, double-blind, controlled clinical trial. Am J Psychiatry 2005;162:1281–90.
19. Calabrese JR et al. Clozapine for treatment-refractory mania. Am J Psychiatry 1996;153:759–64.
20. Green AI et al. Clozapine in the treatment of refractory psychotic mania. Am J Psychiatry 2000; 157:982–6.
21. Kimmel SE et al. Clozapine in treatment-refractory mood disorders. J Clin Psychiatry 1994;55(Suppl B): 91–3.
22. Chang JS et al. The effects of long-term clozapine add-on therapy on the rehospitalization rate and the mood polarity patterns in bipolar disorders. J Clin Psychiatry 2006;67:461–7.
23. Segal J et al. Risperidone compared with both lithium and haloperidol in mania: a double-blind randomized controlled trial. Clin Neuropharmacol 1998;21:176–80.
24. Vieta E et al. Risperidone in the treatment of mania: efficacy and safety results from a large, multicentre, open study in Spain. J Affect Disord 2002;72:15–19.
25. Ghaemi SN et al. The use of quetiapine for treatment-resistant bipolar disorder: a case series. Ann Clin Psychiatry 1999;11:137–40.
26. Sachs G et al. Quetiapine with lithium or divalproex for the treatment of bipolar mania: a randomized, double-blind, placebo-controlled study. Bipolar Disord 2004;6:213–23.
27. Altamura AC et al. Efficacy and tolerability of quetiapine in the treatment of bipolar disorder: preliminary evidence from a 12-month open label study. J Affect Disord 2003;76:267–71.
28. Pariante CM et al. [Multiple sclerosis and major depression resistant to treatment. Case of a patient with antidepressive therapy-induced mood disorder, associated with manic features]. Clin Ter 1995;146: 449–52.
29. Amann B et al. Zotepine loading in acute and severely manic patients: a pilot study. Bipolar Disord 2005;7:471–6.
30. Sachs G et al. Aripiprazole in the treatment of acute manic or mixed episodes in patients with bipolar I disorder: a 3-week placebo-controlled study. J Psychopharmacol 2006;20:536–46.
31. Vieta E et al. Effectiveness of aripiprazole v. haloperidol in acute bipolar mania: double-blind, randomised, comparative 12-week trial. Br J Psychiatry 2005;187:235–42.
32. Cipriani A et al. Haloperidol alone or in combination for acute mania. Cochrane Database Syst Rev 2006;3:CD004362.

Bipolar depression

Bipolar depression is a common and debilitating disorder which differs from unipolar disorder in severity, timecourse, recurrence and response to drug treatment. Episodes of bipolar depression are, compared with unipolar depression, more rapid in onset, more frequent, more severe, shorter and more likely to involve reverse neurovegetative symptoms such as hyperphagia and hypersomnia[1,2]. Around 15% of people with bipolar disorder commit suicide[3], a statistic which aptly reflects the severity and frequency of depressive episodes. Bipolar depression entails greater socioeconomic burden than both mania and unipolar depression[4].

The drug treatment of bipolar depression is somewhat controversial for two reasons. First, there is a dearth of well-conducted, randomised, controlled trials reported in the literature and secondly, the condition entails consideration of lifelong outcome rather than discrete episode response[5]. We have some knowledge of the therapeutic effects of drugs in depressive episodes but more limited awareness of the therapeutic or deleterious effects of drugs in the longer term. In the UK, NICE recommends the initial use of an SSRI (in addition to an antimanic drug) or quetiapine (assuming an antipsychotic is not already prescribed)[6]. Second-line treatment is to switch to mirtazapine or venlafaxine or to add quetiapine, olanzapine or lithium to the antidepressant. The tables below give some broad guidance on treatment options in bipolar depression.

Table Established treatments

Drug/regimen	Comments
Lithium[1,7–10]	Lithium is probably effective in treating bipolar depression but supporting data are confounded by cross-over designs incorporating abrupt switching to placebo. There is some evidence that lithium prevents depressive relapse but its effects on manic relapse are considered more robust. Fairly strong support for lithium in reducing suicidality in bipolar disorder[11,12]
Lithium and antidepressant[13–20]	Antidepressants are widely used in bipolar depression, particularly for breakthrough episodes occurring in those on mood stabilisers. They appear to be effective, although there is a risk of cycle acceleration and/or switching. Tricyclics and MAOIs are usually avoided. SSRIs are generally recommended. Venlafaxine and bupropion (amfebutamone) have also been used. Venlafaxine may be more likely to induce a switch to mania[21,22]. There is limited evidence that antidepressants are effective only when lithium plasma levels are below 0.8 mmol/l
	Continuing antidepressant treatment after resolution of symptoms may protect against depressive relapse, although this is controversial
Lamotrigine[1,8,23–28]	Lamotrigine appears to be effective both as a treatment for bipolar depression and as prophylaxis against further episodes. It does not induce switching or rapid cycling. It is as effective as citalopram and causes less weight gain than lithium
	Treatment is complicated by the risk of rash, which is associated with speed of dose titration. The necessity for titration may limit clinical utility
	A further complication is the question of dose: 50 mg/day has efficacy, but 200 mg/day is probably better. In the USA doses of up to 1200 mg/day have been used (mean around 250 mg/day)
Olanzapine and fluoxetine[8,14,29–31]	This combination ('zyp-zac') is more effective than both placebo and olanzapine alone in treating bipolar depression. The dose is 6 and 25 mg or 12 and 50 mg/day (so presumably 5/20 mg and 10/40 mg are effective). May be more effective than lamotrigine. Reasonable evidence of prophylactic effect
Quetiapine[14,32–35]	Two large RCTs have demonstrated clear efficacy for doses of 300 mg and 600 mg daily (as monotherapy) in bipolar I and bipolar II depression. An anxiolytic effect has also been shown
	As expected, quetiapine appears not to be associated with switching to mania; longer-term data are limited

Table Bipolar depression–alternative treatments – refer to primary literature before using

Drug/regimen	Comments
Pramipexole[36,37]	Pramipexole is a dopamine agonist which is widely used in Parkinson's disease. Two small placebo-controlled trials suggest useful efficacy in bipolar depression. Effective dose averages around 1.7 mg/day. Both studies used pramipexole as an adjunct to existing mood stabiliser treatment. Neither study detected an increased risk of switching to mania/hypomania (a theoretical consideration) but data are insufficient to exclude this possibility. Probably best reserved for specialist centres
Valproate[1,8,38–40]	Limited evidence of efficacy as monotherapy but recommended in some guidelines. Probably protects against depressive relapse but database is small
Carbamazepine[1,8,39,41]	Occasionally recommended but database is poor and effect modest. May have useful activity when added to other mood stabilisers
Antidepressants[42–50]	'Unopposed' antidepressants (i.e. without mood stabiliser protection) are generally avoided in bipolar depression because of the risk of switching. There is also evidence that they are relatively less effective in bipolar depression than in unipolar depression. Nonetheless, short-term use of fluoxetine, venlafaxine and moclobemide seems reasonably effective and safe even as monotherapy. Overall, however, unopposed antidepressant treatment should probably be avoided, especially in bipolar I disorder

Table Other possible treatments – seek specialist advice before using

Drug/regimen	Comments
Aripiprazole[51]	Limited support from an open study
Gabapentin[1,52,53]	Open studies suggest modest effect when added to mood stabilisers or antipsychotics. Doses average around 1750 mg/day. Anxiolytic effect may account for apparent effect in bipolar depression
Inositol[54]	Small, randomised, pilot study suggests that 12 g/day inositol is effective in bipolar depression
Riluzole[55]	Riluzole shares some pharmacological characteristics with lamotrigine. Database is limited to a single case report supporting use in bipolar depression
Thyroxine[56]	Limited evidence of efficacy as augmentation. Doses average around 300 μg/day
Mifepristone[57]	Some evidence of mood-elevating properties in bipolar depression. May also improve cognitive function. Dose is 600 mg/day
Zonisamide[58,59]	Supported by two small RCTs. Dose is 100–300 mg/day.

Bipolar disorder

References

1. Malhi GS et al. Bipolar depression: management options. CNS Drugs 2003;17:9–25.
2. Perlis RH et al. Clinical features of bipolar depression versus major depressive disorder in large multi-center trials. Am J Psychiatry 2006;163:225–31.
3. Haddad P et al. Pharmacological management of bipolar depression. Acta Psychiatr Scand 2002; 105:401–3.
4. Hirschfeld RM. Bipolar depression: the real challenge. Eur Neuropsychopharmacol 2004;14(Suppl 2): S83–8.
5. Baldassano CF et al. Rethinking the treatment paradigm for bipolar depression: the importance of long-term management. CNS Spectr 2004;9:11–18.
6. National Institute for Clinical Excellence. Bipolar disorder. The management of bipolar disorder in adults, children and adolescents, in primary and secondary care. Clinical Guidance 38. http://www.nice.org.uk. 2006.
7. Geddes JR et al. Long-term lithium therapy for bipolar disorder: systematic review and meta-analysis of randomized controlled trials. Am J Psychiatry 2004;161:217–22.
8. Yatham LN et al. Bipolar depression: criteria for treatment selection, definition of refractoriness, and treatment options. Bipolar Disord 2003;5:85–97.
9. Calabrese JR et al. A placebo-controlled 18-month trial of lamotrigine and lithium maintenance treatment in recently depressed patients with bipolar I disorder. J Clin Psychiatry 2003;64:1013–24.
10. Prien RF et al. Lithium carbonate and imipramine in prevention of affective episodes. A comparison in recurrent affective illness. Arch Gen Psychiatry 1973;29:420–5.
11. Goodwin FK et al. Suicide risk in bipolar disorder during treatment with lithium and divalproex. JAMA 2003;290:1467–73.
12. Kessing LV et al. Suicide risk in patients treated with lithium. Arch Gen Psychiatry 2005;62:860–6.
13. Montgomery SA et al. Pharmacotherapy of depression and mixed states in bipolar disorder. J Affect Disord 2000;59(Suppl 1):S39–56.
14. Calabrese JR et al. International Consensus Group on Bipolar I Depression Treatment Guidelines. J Clin Psychiatry 2004;65:571–9.
15. Nemeroff CB et al. Double-blind, placebo-controlled comparison of imipramine and paroxetine in the treatment of bipolar depression. Am J Psychiatry 2001;158:906–12.
16. Vieta E et al. A randomized trial comparing paroxetine and venlafaxine in the treatment of bipolar depressed patients taking mood stabilizers. J Clin Psychiatry 2002;63:508–12.
17. Young LT et al. Double-blind comparison of addition of a second mood stabilizer versus an antidepressant to an initial mood stabilizer for treatment of patients with bipolar depression. Am J Psychiatry 2000;157:124–6.
18. Fawcett JA. Lithium combinations in acute and maintenance treatment of unipolar and bipolar depression. J Clin Psychiatry 2003;64(Suppl 5):32–7.
19. Altshuler L et al. The impact of antidepressant discontinuation versus antidepressant continuation on 1-year risk for relapse of bipolar depression: a retrospective chart review. J Clin Psychiatry 2001; 62:612–16.
20. Erfurth A et al. Bupropion as add-on strategy in difficult-to-treat bipolar depressive patients. Neuropsychobiology 2002;45 (Suppl 1):33–6.
21. Post RM et al. Mood switch in bipolar depression: comparison of adjunctive venlafaxine, bupropion and sertraline. Br J Psychiatry 2006;189:124–31.
22. Leverich GS et al. Risk of switch in mood polarity to hypomania or mania in patients with bipolar depression during acute and continuation trials of venlafaxine, sertraline, and bupropion as adjuncts to mood stabilizers. Am J Psychiatry 2006;163:232–9.
23. Baldassano CF et al. What drugs are best for bipolar depression? Ann Clin Psychiatry 2003;15:225–32.
24. Calabrese JR et al. A double-blind placebo-controlled study of lamotrigine monotherapy in outpatients with bipolar I depression. Lamictal 602 Study Group. J Clin Psychiatry 1999;60:79–88.
25. Bowden CL et al. Lamotrigine in the treatment of bipolar depression. Eur Neuropsychopharmacol 1999;9 (Suppl 4):S113–17.
26. Marangell LB et al. Lamotrigine treatment of bipolar disorder: data from the first 500 patients in STEP-BD. Bipolar Disord 2004;6:139–43.
27. Schaffer A et al. Randomized, double-blind pilot trial comparing lamotrigine versus citalopram for the treatment of bipolar depression. J Affect Disord 2006;96:95–9.
28. Bowden CL et al. Impact of lamotrigine and lithium on weight in obese and nonobese patients with bipolar I disorder. Am J Psychiatry 2006;163:1199–201.
29. Tohen M et al. Efficacy of olanzapine and olanzapine–fluoxetine combination in the treatment of bipolar I depression. Arch Gen Psychiatry 2003;60:1079–88.
30. Brown EB et al. A 7-week, randomized, double-blind trial of olanzapine/fluoxetine combination versus lamotrigine in the treatment of bipolar I depression. J Clin Psychiatry 2006;67:1025–33.
31. Corya SA et al. A 24-week open-label extension study of olanzapine–fluoxetine combination and olanzapine monotherapy in the treatment of bipolar depression. J Clin Psychiatry 2006;67:798–806.
32. Calabrese JR et al. A randomized, double-blind, placebo-controlled trial of quetiapine in the treatment of bipolar I or II depression. Am J Psychiatry 2005;162:1351–60.
33. Thase ME et al. Efficacy of quetiapine monotherapy in bipolar I and II depression: a double-blind, placebo-controlled study (the BOLDER II study). J Clin Psychopharmacol 2006;26:600–9.

34. Hirschfeld RM et al. Quetiapine in the treatment of anxiety in patients with bipolar I or II depression: a secondary analysis from a randomized, double-blind, placebo-controlled study. J Clin Psychiatry 2006;67:355–62.
35. Milev R et al. Add-on quetiapine for bipolar depression: a 12-month open-label trial. Can J Psychiatry 2006;51:523–30.
36. Goldberg JF et al. Preliminary randomized, double-blind, placebo-controlled trial of pramipexole added to mood stabilizers for treatment-resistant bipolar depression. Am J Psychiatry 2004;161:564–6.
37. Zarate CA Jr et al. Pramipexole for bipolar II depression: a placebo-controlled proof of concept study. Biol Psychiatry 2004;56:54–60.
38. Goodwin GM et al. The British Association for Psychopharmacology guidelines for treatment of bipolar disorder: a summary. J Psychopharmacol 2003;17:3–6.
39. Goodwin GM. Evidence-based guidelines for treating bipolar disorder: recommendations from the British Association for Psychopharmacology. J Psychopharmacol 2003;17:149–73.
40. Davis LL et al. Divalproex in the treatment of bipolar depression: a placebo-controlled study. J Affect Disord 2005;85:259–66.
41. Dilsaver SC et al. Treatment of bipolar depression with carbamazepine: results of an open study. Biol Psychiatry 1996;40:935–7.
42. Amsterdam JD et al. Short-term fluoxetine monotherapy for bipolar type II or bipolar NOS major depression – low manic switch rate. Bipolar Disord 2004;6:75–81.
43. Amsterdam JD et al. Efficacy and safety of fluoxetine in treating bipolar II major depressive episode. J Clin Psychopharmacol 1998;18:435–40.
44. Amsterdam J. Efficacy and safety of venlafaxine in the treatment of bipolar II major depressive episode. J Clin Psychopharmacol 1998;18:414–17.
45. Amsterdam JD et al. Venlafaxine monotherapy in women with bipolar II and unipolar major depression. J Affect Disord 2000;59:225–9.
46. Silverstone T. Moclobemide vs. imipramine in bipolar depression: a multicentre double-blind clinical trial. Acta Psychiatr Scand 2001;104:104–9.
47. Ghaemi SN et al. Antidepressant treatment in bipolar versus unipolar depression. Am J Psychiatry 2004;161:163–5.
48. Post RM et al. A re-evaluation of the role of antidepressants in the treatment of bipolar depression: data from the Stanley Foundation Bipolar Network. Bipolar Disord 2003;5:396–406.
49. Amsterdam JD et al. Comparison of fluoxetine, olanzapine, and combined fluoxetine plus olanzapine initial therapy of bipolar type I and type II major depression – lack of manic induction. J Affect Disord 2005;87:121–30.
50. Amsterdam JD et al. Fluoxetine monotherapy of bipolar type II and bipolar NOS major depression: a double-blind, placebo-substitution, continuation study. Int Clin Psychopharmacol 2005;20:257–64.
51. Ketter TA et al. Adjunctive aripiprazole in treatment-resistant bipolar depression. Ann Clin Psychiatry 2006;18:169–72.
52. Wang PW et al. Gabapentin augmentation therapy in bipolar depression. Bipolar Disord 2002;4:296–301.
53. Ashton H et al. GABA-ergic drugs: exit stage left, enter stage right. J Psychopharmacol 2003; 17:174–8.
54. Chengappa KN et al. Inositol as an add-on treatment for bipolar depression. Bipolar Disord 2000;2: 47–55.
55. Singh J et al. Case report: successful riluzole augmentation therapy in treatment-resistant bipolar depression following the development of rash with lamotrigine. Psychopharmacology 2004;173:227–8.
56. Bauer M. Thyroid hormone augmentation with levothyroxine in bipolar depression. Bipolar Disord 2002;4(Suppl 1):109–10.
57. Young AH et al. Improvements in neurocognitive function and mood following adjunctive treatment with mifepristone (RU-486) in bipolar disorder. Neuropsychopharmacology 2004;29:1538–45.
58. Ghaemi SN et al. An open prospective study of zonisamide in acute bipolar depression. J Clin Psychopharmacol 2006;26:385–8.
59. Anand A et al. A preliminary open-label study of zonisamide treatment for bipolar depression in 10 patients. J Clin Psychiatry 2005;66:195–8.

Further reading

Silverstone PH et al. A review of acute treatments for bipolar depression. Int Clin Psychopharmacol 2004;19:113–24.

Rapid-cycling bipolar affective disorder

Rapid-cycling is usually defined as bipolar disorder in which four or more episodes of (hypo) mania or depression occur in a 12-month period. It is generally held to be less responsive to drug treatment than non-rapid-cycling bipolar illness[1,2] and entails considerable depressive morbidity and suicide risk[3]. The following table outlines a treatment strategy for rapid cycling based on rather limited data and very few direct comparisons of drugs[4]. This strategy is broadly in line with UK NICE guidelines[5] which suggest a combination of lithium and valproate as first-line treatment and (somewhat bizarrely) lithium alone 'as second-line treatment'.

In practice, response to treatment is sometimes idiosyncratic: individuals sometimes show significant response only to one or two drugs. Spontaneous or treatment-related remissions occur in around a third of rapid-cyclers[6].

Step	Suggested treatment	References
Step 1	Withdraw antidepressants	7–9
Step 2	Evaluate possible precipitants (e.g. alcohol, thyroid dysfunction, external stressors)	2, 9
Step 3	Optimise mood stabiliser treatment (see page 159)	11, 12
	Consider combining mood stabilisers, e.g. lithium + valproate	
	Lithium may be relatively less effective but this is not certain[10]	
Step 4	Consider other (usually adjunct) treatment options: (alphabetical order)	13–24
	Clozapine (usual doses) Lamotrigine (up to 225 mg/day) Levetiracetam (up to 2000 mg/day) Nimodipine (180 mg/day) Olanzapine (usual doses) Quetiapine (300–600 mg/day) Risperidone (up to 6 mg/day) Thyroxine (150–400 μg/day) Topiramate (up to 300 mg/day)	
	Choice of drug determined by patient factors – no comparative efficacy data to guide choice	

References

1. Calabrese JR et al. Current research on rapid cycling bipolar disorder and its treatment. J Affect Disord 2001;67:241–55.
2. Kupka RW et al. Rapid and non-rapid cycling bipolar disorder: a meta-analysis of clinical studies. J Clin Psychiatry 2003;64:1483–94.
3. Coryell W et al. The long-term course of rapid-cycling bipolar disorder. Arch Gen Psychiatry 2003;60:914–20.
4. Tondo L et al. Rapid-cycling bipolar disorder: effects of long-term treatments. Acta Psychiatr Scand 2003;108:4–14.
5. National Institute for Clinical Excellence. Bipolar disorder. The management of bipolar disorder in adults, children and adolescents, in primary and secondary care. Clinical Guidance 38. http://www.nice.org.uk. 2006.
6. Koukopoulos A et al. Duration and stability of the rapid-cycling course: a long-term personal follow-up of 109 patients. J Affect Disord 2003;73:75–85.
7. Wehr TA et al. Can antidepressants cause mania and worsen the course of affective illness? Am J Psychiatry 1987;144:1403–11.
8. Altshuler LL et al. Antidepressant-induced mania and cycle acceleration: a controversy revisited. Am J Psychiatry 1995;152:1130–8.
9. American Psychiatric Association. Practice guideline for the treatment of patients with bipolar disorder. Am J Psychiatry 2002;159:1–50.
10. Calabrese JR et al. A 20-month, double-blind, maintenance trial of lithium versus divalproex in rapid-cycling bipolar disorder. Am J Psychiatry 2005;162:2152–61.
11. Calabrese JR et al. A medication algorithm for treatment of bipolar rapid cycling? J Clin Psychiatry 1995;56(Suppl 3):11–18.
12. Taylor DM et al. Treatment options for rapid-cycling bipolar affective disorder. Psychiatr Bull 1996;20:601–3.
13. Sanger TM et al. Olanzapine in the acute treatment of bipolar I disorder with a history of rapid cycling. J Affect Disord 2003;73:155–61.
14. Calabrese JR et al. Clozapine prophylaxis in rapid cycling bipolar disorder. J Clin Psychopharmacol 1991;11:396–7.
15. Vieta E et al. Quetiapine in the treatment of rapid cycling bipolar disorder. Bipolar Disord 2002; 4:335–40.
16. Goodnick PJ. Nimodipine treatment of rapid cycling bipolar disorder. J Clin Psychiatry 1995;56:330.
17. Pazzaglia PJ et al. Preliminary controlled trial of nimodipine in ultra-rapid cycling affective dysregulation. Psychiatry Res 1993;49:257–72.
18. Bauer MS et al. Rapid cycling bipolar affective disorder. Arch Gen Psychiatry 1990;47:435–40.
19. Fatemi SH et al. Lamotrigine in rapid-cycling bipolar disorder. J Clin Psychiatry 1997;58:522–7.
20. Calabrese JR et al. A double-blind, placebo-controlled, prophylaxis study of lamotrigine in rapid- cycling bipolar disorder. Lamictal 614 Study Group. J Clin Psychiatry 2000;61:841–50.
21. Braunig P et al. Levetiracetam in the treatment of rapid cycling bipolar disorder. J Psychopharmacol 2003; 17:239–41.
22. Vieta E et al. Treatment of refractory rapid cycling bipolar disorder with risperidone. J Clin Psychopharmacol 1998;18:172–4.
23. Jacobsen FM. Risperidone in the treatment of affective illness and obsessive-compulsive disorder. J Clin Psychiatry 1995;56:423–9.
24. Chen CK et al. Combination treatment of clozapine and topiramate in resistant rapid-cycling bipolar disorder. Clin Neuropharmacol 2005;28:136–8.

Bipolar disorder

173

Prophylaxis in bipolar disorder

NICE recommends that a mood stabiliser should be prescribed as prophylaxis (1) after a single manic episode that was associated with significant risk and adverse consequences or (2), in the case of bipolar I illness, after two or more acute episodes or (3), in the case of bipolar II illness, if there is significant functional impairment, frequent episodes or significant risk of suicide[1]. Most evidence supports the efficacy of lithium[2,3]. Carbamazepine is somewhat effective[3] and the long-term efficacy of valproate is uncertain[4–6]. Lithium has the advantage of an accepted antisuicidal effect[7–9] but the disadvantage of a worsened outcome following abrupt discontinuation[10,11]. Conventional antipsychotics have traditionally been used and are perceived to be effective although the objective evidence base is, again, weak[12,13]. Emerging evidence supports the efficacy of some second-generation antipsychotics, particularly olanzapine[1,5]. Whether atypicals are more effective than typicals or are truly associated with a reduced overall side-effect burden remains untested.

Bipolar disorder

NICE recommends[1]

- Lithium, olanzapine or valproate as first-line prophylactic agents
- Treatment for at least 2 years (longer in high-risk patients)
- Antidepressants (SSRIs are preferred) may be used in combination with a mood stabiliser to treat acute episodes of depression but should not be routinely used for prophylaxis
- Chronic or recurrent depression may be treated with an SSRI or CBT in combination with a mood stabiliser or quetiapine or lamotrigine
- Combined lithium and valproate for the prophylaxis of rapid-cycling illness.

*Note that valproate is teratogenic and should not be routinely used in women of childbearing age (see page 144).

A significant proportion of patients with bipolar illness fail to respond adequately to a single mood stabiliser, so combinations of mood stabilisers[14,15] or a mood stabiliser and an antipsychotic[15,16] may improve outcome. This needs to be balanced against the likely increased side-effect burden associated with polypharmacy. Combinations of two drugs chosen from lithium, olanzapine and valproate are recommended by NICE[1]. Carbamazepine is considered to be third line. Lamotrigine may be useful in bipolar II disorder[1] and seems to prevent recurrence of depression[17]. The patient's views about 'acceptable risk' of recurrence versus 'acceptable side-effect burden' are paramount.

References

1. National Institute for Clinical Excellence. Bipolar disorder. The management of bipolar disorder in adults, children and adolescents, in primary and secondary care. Clinical Guidance 38. http://www.nice.org.uk. 2006.
2. Geddes JR et al. Long-term lithium therapy for bipolar disorder: systematic review and meta-analysis of randomized controlled trials. Am J Psychiatry 2004;161:217–22.
3. Hartong EG et al. Prophylactic efficacy of lithium versus carbamazepine in treatment-naive bipolar patients. J Clin Psychiatry 2003;64:144–51.
4. Bowden CL et al. A randomized, placebo-controlled 12-month trial of divalproex and lithium in treatment of outpatients with bipolar I disorder. Divalproex Maintenance Study Group. Arch Gen Psychiatry 2000;57:481–9.
5. Tohen M et al. Olanzapine versus divalproex sodium for the treatment of acute mania and maintenance of remission: a 47-week study. Am J Psychiatry 2003;160:1263–71.
6. Macritchie KA et al. Valproic acid, valproate and divalproex in the maintenance treatment of bipolar disorder. Cochrane Database Syst Rev 2001;CD003196.
7. Cipriani A et al. Lithium in the prevention of suicidal behavior and all-cause mortality in patients with mood disorders: a systematic review of randomized trials. Am J Psychiatry 2005;162:1805–19.
8. Kessing LV et al. Suicide risk in patients treated with lithium. Arch Gen Psychiatry 2005;62:860–6.
9. Young AH et al. Lithium in maintenance therapy for bipolar disorder. J Psychopharmacol 2006;20:17–22.
10. Mander AJ et al. Rapid recurrence of mania following abrupt discontinuation of lithium. Lancet 1988;2:15–17.
11. Faedda GL et al. Outcome after rapid vs gradual discontinuation of lithium treatment in bipolar disorders. Arch Gen Psychiatry 1993;50:448–55.
12. Gao K et al. Typical and atypical antipsychotics in bipolar depression. J Clin Psychiatry 2005;66:1376–85.
13. Hellewell JS. A review of the evidence for the use of antipsychotics in the maintenance treatment of bipolar disorders. J Psychopharmacol 2006;20:39–45.
14. Freeman MP et al. Mood stabilizer combinations: a review of safety and efficacy. Am J Psychiatry 1998;155:12–21.
15. Muzina DJ et al. Maintenance therapies in bipolar disorder: focus on randomized controlled trials. Aust N Z J Psychiatry 2005;39:652–61.
16. Tohen M et al. Relapse prevention in bipolar I disorder: 18-month comparison of olanzapine plus mood stabiliser v. mood stabiliser alone. Br J Psychiatry 2004;184:337–45.
17. Bowden CL et al. A placebo-controlled 18-month trial of lamotrigine and lithium maintenance treatment in recently manic or hypomanic patients with bipolar I disorder. Arch Gen Psychiatry 2003;60:392–400.

Further reading

American Psychiatric Association. Practice guidelines for the treatment of patients with bipolar disorder. Am J Psychiatry 2002;159(Suppl):1–50.
Goodwin GM et al. The British Association for Psychopharmacology guidelines for treatment of bipolar disorder: a summary. J Psychopharmacol 2003;17:3–6.
Sachs GS. Decision tree for the treatment of bipolar disorder. J Clin Psychiatry 2003;64:35–40.

chapter 4

Depression and anxiety

Antidepressant drugs – tricyclics*

Tricyclic	Licensed indication	Licensed doses (elderly doses not included)	Main adverse effects	Major interactions	Approx. half-life (h)	Cost (£)
Amitriptyline	Depression	30–200 mg/day	Sedation, often with hangover; postural hypotension; tachycardia, arrhythmia; dry mouth, blurred vision, constipation, urinary retention	SSRIs (except citalopram), phenothiazines, cimetidine – ↑plasma levels of TCAs Alcohol Antimuscarinics Antipsychotics, MAOIs	9–25	0.04/50 mg
	Nocturnal enuresis in children	7–10 yr: 10–20 mg 11–16 yr: 25–50 mg at night for 3 months			18–96 Active metabolite (nortriptyline)	
Clomipramine	Depression Phobic and obsessional states	10–250 mg/day 10–150 mg/day	As for amitriptyline	As for amitriptyline	19–37	0.18/50 mg
	Adjunctive treatment of cataplexy associated with narcolepsy	10–75 mg/day			54–77 Active metabolite (desmethyl-clomipramine)	
Dosulepin (dothiepin)	Depression	75–225 mg/day	As for amitriptyline	As for amitriptyline	11–40 22–60 Active metabolite (desmethyl-dosulepin)	0.08/75 mg

Doxepin	Depression	10–300 mg/day (up to 100 mg as a single dose)	As for amitriptyline	As for amitriptyline	8–25 28–52 Active metabolite (desmethyl-doxepin)	0.05/50 mg
Imipramine	Depression Nocturnal enuresis in children	10–200 mg/day (up to 100 mg as a single dose; up to 300 mg in hospital patients) 7 yr: 25 mg 8–11 yr: 25–50 mg >11 yr: 50–75 mg at night for 3 months	As for amitriptyline but less sedative	As for amitriptyline	4–18 12–24 Active metabolite (desipramine)	0.07/25 mg
Lofepramine	Depression	140–210 mg/day	As for amitriptyline but less sedative, anticholinergic, cardiotoxic. Constipation common	As for amitriptyline	1.5–6 12–24 Active metabolite (desipramine)	0.46/70 mg
Nortriptyline	Depression Nocturnal enuresis in children	30–150 mg/day 7 yr: 10 mg 8–11 yrs: 10–20 mg >11 yr: 25–35 mg at night for 3 months	As for amitriptyline but less sedative, anticholinergic, hypotensive. Constipation may be problematic	As for amitriptyline	18–96	0.21/25 mg
Trimipramine	Depression	30–300 mg/day	As for amitriptyline but more sedative	As for amitriptyline Safer with MAOIs than other tricyclics	7–23	0.28/50 mg

*For full details refer to the manufacturer's information.

Antidepressant drugs – SSRIs*

SSRI	Licensed indication	Licensed doses (elderly doses not included)	Main adverse effects	Major interactions	Approx. half-life (h)	Cost (£)
Citalopram	Depression – treatment of the initial phase and as maintenance therapy against potential relapse or recurrence	20–60 mg/day Use lowest dose – evidence for higher doses poor	Nausea, vomiting, dyspepsia, abdominal pain, diarrhoea, rash, sweating, agitation, anxiety, headache, insomnia, tremor, sexual dysfunction (male and female), hyponatraemia, cutaneous bleeding disorders Discontinuation symptoms may occur. (See page 240)	Not a potent inhibitor of most cytochrome enzymes MAOIs – avoid Avoid – St John's wort Caution with alcohol (although no interaction seen), NSAIDs, tryptophan, warfarin	33 Has weak active metabolites	0.12/20 mg (generic available – price may vary) Drops 0.67/16 mg/ 8 drops (= 20 mg tablet)
	Panic disorder ± agoraphobia	10 mg for 1 week, increasing up to 60 mg/day				
Escitalopram	Depression Panic disorder ± agoraphobia	10–20 mg/day 5 mg/day for 1 week, increasing up to 20 mg/day	As for citalopram	As for citalopram	~30 Has weak active metabolites	0.53/10 mg
	Social anxiety Generalised anxiety disorder	20 mg/day 10–20 mg/day				
Fluoxetine	Depression ± anxiety	20 mg/day	As for citalopram but insomnia and agitation possibly more common Rash may occur more frequently May alter insulin requirements (see page 218)	Inhibits CYP2D6, CYP3A4. Increases plasma levels of some antipsychotics, some benzos, carbamazepine, ciclosporin, phenytoin, tricyclics MAOIs – never Avoid: selegiline, St John's wort Caution – alcohol (although no interaction seen), NSAIDs, tryptophan, warfarin	2–3 days 4–16 days Active metabolite (norfluoxetine)	0.05/20 mg (generic – price may vary)
	OCD	20–60 mg/day				
	Bulimia nervosa	60 mg/day				Liquid 0.92/20 mg/5 ml
		Higher doses possible – see SPC				

Drug	Indication	Dose	Side effects	Interactions	Half-life	Price
Fluvoxamine	Depression	100–300 mg/day b.d. if >100 mg	As for citalopram but nausea more common	Inhibits CYP1A2/2C9/3A4 Increases plasma levels of some benzos, carbamazepine, ciclosporin, methadone, olanzapine, phenytoin, propranolol, theophylline, some tricyclics, warfarin MAOIs – never Caution: alcohol, lithium, NSAIDs, St John's wort, tryptophan, warfarin	17–22	0.39/100 mg
	OCD	100–300 mg/day b.d. if >100 mg				
Paroxetine	Depression ± anxiety	20–50 mg/day Use lowest dose – evidence for higher doses poor	As for citalopram but antimuscarinic effects, sedation more common Extrapyramidal symptoms more common, but rare Discontinuation symptoms common – withdraw slowly	Potent inhibitor of CYP2D6 Increases plasma level of some antipsychotics, and tricyclics MAOIs – never Avoid: St John's wort Caution: alcohol, lithium, NSAIDs, tryptophan, warfarin	~24 (non-linear kinetics)	0.20/20 mg (generic – price may vary) Liquid 0.63/20 mg/ 10 ml
	OCD	20–60 mg/day				
	Panic disorder ± agoraphobia	10–50 mg/day				
	Social phobia	20–50 mg/day				
	PTSD	20–50 mg/day				
	Generalised anxiety disorder	20 mg/day				
Sertraline	Depression ± anxiety and prevention of relapse or recurrence of depression ±anxiety	50–200 mg/day Use 50–100 mg – evidence for higher doses poor	As for citalopram	Inhibits CYP2D6 (more likely to occur at doses ≥100 mg/day) Increases plasma levels of some antipsychotics, tricyclics Avoid: St John's wort Caution: alcohol (although no interaction seen), lithium, NSAIDs, tryptophan, warfarin	~26 Has a weak active metabolite	0.09/100 mg generic – price may vary
	OCD (under specialist supervision in children)	50–200 mg/day (adults) 6–12 yr: 25–50 mg/day, may be increased in steps of 50 mg at intervals of 1 week 13–17 yr: 50–200 mg/day				
	PTSD in women	25–50 mg/day				

*For full details refer to the manufacturer's information.

Antidepressant drugs – MAOIs*

MAOI	Licensed indication	Licensed doses (elderly doses not included)	Main adverse effects	Major interactions	Approx. half-life (h)	Cost (£)
Phenelzine	Depression	15 mg t.d.s. – q.i.d. (hospital patients: max. 30 mg t.d.s.) Consider reducing to lowest possible maintenance dose	Postural hypotension, dizziness, drowsiness, insomnia, headaches, oedema, anticholinergic effects, weight gain, hepatotoxicity, leucopenia, hypertensive crisis	Tyramine in food, opioids, antidepressants, levodopa, $5HT_1$ aganists, sympathomimetics, alcohol. Probably safest MAOI in antidepressant combinations	1.5	0.20/15 mg
Tranylcypromine	Depression	10 mg b.d. Doses >30 mg/day under close supervision only Usual maintenance: 10 mg/day Last dose no later than 3 pm	As for phenelzine but insomnia, nervousness, hypertensive crisis more common than with other MAOIS; hepatotoxicity less common Mild dependence as amfetamine-like structure	As for phenelzine but interactions more severe. Never use in combination therapy with other antidepressants	2.5	0.24/10 mg

Moclobemide (reversible inhibitor of MAO-A)	Depression	150–600 mg/day b.d. after food	Sleep disturbances, nausea, agitation, confusion Hypertension reported – may be related to tyramine ingestion	Tyramine interactions rare and mild but possible if high doses (>600 mg/day) used or if large quantities of tyramine ingested. CNS excitation/ depression with dextromethorphan and pethidine. Avoid: clomipramine, levodopa, selegiline, sympathomimetics, SSRIs. Caution with fentanyl, morphine, tricylics. Cimetidine – use half-dose of moclobemide	2–4	0.11/150 mg
	Social phobia	300–600 mg/day b.d. after food Last dose before 3 pm				

*For full details refer to the manufacturer's information.

Antidepressant drugs – others*

Antidepressant	Licensed indication	Licensed doses (elderly doses not included)	Main adverse effects	Major interactions	Approx. half-life (h)	Cost (£)
Duloxetine	Depression (and other non-psychiatric indications)	60–120 mg/day Limited data to support advantage of doses above 60 mg/day	Nausea, insomnia, dizziness, dry mouth, somnolence, constipation, anorexia. Very small increases in heart rate and blood pressure, including hypertensive crisis	Metabolised by CYP1A2 and CYP2D6. Inhibitor of CYP2D6. Caution with drugs acting on either. MAOIs – avoid Caution: alcohol (although no interaction seen)	12 (metabolites inactive)	0.99/60 mg
Mianserin	Depression	30–90 mg daily	Sedation, rash; rarely: blood dyscrasia, jaundice, arthralgia No anticholinergic effects. Sexual dysfunction uncommon. Low cardiotoxicity	Other sedatives, alcohol MAOIs: avoid Effect on hepatic enzymes unclear, so caution is required	10–20 2-desmethyl-mianserin is major metabolite (?activity)	0.14/30 mg
Mirtazapine	Depression	15–45 mg/day	Increased appetite, weight gain, drowsiness, oedema, dizziness, headache, ?blood dyscrasia Nausea/sexual dysfunction relatively uncommon	Minimal effect on CYP2D6/1A2/3A Caution: alcohol/sedatives	20–40 25 Active metabolite (demethyl-mirtazapine)	0.40/30 mg (generic available – price may vary)

Reboxetine	Depression – acute and maintenance	4–6 mg b.d.	Insomnia, sweating, dizziness, dry mouth, constipation, tachycardia, urinary hesitancy Erectile dysfunction may occur rarely	Metabolised by CYP3A4 – avoid drugs inhibiting this enzyme (e.g. erythromycin, ketoconazole). Minimal effect on CYP2D6/3A4 MAOIs: avoid No interaction with alcohol	13	0.32/4 mg
Trazodone	Depression ± anxiety	150–300 mg/day (up to 600 mg/day in hospitalised patients) b.d. dosing above 300 mg/day	Sedation, dizziness, headache, nausea, vomiting, tremor, postural hypotension, tachycardia, priapism Not anticholinergic, less cardiotoxic than tricyclics	Caution: sedatives/ alcohol/other antidepressants/ digoxin/ phenytoin MAOIs: avoid	5–13 (biphasic) 4–9 Active metabolite (mCPP)	0.44/100 mg Liquid 0.71/100 mg/ 10 ml
	Anxiety	75–300 mg/day				
Venlafaxine	Depression ± anxiety and prevention of relapse or recurrence of depression	75–375 mg/day (b.d.) with food 75–225 mg XL/day (o.d.) with food	Nausea, insomnia, dry mouth, somnolence, dizziness, sweating, nervousness, headache, sexual dysfunction	Metabolised by CYP2D6/3A4 – caution with drugs known to inhibit either Minimal effects on CYP2D6 No effects on CYP1A2/2C9/3A4 MAOIs: avoid Caution: alcohol (although no interaction seen)/cimetidine/ clozapine/ warfarin	5 11 Active metabolite (O-desmethyl- venlafaxine)	0.70/75 mg 0.84/75 mg XL
	Generalised anxiety disorder (XL prep only)	75 mg XL/day (discontinue if no response after 8 weeks)	Elevation of blood pressure at higher doses. Avoid if at risk of arrhythmia. Discontinuation symptoms common – withdraw slowly			

*For full details refer to the manufacturer's information.

Treatment of affective illness – depression

Basic principles of prescribing in depression

- Discuss with the patient choice of drug and utility/availability of other, non-pharmacological treatments.
- Discuss with the patient likely outcomes, such as gradual relief from depressive symptoms over several weeks.
- Prescribe a dose of antidepressant (after titration, if necessary) that is likely to be effective.
- For a single episode, continue treatment for at least 4–6 months after resolution of symptoms (multiple episodes may require longer).
- Withdraw antidepressants gradually; always inform patients of the risk and nature of discontinuation symptoms.

Official guidance on the treatment of depression

NICE guidelines[1] – a summary

- Antidepressants are not recommended in mild depression – watchful waiting, problem-solving and exercise are preferred.
- When an antidepressant is prescribed, a generic SSRI is recommended.
- All patients should be informed about the withdrawal effects of antidepressants.
- For severe or resistant depression a combination of antidepressant and CBT is recommended.
- Patients with two prior episodes and functional impairment should be treated for at least 2 years.

MHRA/CSM Expert Working Group on SSRIs[2] – a summary

- Use the lowest possible dose.
- Monitor closely in early stages for restlessness, agitation and suicidality. This is particularly important in young people (<30 years).
- Doses should be tapered gradually on stopping.
- Venlafaxine use was originally restricted but this guidance has now been partly reversed (venlafaxine is probably not cardiotoxic[3,4], but has a less favourable profile in overdose than SSRIs) (see page 228).

References

1. National Institute of Clinical Excellence. Depression: management of depression in primary and secondary care – clinical guidance. http://www.nice.org.uk. 2004.
2. Committee on Safety of Medicines. Report of the CSM expert working group on the safety of selective serotonin reuptake inhibitor antidepressants. http://www.mhra.gov.uk. 2004.
3. Taylor D et al. Volte-face on venlafaxine–reasons and reflections. J Psychopharmacol 2006;20:597–601.
4. Medicines and Healthcare Products Regulatory Agency. Venlafaxine (Efexor) Summary of Basis for Regulatory Position. http://www.mhra.gov.uk. 2006.

Depression & anxiety

Drug treatment of depression

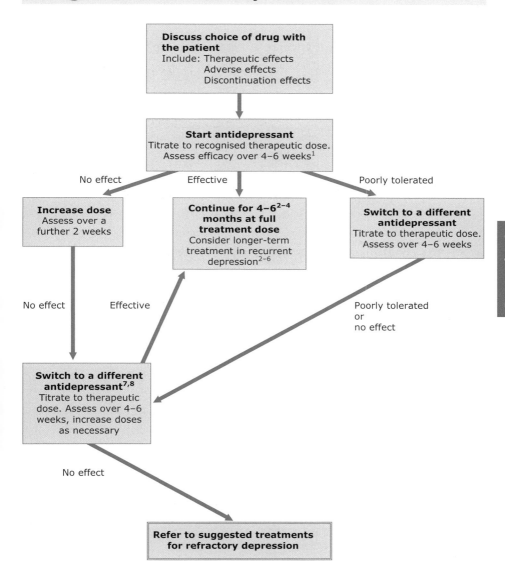

Discuss choice of drug with the patient
Include: Therapeutic effects
Adverse effects
Discontinuation effects

Start antidepressant
Titrate to recognised therapeutic dose.
Assess efficacy over 4–6 weeks[1]

No effect

Effective

Poorly tolerated

Increase dose
Assess over a further 2 weeks

Continue for 4–6[2–4] months at full treatment dose
Consider longer-term treatment in recurrent depression[2–6]

Switch to a different antidepressant
Titrate to therapeutic dose.
Assess over 4–6 weeks

No effect

Effective

Poorly tolerated
or
no effect

Switch to a different antidepressant[7,8]
Titrate to therapeutic dose. Assess over 4–6 weeks, increase doses as necessary

No effect

Refer to suggested treatments for refractory depression

Depression & anxiety

Notes
- Tools such as the Montgomery–Asberg Depression Rating Scale[9] and the Hamilton Depression Rating Scale[10] are recommended to assess drug effect.
- Switching between drug classes in cases of poor tolerability is not well supported by published studies but has a strong theoretical basis. In cases of

non-response, there is some evidence that switching within a drug class can be effective[8,11-13], but switching between classes is, in practice, the most common option (see page 193).

- There is minimal evidence to support increasing the dose of SSRIs in depression[14].
- Switch treatments early if adverse effects intolerable or if no improvement is seen by 3-4 weeks.

References

1. Snow V et al. Pharmacologic treatment of acute major depression and dysthymia. American College of Physicians – American Society of Internal Medicine. Ann Intern Med 2000;132:738-42.
2. Anderson IM et al. Evidence-based guidelines for treating depressive disorders with antidepressants: a revision of the 1993 British Association for Psychopharmacology guidelines. British Association for Psychopharmacology. J Psychopharmacol 2000;14:3-20.
3. Crismon ML et al. The Texas Medication Algorithm Project: report of the Texas Consensus Conference Panel on Medication Treatment of Major Depressive Disorder. J Clin Psychiatry 1999;60:142-56.
4. American Psychiatric Association. Practice guideline for major depressive disorder in adults. Am J Psychiatry 1993;150:1-26.
5. Kocsis JH et al. Maintenance therapy for chronic depression. A controlled clinical trial of desipramine. Arch Gen Psychiatry 1996;53:769-74.
6. Dekker J et al. The use of antidepressants after recovery from depression. Eur Psychiatry 2000; 14:207-12.
7. Nelson JC. Treatment of antidepressant nonresponders: augmentation or switch? J Clin Psychiatry 1998;59(Suppl 15):35-41.
8. Joffe RT. Substitution therapy in patients with major depression. CNS Drugs 1999;11:175-80.
9. Montgomery SA et al. A new depression scale designed to be sensitive to change. Br J Psychiatry 1979;134:382-9.
10. Hamilton M. Development of a rating scale for primary depressive illness. Br J Soc Clin Psychol 1967;6:278-96.
11. Thase ME et al. Citalopram treatment of fluoxetine nonresponders. J Clin Psychiatry 2001;62:683-7.
12. Rush AJ et al. Bupropion-SR, sertraline, or venlafaxine-XR after failure of SSRIs for depression. N Engl J Med 2006;354:1231-42.
13. Ruhe HG et al. Switching antidepressants after a first selective serotonin reuptake inhibitor in major depressive disorder: a systematic review. J Clin Psychiatry 2006;67:1836-55.
14. Adli M et al. Is dose escalation of antidepressants a rational strategy after a medium-dose treatment has failed? A systematic review. Eur Arch Psychiatry Clin Neurosci 2005;255:387-400.

Further reading

Barbui C et al. Amitriptyline v. the rest: still the leading antidepressant after 40 years of randomised controlled trials. Br J Psychiatry 2001;178:129-44.
Rubinow DR. Treatment strategies after SSRI failure – good news and bad news. N Engl J Med 2006;354:1305-7.
Smith D et al. Efficacy and tolerability of venlafaxine compared with selective serotonin reuptake inhibitors and other antidepressants: a meta-analysis. Br J Psychiatry 2002;180:396-404.
Trivedi MH et al. Clinical results for patients with major depressive disorder in the Texas Medication Algorithm Project. Arch Gen Psychiatry 2004;61:669-80.

Recognised minimum effective doses – antidepressants

Tricyclics

Tricyclics	Unclear; at least 75–100 mg/day[1], possibly 125 mg/day[2]
Lofepramine	140 mg/day[3]

SSRIs

Citalopram	20 mg/day[4]
Escitalopram	10 mg/day[5]
Fluoxetine	20 mg/day[6]
Fluvoxamine	50 mg/day[7]
Paroxetine	20 mg/day[8]
Sertraline	50 mg/day[9]

Others

Duloxetine	60 mg/day[10,11]
Mirtazapine	30 mg/day[12]
Moclobemide	300 mg/day[13]
Reboxetine	8 mg/day[14]
Trazodone	150 mg/day[15]
Venlafaxine	75 mg/day[16]

Depression & anxiety

References

1. Furukawa TA et al. Meta-analysis of effects and side effects of low dosage tricyclic antidepressants in depression: systematic review. BMJ 2002;325:991.
2. Donoghue J et al. Suboptimal use of antidepressants in the treatment of depression. CNS Drugs 2000;13:365–8.
3. Lancaster SG et al. Lofepramine. A review of its pharmacodynamic and pharmacokinetic properties, and therapeutic efficacy in depressive illness. Drugs 1989;37:123–40.
4. Montgomery SA et al. The optimal dosing regimen for citalopram – a meta-analysis of nine placebo-controlled studies. Int Clin Psychopharmacol 1994;9(Suppl 1):35–40.
5. Burke WJ et al. Fixed-dose trial of the single isomer SSRI escitalopram in depressed outpatients. J Clin Psychiatry 2002;63:331–6.
6. Altamura AC et al. The evidence for 20mg a day of fluoxetine as the optimal dose in the treatment of depression. Br J Psychiatry Suppl 1988;109–12.
7. Walczak DD et al. The oral dose–effect relationship for fluvoxamine: a fixed-dose comparison against placebo in depressed outpatients. Ann Clin Psychiatry 1996;8:139–51.
8. Dunner DL et al. Optimal dose regimen for paroxetine. J Clin Psychiatry 1992;53(Suppl):21–6.
9. Moon CAL et al. A double-blind comparison of sertraline and clomipramine in the treatment of major depressive disorder and associative anxiety in general practice. J Psychopharmacol 1994;8:171–6.
10. Goldstein DJ et al. Duloxetine in the treatment of depression: a double-blind placebo-controlled comparison with paroxetine. J Clin Psychopharmacol 2004;24:389–99.
11. Detke MJ et al. Duloxetine, 60 mg once daily, for major depressive disorder: a randomized double-blind placebo-controlled trial. J Clin Psychiatry 2002;63:308–15.
12. van Moffaert M et al. Mirtazapine is more effective than trazodone: a double-blind controlled study in hospitalized patients with major depression. Int Clin Psychopharmacol 1995;10:3–9.
13. Priest RG et al. Moclobemide in the treatment of depression. Rev Contemp Pharmacother 1994;5:35–43.
14. Schatzberg AF. Clinical efficacy of reboxetine in major depression. J Clin Psychiatry 2000;61(Suppl 10):31–8.
15. Brogden RN et al. Trazodone: a review of its pharmacological properties and therapeutic use in depression and anxiety. Drugs 1981;21:401–29.
16. Feighner JP et al. Efficacy of once-daily venlafaxine extended release (XR) for symptoms of anxiety in depressed outpatients. J Affect Disord 1998;47:55–62.

Antidepressant prophylaxis

First episode

A single episode of depression should be treated for 4–6 months after recovery (i.e. a total of 9 months in all)[1,2]. If antidepressant therapy is stopped immediately on recovery, 50% of patients experience a return of their depressive symptoms[1].

Recurrent depression

Of those patients who have one episode of major depression, 50–85% will go on to have a second episode, and 80–90% of those who have a second episode will go on to have a third[3]. Many factors are known to increase the risk of recurrence, including a family history of depression, recurrent dysthymia, concurrent non-affective psychiatric illness, chronic medical illness and social factors (e.g. lack of confiding relationships and psychosocial stressors). Some prescription drugs may precipitate depression[4]. Up to 15% of people with depression take their own life[3].

The figure below outlines the risk of recurrence for multiple-episode patients: those recruited to the study had already experienced at least three episodes of depression with 3 years or less between episodes[5,6].

A meta-analysis of antidepressant continuation studies[7] concluded that continuing treatment with antidepressants reduces the odds of depressive relapse by around two-thirds, which is approximately equal to halving the absolute risk. This benefit persisted at 36 months and seemed to be similar across heterogeneous patient groups (first episode, multiple episode and chronic), although none of the studies included first-episode patients only. Specific studies in first-episode patients are required to confirm that treatment beyond 6–9 months confers additional benefit in this patient group.

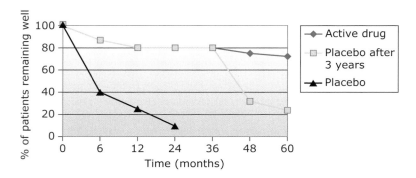

NICE recommend that[8]:
- Patients who have had two or more episodes of depression in the recent past and who have experienced significant functional impairment during these episodes, should be advised to continue antidepressants for 2 years.
- Patients on maintenance treatment should be re-evaluated, taking into account age, co-morbid conditions and other risk factors in the decision to continue maintenance treatment beyond 2 years.

Dose for prophylaxis

Adults should receive the same dose as used for acute treatment[8]. There is very limited evidence that lower doses are effective[9,10]. There is some evidence to support the use of lower doses in elderly patients: dosulepin 75 mg/day offers effective prophylaxis[9]. There is no evidence to support the use of lower than standard doses of SSRIs[11].

Relapse rates after ECT are similar to those after stopping antidepressants[12]. Antidepressant prophylaxis will be required, ideally with a different drug from the one that failed to get the patient well in the first instance, although good data in this area are lacking.

Lithium also has some efficacy in the prophylaxis of unipolar depression; efficacy relative to antidepressants is unknown[13]. NICE recommend that lithium should not be used as the sole prophylactic drug[8]. There is some support for the use of a combination of lithium and nortriptyline[14].

Key points that patients should know

- A single episode of depression should be treated for 6 months after recovery.
- The risk of recurrence of depressive illness is high and increases with each episode.
- Those who have had multiple episodes may require treatment for many years.
- The chances of staying well are greatly increased by taking antidepressants.
- Antidepressants are:
  - effective
  - not addictive
  - not known to lose their efficacy over time
  - not known to cause new long-term side-effects.
- Medication needs to be continued at the treatment dose. If side-effects are intolerable, it may be possible to find a more suitable alternative.
- If patients decide to stop their medication, this must not be done suddenly, as this may lead to unpleasant discontinuation effects (see page XXX). The medication needs to be reduced slowly under the supervision of a doctor.

Depression & anxiety

References

1. Loonen AJ et al. Continuation and maintenance therapy with antidepressive agents. Meta-analysis of research. Pharm Weekly Sci 1991;13:167–75.
2. Reimherr FW et al. Optimal length of continuation therapy in depression: a prospective assessment during long-term fluoxetine treatment. Am J Psychiatry 1998;155:1247–53.
3. Forshall S et al. Maintenance pharmacotherapy of unipolar depression. Psychiatr Bull 1999;23:370–3.
4. Patten SB et al. Drug-induced depression. Psychother Psychosom 1997;66:63–73.
5. Frank E et al. Three-year outcomes for maintenance therapies in recurrent depression. Arch Gen Psychiatry 1990;47:1093–9.
6. Kupfer DJ et al. Five-year outcome for maintenance therapies in recurrent depression. Arch Gen Psychiatry 1992;49:769–73.
7. Geddes JR et al. Relapse prevention with antidepressant drug treatment in depressive disorders: a systematic review. Lancet 2003;361:653–61.
8. National Institute for Clinical Excellence. Depression: management of depression in primary and secondary care – clinical guidance. http://www.nice.org.uk. 2004.
9. Frank E et al. Comparison of full-dose versus half-dose pharmacotherapy in the maintenance treatment of recurrent depression. J Affect Disord 1993;27:139–45.
10. Old Age Depression Interest Group. How long should the elderly take antidepressants? A double-blind placebo-controlled study of continuation/prophylaxis therapy with dothiepin. Br J Psychiatry 1993;162: 175–82.
11. Franchini L et al. Dose–response efficacy of paroxetine in preventing depressive recurrences: a randomized, double-blind study. J Clin Psychiatry 1998;59:229–32.
12. Nobler MS, Sackeim HA. Refractory depression and electroconvulsive therapy. In Nolen WA, Zohar J, Roose SP, eds. Refractory depression: current strategies and future directions. Chichester: John Wiley & Sons, 1994;69–81.
13. Cipriani A et al. Lithium versus antidepressants in the long-term treatment of unipolar affective disorder. Cochrane Database Syst Rev 2006;CD003492.
14. Sackeim HA et al. Continuation pharmacotherapy in the prevention of relapse following electroconvulsive therapy: a randomized controlled trial. JAMA 2001;285:1299–307.

Further reading

Jackson GA et al. Psychiatrist's attitudes to maintenance drug treatment in depression. Psychiatr Bull 1999;23:74–7.

Depression &
anxiety

Treatment of refractory depression

Refractory depression is difficult to treat successfully and outcomes are poor[1] especially if evidence-based protocols are not followed[2]. The evidence base has been substantially improved by publication of results of the STAR*D programme (Sequenced Treatment Alternatives to Relieve Depression). This was a pragmatic effectiveness study which used remission of symptoms as its main outcome. At stage 1[3], 2786 subjects received citalopram (mean dose 41.8 mg/day) for 14 weeks; remission was seen in 28% – response (50% reduction in symptoms score) 47%. Subjects who failed to remit were entered into the continued study of sequential treatments[4–8]. Remission rates are given in the figure below. Very few statistically significant differences were noted from this point on. At stage 3[7], tri-iodothyronine (T_3) was found to be significantly better tolerated than lithium. At stage 4[8], tranylcypromine was less effective and less well tolerated than the mirtazapine/venlafaxine combination. Overall, remission rates, as can be seen, were worryingly low.

STAR*D shows that the treatment of refractory depression requires a flexible approach and that response to a particular treatment option is not readily predicted by pharmacology or previous treatments. The programme has established bupropion and buspirone augmentation as worthwhile options and resurrected from obscurity the use of T_3 augmentation and of nortriptyline.

Figure   Remission rates in STAR*D

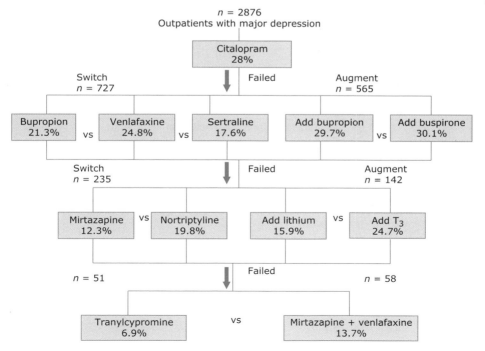

193

Table First choice: commonly used treatments generally well supported by published literature (no preference implied by order)

Treatment	Advantages	Disadvantages	Refs
Add **lithium** Aim for plasma level of 0.4–1.0 mmol/l	• Well established • Well supported in the literature • Recommended by NICE	• Sometimes poorly tolerated • Potentially toxic (NICE recommend ECG) • Usually needs specialist referral • Plasma monitoring is essential	7,9–11
ECT	• Well established • Effective • Well supported in the literature	• Poor reputation in public domain • Necessitates general anaesthetic • Needs specialist referral • Usually reserved for last-line treatment • Usually combined with other treatments	12–14
Venlafaxine (high dose) (>200 mg/day) *(note use with mirtazapine below)*	• Usually well tolerated • Can be initiated in primary care • Recommended by NICE • Supported by STAR*D	• Nausea and vomiting more common • Discontinuation reactions common • Blood pressure monitoring essential	4,15–17
Add **tri-iodothyronine** (20–50 μg/day)	• Usually well tolerated • Good literature support (including by STAR*D)	• TFT monitoring required • Usually needs specialist referral • Some negative studies	7,18–21
SSRI + bupropion Up to 400 mg/day	• Supported by STAR*D • Well tolerated	• Not licensed for depression in the UK	5,22–26
SSRI + buspirone Up to 60 mg/day	• Supported by STAR*D	• Higher doses required poorly tolerated	5,27–29
SSRI or venlafaxine + mianserin or **mirtazapine**	• Recommended by NICE • Usually well tolerated • Reasonable literature support • Becoming more widely used	• Risk of serotonin syndrome (inform patient) • Risk of blood dyscrasia with mianserin	8,30–32

Note: Data relating to augmentation or switching strategies in refractory depression are poor by evidence-based standards[33,34]. Recommendations are therefore partly based on clinical experience and expert consensus.

Always consider non-drug approaches (e.g. CBT).

References

1. Dunner DL et al. Prospective, long-term, multicenter study of the naturalistic outcomes of patients with treatment-resistant depression. J Clin Psychiatry 2006;67:688–95.
2. Trivedi MH et al. Clinical results for patients with major depressive disorder in the Texas Medication Algorithm Project. Arch Gen Psychiatry 2004;61:669–80.
3. Trivedi MH et al. Evaluation of outcomes with citalopram for depression using measurement-based care in STAR*D: implications for clinical practice. Am J Psychiatry 2006;163:28–40.
4. Rush AJ et al. Bupropion-SR, sertraline, or venlafaxine-XR after failure of SSRIs for depression. N Engl J Med 2006;354:1231–42.
5. Trivedi MH et al. Medication augmentation after the failure of SSRIs for depression. N Engl J Med 2006;354:1243–52.
6. Fava M et al. A comparison of mirtazapine and nortriptyline following two consecutive failed medication treatments for depressed outpatients: a STAR*D report. Am J Psychiatry 2006;163:1161–72.
7. Nierenberg AA et al. A comparison of lithium and T(3) augmentation following two failed medication treatments for depression: a STAR*D report. Am J Psychiatry 2006;163:1519–30.
8. McGrath PJ et al. Tranylcypromine versus venlafaxine plus mirtazapine following three failed antidepressant medication trials for depression: a STAR*D report. Am J Psychiatry 2006;163:1531–41.
9. Fava M et al. Lithium and tricyclic augmentation of fluoxetine treatment for resistant major depression: a double-blind, controlled study. Am J Psychiatry 1994;151:1372–4.
10. Dinan TG. Lithium augmentation in sertraline-resistant depression: a preliminary dose–response study. Acta Psychiatr Scand 1993;88:300–1.
11. Bauer M et al. Lithium augmentation in treatment-resistant depression: meta-analysis of placebo-controlled studies. J Clin Psychopharmacol 1999;19:427–34.
12. Folkerts HW et al. Electroconvulsive therapy vs. paroxetine in treatment-resistant depression – a randomized study. Acta Psychiatr Scand 1997;96:334–42.
13. Gonzalez-Pinto A et al. Efficacy and safety of venlafaxine-ECT combination in treatment-resistant depression. J Neuropsychiatry Clin Neurosci 2002;14:206–9.
14. Eranti S et al. A randomized, controlled trial with 6-month follow-up of repetitive transcranial magnetic stimulation and electroconvulsive therapy for severe depression. Am J Psychiatry 2007; 164:73–81.
15. Poirier MF et al. Venlafaxine and paroxetine in treatment-resistant depression. Double-blind, randomised comparison. Br J Psychiatry 1999;175:12–16.
16. Nierenberg AA et al. Venlafaxine for treatment-resistant unipolar depression. J Clin Psychopharmacol 1994;14:419–23.
17. Smith D et al. Efficacy and tolerability of venlafaxine compared with selective serotonin reuptake inhibitors and other antidepressants: a meta-analysis. Br J Psychiatry 2002;180:396–404.
18. Joffe RT et al. A comparison of triiodothyronine and thyroxine in the potentiation of tricyclic antidepressants. Psychiatry Res 1990;32:241–51.
19. Anderson IM. Drug treatment of depression: reflections on the evidence. Adv Psychiatr Treat 2003; 9:11–20.
20. Iosifescu DV et al. An open study of triiodothyronine augmentation of selective serotonin reuptake inhibitors in treatment-resistant major depressive disorder. J Clin Psychiatry 2005;66: 1038–42.
21. Abraham G et al. T3 augmentation of SSRI resistant depression. J Affect Disord 2006;91:211–15.
22. Zisook S et al. Use of bupropion in combination with serotonin reuptake inhibitors. Biol Psychiatry 2006;59:203–10.
23. Fatemi SH et al. Venlafaxine and bupropion combination therapy in a case of treatment-resistant depression. Ann Pharmacother 1999;33:701–3.
24. Pierre JM et al. Bupropion–tranylcypromine combination for treatment-refractory depression. J Clin Psychiatry 2000;61:450–1.
25. Lam RW et al. Citalopram and bupropion-SR: combining versus switching in patients with treatment-resistant depression. J Clin Psychiatry 2004;65:337–40.
26. Papakostas GI et al. The combination of duloxetine and bupropion for treatment-resistant major depressive disorder. Depress Anxiety 2006;23:178–81.
27. Bakish D. Fluoxetine potentiation by buspirone: three case histories. Can J Psychiatry 1991;36: 749–50.
28. Onder E et al. Faster response in depressive patients treated with fluoxetine alone than in combination with buspirone. J Affect Disord 2003;76:223–7.
29. Appelberg BG et al. Patients with severe depression may benefit from buspirone augmentation of selective serotonin reuptake inhibitors: results from a placebo-controlled, randomized, double-blind, placebo wash-in study. J Clin Psychiatry 2001;62:448–52.
30. Carpenter LL et al. A double-blind, placebo-controlled study of antidepressant augmentation with mirtazapine. Biol Psychiatry 2002;51:183–8.
31. Carpenter LL et al. Mirtazapine augmentation in the treatment of refractory depression. J Clin Psychiatry 1999;60:45–9.

32. Ferreri M et al. Benefits from mianserin augmentation of fluoxetine in patients with major depression non-responders to fluoxetine alone. Acta Psychiatr Scand 2001;103:66–72.
33. Lam RW et al. Combining antidepressants for treatment-resistant depression: a review. J Clin Psychiatry 2002;63:685–93.
34. Stimpson N et al. Randomised controlled trials investigating pharmacological and psychological interventions for treatment-refractory depression. Systematic review. Br J Psychiatry 2002;181: 284–94.

Treatment of refractory depression

Table Second choice: less commonly used, variably supported by published evaluations (no preference implied by order)

Treatment	Advantages	Disadvantages	Refs
Add **lamotrigine** (aim for 200 mg/day but lower doses may be effective)	• Reasonably well researched • Quite widely used • Probably more robust data for bipolar depression	• Slow titration • Risk of rash • Appropriate dosing unclear (higher doses used)	1–5
Add **pindolol** (5 mg t.d.s. or 7.5 mg once daily)	• Well tolerated • Can be initiated in primary care • Reasonably well researched (but combined with SSRIs, trazodone, venlafaxine only)	• Data mainly relate to acceleration of response • Refractory data contradictory – some negative studies • Appropriate dosing unclear – higher doses may be more effective	6–10
Combine **olanzapine** and **fluoxetine** (12.5 mg + 50 mg daily)	• Well researched • Usually well tolerated	• Expensive • Risk of weight gain • Limited clinical experience in UK	11–15
Combine **MAOI** and **TCA** (e.g. trimipramine + phenelzine)	• Widely used in 1960s and 1970s • Inexpensive	• Potential for severe interaction • Needs specialist referral • Becoming less popular	16,17
Add **tryptophan** 2–3 g t.d.s.	• Usually well tolerated • Established treatment option	• Theoretical risk of eosinophilia – myalgia syndrome • Data relate mainly to combination with tricyclics/MAOIs • Risk of serotonin syndrome • Becoming less popular	18–22

Depression & anxiety

References

1. Calabrese JR et al. A double-blind placebo-controlled study of lamotrigine monotherapy in outpatients with bipolar I depression. Lamictal 602 Study Group. J Clin Psychiatry 1999;60:79–88.
2. Maltese TM. Adjunctive lamotrigine treatment for major depression. Am J Psychiatry 1999;156:1833.
3. Normann C et al. Lamotrigine as adjunct to paroxetine in acute depression: a placebo-controlled, double-blind study. J Clin Psychiatry 2002;63:337–44.
4. Barbee JG et al. Lamotrigine as an augmentation agent in treatment-resistant depression. J Clin Psychiatry 2002;63:737–41.
5. Barbosa L et al. A double-blind, randomized, placebo-controlled trial of augmentation with lamotrigine or placebo in patients concomitantly treated with fluoxetine for resistant major depressive episodes. J Clin Psychiatry 2003;64:403–7.
6. Rabiner EA et al. Pindolol augmentation of selective serotonin reuptake inhibitors: PET evidence that the dose used in clinical trials is too low. Am J Psychiatry 2001;158:2080–2.
7. McAskill R et al. Pindolol augmentation of antidepressant therapy. Br J Psychiatry 1998;173:203–8.
8. Räsänen P et al. Mitchell B. Balter Award – 1998. Pindolol and major affective disorders: a three-year follow-up study of 30,485 patients. J Clin Psychopharmacol 1999;19:297–302.
9. Perry EB et al. Pindolol augmentation in depressed patients resistant to selective serotonin reuptake inhibitors: a double-blind, randomized, controlled trial. J Clin Psychiatry 2004;65:238–43.
10. Sokolski KN et al. Once-daily high-dose pindolol for SSRI-refractory depression. Psychiatry Res 2004; 125:81–6.
11. Dube S et al. Meta-analysis of olanzapine/fluoxetine use in treatment-resistant depression. Poster presented at: 15th European College of Neuropsychopharmacology, 5–9 October 2002, Barcelona, Spain.
12. Corya SA et al. Long-term antidepressant efficacy and safety of olanzapine/fluoxetine combination: a 76-week open-label study. J Clin Psychiatry 2003;64:1349–56.
13. Corya SA et al. Safety meta-analysis of olanzapine/fluoxetine combination versus fluoxetine. Poster presented at: 15th European College of Neuropsychopharmacology, 5–9 October 2002, Barcelona, Spain.
14. Shelton RC et al. Olanzapine/fluoxetine combination for treatment-resistant depression: a controlled study of SSRI and nortriptyline resistance. J Clin Psychiatry 2005;66:1289–97.
15. Corya SA et al. A randomized, double-blind comparison of olanzapine/fluoxetine combination, olanzapine, fluoxetine, and venlafaxine in treatment-resistant depression. Depress Anxiety 2006;23:364–72.
16. White K et al. The combined use of MAOIs and tricyclics. J Clin Psychiatry 1984;45:67–9.
17. Kennedy N et al. Treatment and response in refractory depression: results from a specialist affective disorders service. J Affect Disord 2004;81:49–53.
18. Angst J et al. The treatment of depression with L-5-hydroxytryptophan versus imipramine. Results of two open and one double-blind study. Arch Psychiatr Nervenkr 1977;224:175–86.
19. Alino JJ et al. 5-Hydroxytryptophan (5-HTP) and a MAOI (nialamide) in the treatment of depressions. A double-blind controlled study. Int Pharmacopsychiatry 1976;11:8–15.
20. Hale AS et al. Clomipramine, tryptophan and lithium in combination for resistant endogenous depression: seven case studies. Br J Psychiatry 1987;151:213–17.
21. Young SN. Use of tryptophan in combination with other antidepressant treatments: a review. J Psychiatry Neurosci 1991;16:241–6.
22. Dursun SM et al. The 'dalhousie serotonin cocktail' for treatment-resistant major depressive disorder. J Psychopharmacol 2001;15:136–8.

Depression & anxiety

Treatment of refractory depression

Table Other reported treatments (alphabetical order – no preference implied). Prescribers must familiarise themselves with the primary literature before using these strategies.

Treatment	Comments	References
Add amantadine up to 300 mg/day	Limited data	1
Add aripiprazole 2.5–15 mg/day	Developing database. No RCTs	2–4
Add carbergoline 2 mg/day	Very limited data	5
Add clonazepam 0.5–1.0 mg/day	Use of benzodiazepines is widespread but not well supported	6
Add metyrapone 1 g/day	Data relate to non-refractory illness	7
Add quetiapine around 300 mg/day	Few data, but effective in bipolar depression	8
Add reboxetine 2–8 mg/day	Reasonably well supported augmentation strategy	9–12
Add risperidone 0.5–1.0 mg/day	Limited data but becoming more widely used	13–15
Add yohimbine up to 30 mg/day	Data relate to non-refractory illness	16
Add ziprasidone up to 160 mg/day	Reasonably well supported	17
Dexamethasone 3–4 mg/day	Use for 4 days only. Limited data	18,19
Ketoconazole 400–800 mg/day	Rarely used. Risk of hepatotoxicity	20
Modafanil 100–400 mg/day	Data mainly relate to non-refractory illness. Usually added to antidepressant treatment. May worsen anxiety	21–24
Nortriptyline ± lithium	Re-emergent treatment option	25–28
Oestrogens various regimens	Limited data	29
Omega–3 triglycerides EPA 1–2 g/day	Developing database. Usually added to antidepressant treatment	30–32

Depression & anxiety

Table   (Cont.)

Treatment	Comments	References
Pramipexole 0.125–5 mg/day	Few data in refractory unipolar depression	33
Riluzole 100–200 mg/day	Very limited data	34
S-adenosyl-L-methionine 400 mg/day IM; 1600 mg/day oral	Limited data in refractory depression	35,36
SSRI + TCA	Formerly widely used	37
rTMS	Developing database	38–41
TCA – high dose	Formerly widely used	42
Testosterone gel	Effective in those with low testosterone levels	43
Vagus nerve stimulation	Developing database	44–47
Venlafaxine – high dose up to 600 mg/day	Cardiac monitoring essential	48
Venlafaxine + IV clomipramine	Cardiac monitoring essential	49

References

1. Stryjer R et al. Amantadine as augmentation therapy in the management of treatment-resistant depression. Int Clin Psychopharmacol 2003;18:93–6.
2. Simon JS et al. Aripiprazole augmentation of antidepressants for the treatment of partially responding and nonresponding patients with major depressive disorder. J Clin Psychiatry 2005;66:1216–20.
3. Papakostas GI et al. Aripiprazole augmentation of selective serotonin reuptake inhibitors for treatment-resistant major depressive disorder. J Clin Psychiatry 2005;66:1326–30.
4. Patkar AA et al. An open-label, rater-blinded, augmentation study of aripiprazole in treatment-resistant depression. Prim Care Companion J Clin Psychiatry 2006;8:82–7.
5. Takahashi H et al. Addition of a dopamine agonist, cabergoline, to a serotonin-noradrenalin reuptake inhibitor, milnacipran as a therapeutic option in the treatment of refractory depression: two case reports. Clin Neuropharmacol 2003;26:230–2.
6. Smith WT et al. Short-term augmentation of fluoxetine with clonazepam in the treatment of depression: a double-blind study. Am J Psychiatry 1998;155:1339–45.
7. Jahn H et al. Metyrapone as additive treatment in major depression: a double-blind and placebo-controlled trial. Arch Gen Psychiatry 2004;61:1235–44.
8. Sagud M et al. Quetiapine augmentation in treatment-resistant depression: a naturalistic study. Psychopharmacology 2006;187:511–14.
9. Dursun SM et al. The 'dalhousie serotonin cocktail' for treatment-resistant major depressive disorder. J Psychopharmacol 2001;15:136–8.
10. Devarajan S et al. Citalopram plus reboxetine in treatment-resistant depression. Can J Psychiatry 2000;45:489–90.
11. Rubio G et al. Reboxetine adjunct for partial or nonresponders to antidepressant treatment. J Affect Disord 2004;81:67–72.
12. Lopez-Munoz F et al. Reboxetine addition in patients with mirtazapine-resistant depression: a case series. Clin Neuropharmacol 2006;29:192–6.

13. Ostroff RB et al. Risperidone augmentation of selective serotonin reuptake inhibitors in major depression. J Clin Psychiatry 1999;60:256–9.
14. Stoll AL et al. Tranylcypromine plus risperidone for treatment-refractory major depression. J Clin Psychopharmacol 2000;20:495–6.
15. Rapaport MH et al. Effects of risperidone augmentation in patients with treatment-resistant depression: results of open-label treatment followed by double-blind continuation. Neuropsychopharmacology 2006;31:2505–13.
16. Sanacora G et al. Addition of the alpha2-antagonist yohimbine to fluoxetine: effects on rate of antidepressant response. Neuropsychopharmacology 2004;29:1166–71.
17. Papakostas GI et al. Ziprasidone augmentation of selective serotonin reuptake inhibitors (SSRIs) for SSRI-resistant major depressive disorder. J Clin Psychiatry 2004;65:217–21.
18. Dinan TG et al. Dexamethasone augmentation in treatment-resistant depression. Acta Psychiatr Scand 1997;95:58–61.
19. Bodani M et al. The use of dexamethasone in elderly patients with antidepressant-resistant depressive illness. J Psychopharmacol 1999;13:196–7.
20. Wolkowitz OM et al. Antiglucocorticoid treatment of depression: double-blind ketoconazole. Biol Psychiatry 1999;45:1070–4.
21. DeBattista C et al. A prospective trial of modafinil as an adjunctive treatment of major depression. J Clin Psychopharmacol 2004;24:87–90.
22. Ninan PT et al. Adjunctive modafinil at initiation of treatment with a selective serotonin reuptake inhibitor enhances the degree and onset of therapeutic effects in patients with major depressive disorder and fatigue. J Clin Psychiatry 2004;65:414–20.
23. Menza MA et al. Modafinil augmentation of antidepressant treatment in depression. J Clin Psychiatry 2000;61:378–81.
24. Taneja I et al. A randomized, double-blind, crossover trial of modafinil on mood. J Clin Psychopharmacol 2007;27:76–8.
25. Nierenberg AA et al. Nortriptyline for treatment-resistant depression. J Clin Psychiatry 2003;64:35–9.
26. Nierenberg AA et al. Lithium augmentation of nortriptyline for subjects resistant to multiple antidepressants. J Clin Psychopharmacol 2003;23:92–5.
27. Fava M et al. A comparison of mirtazapine and nortriptyline following two consecutive failed medication treatments for depressed outpatients: a STAR*D report. Am J Psychiatry 2006;163:1161–72.
28. Shelton RC et al. Olanzapine/fluoxetine combination for treatment-resistant depression: a controlled study of SSRI and nortriptyline resistance. J Clin Psychiatry 2005;66:1289–97.
29. Stahl SM. Basic psychopharmacology of antidepressants, part 2. Oestrogen as an adjunct to antidepressant treatment. J Clin Psychiatry 1998;59(Suppl 4):15–24.
30. Peet M et al. A dose-ranging exploratory study of the effects of ethyl-eicosapentaenoate in patients with persistent schizophrenic symptoms. J Psychiatr Res 2002;36:7–18.
31. Su KP et al. Omega-3 fatty acids as a psychotherapeutic agent for a pregnant schizophrenic patient. Eur Neuropsychopharmacol 2001;11:295–9.
32. Nemets B et al. Addition of omega-3 fatty acid to maintenance medication treatment for recurrent unipolar depressive disorder. Am J Psychiatry 2002;159:477–9.
33. Whiskey E et al. Pramipexole in unipolar and bipolar depression. Psychiatr Bull 2004;28:438–40.
34. Zarate CA, Jr. et al. An open-label trial of riluzole in patients with treatment-resistant major depression. Am J Psychiatry 2004;161:171–4.
35. Pancheri P et al. A double-blind, randomized parallel-group, efficacy and safety study of intramuscular S-adenosyl-L-methionine 1,4-butanedisulphonate (SAMe) versus imipramine in patients with major depressive disorder. Int J Neuropsychopharmacol 2002;5:287–94.
36. Alpert JE et al. S-adenosyl-L-methionine (SAMe) as an adjunct for resistant major depressive disorder: an open trial following partial or nonresponse to selective serotonin reuptake inhibitors or venlafaxine. J Clin Psychopharmacol 2004;24:661–4.
37. Taylor D. Selective serotonin reuptake inhibitors and tricyclic antidepressants in combination – interactions and therapeutic uses. Br J Psychiatry 1995;167:575–80.
38. Huang CC et al. An open trial of daily left prefrontal cortex repetitive transcranial magnetic stimulation for treating medication-resistant depression. Eur Psychiatry 2004;19:523–4.
39. Su TP et al. Add-on rTMS for medication-resistant depression: a randomized, double-blind, sham-controlled trial in Chinese patients. J Clin Psychiatry 2005;66:930–7.
40. Fitzgerald PB et al. A randomized trial of low-frequency right-prefrontal-cortex transcranial magnetic stimulation as augmentation in treatment-resistant major depression. Int J Neuropsychopharmacol 2006;9:655–66.
41. Fitzgerald PB et al. A randomized, controlled trial of sequential bilateral repetitive transcranial magnetic stimulation for treatment-resistant depression. Am J Psychiatry 2006;163:88–94.
42. Malhi GS et al. Management of resistant depression. Int J Psychiatry Clin Pract 1997;1:269–76.
43. Pope HG Jr. et al. Testosterone gel supplementation for men with refractory depression: a randomized, placebo-controlled trial. Am J Psychiatry 2003;160:105–11.
44. Matthews K et al. Vagus nerve stimulation and refractory depression: please can you switch me on doctor? Br J Psychiatry 2003;183:181–3.
45. George MS et al. Vagus nerve stimulation for the treatment of depression and other neuropsychiatric disorders. Expert Rev Neurother 2007;7:63–74.

Depression & anxiety

46. Corcoran CD et al. Vagus nerve stimulation in chronic treatment-resistant depression: preliminary findings of an open-label study. Br J Psychiatry 2006;189:282–3.
47. Nemeroff CB et al. VNS therapy in treatment-resistant depression: clinical evidence and putative neurobiological mechanisms. Neuropsychopharmacology 2006;31:1345–55.
48. Harrison CL et al. Tolerability of high-dose venlafaxine in depressed patients. J Psychopharmacol 2004;18:200–4.
49. Fountoulakis KN et al. Combined oral venlafaxine and intravenous clomipramine-A: successful temporary response in a patient with extremely refractory depression. Can J Psychiatry 2004;49:73–4.

Psychotic depression

Although TCAs are probably more effective than newer antidepressants in the treatment of psychotic depression[1], the response rate is poorer than in patients with non-psychotic major depression: one meta-analysis found rates to be 35% and 67%, respectively[2]. A combination of an antidepressant and an antipsychotic is more effective than an antipsychotic alone but it is not clear if it is more effective than an antidepressant alone[1].

There are few studies of newer antidepressants and atypical antipsychotics, either alone or in combination, specifically for psychotic depression. A large RCT showed response rates of 64% for combined olanzapine and fluoxetine compared with 35% for olanzapine alone and 28% for placebo[3]. There was no fluoxetine-alone group.

Long-term outcome is generally poorer for psychotic than non-psychotic depression[4]. Patients with psychotic depression may also have a poorer response to combined pharmacological and psychological treatment than those with non-psychotic depression[5].

Psychotic depression is one of the indications for ECT. Not only is ECT effective, but also it may be more protective against relapse in psychotic depression than in non psychotic depression[6].

Novel approaches being developed include those based on antiglucocorticoid strategies; one small open study found rapid effects of the glucocorticoid receptor antagonist mifepristone[7], although these findings have been criticised[8].

There is no specific indication for other therapies or augmentation strategies in psychotic depression over and above that for resistant depression or psychosis described elsewhere.

References

1. Wijkstra JAAP et al. Pharmacological treatment for unipolar psychotic depression: systematic review and meta-analysis. Br J Psychiatry 2006;188:410–15.
2. Chan CH et al. Response of psychotic and nonpsychotic depressed patients to tricyclic antidepressants. J Clin Psychiatry 1987;48:197–200.
3. Rothschild AJ et al. A double-blind, randomized study of olanzapine and olanzapine/fluoxetine combination for major depression with psychotic features. J Clin Psychopharmacol 2004;24:365–73.
4. Flint AJ et al. Two-year outcome of psychotic depression in late life. Am J Psychiatry 1998;155:178–83.
5. Gaudiano BA et al. Differential response to combined treatment in patients with psychotic versus nonpsychotic major depression. J Nerv Ment Dis 2005;193:625–8.
6. Birkenhager TK et al. One-year outcome of psychotic depression after successful electroconvulsive therapy. J ECT 2005;21:221–6.
7. Belanoff JK et al. An open label trial of C-1073 (mifepristone) for psychotic major depression. Biol Psychiatry 2002;52:386–92.
8. Rubin RT. Dr. Rubin replies (Letter). Am J Psychiatry 2004;161:1722.

Further reading

Tyrka AR et al. Psychotic major depression: a benefit–risk assessment of treatment options. Drug Saf 2006;29:491–508.

Depression & anxiety

Electroconvulsive therapy (ECT) and psychotropics

The table below summarises the effect of various psychotropics on seizure duration during ECT. Note that there are few well-controlled studies in this area and so recommendations should be viewed with this in mind. Note also that choice of anaesthetic agent profoundly affects seizure duration[1-5].

Drug	Effect on ECT seizure duration	Comments[6-21]
Benzodiazepines	Reduced	All may raise seizure threshold and so should be avoided where possible. Many are long-acting and may need to be discontinued some days before ECT. Benzodiazepines may also complicate anaesthesia
		If sedation is required, consider hydroxyzine. If very long term and essential, continue benzodiazepine and use higher stimulus
SSRIs	Minimal effect; small increase possible	Generally considered safe to use during ECT. Beware complex pharmacokinetic interactions with anaesthetic agents
Venlafaxine	Minimal effect at standard doses	Limited data suggest no effect on seizure duration but possibility of increased risk of asystole with doses above 300 mg/day. Clearly epileptogenic in higher doses. ECG advised
TCAs	Possibly increased	Few data relevant to ECT but many TCAs lower seizure threshold. TCAs are associated with arrhythmia following ECT and should be avoided in elderly patients and those with cardiac disease. In others, it is preferable to continue TCA treatment during ECT. Close monitoring is essential. Beware hypotension
MAOIs	Minimal effect	Data relating to ECT very limited but long history of ECT use during MAOI therapy
		MAOIs probably do not affect seizure duration but interactions with sympathomimetics used in anaesthesia are possible and may lead to hypertensive crisis
		MAOIs may be continued during ECT but the anaesthetist must be informed. Beware hypotension

Drug	Effect on ECT seizure duration	Comments[6-21]
Lithium	Possibly increased	Conflicting data on lithium and ECT. The combination may be more likely to lead to delirium and confusion, and some authorities suggest stopping lithium 48 hours before ECT. In the UK, ECT is often used during lithium therapy but starting with a low stimulus and with very close monitoring. The combination is generally well tolerated
		Note that lithium potentiates the effects of non-depolarising neuromuscular blockers such as suxamethonium
Antipsychotics	Variable – increased with phenothiazines	Few published data but widely used. Phenothiazines and clozapine are perhaps most likely to prolong seizures, and some suggest withdrawal before ECT. However, safe concurrent use has been reported. ECT and antipsychotics appear generally to be a safe combination
Anticonvulsants	Reduced	If used as a mood stabiliser, continue but be prepared to use higher energy stimulus (not always required). If used for epilepsy, their effect is to normalise seizure threshold. Interactions are possible. Valproate may prolong the effect of thiopental; carbamazepine may inhibit neuromuscular blockade
Barbiturates	Reduced	All barbiturates reduce seizure duration in ECT but are widely used as sedative anaesthetic agents
		Thiopental and methohexital may be associated with cardiac arrhythmia

Depression & anxiety

For drugs known to lower seizure threshold, treatment is best begun with a low-energy stimulus (50 mC). Staff should be alerted to the possibility of prolonged seizures and IV diazepam should be available. With drugs known to elevate seizure threshold, higher stimuli may, of course, be required. Methods are available to lower seizure threshold or prolong seizures[22], but discussion of these is beyond the scope of this book.

ECT frequently causes confusion and disorientation; more rarely, it causes delirium. Close observation is essential. Very limited data support the use of thiamine (200 mg daily) in reducing post-ECT confusion[23]. Ibuprofen may be used to prevent headache[24].

References

1. Avramov MN et al. The comparative effects of methohexital, propofol, and etomidate for electroconvulsive therapy. Anesth Analg 1995;81:596–602.
2. Stadtland C et al. A switch from propofol to etomidate during an ECT course increases EEG and motor seizure duration. J ECT 2002;18:22–5.
3. Gazdag G et al. Etomidate versus propofol for electroconvulsive therapy in patients with schizophrenia. J ECT 2004;20:225–9.
4. Conca A et al. Etomidate vs. thiopentone in electroconvulsive therapy. An interdisciplinary challenge for anesthesiology and psychiatry. Pharmacopsychiatry 2003;36:94–7.
5. Rasmussen KG et al. Seizure length with sevoflurane and thiopental for induction of general anesthesia in electroconvulsive therapy: a randomized double-blind trial. J ECT 2006; 22:240–2.
6. Bazire S. Psychotropic Drug Directory: The Professionals' Pocket Handbook and Aide Memoire. Salisbury: Fivepin, 2005.
7. Curran S, Freeman CP. ECT and drugs. In Freeman CP, ed. The ECT Handbook – The Second Report of the Royal College of Psychiatrists' Special Committee on ECT, Dorchester: Henry Ling, 1995.
8. Jarvis MR et al. Novel antidepressants and maintenance electroconvulsive therapy: a review. Ann Clin Psychiatry 1992;4:275–84.
9. Kellner CH et al. ECT–drug interactions: a review. Psychopharmacol Bull 1991;27:595–609.
10. Maidment I. The interaction between psychiatric medicines and ECT. Hosp Pharm 1997;4:102–5.
11. Welch CA. Electroconvulsive therapy. In Ciraulo DA, Shader RI, Greenblatt DJ, eds. Drug Interactions in Psychiatry, Baltimore: Williams and Wilkins, 1995:399–414.
12. Gonzalez-Pinto A et al. Efficacy and safety of venlafaxine–ECT combination in treatment-resistant depression. J Neuropsychiatry Clin Neurosci 2002;14:206–9.
13. Naguib M et al. Interactions between psychotropics, anaesthetics and electroconvulsive therapy: implications for drug choice and patient management. CNS Drugs 2002;16:229–47.
14. Jha AK et al. Negative interaction between lithium and electroconvulsive therapy – a case-control study. Br J Psychiatry 1996;168:241–3.
15. Dolenc TJ et al. Electroconvulsive therapy in patients taking monoamine oxidase inhibitors. J ECT 2004;20:258–61.
16. Papakostas YG et al. Administration of citalopram before ECT: seizure duration and hormone responses. J ECT 2000;16:356–60.
17. Dursun SM et al. Effects of antidepressant treatments on first-ECT seizure duration in depression. Prog Neuropsychopharmacol Biol Psychiatry 2001;25:437–43.
18. Baghai TC et al. The influence of concomitant antidepressant medication on safety, tolerability and clinical effectiveness of electroconvulsive therapy. World J Biol Psychiatry 2006;7: 82–90.
19. Nothdurfter C et al. The influence of concomitant neuroleptic medication on safety, tolerability and clinical effectiveness of electroconvulsive therapy. World J Biol Psychiatry 2006;7:162–70.
20. Gazdag G et al. The impact of neuroleptic medication on seizure threshold and duration in electroconvulsive therapy. Ideggyogy Sz 2004;57:385–90.
21. Penland HR et al. Combined use of lamotrigine and electroconvulsive therapy in bipolar depression: a case series. J ECT 2006;22:142–7.
22. Datto C et al. Augmentation of seizure induction in electroconvulsive therapy: a clinical reappraisal. J ECT 2002;18:118–25.
23. Linton CR et al. Using thiamine to reduce post-ECT confusion. Int J Geriatr Psychiatry 2002;17:189–92.
24. Leung M et al. Pretreatment with ibuprofen to prevent electroconvulsive therapy-induced headache. J Clin Psychiatry 2003;64:551–3.

Further reading

National Institute for Clinical Excellence. The clinical effectiveness and cost effectiveness of electroconvulsive therapy (ECT) for depressive illness, schizophrenia, catatonia and mania. Technology Appraisal 59, April 2003.

Patra KK et al. Implications of herbal alternative medicine for electroconvulsive therapy. J ECT 2004; 20:186–94.

Stimulants in depression

Psychostimulants reduce fatigue, promote wakefulness and are mood elevating (as distinct from antidepressant). Amfetamines have been used as treatments for depression since the 1930s[1] and modafinil has been evaluated as an adjunct to standard antidepressants[2]. Amfetamines are now rarely used in depression because of their propensity for the development of tolerance and dependence. Prolonged use of high doses is associated with paranoid psychosis[3]. Modafinil seems not to induce tolerance, dependence or psychosis but lacks the euphoric effects of amfetamines.

Psychostimulants differ importantly from standard antidepressants in that their effects are usually seen within a few hours. Amfetamines may thus be useful where a prompt effect is required and where dependence would not be problematic (e.g. in depression associated with terminal illness). Their use might also be justified in severe, prolonged depression unresponsive to standard treatments (e.g. in those considered for psychosurgery). Modafinil might justifiably be used as an adjunct to antidepressants in a wider range of patients and as a specific treatment for hypersomnia and fatigue.

The table below outlines support (or the absence of it) for the use of psychostimulants in various clinical situations. Careful consideration should be given to the use of any psychostimulant in depression since their short and long-term safety have not been clearly established. The table below should not in itself be considered a recommendation for their use.

Clinical use	Regimens evaluated	Comments	Recommendations
Monotherapy in uncomplicated depression	Modafinil 100–200 mg a day[4,5] Methylphenidate 20–40mg a day[6,7] Dexamphetamine 20mg a day[6]	Case reports only – efficacy unproven Minimal efficacy Minimal efficacy	Standard antidepressants preferred. Avoid psychostimulants as monotherapy in uncomplicated depression
Adjunctive therapy to accelerate response	SSRI + methyl-phenidate 10–20mg a day[8,9] Tricyclic + methyl-phenidate 5–15mg a day[10]	No clear effect on time to response Single open-label trial suggests faster response	Data very limited. Psychostimulants not recommended
Adjunctive therapy in refractory depression	SSRI + modafinil 100–400mg a day[11–15] MAOI + dexamfetamine 7.5–40mg a day[16]	Effect mainly on fatigue and daytime sleepiness. Support by single case series	Data limited. Only modafinil can be recommended and only for specific symptoms
Monotherapy in late-stage terminal cancer	Methylphenidate 5–30mg a day[17–21] Dexamfetamine 2.5–20mg a day[22,23]	Case series and open prospective studies. Beneficial effects seen on mood, fatigue and pain	Useful treatment options in those expected to live only for a few weeks. Best reserved for hospices and other specialist units
Monotherapy for depression in the very old	Methylphenidate 1.25–20mg a day[24,25]	Use supported by two placebo-controlled studies. Rapid effect observed on mood and activity	Recommended only where patients fail to tolerate standard antidepressants or where contra-indications apply
Monotherapy in post-stroke depression	Methylphenidate 5–40mg a day[26–28] Modafinil 100mg/day[29]	Variable support but including a placebo-controlled trial[26]. Effect on mood evident after a few days Single case report	Standard antidepressants preferred. Further investigation required: stimulants may improve cognition and motor function
Monotherapy in depression secondary to medical illness	Methylphenidate 5–20mg/day[30] Dexamfetamine 2.5–30mg/day[31,32]	Limited data	Psychostimulants now not appropriate therapy. Standard antidepressant preferred
Monotherapy in depression and fatigue associated with HIV	Dexamfetamine 2.5–40mg/day[33,34]	Supported by one good, controlled study[34] Beneficial effect on mood and fatigue	Possible treatment option where fatigue is not responsive to standard antidepressants

References

1. Satel SL et al. Stimulants in the treatment of depression: a critical overview. J Clin Psychiatry 1989;50: 241–9.
2. Menza MA et al. Modafinil augmentation of antidepressant treatment in depression. J Clin Psychiatry 2000;61:378–81.
3. Warneke L. Psychostimulants in psychiatry. Can J Psychiatry 1990;35:3–10.
4. Lundt L. Modafinil treatment in patients with measonal affective disorder/ winter depression: An open-label pilot study. J Affect Disord 2004;81:173–8.
5. Kaufman KR et al. Modafinil monotherapy in depression. Eur Psychiatry 2002;17:167–9.
6. Little KY. d-Amphetamine versus methylphenidate effects in depressed inpatients. J Clin Psychiatry 1993;54:349–55.
7. Robin AA et al. A controlled trial of methylphenidate (ritalin) in the treatment of depressive states. J Neurol Neurosurg Psychiatry 1958;21:55–7.
8. Lavretsky H et al. Combined treatment with methylphenidate and citalopram for accelerated response in the elderly: An open trial. J Clin Psychiatry 2003;64:1410–4.
9. Postolache TT et al. Early augmentation of sertraline with methylphenidate. J Clin Psychiatry 1999; 60:123–4.
10. Gwirtsman HE et al. The antidepressant response to tricyclics in major depressives is accelerated with adjunctive use of methylphenidate. Psychopharmacol Bull 1994;30:157–64.
11. DeBattista C et al. Adjunct modafinil for the short-term treatment of fatigue and sleepiness in patients with major depressive disorder: A preliminary double-blind, placebo-controlled study. J Clin Psychiatry 2003;64:1057–64.
12. Fava M et al. A multicenter, placebo-controlled study of modafinil augmentation in partial responders to selective serotonin reuptake inhibitors with persistent fatigue and sleepiness. J Clin Psychiatry 2005;66:85–93.
13. Rasmussen NA et al. Modafinil augmentation in depressed patients with partial response to antidepressants: A pilot study on self-reported symptoms covered by the major depression inventory (MDI) and the symptom checklist (SCL-92). Nord J Psychiatry 2005;59:173–8.
14. DeBattista C et al. A prospective trial of modafinil as an adjunctive treatment of major depression. J Clin Psychopharmacol 2004;24:87–90.
15. Markovitz PJ et al. An open-label trial of modafinil augmentation in patients with partial response to antidepressant therapy. J Clin Psychopharmacol 2003;23:207–9.
16. Fawcett J et al. CNS stimulant potentiation of monoamine oxidase inhibitors in treatment refractory depression. J Clin Psychopharmacol 1991;11:127–32.
17. Fernandez F et al. Methylphenidate for depressive disorders in cancer patients. Psychosomatics 1987; 28:455–61.
18. Macleod AD. Methylphenidate in terminal depression. J Pain Symptom Manage 1998;16:193–8.
19. Homsi J et al. Methylphenidate for depression in hospice practice. Am J Hosp Palliat Care 2000;17: 393–8.
20. Sarhill N et al. Methylphenidate for fatigue in advanced cancer: A prospective open-label pilot study. Am J Hosp Palliat Care 2001;18:187–92.
21. Homsi J et al. A phase II study of methylphenidate for depression in advanced cancer. Am J Hosp Palliat Care 2001;18:403–7.
22. Burns MM et al. Dextroamphetamine treatment for depression in terminally ill patients. Psychosomatics 1994;35:80–3.
23. Olin J et al. Psychostimulants for depression in hospitalized cancer patients. Psychosomatics 1996;37: 57–62.
24. Kaplitz SE. Withdrawn, apathetic geriatric patients responsive to methylphenidate. J Am Geriatr Soc 1975;23:271–6.
25. Wallace AE et al. Double-blind, placebo-controlled trial of methylphenidate in older, depressed, medically ill patients. Am J Psychiatry 1995;152:929–31.
26. Grade C et al. Methylphenidate in early poststroke recovery: A double-blind, placebo-controlled study. Arch Phys Med Rehabil 1998;79:1047–50.
27. Lazarus LW et al. Efficacy and side effects of methylphenidate for poststroke depression. J Clin Psychiatry 1992;53:447–9.
28. Lingam VR et al. Methylphenidate in treating poststroke depression. J Clin Psychiatry 1988;49:151–3.
29. Sugden SG et al. Modafinil monotherapy in poststroke depression. Psychosomatics 2004;45:80–1.
30. Rosenberg PB et al. Methylphenidate in depressed medically ill patients. J Clin Psychiatry 1991;52:263–7.
31. Woods SW et al. Psychostimulant treatment of depressive disorders secondary to medical illness. J Clin Psychiatry 1986;47:12–5.
32. Kaufmann MW et al. The use of d-amphetamine in medically ill depressed patients. J Clin Psychiatry 1982;43:463–4.
33. Wagner GJ et al. Dexamphetamine as a treatment for depression and low energy in AIDS patients: A pilot study. J Psychosom Res 1997;42:407–11.
34. Wagner GJ et al. Effects of dextroamphetamine on depression and fatigue in men with HIV: A double-blind, placebo-controlled trial. J Clin Psychiatry 2000;61:436–40.

Depression & anxiety

209

Antidepressant-induced hyponatraemia

Most antidepressants have been associated with hyponatraemia. The mechanism of this adverse effect is probably the syndrome of inappropriate secretion of antidiuretic hormone (SIADH). Hyponatraemia is a potentially serious adverse effect of antidepressants that demands careful monitoring, particularly in those patients at greatest risk (see table below).

Table Risk factors[1–5]

Old age

Female sex

Low body weight

Low baseline sodium concentration

Some drug treatments (e.g. *diuretics, NSAIDs, carbamazepine, cancer chemotherapy*)

Reduced renal function (*especially acute and chronic renal failure*)

Medical co-morbidity (e.g. *hypothyroidism, diabetes, COPD, hypertension, head injury, CVA, various cancers*)

Warm weather (summer)

Antidepressants

No antidepressant has been shown *not* to be associated with hyponatraemia and most have a reported association[6]. It has been suggested that serotonergic drugs are relatively more likely to cause hyponatraemia[7,8], although this is disputed[9]. None of the newer serotonergic drugs are free of this effect – cases of hyponatraemia have been described with mirtazapine[10,11], escitalopram[12,13] and duloxetine[14]. Noradrenergic antidepressants are clearly linked to hyponatraemia[15–19] but there are notably few reports linking MAOIs to hyponatraemia[20,21].

Monitoring

All patients taking antidepressants should be observed for signs of hyponatraemia (dizziness, nausea, lethargy, confusion, cramps, seizures). Serum sodium should be determined (at baseline and 2 and 4 weeks, and then 3-monthly[22]) for those at high risk of drug-induced hyponatraemia. The high-risk factors are as follows:

- extreme old age (>80 years)
- history of hyponatraemia
- co-therapy with other drugs known to be associated with hyponatraemia (as above)

Depression & anxiety

- reduced renal function (GFR <50 ml/min)
- medical co-morbidity (as above).

Note that hyponatraemia is common in elderly patients, so monitoring is essential[23,24].

Treatment[25]

Withdraw antidepressants immediately (note risk of discontinuation effects which may complicate clinical picture):

- If serum sodium is >125 mmol/l – monitor sodium daily until normal.
- If serum sodium is <125 mmol/l – refer to specialist medical care.

Restarting treatment

- Consider ECT.
- Prescribe a drug from a different class. Consider noradrenergic drugs such as reboxetine and lofepramine or an MAOI such as moclobemide. Begin with a low dose, increasing slowly, and monitor closely. If hyponatraemia recurs and continued antidepressant use is essential, consider water restriction and/or careful use of demeclocycline (see *BNF*).

Other psychotropics

Carbamazepine has a well-known association with SIADH. Note also that antipsychotic use has been linked to hyponatraemia[26–28] (see page 137).

References

1. Spigset O et al. Hyponatremia in relation to treatment with antidepressants: a survey of reports in the World Health Organization data base for spontaneous reporting of adverse drug reactions. Pharmacotherapy 1997;17:348–52.
2. Madhusoodanan S et al. Hyponatraemia associated with psychotropic medications. A review of the literature and spontaneous reports. Adverse Drug React Toxicol Rev 2002;21:17–29.
3. Wilkinson TJ et al. Incidence and risk factors for hyponatraemia following treatment with fluoxetine or paroxetine in elderly people. Br J Clin Pharmacol 1999;47:211–17.
4. McAskill R et al. Psychotropics and hyponatraemia. Psychiatr Bull 1997;21:33–5.
5. Jacob S et al. Hyponatremia associated with selective serotonin-reuptake inhibitors in older adults. Ann Pharmacother 2006;40:1618–22.
6. Thomas A et al. Hyponatraemia and the syndrome of inappropriate antidiuretic hormone secretion associated with drug therapy in psychiatric patients. CNS Drugs 1995;5:357–69.
7. Movig KL et al. Serotonergic antidepressants associated with an increased risk for hyponatraemia in the elderly. Eur J Clin Pharmacol 2002;58:143–8.
8. Movig KL et al. Association between antidepressant drug use and hyponatraemia: a case-control study. Br J Clin Pharmacol 2002;53:363–9.
9. Kirby D et al. Hyponatraemia and selective serotonin re-uptake inhibitors in elderly patients. Int J Geriatr Psychiatry 2001;16:484–93.
10. Bavbek N et al. Recurrent hyponatremia associated with citalopram and mirtazapine. Am J Kidney Dis 2006;48:e61–e62.
11. Ladino M et al. Mirtazapine-induced hyponatremia in an elderly hospice patient. J Palliat Med 2006; 9:258–60.
12. Grover S et al. Escitalopram-associated hyponatremia. Psychiatry Clin Neurosci 2007;61:132–3.
13. Covyeou JA et al. Hyponatremia associated with escitalopram. N Engl J Med 2007;356:94–5.
14. Kruger S et al. Duloxetine and hyponatremia: a report of 5 cases. J Clin Psychopharmacol 2007;27: 101–4.
15. O'Sullivan D et al. Hyponatraemia and lofepramine. Br J Psychiatry 1987;150:720–1.
16. Wylie KR et al. Lofepramine-induced hyponatraemia. Br J Psychiatry 1989;154:419–20.
17. Ranieri P et al. Reboxetine and hyponatremia. N Engl J Med 2000;342:215–16.
18. Miller MG. Tricyclics as a possible cause of hyponatremia in psychiatric patients. Am J Psychiatry 1989;146:807.
19. Colgate R. Hyponatraemia and inappropriate secretion of antidiuretic hormone associated with the use of imipramine. Br J Psychiatry 1993;163:819–22.
20. Mercier S et al. Severe hyponatremia induced by moclobemide (in French). Therapie 1997;52:82–3.
21. Peterson JC et al. Inappropriate antidiuretic hormone secondary to a monamine oxidase inhibitor. JAMA 1978;239:1422–3.
22. Arinzon ZH et al. Delayed recurrent SIADH associated with SSRIs. Ann Pharmacother 2002;36: 1175–7.
23. Fabian TJ et al. Paroxetine-induced hyponatremia in older adults: a 12-week prospective study. Arch Intern Med 2004;164:327–32.
24. Fabian TJ et al. Paroxetine-induced hyponatremia in the elderly due to the syndrome of inappropriate secretion of antidiuretic hormone (SIADH). J Geriatr Psychiatry Neurol 2003;16:160–4.
25. Sharma H et al. Antidepressant-induced hyponatraemia in the aged. Avoidance and management strategies. Drugs Aging 1996;8:430–5.
26. Ohsawa H et al. An epidemiological study on hyponatremia in psychiatric patients in mental hospitals in Nara Prefecture. Jpn J Psychiatry Neurol 1992;46:883–9.
27. Leadbetter RA et al. Differential effects of neuroleptics and clozapine on polydipsia and intermittent hyponatremia. J Clin Psychiatry 1994;55(Suppl B):110–13.
28. Collins A et al. SIADH induced by two atypical antipsychotics. Int J Geriat Psychiatry 2000;15:282–3.

Depression & anxiety

Post-stroke depression

Post-stroke depression is a common problem seen in at least 30–40% of survivors of intracerebral haemorrhage[1,2]. Depression probably slows functional rehabilitation[3], but antidepressants may be beneficial through relieving depressive symptoms and allowing faster rehabilitation[4].

Prophylaxis

The high incidence of depression after stroke makes prophylaxis worthy of consideration. Nortriptyline, fluoxetine and sertraline may prevent post-stroke depression[5,6], but data are very limited. Mianserin seems ineffective[7] but mirtazapine may protect against depressive episodes and treat them[8]. Amitriptyline appears to prevent central post-stroke pain[9].

Treatment

Treatment is complicated by medical co-morbidity and by the potential for interaction with other co-prescribed drugs (especially warfarin). Contrain-dication to antidepressant treatment seems to be substantially more likely with tricyclics than with SSRIs[10]. Fluoxetine[11], citalopram[12] and nortriptyline[13] are probably the most studied and seem to be effective. SSRIs and nortripty-line are widely recommended for post-stroke depression. Reboxetine may also be effective and well tolerated[14]. Despite early fears, SSRIs seem not to increase risk of stroke[15], although some doubt remains[16]. (Stroke can be embolic or haemorrhagic – SSRIs may protect against the former and provoke the latter.) Antidepressants are clearly effective in post-stroke depression[17] and treatment should not usually be withheld.

Post-stroke depression – recommended drugs

> **SSRIs***
> **Nortriptyline**

* If patient is also taking warfarin, suggest citalopram[18].

References

1. Gainotti G et al. Relation between depression after stroke, antidepressant therapy, and functional recovery. J Neurol Neurosurg Psychiatry 2001;71:258–61.
2. Hayee MA et al. Depression after stroke – analysis of 297 stroke patients. Bangladesh Med Res Counc Bull 2001;27:96–102.
3. Paolucci S et al. Post-stroke depression, antidepressant treatment and rehabilitation results. A case-control study. Cerebrovasc Dis 2001;12:264–71.
4. Gainotti G et al. Determinants and consequences of post-stroke depression. Curr Opin Neurol 2002; 15:85–9.
5. Narushima K et al. Preventing poststroke depression: a 12-week double-blind randomized treatment trial and 21-month follow-up. J Nerv Ment Dis 2002;190:296–303.
6. Rasmussen A et al. A double-blind, placebo-controlled study of sertraline in the prevention of depression in stroke patients. Psychosomatics 2003;44:216–21.
7. Palomaki H et al. Prevention of poststroke depression: 1 year randomised placebo controlled double blind trial of mianserin with 6 month follow up after therapy. J Neurol Neurosurg Psychiatry 1999;66:490–4.
8. Niedermaier N et al. Prevention and treatment of poststroke depression with mirtazapine in patients with acute stroke. J Clin Psychiatry 2004;65:1619–23.
9. Lampl C et al. Amitriptyline in the prophylaxis of central poststroke pain. Preliminary results of 39 patients in a placebo-controlled, long-term study. Stroke 2002;33:3030–2.
10. Cole MG et al. Feasibility and effectiveness of treatments for post-stroke depression in elderly inpatients: systematic review. J Geriatr Psychiatry Neurol 2001;14:37–41.
11. Wiart L et al. Fluoxetine in early poststroke depression: a double-blind placebo-controlled study. Stroke 2000;31:1829–32.
12. Andersen G et al. Effective treatment of poststroke depression with the selective serotonin reuptake inhibitor citalopram. Stroke 1994;25:1099–104.
13. Robinson RG et al. Nortriptyline versus fluoxetine in the treatment of depression and in short-term recovery after stroke: a placebo-controlled, double-blind study. Am J Psychiatry 2000;157:351–9.
14. Rampello L et al. An evaluation of efficacy and safety of reboxetine in elderly patients affected by "retarded" post-stroke depression. A random, placebo-controlled study. Arch Gerontol Geriatr 2005; 40:275–85.
15. Bak S et al. Selective serotonin reuptake inhibitors and the risk of stroke: a population-based case-control study. Stroke 2002;33:1465–73.
16. Ramasubbu R. SSRI treatment-associated stroke: causality assessment in two cases. Ann Pharmacother 2004;38:1197–201.
17. Chen Y et al. Treatment effects of antidepressants in patients with post-stroke depression: a meta-analysis. Ann Pharmacother 2006;40:2115–22.
18. Sayal KS et al. Psychotropic interactions with warfarin. Acta Psychiatr Scand 2000;102:250–5.

Depression & anxiety

SSRIs and bleeding

Serotonin is released from platelets in response to vascular injury and promotes vasoconstriction and morphological changes in platelets that lead to aggregation[1]. Serotonin is a relatively weak platelet aggregator on its own: the presence of epinephrine, collagen and adenosine diphosphate are required for effective clotting[2]. Platelets cannot synthesise serotonin – it is taken up by active transport. Selective serotonin reuptake inhibitors (SSRIs) inhibit the serotonin transporter, which is responsible for the uptake of serotonin into platelets. It might thus be predicted that SSRIs will deplete platelet serotonin, leading to a reduced ability to form clots and a subsequent increase in the risk of bleeding.

Database studies have found that patients who take SSRIs are at three-fold increased risk of being admitted to hospital with an upper gastrointestinal (GI) bleed compared with age- and sex-matched controls[3,4]. The risk is greatest with SSRIs that have a high affinity for the serotonin transporter[5]. Risk decreases to the same level as controls in past users of SSRIs, indicating that bleeding is likely to be associated with treatment rather than some inherent characteristic of the patients being treated[4]. The association also holds when age, gender and the effects of other drugs such as aspirin and non-steroidal anti-inflammatory drugs (NSAIDs) are controlled for. Co-prescription of low-dose aspirin doubles the risk associated with SSRIs alone and co-prescription of NSAIDs quadruples risk[5]. The elderly and those with a history of GI bleeding are at greatest risk[6].

The excess risk of bleeding is not confined to upper GI bleeds. The risk of lower GI bleeds may also be increased[7] and an increased risk of uterine bleeding has also been reported[8].

One study[9] found that patients prescribed SSRIs who underwent orthopaedic surgery had an almost four-fold risk of requiring a blood transfusion. This equated to one additional patient requiring transfusion for every 10 SSRI patients undergoing surgery and was double the risk of patients who were taking NSAIDs alone. It should be noted in this context that treatment with SSRIs has been associated with a 2.4-fold increase in the risk of hip fracture[10] and a two-fold increase of fracture in old age[11]. The combination of advanced age, SSRI treatment, orthopaedic surgery and NSAIDs clearly presents a very high risk.

SSRIs should be used cautiously in patients with cirrhosis or other risk factors for internal bleeding[12].

It is likely that SSRIs are responsible for an additional three episodes of bleeding in every 1000 patient-years of treatment over the normal background incidence[4,8], but this figure masks large variations in risk: for example, 1 in 85 patients with a history of GI bleed will have a further bleed attributable to treatment with a SSRI[6].

Gastroprotective agents such as ranitidine and omeprazole have not been shown to reduce the risk of bleeds associated with SSRIs. No studies have been done. However, lack of evidence for gastroprotective drugs in reducing NSAID-associated bleeds does not prevent them being recommended in high-risk patients. Until studies are conducted, it would seem reasonable to add SSRIs to the list of drugs that increase the risk of NSAID-induced bleeds and to consider the use of gastroprotection in these patients.

Some studies have been prompted by the hypothesis that the increased risk of upper GI bleeds associated with SSRIs may be balanced by a decreased risk of embolic events. One database study failed to find a reduction in the risk of a first myocardial infarction (MI) in SSRI-treated patients compared with controls[13], while another[14] found a reduction in the risk of being admitted to hospital with a first MI in smokers on SSRIs. The effect size in the second study was large: approximately 1 in 10 hospitalisations were avoided in SSRI-treated patients[14]. This is similar to the effect size of other antiplatelet therapies such as aspirin[15]. Two large database studies have failed to find a reduction in the risk of an ischaemic stroke (or increase in the risk of haemorrhagic stroke) in SSRI users[16,17].

Summary

- SSRIs increase the risk of bleeding.
- The effect is additive to that produced by aspirin and NSAIDs.
- Gastroprotective acid-reducing drugs should be considered in those patients taking SSRIs with other risk factors for bleeding.

References

1. Skop BP et al. Potential vascular and bleeding complications of treatment with selective serotonin reuptake inhibitors. Psychosomatics 1996;37:12–16.
2. Hergovich N et al. Paroxetine decreases platelet serotonin storage and platelet function in human beings. Clin Pharmacol Ther 2000;68:435–42.
3. de Abajo FJ et al. Association between selective serotonin reuptake inhibitors and upper gastrointestinal bleeding: population based case-control study. BMJ 1999;319:1106–9.
4. Dalton SO et al. Use of selective serotonin reuptake inhibitors and risk of upper gastrointestinal tract bleeding: a population-based cohort study. Arch Intern Med 2003;163:59–64.
5. Paton C et al. SSRIs and gastrointestinal bleeding. BMJ 2005;331:529–30.
6. van Walraven C et al. Inhibition of serotonin reuptake by antidepressants and upper gastrointestinal bleeding in elderly patients: retrospective cohort study. BMJ 2001;323:655–8.
7. Wessinger S et al. Increased use of selective serotonin reuptake inhibitors in patients admitted with gastrointestinal haemorrhage: a multicentre retrospective analysis. Aliment Pharmacol Ther 2006; 23:937–44.
8. Meijer WE et al. Association of risk of abnormal bleeding with degree of serotonin reuptake inhibition by antidepressants. Arch Intern Med 2004;164:2367–70.
9. Movig KL et al. Relationship of serotonergic antidepressants and need for blood transfusion in orthopedic surgical patients. Arch Intern Med 2003;163:2354–8.
10. Liu B et al. Use of selective serotonin-reuptake inhibitors of tricyclic antidepressants and risk of hip fractures in elderly people. Lancet 1998;351:1303–7.
11. Richards JB et al. Effect of selective serotonin reuptake inhibitors on the risk of fracture. Arch Intern Med 2007;167:188–94.
12. Weinrieb RM et al. A critical review of selective serotonin reuptake inhibitor-associated bleeding: balancing the risk of treating hepatitis C-infected patients. J Clin Psychiatry 2003;64:1502–10.
13. Meier CR et al. Use of selective serotonin reuptake inhibitors and risk of developing first-time acute myocardial infarction. Br J Clin Pharmacol 2001;52:179–84.
14. Sauer WH et al. Selective serotonin reuptake inhibitors and myocardial infarction. Circulation 2001; 104:1894–8.
15. Antiplatelet Trialists' Collaboration. Collaborative overview of randomised trials of antiplatelet therapy – I: prevention of death, myocardial infarction, and stroke by prolonged antiplatelet therapy in various categories of patients. BMJ 1994;308:81–106.
16. Bak S et al. Selective serotonin reuptake inhibitors and the risk of stroke: a population-based case-control study. Stroke 2002;33:1465–73.
17. Barbui C et al. Past use of selective serotonin reuptake inhibitors and the risk of cerebrovascular events in the elderly. Int Clin Psychopharmacol 2005;20:169–71.

Further reading

Dalton SO et al. SSRIs and upper gastrointestinal bleeding: what is known and how should it influence prescribing? CNS Drugs 2006;20:143–51.

Antidepressants and diabetes mellitus

Depression and diabetes

There is an established link between diabetes and depression. Prevalence rates of co-morbid depressive symptoms in diabetic patients have been reported to range from 9% to 60%, depending on the screening method[1]. Similarly, the findings of a meta-analysis suggest that having diabetes doubles the odds of co-morbid depression[2]. Patients with depression and diabetes have a high number of cardiovascular risk factors and increased mortality[3,4]. A recent review concluded that the presence of depression has a negative impact on metabolic control, and likewise poor metabolic control may worsen depression[5]. Considering all of the above, the treatment of co-morbid depression in patients with diabetes is of vital importance, and drug choice should take into account likely effects on metabolic control (see table).

Effect of antidepressants on glucose homeostasis and weight	
Antidepressant class	**Effect on glucose homeostasis and weight**
SSRIs[6-9]	• Studies indicate that SSRIs have a favourable effect on diabetic parameters in patients with type 2 diabetes • Fluoxetine has been associated with improvement in HbA_{1c} levels, reduced insulin requirements, weight loss and enhanced insulin sensitivity. Its effect on insulin sensitivity is independent of its effect on weight loss • Most evidence with fluoxetine, but evidence for sertraline also looks promising
TCAs[10,11]	• TCAs are associated with increased appetite, weight gain and hyperglycaemia • Nortriptyline improved depression but worsened glycaemic control in diabetic patients in one study. Overall improvement in depression had a beneficial effect on HbA_{1c}
MAOIs[12,13]	• Irreversible MAOIs have a tendency to cause extreme hypoglycaemic episodes and weight gain • No known effects with moclobemide
SNRIs[11,14]	• SNRIs do not appear to disrupt glycaemic control and have minimal impact on weight • Studies of duloxetine in the treatment of diabetic neuropathy show that it has little influence on glycaemic control. No data for depression and diabetes • Limited data on venlafaxine
Mirtazapine, reboxetine and trazodone[1,15]	• Mirtazapine is associated with weight gain, but little is known about its effect in diabetic patients • Mirtazapine does not appear to impair glucose tolerance in non-diabetic depressed patients • No data with trazodone and reboxetine

Recommendations

- All patients with a diagnosis of depression should be screened for diabetes.

In those who are diabetic

- Use SSRIs as first-line treatment; most data support fluoxetine.
- SNRIs are also likely to be safe, but there are fewer supporting data.
- Avoid TCAs and MAOIs if possible, due to their effects on weight and glucose homeostasis.
- Monitor blood glucose carefully when antidepressant treatment is initiated, the dose is changed and after discontinuation.

References

1. Musselman DL et al. Relationship of depression to diabetes types 1 and 2: epidemiology, biology, and treatment. Biol Psychiatry 2003;54:317–29.
2. Anderson RJ et al. The prevalence of comorbid depression in adults with diabetes: a meta-analysis. Diabetes Care 2001;24:1069–78.
3. Katon WJ et al. Cardiac risk factors in patients with diabetes mellitus and major depression. J Gen Intern Med 2004;19:1192–9.
4. Katon WJ et al. The association of comorbid depression with mortality in patients with type 2 diabetes. Diabetes Care 2005;28:2668–72.
5. Lustman PJ et al. Depression in diabetic patients: the relationship between mood and glycemic control. J Diabetes Complications 2005;19:113–22.
6. Maheux P et al. Fluoxetine improves insulin sensitivity in obese patients with non-insulin-dependent diabetes mellitus independently of weight loss. Int J Obes Relat Metab Disord 1997;21:97–102.
7. Gulseren L et al. Comparison of fluoxetine and paroxetine in type II diabetes mellitus patients. Arch Med Res 2005;36:159–65.
8. Lustman PJ et al. Sertraline for prevention of depression recurrence in diabetes mellitus: a randomized, double-blind, placebo-controlled trial. Arch Gen Psychiatry 2006;63:521–9.
9. Gray DS et al. A randomized double-blind clinical trial of fluoxetine in obese diabetics. Int J Obes Relat Metab Disord 1992;16(Suppl 4):S67–S72.
10. Lustman PJ et al. Effects of nortriptyline on depression and glycemic control in diabetes: results of a double-blind, placebo-controlled trial. Psychosom Med 1997;59:241–50.
11. McIntyre RS et al. The effect of antidepressants on glucose homeostasis and insulin sensitivity: synthesis and mechanisms. Expert Opin Drug Saf 2006;5:157–68.
12. Goodnick PJ. Use of antidepressants in treatment of comorbid diabetes mellitus and depression as well as in diabetic neuropathy. Ann Clin Psychiatry 2001;13:31–41.
13. McIntyre RS et al. Mood and psychotic disorders and type 2 diabetes: a metabolic triad. Can J Diab 2005;29:122–32.
14. Raskin J et al. Duloxetine versus routine care in the long-term management of diabetic peripheral neuropathic pain. J Palliat Med 2006;9:29–40.
15. Himmerich H et al. Changes in weight and glucose tolerance during treatment with mirtazapine. Diabetes Care 2006;29:170.

Depression & anxiety

Treatment of depression in the elderly

The prevalence of most physical illnesses increases with age. Many physical problems such as cardiovascular disease, chronic pain and Parkinson's disease are associated with a high risk of depressive illness[1]. The morbidity and mortality associated with depression are increased, as the elderly are more physically frail and therefore more likely to suffer serious consequences from self-neglect (e.g. life-threatening dehydration or hypothermia) and immobility (e.g. venous stasis). Almost 20% of completed suicides occur in the elderly[2].

In common with placebo-controlled studies in younger adults, at least some adequately powered studies in elderly patients have failed to find 'active' antidepressants to be more effective than placebo[3], although it is commonly perceived that the elderly may take longer to respond to antidepressants than younger adults[4]. It may be possible to identify non-responders as early as 4 weeks into treatment[5]. Two studies have found that of elderly people who had recovered from an episode of depression and had received antidepressants for 2 years, 60% relapsed within 2 years if antidepressant treatment was withdrawn[6,7]. This finding held true for first-episode patients. Lower doses of antidepressants may be effective as prophylaxis. Dosulepin (dothiepin) 75 mg/day has been shown to be effective in this regard[8]. There is no evidence to suggest that the response to antidepressants is reduced in the physically ill[9], although outcome in the elderly in general is often suboptimal[10,11].

There is no ideal antidepressant. All are associated with problems (see table on page 222). SSRIs are generally better tolerated than TCAs[12]; they do, however, increase the risk of GI bleeding, particularly in the very elderly and those with established risk factors such as a history of bleeds or treatment with an NSAID[13]. (See page 215.) Ultimately, choice is determined by the individual clinical circumstances of each patient, particularly physical co-morbidity and concomitant medication (both prescribed and 'over the counter').

References

1. Katona C et al. Impact of screening old people with physical illness for depression? Lancet 2000; 356:91–2.
2. Cattell H et al. One hundred cases of suicide in elderly people. Br J Psychiatry 1995;166:451–7.
3. Schatzberg A et al. A double-blind, placebo-controlled study of venlafaxine and fluoxetine in geriatric outpatients with major depression. Am J Geriatr Psychiatry 2006;14:361–70.
4. Paykel ES et al. Residual symptoms after partial remission: an important outcome in depression. Psychol Med 1995;25:1171–80.
5. Mulsant BH et al. What is the optimal duration of a short-term antidepressant trial when treating geriatric depression? J Clin Psychopharmacol 2006;26:113–20.
6. Flint AJ et al. Recurrence of first-episode geriatric depression after discontinuation of maintenance antidepressants. Am J Psychiatry 1999;156:943–5.
7. Reynolds CF III et al. Maintenance treatment of major depression in old age. N Engl J Med 2006; 354:1130–8.
8. Old Age Depression Interest Group. How long should the elderly take antidepressants? A double-blind placebo-controlled study of continuation/prophylaxis therapy with dothiepin. Br J Psychiatry 1993; 162:175–82.
9. Evans M et al. Placebo-controlled treatment trial of depression in elderly physically ill patients. Int J Geriatr Psychiatry 1997;12:817–24.
10. Heeren TJ et al. Treatment, outcome and predictors of response in elderly depressed in-patients. Br J Psychiatry 1997;170:436–40.
11. Tuma TA. Outcome of hospital-treated depression at 4.5 years. An elderly and a younger adult cohort compared. Br J Psychiatry 2000;176:224–8.
12. Mottram P et al. Antidepressants for depressed elderly. Cochrane Database Syst Rev 2006;CD003491.
13. Paton C et al. SSRIs and gastrointestinal bleeding. BMJ 2005;331:529–30.

Further reading

Juurlink DN et al. The risk of suicide with selective serotonin reuptake inhibitors in the elderly. Am J Psychiatry 2006;163:813–21.

Movig KL et al. Serotonergic antidepressants associated with an increased risk of hyponatraemia in the elderly. Eur J Clin Pharmacol 2002;58:143–8.

National Service Framework for Older People. London: Department of Health (a whole supplement dedicated to the use of medicines in older people), 2001.

Pacher P et al. Selective serotonin reuptake inhibitor antidepressants increase the risk of falls and hip fractures in elderly people by inhibiting cardiovascular ion channels. Med Hypotheses 2001;57:469–71.

Spina E et al. Clinically significant drug interactions with antidepressants in the elderly. Drugs Aging 2002;19:299–320.

Van der Wurff FB et al. Electroconvulsive therapy for the depressed elderly. Cochrane Database Syst Rev 2003;CD003593.

Table Antidepressants and the elderly

	Anticholinergic side-effects (urinary retention, dry mouth, blurred vision, constipation)	Postural hypotension	Sedation
Older tricyclics	Variable: moderate with nortriptyline, imipramine and dosulepin (dothiepin). Marked with others	All can cause postural hypotension Dosage titration is required	Variable: from minimal with imipramine to profound with trimipramine
Lofepramine	Moderate, although constipation/sweating can be severe	Can be a problem but generally better tolerated than the older tricyclics	Minimal
SSRIs	Dry mouth can be a problem with paroxetine	Much less of a problem, but an increased risk of falls is documented with SSRIs	Can be a problem with paroxetine Unlikely wth the other SSRIs
Others	Minimal with mirtazapine and venlafaxine. Can be rarely a problem with reboxetine Duloxetine – few effects	Hypotension not a problem with venlafaxine but it can increase BP at higher doses	Mirtazapine, mianserin and trazodone are sedative Duloxetine – neutral effects

Further reading

Pinquart M et al. Treatments for later-life depressive conditions: a meta-analytic comparison of pharma-

Weight gain	Safety in overdose	Other side-effects	Drug interactions
All tricyclics can cause weight gain	Dosulepin and amitriptyline are the most toxic (seizures and cardiac arrhythmia)	Seizures, anticholinergic-induced cognitive impairment	Mainly pharmacodynamic: increased sedation with benzodiazepines, increased hypotension with diuretics, increased constipation with other anticholinergic drugs, etc.
Few data, but lack of spontaneous reports may indicate less potential than the older tricyclics	Relatively safe	Raised LFTs	
Paroxetine and possibly citalopram may cause weight gain Others are weight neutral	Safe with the possible exception of citalopram (one minor metabolite is possibly cardiotoxic)	GI effects and headaches, hyponatraemia, increased risk of GI bleeds in the elderly, orofacial dyskinesia with paroxetine	Fluvoxamine, fluoxetine and paroxetine are potent inhibitors of several hepatic cytochrome enzymes (see page 247). Sertraline is safer and citalopram is the safest
Greatest problem is with mirtazapine	Venlafaxine is more toxic in overdose than SSRIs, but safer than TCAs. Others are relatively safe	Insomnia and hypokalaemia with reboxetine	Duloxetine inhibits CYP2D6 Moclobemide and venlafaxine inhibit CYP450 enzymes Check for potential interactions Reboxetine is safe

cotherapy and psychotherapy. Am J psychiatry 2006;163:1493–501.

Cardiac effects of antidepressants

Drug	Heart rate	Blood pressure	QTc
Tricyclics[1-3]	Increase in heart rate	Postural hypotension	Prolongation of QTc interval
Lofepramine[1,4]	Modest increase in heart rate	Less decrease in postural blood pressure compared with other TCAs	Can possibly prolong QTc interval at higher doses (*desipramine is main metabolite*)
MAOIs[1]	Decrease in heart rate	Postural hypotension. Risk of hypertensive crisis	Unclear but may shorten QTc interval
Fluoxetine[5-7]	Small decrease in mean heart rate	Minimal effect on blood pressure	No effect on QTc interval
Paroxetine[8,9]	Small decrease in mean heart rate	Minimal effect on blood pressure	No effect on QTc interval
Sertraline[10-12]	Minimal effect on heart rate	Minimal effect on blood pressure	No effect on QTc interval
Citalopram[13-15] (assume same for escitalopram)	Small decrease in heart rate	Slight drop in systolic blood pressure	No effect on QTc interval in normal doses. Prolongation in overdose
Fluvoxamine[16]	Minimal effect on heart rate	Small drops in systolic blood pressure	No significant effect on QTc
Venlafaxine[17-20]	Marginally increased	Some increase in postural blood pressure. At higher doses increase in blood pressure	Possible prolongation in overdose
Duloxetine[21-23]	Slight increase	Important effect (see SPC). Caution in hypertension	No effect on QTc
Mirtazapine[24]	Minimal change in heart rate	Minimal effect on blood pressure	No effect on QTc
Reboxetine[25-27]	Significant increase in heart rate	Marginal increase in both systolic and diastolic blood pressure. Postural decrease at higher doses	No effect on QTc
Moclobemide[28-30]	Marginal decrease in heart rate	Minimal effect on blood pressure. Isolated cases of hypertensive episodes	No effect on QTc interval in normal doses. Prolongation in overdose
Trazodone[1]	Decrease in heart rate more common, although increase can also occur	Can cause significant postural hypotension	Can prolong QTc interval

Notes: SSRIs are generally recommended in cardiac disease but beware cytochrome-medicated interactions with co-administered cardiac drugs. SSRIs may protect against myocardial infarction[31], and untreated depression worsens prognosis in cardiovascular disease[32]. Treatment of depression with SSRIs should not therefore be withheld post-MI. Protective effects of treatment of depression post-MI

Depression & anxiety

Arrhythmia	Conduction disturbance	Licensed restrictions post-MI	Comments
Class 1 anti-arrhythmic activity. Ventricular arrhythmia common in overdose	Slows down cardiac conduction – blocks cardiac Na/K channels	CI in patients with recent MI	TCAs affect cardiac contractility. Some TCAs linked to ischaemic heart disease. Association with sudden cardiac death
May occur at higher doses	Benign effect on cardiac conduction	CI in patient with recent MI	Less cardiotoxic than other TCAs. Reasons unclear
May cause arrhythmia and decrease LVF	No clear effect on cardiac conduction	Use with caution in patients with cardiovascular disease	
Few cases reported in literature	None	Caution. Clinical experience is limited	Probably safe post MI
None	None	General caution in cardiac patients	Probably safe post MI
None	None	None – drug of choice	Safe post MI
None	None	Caution, although no ECG changes	Minor metabolite which may ↑ QTc interval. Has been used post MI
None	None	Caution	Limited changes in ECG have been observed
Rare reports of cardiac arrhythima in overdose	Rare reports of conduction abnormalities	Has not been evaluated in post-MI patients. Avoid	Evidence for arrhythmogenic potential is slim
None	None	Caution in patients with recent MI	Limited clinical experience
None	None	Caution in patients with recent MI	
Rhythm abnormalities may occur	Atrial and ventricular ectopic beats, especially in the elderly	Caution in patient with cardiac disease	
None	None	None	Possibly arrhythmogenic in overdose
Several case reports of arrhythmia	May have a minimal effect on cardiac conduction	Care in patients with severe cardiac disease	May be arrhythmogenic in patients with pre-existing cardiac disease

appear to relate to antidepressant administration. CBT may be ineffective in this respect[33]. Note that the mild anticoagulant effect of SSRIs may have adverse consequences too: upper GI bleeding is more common in those taking SSRIs[34].

References

1. Warrington SJ et al. The cardiovascular effects of antidepressants. Psychol Med Monogr Suppl 1989; 16:i–40.
2. Hippisley-Cox J et al. Antidepressants as a risk factor for ischaemic heart disease: case-control study in primary care. BMJ 2001;323:666–9.
3. Whyte IM et al. Relative toxicity of venlafaxine and selective serotonin reuptake inhibitors in overdose compared to tricyclic antidepressants. QJM 2003;96:369–74.
4. Stern H et al. Cardiovascular effects of single doses of the antidepressants amitriptyline and lofepramine in healthy subjects. Pharmacopsychiatry 1985;18:272–7.
5. Fisch C. Effect of fluoxetine on the electrocardiogram. J Clin Psychiatry 1985;46:42–4.
6. Ellison JM et al. Fluoxetine-induced bradycardia and syncope in two patients. J Clin Psychiatry 1990;51:385–6.
7. Roose SP et al. Cardiovascular effects of fluoxetine in depressed patients with heart disease. Am J Psychiatry 1998;155:660–5.
8. Kuhs H et al. Cardiovascular effects of paroxetine. Psychopharmacology 1990;102:379–82.
9. Roose SP et al. Comparison of paroxetine and nortriptyline in depressed patients with ischemic heart disease. JAMA 1998;279:287–91.
10. Shapiro PA et al. An open-label preliminary trial of sertraline for treatment of major depression after acute myocardial infarction (the SADHAT Trial). Sertraline Anti-Depressant Heart Attack Trial. Am Heart J 1999;137:1100–6.
11. Glassman AH et al. Sertraline treatment of major depression in patients with acute MI or unstable angina. JAMA 2002;288:701–9.
12. Winkler D et al. Trazodone-induced cardiac arrhythmias: a report of two cases. Hum Psychopharmacol 2006;21:61–2.
13. Rasmussen SL et al. Cardiac safety of citalopram: prospective trials and retrospective analyses. J Clin Psychopharmacol 1999;19:407–15.
14. Catalano G et al. QTc interval prolongation associated with citalopram overdose: a case report and literature review. Clin Neuropharmacol 2001;24:158–62.
15. Lesperance F et al. Effects of citalopram and interpersonal psychotherapy on depression in patients with coronary artery disease: the Canadian Cardiac Randomized Evaluation of Antidepressant and Psychotherapy Efficacy (CREATE) trial. JAMA 2007;297:367–79.
16. Strik JJ et al. Cardiac side-effects of two selective serotonin reuptake inhibitors in middle-aged and elderly depressed patients. Int Clin Psychopharmacol 1998;13:263–7.
17. Wyeth Pharmaceuticals. Efexor. Summary of Product Characteristics. www.medicines.org.uk. 2006.
18. Khawaja IS et al. Cardiovascular effects of selective serotonin reuptake inhibitors and other novel antidepressants. Heart Dis 2003;5:153–60.
19. Letsas K et al. QT interval prolongation associated with venlafaxine administration. Int J Cardiol 2006;109:116–17.
20. Taylor D et al. Volte-face on venlafaxine – reasons and reflections. J Psychopharmacol 2006;20:597–601.
21. Sharma A et al. Pharmacokinetics and safety of duloxetine, a dual-serotonin and norepinephrine reuptake inhibitor. J Clin Pharmacol 2000;40:161–7.
22. Schatzberg AF. Efficacy and tolerability of duloxetine, a novel dual reuptake inhibitor, in the treatment of major depressive disorder. J Clin Psychiatry 2003;64(Suppl 13):30–7.
23. Detke MJ et al. Duloxetine, 60 mg once daily, for major depressive disorder: a randomized double-blind placebo-controlled trial. J Clin Psychiatry 2002;63:308–15.
24. Montgomery SA. Safety of mirtazapine: a review. Int Clin Psychopharmacol 1995;10(Suppl 4):37–45.
25. Mucci M. Reboxetine: a review of antidepressant tolerability. J Psychopharmacol 1997;11:S33–S37.
26. Holm KJ et al. Reboxetine: a review of its use in depression. CNS Drugs 1999;12:65–83.
27. Fleishaker JC et al. Lack of effect of reboxetine on cardiac repolarization. Clin Pharmacol Ther 2001;70:261–9.
28. Moll E et al. Safety and efficacy during long-term treatment with moclobemide. Clin Neuropharmacol 1994;17(Suppl 1):S74–S87.
29. Hilton S et al. Moclobemide safety: monitoring a newly developed product in the 1990s. J Clin Psychopharmacol 1995;15:76S–83S.
30. Downes MA et al. QTc abnormalities in deliberate self-poisoning with moclobemide. Intern Med J 2005;35:388–91.
31. Sauer WH et al. Selective serotonin reuptake inhibitors and myocardial infarction. Circulation 2001;104:1894–8.
32. Davies SJ et al. Treatment of anxiety and depressive disorders in patients with cardiovascular disease. BMJ 2004;328:939–43.
33. Berkman LF et al. Effects of treating depression and low perceived social support on clinical events after myocardial infarction: the Enhancing Recovery in Coronary Heart Disease Patients (ENRICHD) Randomized Trial. JAMA 2003;289:3106–16.
34. Dalton SO et al. Use of selective serotonin reuptake inhibitors and risk of upper gastrointestinal tract bleeding: a population-based cohort study. Arch Intern Med 2003;163:59–64.

Depression & anxiety

Further reading

Alvarez W et al. Safety of antidepressant drugs in the patient with cardiac disease. A review of the literature. Pharmacotherapy 2003;23:754–71.

Roose SP. Treatment of depression in patients with heart disease. Biol Psychiatry 2003;54:262–8.

Von Kanel R. Platelet hyperactivity in clinical depression and the beneficial effect of antidepressant drug treatment: how strong is the evidence? Acta Psychiatr Scand 2004;110:163–77.

Depression & anxiety

227

Antidepressant-induced arrhythmia

Tricyclic antidepressants (TCAs) have established arrhythmogenic activity that arises as a result of potent blockade of cardiac sodium channels and variable activity at potassium channels[1]. ECG changes produced include PR, QRS and QT prolongation. In patients taking tricyclics, ECG monitoring is a more accurate and useful measure of toxicity than plasma level monitoring. **Lofepramine**, for reasons unknown, seems to lack the arrhythmogenicity of other TCAs. There is limited evidence that **venlafaxine** is a sodium channel antagonist[2] and a weak antagonist at hERG potassium channels. Arrhythmia is a rare occurrence even after massive overdose[3–5] and ECG changes are no more common than with SSRIs[6]. No ECG changes are seen in therapeutic dosing[7]. **Moclobemide**[8], **citalopram**[9,10], **bupropion** (amfebutamone)[11] and **sertraline**[12] have been reported to prolong the QTc interval in overdose but the consequences of this are uncertain. There is clear evidence, uniquely, for sertraline's safety in subjects at risk of arrhythmia following myocardial infarction[13]. Another recent study supports the safety of citalopram in patients with coronary artery disease[14].

Relative cardiotoxicity of antidepressants is difficult to establish with any precision. Yellow Card (ADROIT) data suggest that all marketed antidepressants are associated with arrhythmia (ranging from clinically insignificant to life threatening) and sudden cardiac death. For a substantial proportion of drugs these figures are more likely to reflect coincidence rather than causation. The Fatal Toxicity Index (FTI) may provide some means for comparison. This is a measure of the number of overdose deaths per million (FP10) prescriptions issued. FTI figures suggest high toxicity for tricyclic drugs (especially dosulepin but not lofepramine), medium toxicity for venlafaxine and moclobemide, and low toxicity for SSRIs, mirtazapine and reboxetine[15–19]. However, FTI does not necessarily reflect only cardiotoxicity (antidepressants variously cause serotonin syndrome, seizures and coma) and is, in any case, open to other influences. This is best evidenced in the change in FTI over time. A good example here is nortriptyline, the FTI of which has been estimated at 0.6[16] and 39.2[12] and several values in between[15,16,18]. This change probably reflects changes in the type of patient prescribed nortriptyline. There is good evidence that venlafaxine is relatively more often prescribed to patients with more severe depression and who are relatively more likely to attempt suicide[20,21]. This is likely to inflate venlafaxine's FTI and erroneously suggest greater inherent toxicity.

Summary

- Sertraline is recommended post MI, but other SSRIs are also likely to be safe.
- Bupropion, citalopram, moclobemide, lofepramine and venlafaxine should be used with caution (preferably avoided) in those at risk of serious arrhythmia (those with heart failure, left ventricular hypertrophy; previous arrhythmia or MI). An ECG should be performed at baseline and 1 week after every increase in dose in high risk patients.
- TCAs (with the exception of lofepramine) are best avoided completely in patients at risk of serious arrhythmia. If use of a TCA cannot be avoided, an ECG should be performed at baseline, 1 week after each increase in dose and periodically throughout treatment. Frequency will be determined by the stability of the cardiac disorder and the TCA (and dose) being used; advice from cardiology should be sought.
- The arrhythmogenic potential of TCAs is dose-related. Consideration should be given to ECG monitoring of all patients prescribed doses towards the top of the licensed range and those who are prescribed other drugs that, through pharmacokinetic (e.g. fluoxetine) or pharmacodynamic (e.g. diuretics) mechanisms, may add to the risk posed by the TCA.

Depression & anxiety

References

1. Thanacoody HK et al. Tricyclic antidepressant poisoning: cardiovascular toxicity. Toxicol Rev 2005; 24:205–14.
2. Khalifa M et al. Mechanism of sodium channel block by venlafaxine in guinea pig ventricular myocytes. J Pharmacol Exp Ther 1999;291:280–4.
3. Colbridge MG et al. Venlafaxine in overdose – experience of the National Poisons Information Service (London centre). J Toxicol Clin Toxicol 1999;37:383.
4. Blythe D et al. Cardiovascular and neurological toxicity of venlafaxine. Hum Exp Toxicol 1999; 18:309–13.
5. Combes A et al. Conduction disturbances associated with venlafaxine. Ann Intern Med 2001;134:166–7.
6. Whyte IM et al. Relative toxicity of venlafaxine and selective serotonin reuptake inhibitors in overdose compared to tricyclic antidepressants. QJM 2003;96:369–74.
7. Feighner JP. Cardiovascular safety in depressed patients: focus on venlafaxine. J Clin Psychiatry 1995;56:574–9.
8. Downes MA et al. QTc abnormalities in deliberate self-poisoning with moclobemide. Intern Med J 2005;35:388–91.
9. Kelly CA et al. Comparative toxicity of citalopram and the newer antidepressants after overdose. J Toxicol Clin Toxicol 2004;42:67–71.
10. Grundemar L et al. Symptoms and signs of severe citalopram overdose. Lancet 1997;349:1602.
11. Isbister GK et al. Bupropion overdose: QTc prolongation and its clinical significance. Ann Pharmacother 2003;37:999–1002.
12. de Boer RA et al. QT interval prolongation after sertraline overdose: a case report. BMC Emerg Med 2005;5:5.
13. Glassman AH et al. Sertraline treatment of major depression in patients with acute MI or unstable angina. JAMA 2002;288:701–9.
14. Lesperance F et al. Effects of citalopram and interpersonal psychotherapy on depression in patients with coronary artery disease: the Canadian Cardiac Randomized Evaluation of Antidepressant and Psychotherapy Efficacy (CREATE) trial. JAMA 2007;297:367–79.
15. Crome P. The toxicity of drugs used for suicide. Acta Psychiatr Scand Suppl 1993;371:33–7.
16. Cheeta S et al. Antidepressant-related deaths and antidepressant prescriptions in England and Wales, 1998–2000. Br J Psychiatry 2004;184:41–7.
17. Buckley NA et al. Fatal toxicity of serotoninergic and other antidepressant drugs: analysis of United Kingdom mortality data. BMJ 2002;325:1332–3.

18. Buckley NA et al. Greater toxicity in overdose of dothiepin than of other tricyclic antidepressants. Lancet 1994;343:159–62.
19. Morgan O et al. Fatal toxicity of antidepressants in England and Wales, 1993–2002. Health Stat Q 2004;18–24.
20. Egberts A et al. Channeling of three newly introduced antidepressants to patients not responding satisfactorily to previous treatment. J Clin Psychopharmacol 1997;17:149–55.
21. Mines D et al. Prevalence of risk factors for suicide in patients prescribed venlafaxine, fluoxetine, and citalopram. Pharmacoepidemiol Drug Saf 2005;14:367–72.

Antidepressants and sexual dysfunction

Primary sexual disorders are common, although reliable normative data are lacking[1]. Reported prevalence rates vary depending on the method of data collection (low numbers with spontaneous reports, increasing with confidential questionnaires and further still with direct questioning)[1,2]. Physical illness, psychiatric illness, substance misuse and prescribed drug treatment can all cause sexual dysfunction[1,2]. Baseline sexual functioning should be determined, if possible (questionnaires may be useful), because sexual function can affect quality of life and compliance (sexual dysfunction is one of the major causes of treatment dropout[3]). Complaints of sexual dysfunction may also indicate progression or inadequate treatment of underlying medical or psychiatric conditions. It may also be the result of drug treatment and intervention may greatly improve quality of life[4]. The normal human sexual response is described on page 131.

Effects of depression

Both depression and the drugs used to treat it can cause disorders of desire, arousal and orgasm. The precise nature of the sexual dysfunction may indicate whether depression or treatment is the more likely cause. For example, 40–50% of people with depression report diminished libido and problems regarding sexual arousal in the month before diagnosis, compared with only 15–20% who experience orgasm problems prior to taking an antidepressant[5]. In some patients reporting sexual dysfunction before or at diagnosis, sexual functioning improves on treatment with antidepressants[6]. In any cohort of people with depression there will be some who do not have sexual dysfunction; some, but not all, will develop sexual dysfunction on antidepressants. Amongst those patients presenting with sexual dysfunction, some will see an improvement, some no change and some a worsening when taking an antidepressant[7].

Effects of antidepressant drugs

Antidepressants can cause sedation, hormonal changes, disturbance of cholinergic/adrenergic balance, peripheral alpha-adrenergic antagonism, inhibition of nitric oxide and increased serotonin neurotransmission, all of which can result in sexual dysfunction[8]. Sexual dysfunction has been reported as a side-effect of all antidepressants, although rates vary (see table below). Individual susceptibility also varies and all effects are reversible.

Not all of the sexual side-effects of antidepressants are undesirable[1]: serotonergic antidepressants are effective in the treatment of premature ejaculation and may also be beneficial in paraphilias.

Depression & anxiety

Table Sexual adverse effects of antidepressant drugs

Drug	Approximate prevalence	Type of problem
Tricyclics[9-12]	30%	Decreased libido, erectile dysfunction, delayed orgasm, impaired ejaculation. Prevalence of delayed orgasm with clomipramine may be double that with other TCAs. Painful ejaculation reported rarely
Trazodone[3,13-15]	Unknown	Impaired ejaculation and both increases and decreases in libido reported. Used in some cases to promote erection. Priapism occurs in approximately 0.01%
MAOIs[3,16]	40%	Similar to TCAs, although prevalence may be higher[1]. Moclobemide much less likely to cause problems than older MAOIs (4% vs 40%)
SSRIs[3,17-20]	60–70%	Decreased libido and delayed orgasm. Paroxetine is associated with more erectile dysfunction and decreased vaginal lubrication than the other SSRIs. High prevalence with SSRIs may be due to selective reporting. Difficult to determine relative prevalence but there is evidence that ejaculatory delay is worse with paroxetine than citalopram[21] Penile anaesthesia has been reported rarely with fluoxetine
Venlafaxine[3]	70%	Decreased libido and delayed orgasm common. Erectile dysfunction less common
Mirtazapine[3,18]	25%	Decreased libido and delayed orgasm possible. Erectile dysfunction less common
Reboxetine[22]	5–10%	Various abnormalities of orgasmic function
Duloxetine[23]	46%	Any sexual dysfunction with a score ≥5 on the ASEX scale, with a statistical significance seen for the specific item 'ease of orgasm' in male patients

Treatment

Spontaneous remission occurs in approximately 10% of cases and partial remission in a further 11%[3]. If this does not happen, the dose may be reduced or the antidepressant discontinued where appropriate.

Drug 'holidays' or delayed dosing may be used[24]. This approach is problematic as the patient may relapse or experience antidepressant discontinuation symptoms. More logical is a switch to a different drug that is less likely to cause the specific sexual problem experienced (see table above). Note that amfebutamone (buproprion – not licensed for depression in UK) may have the lowest risk of sexual dysfunction[25,26] among newer antidepressants.

Adjunctive or 'antidote' drugs may also be used (see page 131 for further information).

Sildenafil is more effective than placebo at improving erectile function in men taking serotonin reuptake inhibitors[27].

A Cochrane Review of the 'Strategies for managing sexual dysfunction induced by antidepressant medication' found that the addition of sildenafil, tadalafil or bupropion may improve sexual function but that other augmentation strategies did not[28].

References

1. Baldwin DS et al. Effects of antidepressant drugs on sexual function. Int J Psychiatry Clin Pract 1997; 1:47–58.
2. Pollack MH et al. Genitourinary and sexual adverse effects of psychotropic medication. Int J Psychiatry Med 1992;22:305–27.
3. Montejo AL et al. Incidence of sexual dysfunction associated with antidepressant agents: a prospective multicenter study of 1022 outpatients. Spanish Working Group for the Study of Psychotropic-Related Sexual Dysfunction. J Clin Psychiatry 2001;62(Suppl 3):10–21.
4. Segraves RT. Effects of psychotropic drugs on human erection and ejaculation. Arch Gen Psychiatry 1989;46:275–84.
5. Kennedy SH et al. Sexual dysfunction before antidepressant therapy in major depression. J Affect Disord 1999;56:201–8.
6. Saiz-Ruiz J et al. Assessment of sexual functioning in depressed patients treated with mirtazapine: a naturalistic 6-month study. Hum Psychopharmacol 2005;20:435–40.
7. Werneke U et al. Antidepressants and sexual dysfunction. Acta Psychiatr Scand 2006;114:384–97.
8. Clayton AH. Recognition and assessment of sexual dysfunction associated with depression. J Clin Psychiatry 2001;62(Suppl 3):5–9.
9. Harrison WM et al. Effects of antidepressant medication on sexual function: a controlled study. J Clin Psychopharmacol 1986;6:144–9.
10. Beaumont G. Sexual side-effects of clomipramine (Anafranil). J Int Med Res 1977;5:37–44.
11. Rickels K et al. Nefazodone: aspects of efficacy. J Clin Psychiatry 1995;56(Suppl 6):43–6.
12. Sovner R. Anorgasmia associated with imipramine but not desipramine: case report. J Clin Psychiatry 1983;44:345–6.
13. Gartrell N. Increased libido in women receiving trazodone. Am J Psychiatry 1986;143:781–2.
14. Sullivan G. Increased libido in three men treated with trazodone. J Clin Psychiatry 1988;49:202–3.
15. Thompson JW, Jr. et al. Psychotropic medication and priapism: a comprehensive review. J Clin Psychiatry 1990;51:430–3.
16. Lesko LM et al. Three cases of female anorgasmia associated with MAOIs. Am J Psychiatry 1982;139: 1353–4.
17. Herman JB et al. Fluoxetine-induced sexual dysfunction. J Clin Psychiatry 1990;51:25–7.
18. Gelenberg AJ et al. Mirtazapine substitution in SSRI-induced sexual dysfunction. J Clin Psychiatry 2000;61:356–60.
19. Jacobsen FM. Fluoxetine-induced sexual dysfunction and an open trial of yohimbine. J Clin Psychiatry 1992;53:119–22.
20. Lauerma H. Successful treatment of citalopram-induced anorgasmia by cyproheptadine. Acta Psychiatr Scand 1996;93:69–70.

21. Waldinger MD et al. SSRIs and ejaculation: a double-blind, randomized, fixed-dose study with paroxetine and citalopram. J Clin Psychopharmacol 2001;21:556–60.
22. Haberfellner EM. Sexual dysfunction caused by reboxetine. Pharmacopsychiatry 2002;35:77–8.
23. Delgado PL et al. Sexual functioning assessed in 4 double-blind placebo- and paroxetine-controlled trials of duloxetine for major depressive disorder. J Clin Psychiatry 2005;66:686–92.
24. Rothschild AJ. Selective serotonin reuptake inhibitor-induced sexual dysfunction: efficacy of a drug holiday. Am J Psychiatry 1995;152:1514–16.
25. Clayton AH et al. Prevalence of sexual dysfunction among newer antidepressants. J Clin Psychiatry 2002;63:357–66.
26. Clayton AH et al. Bupropion extended release compared with escitalopram: effects on sexual functioning and antidepressant efficacy in 2 randomized, double-blind, placebo-controlled studies. J Clin Psychiatry 2006;67:736–46.
27. Fava M et al. Efficacy and safety of sildenafil in men with serotonergic antidepressant-associated erectile dysfunction: results from a randomized, double-blind, placebo-controlled trial. J Clin Psychiatry 2006;67:240–6.
28. Rudkin L et al. Strategies for managing sexual dysfunction induced by antidepressant medication. Cochrane Database Syst Rev 2004;CD003382.

Further reading

Fava M et al. Sexual functioning and SSRIs. J Clin Psychiatry 2002;63(Suppl 5):13–16.

Depression &
anxiety

Antidepressants – swapping and stopping

General guidelines

- All antidepressants have the potential to cause withdrawal phenomena. When taken continuously *for 6 weeks or longer*, antidepressants should not be stopped abruptly unless a serious adverse event has occurred (e.g. cardiac arrhythmia with a tricyclic). (See page 228.)
- When changing from one antidepressant to another, abrupt withdrawal should usually be avoided. Cross-tapering is preferred, in which the dose of the ineffective or poorly tolerated drug is slowly reduced while the new drug is slowly introduced.

Example		Week 1	Week 2	Week 3	Week 4
Withdrawing dosulepin	150 mg OD	100 mg OD	50 mg OD	25 mg OD	Nil
Introducing citalopram	Nil	10 mg OD	10 mg OD	20 mg OD	20 mg OD

- The speed of cross-tapering is best judged by monitoring patient tolerability. No clear guidelines are available, so caution is required.
- Note that the co-administration of some antidepressants, even when cross-tapering, is absolutely contraindicated. In other cases, theoretical risks or lack of experience preclude recommending cross-tapering.
- In some cases cross-tapering may not be considered necessary. An example is when switching from one SSRI to another: their effects are so similar that administration of the second drug is likely to ameliorate withdrawal effects of the first.
- Potential dangers of simultaneously administering two antidepressants include pharmacodynamic interactions (serotonin syndrome[1-4], hypotension, drowsiness) and pharmacokinetic interactions (e.g. elevation of tricyclic plasma levels by some SSRIs).

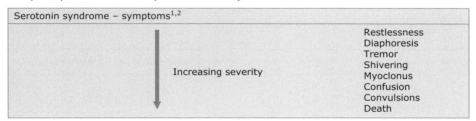

Serotonin syndrome – symptoms[1,2]

Increasing severity

Restlessness
Diaphoresis
Tremor
Shivering
Myoclonus
Confusion
Convulsions
Death

- The advice given in the following table should be treated with caution and patients should be very carefully monitored when switching.

References

1. Sternbach H. The serotonin syndrome. Am J Psychiatry 1991;148:705–13.
2. Mir S et al. Serotonin syndrome. Psychiatr Bull 1999;23:742–7.
3. Pan JJ et al. Serotonin syndrome induced by low-dose venlafaxine. Ann Pharmacother 2003;37:209–11.
4. Houlihan DJ. Serotonin syndrome resulting from coadministration of tramadol, venlafaxine, and mirtazapine. Ann Pharmacother 2004;38:411–13.

Depression & anxiety

Table Antidepressants – swapping and stopping*

To ⟍ From	MAOIs-hydrazines	Tranyl-cypromine[a]	Tricyclics	Citalopram/escitalopram	Fluoxetine	Paroxetine
MAOIs-hydrazines	Withdraw and wait for 2 weeks	Withdraw and wait for 2 weeks	Withdraw and wait for 2 weeks	Withdraw and wait for 2 weeks	Withdraw and wait for 2 weeks	Withdraw and wait for 2 weeks
Tranylcypromine	Withdraw and wait for 2 weeks	–	Withdraw and wait for 2 weeks	Withdraw and wait for 2 weeks	Withdraw and wait for 2 weeks	Withdraw and wait for 2 weeks
Tricyclics	Withdraw and wait for 1 week	Withdraw and wait for 1 week	Cross-taper cautiously	Halve dose and add citalopram then slow withdrawal[c]	Halve dose and add fluoxetine then slow withdrawal[c]	Halve dose and add paroxetine then slow withdrawal[c]
Citalopram/escitalopram	Withdraw and wait for 1 week	Withdraw and wait for 1 week	Cross-taper cautiously[c]	–	Withdraw then start fluoxetine at 10 mg/day	Withdraw and start paroxetine at 10 mg/day
Paroxetine	Withdraw and wait for 2 weeks	Withdraw and wait for 1 week	Cross-taper cautiously with very low dose of tricyclic[c]	Withdraw and start citalopram	Withdraw then start fluoxetine	–
Fluoxetine[d]	Withdraw and wait 5–6 weeks	Withdraw and wait 5–6 weeks	Stop fluoxetine Wait 4–7 days Start tricyclic at very low dose and increase very slowly	Stop fluoxetine Wait 4–7 days Start citalopram at 10 mg/day and increase slowly	–	Stop fluoxetine Wait 4–7 days, then start paroxetine 10 mg/day

*Note: Advice given in this table is partly derived manufacturers' information and partly theoretical. Caution is required in every instance.

Sertraline	Trazodone	Moclobemide	Reboxetine	Venlafaxine	Mirtazapine	Duloxetine
Withdraw and wait for 2 weeks	*Withdraw and wait for 2 weeks*	*Withdraw and wait for 2 weeks*[b]	*Withdraw and wait for 2 weeks*	*Withdraw and wait for 2 weeks*	*Withdraw and wait for 2 weeks*	*Withdraw and wait for 2 weeks*
Withdraw and wait for 2 weeks	*Withdraw and wait for 2 weeks*	*Withdraw and wait for 2 weeks*[b]	*Withdraw and wait for 2 weeks*	*Withdraw and wait for 2 weeks*	*Withdraw and wait for 2 weeks*	*Withdraw and wait for 2 weeks*
Halve dose and add sertraline then slow withdrawal[c]	Halve dose and add trazodone, then slow withdrawal	Withdraw and wait at least 1 week	Cross-taper cautiously	Cross-taper cautiously, starting with venlafaxine 37.5 mg/day	Cross-taper cautiously	Cross-taper cautiously, start at 60 mg alt die Increase slowly
Withdraw and start sertraline at 25 mg/day	Withdraw before starting titration of trazodone	Withdraw and wait at least 2 weeks	Cross-taper cautiously	Cross-taper cautiously Start venlafaxine 37.5 mg/day and increase very slowly	Cross-taper cautiously	Withdraw - start at 60 mg alt die Increase slowly
Withdraw and start sertraline at 25 mg/day	Withdraw before starting titration of trazodone	Withdraw and wait for 1 week	Cross-taper cautiously	Cross-taper cautiously Start venlafaxine 37.5 mg/day and increase very slowly	Cross-taper cautiously	Withdraw, start at 60 mg alt die Increase slowly
Stop fluoxetine Wait 4–7 days, then start sertraline 25 mg/day	Stop fluoxetine Wait 4–7 days, then start low-dose trazodone	Withdraw and at least 5 weeks	Withdraw Start reboxetine at 2 mg b.d. and increase cautiously	Withdraw Start venlafaxine at 37.5 mg/day Increase very slowly	Cross-taper cautiously	Withdraw, wait 4–7 days and start at 60 mg alt die Increase slowly

Table   Antidepressants – swapping and stopping* (Cont.)

To From	MAOIs- hydrazines	Tranyl- cypromine[a]	Tricyclics	Citalopram/ escitalopram	Fluoxetine	Paroxetine
Sertraline	Withdraw and wait for 2 weeks	Withdraw and wait for 2 weeks	Cross-taper cautiously with very low dose of tricyclic[c]	Withdraw, then start citalopram	Withdraw, then start fluoxetine	Withdraw, then start paroxetine
Trazodone	Withdraw and wait at least 1 week	Withdraw and wait at least 1 week	Cross-taper cautiously with very low dose of tricyclic	Withdraw, then start citalopram	Withdraw, then start fluoxetine	Withdraw, then start paroxetine
Moclobemide	Withdraw and wait 24 hours	Withdraw and wait 24 hours	Withdraw and wait 24 hours	Withdraw and wait 24 hours	Withdraw and wait 24 hours	Withdraw and wait 24 hours
Reboxetine	Withdraw and wait at least 1 week	Withdraw and wait at least 1 week	Cross-taper cautiously	Cross-taper cautiously	Cross-taper cautiously	Cross-taper cautiously
Venlafaxine	Withdraw and wait at least 1 week	Withdraw and wait at least 1 week	Cross-taper cautiously with very low dose of tricyclic[c]	Cross-taper cautiously Start with 10 mg/day	Cross-taper cautiously Start with 20 mg every other day	Cross-taper cautiously Start with 10 mg/day
Mirtazapine	Withdraw and wait for 1 week	Withdraw and wait for 1 week	Withdraw, then start tricyclic	Cross-taper cautiously	Cross-taper cautiously	Cross-taper cautiously
Duloxetine	Withdraw and wait 1 week	Withdraw and wait 1 week	Cross-taper cautiously with very low dose of tricyclic	Withdraw, then start citalopram	Withdraw, then start fluoxetine	Withdraw, then start paroxetine
Stopping[e]	Reduce over 4 weeks	Reduce over 4 weeks	Reduce over 4 weeks	Reduce over 4 weeks	At 20 mg/day, just stop At 40 mg day, reduce over 2 weeks	Reduce over 4 weeks or longer, if necessary[f]

Notes
[a] SPC for tranylcypromine suggests at least 1-week gap between cessation of prior drug and starting tranylcypromine.
[b] Abrupt switching is possible but not recommended.
[c] Do not co-administer clomipramine and SSRIs or venlafaxine. Withdraw clomipramine before starting.
[d] Beware: interactions with fluoxetine may still occur for 5 weeks after stopping fluoxetine because of its long half-life.
[e] See general guidelines (page 240).
[f] Withdrawal effects seem to be more pronounced. Slow withdrawal over 1–3 months may be necessary.

Sertraline	Trazodone	Moclobemide	Reboxetine	Venlafaxine	Mirtazapine	Duloxetine
–	Withdraw before starting trazodone	Withdraw and wait at least 2 weeks	Cross-taper cautiously	Cross-taper cautiously Start venlafaxine at 37.5 mg/day	Cross-taper cautiously	Withdraw, start at 60 mg alt die Increase slowly
Withdraw, then start sertraline	–	Withdraw and wait at least 1 week	Withdraw, start reboxetine at 2 mg b.d and increase cautiously	Cross-taper cautiously Start venlafaxine at 37.5 mg/day	Withdraw, then start mirtazapine	Withdraw, start at 60 mg alt die Increase slowly
Withdraw and wait 24 hours	Withdraw and wait 24 hours	–	Withdraw and wait 24 hours	Withdraw and wait 24 hours	Withdraw and wait 24 hours	Withdraw and wait 24 hours
Cross-taper cautiously	Cross-taper cautiously	Withdraw and wait at least 1 week	–	Cross-taper cautiously	Withdraw, then start mirtazapine	Cross-taper cautiously
Cross-taper cautiously Start with 25 mg/day	Cross-taper cautiously	Withdraw and wait at least 1 week	Cross-taper cautiously	–	Cross-taper cautiously	Withdraw, start at 60 mg alt die Increase slowly
Cross-taper cautiously	Withdraw, then start trazodone	Withdraw and wait 1 week	Withdraw, then start reboxetine	Cross-taper cautiously	–	Withdraw, start at 60 mg alt die Increase slowly
Withdraw, then start sertraline	Withdraw, then start trazodone	Withdraw and wait 1 week	Cross-taper cautiously	Withdraw, then start venlafaxine	Withdraw, then start mirtazapine	–
Reduce over 4 weeks	Reduce over 4 weeks	Reduce over 4 weeks	Reduce over 4 weeks	Reduce over 4 weeks or longer, if necessary[f]	Reduce over 4 weeks	–

Antidepressant discontinuation symptoms

What are discontinuation symptoms?

The term 'discontinuation symptoms' is used to describe symptoms experienced on stopping prescribed drugs that are not drugs of dependence. There is an important semantic difference between 'discontinuation' and 'withdrawal' symptoms – the latter implies addiction, the former does not. While this distinction is important for precise medical terminology, it may be irrelevant to patient experience. Discontinuation symptoms may occur after stopping many drugs, including antidepressants, and can sometimes be explained in the context of 'receptor rebound'[1,2] – e.g. an antidepressant with potent anticholinergic side-effects may be associated with diarrhoea on discontinuation.

Discontinuation symptoms may be entirely new or similar to some of the original symptoms of the illness, and so cannot be attributed to other causes. They can be broadly divided into six categories: affective (e.g. irritability); gastrointestinal (e.g. nausea); neuromotor (e.g. ataxia); vasomotor (e.g. diaphoresis); neurosensory (e.g. paraesthesia); and other neurological (e.g. increase dreaming)[2]. Discontinuation symptoms are experienced by at least a third of patients[3–5] and are seen to some extent with all antidepressants[6].

The onset is usually within 5 days of stopping treatment (depending on the half-life of the antidepressant) or occasionally during taper or after missed doses[7,8] (short-half-life drugs only). Symptoms can vary in form and intensity and occur in any combination. They are usually mild and self-limiting, but can occasionally be severe and prolonged. The perception of symptom severity is probably made worse by the absence of forewarnings. Some symptoms are more likely with individual drugs (see below). Symptoms can be quantified using the discontinuation – emergent signs and symptoms (DESS) scale[4].

Table	Antidepressant discontinuation symptoms		
	MAOIs	**TCAs**	**SSRIs and related**
Symptoms	**Common** Agitation, irritability, ataxia, movement disorders, insomnia, somnolence, vivid dreams, cognitive impairment, slowed speech, pressured speech	**Common** Flu-like symptoms (chills, myalgia, excessive sweating, headache, nausea), insomnia, excessive dreaming	**Common** Flu-like symptoms, 'shock-like' sensations, dizziness exacerbated by movement, insomnia, excessive (vivid) dreaming, irritability
	Occasionally Hallucinations, paranoid delusions	**Occasionally** Movement disorders, mania, cardiac arrhythmia	**Occasionally** Movement disorders, problems with concentration and memory

Table	Antidepressant discontinuation symptoms (Cont.)		
	MAOIs	**TCAs**	**SSRIs and related**
Drugs most commonly associated with discontinuation symptoms	All Tranylcypromine is partly metabolised to amfetamine and is therefore associated with a true 'withdrawal syndrome'	Amitriptyline Imipramine	Paroxetine Venlafaxine

Early data from one RCT suggest that agomelatine is associated with low, if any, risk of discontinuation symptoms[9].

Clinical relevance[10]

The symptoms of a discontinuation reaction may be mistaken for a relapse of depressive illness or the emergence of a new physical illness[11], leading to unnecessary investigations or reintroduction of the antidepressant. Symptoms may be severe enough to interfere with daily functioning, and those who have experienced discontinuation symptoms may reason (perhaps appropriately) that antidepressants are 'addictive' and not wish to accept treatment.

Who is most at risk?[10–12]

Although anyone can experience discontinuation symptoms, the risk is increased in those prescribed short-half-life drugs[4,7,13,14] (e.g. paroxetine, venlafaxine), particularly if they do not take them regularly. Two-thirds of patients prescribed antidepressants may skip a few doses from time to time[15], and many patients stop their antidepressant abruptly[3]. The risk is also increased in those who have been taking antidepressants for 8 weeks or longer[16], those who have developed anxiety symptoms at the start of antidepressant therapy (particularly with SSRIs), those receiving other centrally acting medication (e.g. antihypertensives, antihistamines, antipsychotics), children and adolescents, and those who have experienced discontinuation symptoms before.

Antidepressant discontinuation symptoms are common in neonates born to woman taking antidepressants. See page 368.

How to avoid[10–12]

Generally, antidepressant therapy should be discontinued over at least a 4-week period (this is not required with fluoxetine)[7]. The shorter the half-life of the drug, the more important that this rule is followed. The end of the taper may need to be slower, as symptoms may not appear until the reduction in the total daily dosage of the antidepressant is (proportionately) substantial.

Patients receiving MAOIs may need to be tapered over a longer period. Tranylcypromine may be particularly difficult to stop. At-risk patients (see above) may need a slower taper.

Many people suffer symptoms despite slow withdrawal. For these patients the option of abrupt withdrawal should be discussed. Some may prefer to face a week or two of intense symptoms rather than months of less severe discontinuation syndrome.

How to treat[10,11]

There are few systematic studies in this area. Treatment is pragmatic. If symptoms are mild, reassure the patient that these symptoms are common after discontinuing an antidepressant and will pass in a few days. If symptoms are severe, reintroduce the original antidepressant (or another with a longer half-life from the same class) and taper gradually while monitoring for symptoms.

Some evidence supports the use of anticholinergic agents in tricyclic withdrawal[17] and fluoxetine for symptoms associated with stopping clomipramine[18] or venlafaxine[19] – fluoxetine, having a longer plasma half-life, seems to be associated with a lower incidence of discontinuation symptoms than other similar drugs[20].

Key points that patients should know

- Antidepressants are not addictive; a survey of 2000 people across the UK conducted in 1991 found that 78% thought that antidepressants were addictive[21]. It is important to dispel this myth. In order for a drug to be addictive it must also fulfil certain other criteria including tolerance, escalating use, etc. This should be discussed. Note, however, that this semantic and categorical distinction may be lost on many people.
- Patients should be informed that they may experience discontinuation symptoms (and the most likely symptoms associated with the drug that they are taking) when they stop their antidepressant.
- Antidepressants should not be stopped abruptly. The dose should be tapered over at least 4 weeks. Fluoxetine is an exception to this rule[7].
- Discontinuation symptoms may occur after missed doses if the antidepressant prescribed has a short half-life.

References

1. Blier P et al. Physiologic mechanisms underlying the antidepressant discontinuation syndrome. J Clin Psychiatry 2006;67(Suppl 4):8–13.
2. Delgado PL. Monoamine depletion studies: implications for antidepressant discontinuation syndrome. J Clin Psychiatry 2006;67(Suppl 4):22–6.
3. van Geffen EC et al. Discontinuation symptoms in users of selective serotonin reuptake inhibitors in clinical practice: tapering versus abrupt discontinuation. Eur J Clin Pharmacol 2005;61:303–7.
4. Fava M. Prospective studies of adverse events related to antidepressant discontinuation. J Clin Psychiatry 2006;67(Suppl 4):14–21.
5. Perahia DG et al. Symptoms following abrupt discontinuation of duloxetine treatment in patients with major depressive disorder. J Affect Disord 2005;89:207–12.
6. Taylor D et al. Antidepressant withdrawal symptoms – telephone calls to a national medication helpline. J Affect Disord 2006;95:129–33.
7. Rosenbaum JF et al. Selective serotonin reuptake inhibitor discontinuation syndrome: a randomized clinical trial. Biol Psychiatry 1998;44:77–87.
8. Michelson D et al. Interruption of selective serotonin reuptake inhibitor treatment. Double-blind, placebo-controlled trial. Br J Psychiatry 2000;176:363–8.
9. Montgomery SA et al. Absence of discontinuation symptoms with agomelatine and occurrence of discontinuation symptoms with paroxetine: a randomized, double-blind, placebo-controlled discontinuation study. Int Clin Psychopharmacol 2004;19:271–80.
10. Lejoyeux M et al. Antidepressant withdrawal syndrome: recognition, prevention and management. CNS Drugs 1996;5:278–92.
11. Haddad PM. Antidepressant discontinuation syndromes. Drug Saf 2001;24:183–97.
12. Anon. Antidepressant discontinuation syndrome: update on serotonin reuptake inhibitors. J Clin Psychiatry 1997;58(Suppl 7):3–40.
13. Sir A et al. Randomized trial of sertraline versus venlafaxine XR in major depression: efficacy and discontinuation symptoms. J Clin Psychiatry 2005;66:1312–20.
14. Baldwin DS et al. A double-blind, randomized, parallel-group, flexible-dose study to evaluate the tolerability, efficacy and effects of treatment discontinuation with escitalopram and paroxetine in patients with major depressive disorder. Int Clin Psychopharmacol 2006;21:159–69.
15. Meijer WE et al. Spontaneous lapses in dosing during chronic treatment with selective serotonin reuptake inhibitors. Br J Psychiatry 2001;179:519–22.
16. Kramer JC et al. Withdrawal symptoms following dicontinuation of imipramine therapy. Am J Psychiatry 1961;118:549–50.
17. Dilsaver SC et al. Antidepressant withdrawal symptoms treated with anticholinergic agents. Am J Psychiatry 1983;140:249–51.
18. Benazzi F. Fluoxetine for clomipramine withdrawal symptoms. Am J Psychiatry 1999;156:661–2.
19. Giakas WJ et al. Intractable withdrawal from venlafaxine treated with fluoxetine. Psychiatr Ann 1997;27:85–93.
20. Coupland NJ et al. Serotonin reuptake inhibitor withdrawal. J Clin Psychopharmacol 1996;16:356–62.
21. Priest RG et al. Lay people's attitudes to treatment of depression: results of opinion poll for Defeat Depression Campaign just before its launch. BMJ 1996;313:858–9.

Further reading

Blier P et al. Physiologic mechanisms underlying the antidepressant discontinuation syndrome. J Clin Psychiatry 2006;67(Suppl 4):8–13.
Schatzberg AF et al. Antidepressant discontinuation syndrome: consensus panel recommendations for clinical management and additional research. J Clin Psychiatry 2006;67(Suppl 4):27–30.
Shelton RC. The nature of the discontinuation syndrome associated with antidepressant drugs. J Clin Psychiatry 2006;67(Suppl 4):3–7.

St John's wort

St John's wort (SJW) is the popular name for the plant *Hypericum perforatum*. It contains a combination of at least 10 different components, including hypericins, flavonoids and xanthons[1]. Preparations of SJW are often unstandardised and this has complicated the interpretation of clinical trials.

The active ingredient and mechanism of action of SJW are unclear although many hypotheses have been proposed. At one time MAO inhibition was thought to be the most likely mechanism of action but this may account for only a small part of SJW's antidepressant effect[2]. Reuptake inhibition of both norepinephrine and serotonin has been demonstrated, as has the upregulation of serotonin receptors[3]. No firm conclusions can be drawn.

SJW is not a licensed preparation in the UK but is available as a herbal or complementary therapy. (It is licensed in Germany for the treatment of depression.)

Evidence for SJW in the treatment of depression

A number of trials have been published that look at the efficacy of SJW in the treatment of depression. They have been extensively reviewed[4,5] and most authors conclude that SJW is likely to be effective in the treatment of mild-to-moderate depression. Evidence that this may hold true in severe depression is increasing[6]. Some doubt over the efficacy of SJW still remains, however[7].

It should be noted that:

- The active component of SJW for treating depression has not yet been determined. The trials used different preparations of SJW which were standardised according to their total content of hypericins. However, evidence suggests that hypericins alone do not treat depression[8].
- None of the trials has lasted longer than 8 weeks. A Cochrane review concluded that the evidence base is confusing, with some studies demonstrating equivalence with standard antidepressants while others show little benefit over placebo[9]. This is strikingly similar to the primary literature for standard antidepressants where the separation between active drug and placebo is small, particularly in mild depression[5].

On balance, SJW should not be prescribed: we lack understanding of what the active ingredient is or what constitutes a therapeutic dose. SJW is an unlicensed herbal treatment.

Adverse effects

SJW appears to be well tolerated. Pooled data from 35 RCTs show that dropout rates and adverse effects were less than with older antidepressants, slightly less than SSRIs and similar to placebo[10]. The most common, if infrequent, side-effects are dry mouth, nausea, constipation, fatigue, dizziness, headache and restlessness[11–14]. In addition, SJW contains a red pigment that can cause photosensitivity reactions[15]. In common with other antidepressant drugs, SJW has been known to precipitate hypomania in people with bipolar affective disorder[16].

Drug interactions

SJW is an inducer of intestinal and hepatic CYP3A4 and intestinal p-glycoprotein[17,18]. Studies have shown that SJW significantly reduces plasma concentrations of digoxin and indinavir[19,20] (a drug used in the treatment of HIV). According to a number of case reports, SJW has lowered the plasma concentrations of theophylline, ciclosporin, warfarin and the combined oral contraceptive pill and has led to treatment failure[21]. There is a theoretical risk that SJW may interact with some anticonvulsant drugs[22]. Serotonin syndrome has been reported when SJW was taken together with each of sertraline, paroxetine, nefazodone and the triptans[22,23] (a group of serotonin agonists used to treat migraine). SJW should not be taken with any drugs that have a predominantly serotonergic action.

Key points that patients should know

- The evidence so far available suggests that SJW may be effective in the treatment of mild depression, but we do not know enough about how much should be taken or what the side-effects are. There is less evidence of benefit in severe depression.

- SJW is not a licensed medicine.

- SJW can interact with other medicines, resulting in serious side-effects. Some important drugs may be metabolised more rapidly and therefore become ineffective with serious consequences (e.g. increased viral load in HIV, failure of oral contraceptives leading to unwanted pregnancy, reduced anticoagulant effect with warfarin leading to thrombosis).

- The symptoms of depression can sometimes be caused by other physical or mental illness. It is important that these possible causes are investigated.

- It is always best to consult the doctor if any herbal or natural remedy is being taken or the patient is thinking of taking one.

- Many people regard herbal remedies as 'natural' and therefore harmless[24]. They are not aware of the potential of such remedies for causing side-effects or interacting with other drugs. A small US study ($n=22$) found that people tend to take SJW because it is easy to obtain alternative medicines and also because they perceive herbal medicines as being purer and safer than prescription medicines. Few would discuss this medication with their conventional healthcare provider[14]. Clinicians need to be proactive in asking patients if they use such treatments and try to dispel the myth that natural is the same as safe.

References

1. Linde K et al. St John's wort for depression: meta-analysis of randomised controlled trials. Br J Psychiatry 2005;186:99–107.
2. Cott JM. In vitro receptor binding and enzyme inhibition by *Hypericum perforatum* extract. Pharmacopsychiatry 1997;30(Suppl 2):108–12.
3. Muller WE et al. Effects of *Hypericum* extract (LI 160) in biochemical models of antidepressant activity. Pharmacopsychiatry 1997;30(Suppl 2):102–7.
4. Linde K et al. St John's wort for depression: meta-analysis of randomised controlled trials. Br J Psychiatry 2005;186:99–107.
5. National Institute for Clinical Excellence. Depression: management of depression in primary and secondary care – clinical guidance. http://www.nice.org.uk. 2004.
6. Szegedi A et al. Acute treatment of moderate to severe depression with hypericum extract WS 5570 (St John's wort): randomised controlled double blind non-inferiority trial versus paroxetine. BMJ 2005;330:503.
7. Werneke U et al. How effective is St John's Wort? The evidence revisited. J Clin Psychiatry 2004;65: 611–17.
8. Teufel-Mayer R et al. Effects of long-term administration of *Hypericum* extracts on the affinity and density of the central serotonergic 5-HT1 A and 5-HT2 A receptors. Pharmacopsychiatry 1997;30(Suppl 2):113–16.
9. Linde K et al. St John's wort for depression: meta-analysis of randomised controlled trials. Br J Psychiatry 2005;186:99–107.
10. Knuppel L et al. Adverse effects of St. John's Wort: a systematic review. J Clin Psychiatry 2004;65: 1470–9.
11. Volz HP. Controlled clinical trials of *Hypericum* extracts in depressed patients – an overview. Pharmacopsychiatry 1997;30(Suppl 2):72–6.
12. Gaster B et al. St John's wort for depression: a systematic review. Arch Intern Med 2000;160:152–6.
13. Woelk H. Comparison of St John's wort and imipramine for treating depression: randomised controlled trial. BMJ 2000;321:536–9.
14. Wagner PJ et al. Taking the edge off: why patients choose St. John's Wort. J Fam Pract 1999;48: 615–19.
15. Bove GM. Acute neuropathy after exposure to sun in a patient treated with St John's Wort. Lancet 1998;352:1121–2.
16. Nierenberg AA et al. Mania associated with St. John's wort. Biol Psychiatry 1999;46:1707–8.
17. Singh YN. Potential for interaction of kava and St. John's wort with drugs. J Ethnopharmacol 2005;100:108–13.
18. Ernst E. Second thoughts about safety of St John's wort. Lancet 1999;354:2014–6.
19. Johne A et al. Pharmacokinetic interaction of digoxin with an herbal extract from St John's wort (*Hypericum perforatum*). Clin Pharmacol Ther 1999;66:338–45.
20. Piscitelli SC et al. Indinavir concentrations and St John's wort. Lancet 2000;355:547–8.
21. Ernst E. Second thoughts about safety of St John's wort. Lancet 1999;354:2014–16.
22. Anon. Reminder: St John's wort (*Hypericum perforatum*) interactions. Current Problems in Pharmacovigilance 2000;26:6.
23. Lantz MS et al. St. John's wort and antidepressant drug interactions in the elderly. J Geriatr Psychiatry Neurol 1999;12:7–10.
24. Barnes J et al. Different standards for reporting ADRs to herbal remedies and conventional OTC medicines: face-to-face interviews with 515 users of herbal remedies. Br J Clin Pharmacol 1998;45: 496–500.

Further reading

Mills E et al. Interaction of St John's Wort with conventional drugs: systematic review of clinical trials. BMJ 2004;329:27–30.

Drug interactions with antidepressants

Drugs can interact with each other in two different ways:

1. *Pharmacokinetic interactions* where one drug interferes with the absorption, distribution, metabolism or elimination of another drug. This may result in subtherapeutic effect or toxicity. The largest group of pharmacokinetic interactions involves drugs that inhibit or induce hepatic CYP450 enzymes (see the table overleaf). Other enzyme systems include FMO[1] and UGT[2]. While both of these enzyme systems are involved in the metabolism of psychotropic drugs, the potential for drugs to inhibit or induce these enzyme systems has been poorly studied. The clinical consequences of pharmacokinetic interactions in an individual patient can be difficult to predict. The following factors affect outcome of interactions: the degree of enzyme inhibition or induction, the pharmacokinetic properties of the affected drug and other co-administered drugs, the relationship between plasma level and pharmacodynamic effect for the affected drug, and patient-specific factors such as variability in the role of primary and secondary metabolic pathways and the presence of co-morbid physical illness[3].

2. *Pharmacodynamic interactions* where the effects of one drug are altered by another drug via physiological mechanisms such as direct competition at receptor sites (e.g. dopamine agonists with dopamine blockers negate any therapeutic effect), augmentation of the same neurotransmitter pathway (e.g. fluoxetine with tramadol can lead to serotonin syndrome) or an effect on the physiological functioning of an organ/organ system in different ways (e.g. two different antiarrhythmic drugs). Most of these interactions can be easily predicted by a sound knowledge of pharmacology. An up-to-date list of important interactions can be found at the back of the *BNF*.

Pharmacodynamic interactions

Tricyclic antidepressants[4,5]:

- are H_1 blockers (sedative). This effect can be exacerbated by other sedative drugs or alcohol. Beware respiratory depression.

- are anticholinergic (dry mouth, blurred vision, constipation). This effect can be exacerbated by other anticholinergic drugs such as antihistamines or antipsychotics. Beware cognitive impairment and GI obstruction.

- are adrenergic α_1-blockers (postural hypotension). This effect can be exacerbated by other drugs that block α_1-receptors and by antihypertensive drugs in general. Epinephrine, in combination with α_1-blockers, can lead to hypertension.

- are arrhythmogenic. Caution is required with other drugs that can alter cardiac conduction directly (e.g. antiarrhythmics or phenothiazines) or indirectly through a potential to cause electrolyte disturbance (e.g. diuretics). (Also see page 228.)

- lower the seizure threshold. Caution is required with other proconvulsive drugs (e.g. antipsychotics) and particularly if the patient is being treated for epilepsy (higher doses of anticonvulsants may be required).

Depression & anxiety

- may be serotonergic (e.g. amitriptyline, clomipramine). There is the potential for these drugs to interact with other serotonergic drugs (e.g. tramadol, SSRIs, selegiline) to cause serotonin syndrome.

Table Pharmacokinetic interactions[6-10]

p4501A2	*p4502C*	*p4502D6*	*p4503A*
Genetic polymorphism	5–10% of Caucasians lack it	3–5% of Caucasians lack it	60% p450 content
Induced by: cigarette smoke charcoal cooking carbamazepine omeprazole phenobarbital phenytoin	*Induced by:* phenytoin rifampicin	*Induced by:* carbamazepine phenytoin	*Induced by:* carbamazepine phenytoin prednisolone rifampicin
Inhibited by: cimetidine ciprofloxacin erythromycin fluvoxamine paroxetine	*Inhibited by:* cimetidine fluoxetine fluvoxamine sertraline	*Inhibited by:* chlorpromazine duloxetine fluoxetine fluphenazine haloperidol paroxetine sertraline tricyclics	*Inhibited by:* erythromycin fluoxetine fluvoxamine ketoconazole paroxetine sertraline (?) tricyclics
Metabolises: caffeine clozapine haloperidol mirtazapine olanzapine theophylline tricyclics warfarin	*Metabolises:* diazepam omeprazole phenytoin tolbutamide tricyclics warfarin	*Metabolises:* clozapine codeine donepezil haloperidol phenothiazines risperidone TCA secondary amines tramadol trazodone venlafaxine	*Metabolises:* benzodiazepines calcium blockers carbamazepine cimetidine clozapine codeine donepezil erythromycin galantamine methadone mirtazapine risperidone steroids terfenadine tricyclics valproate venlafaxine Z-hypnotics

SSRIs[7,11]:

- increase serotonergic neurotransmission. The main concern is serotonin syndrome (see page 235).

- inhibit platelet aggregation and increase the risk of bleeding, particularly of the upper GI tract. This effect is exacerbated by aspirin and NSAIDs.

MAOIs[12]:

- prevent the destruction of monoamine neurotransmitters. Sympathomimetic and dopaminergic drugs can lead to monoamine overload and hypertensive crisis. Pethidine and fermented foods can have the same effect.

- can interact with serotonergic drugs to cause serotonin syndrome.

Avoid/minimise problems by:

1. avoiding antidepressant polypharmacy

2. avoiding the co-prescription of other drugs with a similar pharmacology but not marketed as antidepressants (e.g. bupropion, sibutramine)

3. knowing your pharmacology (most interactions can be easily predicted).

References

1. Cashman JR. Human flavin-containing monooxygenase: substrate specificity and role in drug metabolism. Curr Drug Metab 2000;1:181–91.
2. Anderson GD. A mechanistic approach to antiepileptic drug interactions. Ann Pharmacother 1998;32: 554–63.
3. Devane CL. Antidepressant-drug interactions are potentially but rarely clinically significant. Neuro-psychopharmacology 2006;31:1594–604.
4. British National Formulary. London: British Medical Association and Royal Pharmaceutical Society of Great Britain, 2002.
5. Watsky EJ et al. Psychotropic drug interactions. Hosp Community Psychiatry 1991;42:247–56.
6. Lin JH et al. Inhibition and induction of cytochrome P450 and the clinical implications. Clin Pharmacokinet 1998;35:361–90.
7. Mitchell PB. Drug interactions of clinical significance with selective serotonin reuptake inhibitors. Drug Saf 1997;17:390–406.
8. Richelson E. Pharmacokinetic interactions of antidepressants. J Clin Psychiatry 1998;59(Suppl 10): 22–6.
9. Greenblatt DJ et al. Drug interactions with newer antidepressants: role of human cytochromes P450. J Clin Psychiatry 1998;59(Suppl 15):19–27.
10. Taylor D. Pharmacokinetic interactions involving clozapine. Br J Psychiatry 1997;171:109–12.
11. Edwards JG et al. Systematic review and guide to selection of selective serotonin reuptake inhibitors. Drugs 1999;57:507–33.
12. Livingston MG et al. Monoamine oxidase inhibitors. An update on drug interactions. Drug Saf 1996; 14:219–27.

Depression & anxiety

Table Antidepressants: relative adverse effects – a rough guide

Drug	Sedation	Hypotension	Anticholinergic effects	Forms available
Tricyclics				
Amitriptyline	+++	+++	+++	tabs/caps, liq, inj
Clomipramine	++	+++	++	tabs/caps, liq
Dosulepin	+++	+++	++	tabs, caps
Doxepin	+++	++	++	caps
Imipramine	++	+++	+++	tabs, liq
Lofepramine	+	+	+	tabs
Nortriptyline	+	++	+	tabs
Trimipramine	+++	+++	++	tabs, caps
Other antidepressants				
Duloxetine	+/−	−	−	caps
Mianserin	++	−	−	tabs
Mirtazapine	+++	−	+	tabs, soluble tabs
Reboxetine	+	−	+	tabs
Trazodone	+++	++	−	caps, liq
Venlafaxine	+/−	−	+	tabs
Selective serotonin reuptake inhibitors (SSRIs)				
Citalopram	+/−	−	−	tabs, liq
Escitalopram	+/−	−	−	tabs
Fluoxetine	−	−	−	caps, liq
Fluvoxamine	+	−	−	tabs
Paroxetine	+	−	+	tabs, liq
Sertraline	−	−	−	tabs
Monoamine oxidase inhibitors (MAOIs)				
Isocarboxazid	+	++	++	tabs
Phenelzine	+	+	+	tabs
Tranylcypromine	−	+	+	tabs
Reversible inhibitor of monoamine oxidase A (RIMA)				
Moclobemide	−	−	−	tabs

KEY: +++ High incidence/severity
  ++ Moderate
  + Low
  − Very low/none

Depression & anxiety

Anxiety spectrum disorders

Anxiety is a normal emotion that is experienced by everyone at some time. Symptoms can be psychological, physical, or a mixture of both. Intervention is required when symptoms become disabling.

There are several disorders within the overall spectrum of anxiety disorders, each with its own characteristic symptoms. These are outlined briefly in the table below. Anxiety disorders can occur on their own, be part of other psychiatric disorders (particularly depression), be a consequence of physical illness such as thyrotoxicosis or be drug-induced (e.g. by caffeine)[1]. Co-morbidity with other psychiatric disorders is very common.

Anxiety spectrum disorders tend to be chronic and treatment is often only partially successful.

Benzodiazepines

Benzodiazepines provide rapid symptomatic relief from acute anxiety states. All guidelines and consensus statements recommend that this group of drugs should only be used to treat anxiety that is severe, disabling, or subjecting the individual to extreme distress. Because of their potential to cause physical dependence and withdrawal symptoms, these drugs should be used at the lowest effective dose for the shortest period of time (maximum 4 weeks), while medium/long-term treatment strategies are put in place. For the majority of patients these recommendations are sensible and should be adhered to. A very small number of patients with severely disabling anxiety may benefit from long-term treatment with a benzodiazepine and these patients should not be denied treatment[2]. NICE recommends that benzodiazepines should not be used to treat panic disorder[3]. They should be used with care in post-traumatic stress disorder (**PTSD**)[4].

SSRI – dose and duration of treatment

When used to treat generalised anxiety disorder (**GAD**), SSRIs should initially be prescribed at half the normal starting dose for the treatment of depression and the dose titrated upwards into the normal antidepressant dosage range as tolerated (initial worsening of anxiety may be seen when treatment is started[5]). Response is usually seen within 6 weeks and continues to increase over time[6]. The optimal duration of treatment has not been determined but should be at least 6 months[7]. Effective treatment of GAD may prevent the development of major depression[8].

When used to treat **panic disorder**, the same starting dose and dosage titration as in GAD should be used. Doses of clomipramine[9], citalopram[10] and sertraline[11] towards the bottom of the antidepressant range give the best balance between efficacy and side-effects, whereas higher doses of paroxetine (40 mg and above) may be required[12]. Higher doses may be effective when standard doses have failed. Onset of action may be as long as 6 weeks.

Women may respond better to SSRIs than men[13]. There is some evidence that augmentation with clonazepam leads to a more rapid response (but not a greater magnitude of response overall)[12,14]. The optimal duration of treatment is unknown, but should be at least 8 months[15], with some authors recommending up to 18 months[16]. Less than 50% of patients are likely to remain well after medication is withdrawn[16].

Lower starting doses are also required in **PTSD**, with high doses (e.g. fluoxetine 60 mg) often being required for full effect. Response is usually seen within 8 weeks, but can take up to 12 weeks[16]. Treatment should be continued for at least 6 months and probably longer[17-19].

Although the doses of SSRIs licensed for the treatment of obsessive compulsive disorder (**OCD**) are higher than those licensed for the treatment of depression (e.g. fluoxetine 60 mg, paroxetine 40–60 mg), lower (standard antidepressant) doses may be effective, particularly for maintenance treatment[20,21]. Initial response is usually slower to emerge than in depression (can take 10–12 weeks). The relapse rate in patients who continue treatment for 2 years is half that of those who stop treatment after initial response (25–40% vs 80%)[22,23].

Body dysmorphic disorder (**BDD**) should be treated initially with CBT. If symptoms are moderate–severe, adding an SSRI may improve outcome[24]. Buspirone may usefully augment the SSRI[24].

Standard antidepressant starting doses are well tolerated in **social phobia**[25-27], and upward-dosage titration may benefit some patients but is not always required. Response is usually seen within 8 weeks and treatment should be continued for at least a year and probably longer[28].

All patients treated with SSRIs should be monitored for the development of akathisia, increased anxiety and the emergence of suicidal ideation; the risk is thought to be greatest in those <30 years, those with co-morbid depression and those already known to be at higher risk of suicide[24].

SSRIs should not be stopped abruptly, as patients with anxiety spectrum disorders are particularly sensitive to discontinuation symptoms (see page XX). The dose should be titrated down as tolerated over several weeks to months.

Psychological approaches

There is good evidence to support the efficacy of some psychological interventions in anxiety spectrum disorders. Examples include exposure therapy in OCD and social phobia. Initial drug therapy may be required to help the patient become more receptive to psychological input, and some studies suggest that optimal outcome is achieved by combining psychological and drug therapies[1,3].

A discussion of the evidence base for psychological interventions is outside the scope of these guidelines. Further information can be found at www.doh.gov.uk[29]. There are often long waiting lists for psychological therapies and some specialist interventions may not be available at all in some areas. The table on the following pages does not list psychological interventions as first-line treatments for these reasons. It is recognised that for many patients their use as a first-line treatment would be appropriate, and indeed this is supported by NICE[3].

Summary of NICE guidelines for the treatment of generalised anxiety disorder, panic disorder[3] and OCD[24]

1. Psychological therapy is more effective than pharmacological therapy and should be used as first line where possible. Details of the types of therapy recommended and their duration can be found in the NICE guidelines.
2. Pharmacological therapy is also effective. Most evidence supports the use of the SSRIs.

Panic disorder
- Benzodiazepines should not be used.
- An SSRI should be used as first line. If SSRIs are contraindicated or there is no response, imipramine or clomipramine can be used.
- Self-help (based on CBT principles) should be encouraged.

Generalised anxiety disorder
- Benzodiazepines should not be used beyond 2–4 weeks.
- An SSRI should be used as first line.
- Self-help (based on CBT principles) should be encouraged.

OCD (where there is moderate or severe functional impairment)
- Use an SSRI or intensive CBT.
- Combine the SSRI and CBT if response to a single strategy is suboptimal.
- Use clomipramine if SSRIs fail.
- If response is still suboptimal, add an antipsychotic or combine clomipramine and citalopram.

	Generalised anxiety disorder[3-7,30-43]	Obsessive compulsive disorder[21-23,25,44-54]
Clinical presentation	• Irrational worries • Motor tension • Hypervigilance • Somatic symptoms (e.g. hyperventilation, tachycardia and sweating)	• Obsessional thinking (e.g. constantly thinking that the door has been left unlocked) • Compulsive behaviour (e.g. constantly going back to check)
Emergency management	Benzodiazepines (normally for short-term use only: max. 2–4 weeks, but see reference 2)	Not usually appropriate
First-line drug treatment Treatment of anxiety may prevent the subsequent development of depression[7]	• SSRIs (although may initially exacerbate symptoms. A lower starting dose is often required) • Venlafaxine • Some TCAs (e.g. imipramine, clomipramine)	• SSRIs • Clomipramine
Other treatments (less well tolerated or weaker evidence base)	• Buspirone (has a delayed onset of action) • Hydroxyzine • β-Blockers (useful for somatic symptoms, particularly tachycardia) • Tiagabine • Pregabalin • Riluzole	• Antipsychotics (evidence for quetiapine and risperidone as antidepressant augmentation, but not haloperidol) • Venlafaxine (not recommended by NICE) • Buspirone • Clomipramine (IV pulse loading) • Clonazepam (benzodiazepines in general are mainly useful in reducing associated anxiety; only careful short-term use supported by NICE) • Mirtazapine augmentation of SSRI • Citalopram augmentation of clomipramine (supported by NICE)
Non-drug treatments *See* www.doh.org.uk and NICE[3]	• Reassurance • Anxiety management, including relaxation training and drug and exposure therapy • CBT	• Exposure therapy • Behavioural therapy • CBT • Combined drug and psychological therapy may be the most effective option

Panic disorder[10–12,14–16,55–62]	Post-traumatic stress disorder[8,17,20,63–74]	Social phobia[26–28,75–79]
• Sudden unpredictable episodes of severe anxiety • Shortness of breath • Fear of suffocation/dying • Urgent desire to flee	• History of a traumatic life event (as perceived by the sufferer) • Emotional numbness or detachment • Intrusive flashbacks or vivid dreams • Disabling fear of re-exposure, causing avoidance of perceived similar situations	• Extreme fear of social situations (e.g. eating in public or public speaking) • Fear of humiliation or embarrassment • Avoidant behaviour (e.g. never eating in restaurants) • Anxious anticipation (e.g. feeling sick on entering a restaurant)
Benzodiazepines *(have a rapid effect, although panic symptoms return quickly if the drug is withdrawn)* NICE do *not* recommend	Not usually appropriate	Benzodiazepines (have a rapid effect and may be useful on a PRN basis)
• SSRIs (therapeutic effect can be delayed and patients can experience an initial exacerbation of panic symptoms) • Some TCAs (e.g. imipramine, clomipramine) • Reboxetine	• SSRIs • Serotonergic TCAs	• SSRIs • MAOIs
• MAOIs • Mirtazapine • Valproate • Inositol • Venlafaxine	• MAOIs • Valproate • Carbamazepine • Clonidine • Tiagabine • Olanzapine • Risperidone • Quetiapine • Mirtazapine • Phenytoin • Venlafaxine	• Moclobemide • Clonazepam • Propranolol (performance anxiety only) • Buspirone (adjunct to SSRIs only) • Venlafaxine • Valproate • Levetiracetam
• CBT • Anxiety management, including relaxation training • Combined drug and psychological therapy may be the most effective option	• Debriefing should be available if desired • Counselling • Anxiety management • CBT, especially for avoidance behaviours or intrusive images	• CBT • Exposure therapy (combined drug and exposure therapy may be more effective)

Depression & anxiety

References

1. Fineberg N et al. Anxiety disorders: drug treatment or behavioural cognitive psychotherapy. CNS Drugs 1995;3:448–66.
2. Royal College of Psychiatrists. Benzodiazepines: risks, benefits and dependence, a re-evaluation. Council Report 59. http://www.rcpsych.ac.uk/ (London). 1997.
3. National Institute for Clinical Excellence. Anxiety: management of anxiety (panic disorder, with or without agoraphobia, and generalized anxiety disorder) in adult in primary, secondary and community care. http://www.nice.org.uk. 2004.
4. Davidson JR. Use of benzodiazepines in social anxiety disorder, generalized anxiety disorder, and post-traumatic stress disorder. J Clin Psychiatry 2004;65(Suppl 5):29–33.
5. Scott A et al. Antidepressant drugs in the treatment of anxiety disorders. Adv Psychiatr Treat 2001;7:275–82.
6. Ballenger JC. Remission rates in patients with anxiety disorders treated with paroxetine. J Clin Psychiatry 2004;65:1696–707.
7. Stocchi F et al. Efficacy and tolerability of paroxetine for the long-term treatment of generalized anxiety disorder. J Clin Psychiatry 2003;64:250–8.
8. Ballenger JC et al. Consensus statement on generalized anxiety disorder from the International Consensus Group on Depression and Anxiety. J Clin Psychiatry 2001;62(Suppl 11):53–8.
9. Goodwin RD et al. Psychopharmacologic treatment of generalized anxiety disorder and the risk of major depression. Am J Psychiatry 2002;159:1935–7.
10. Caillard V et al. Comparative effects of low and high doses of clomipramine and placebo in panic disorder: a double-blind controlled study. French University Antidepressant Group. Acta Psychiatr Scand 1999;99:51–8.
11. Wade AG et al. The effect of citalopram in panic disorder. Br J Psychiatry 1997;170:549–53.
12. Londborg PD et al. Sertraline in the treatment of panic disorder. A multi-site, double-blind, placebo-controlled, fixed-dose investigation. Br J Psychiatry 1998;173:54–60.
13. Clayton AH et al. Sex differences in clinical presentation and response in panic disorder: pooled data from sertraline treatment studies. Arch Womens Ment Health 2006;9:151–7.
14. Pollack MH et al. Combined paroxetine and clonazepam treatment strategies compared to paroxetine monotherapy for panic disorder. J Psychopharmacol 2003;17:276–82.
15. Rickels K et al. Panic disorder: long-term pharmacotherapy and discontinuation. J Clin Psychopharmacol 1998;18:12S–18S.
16. Michelson D et al. Continuing treatment of panic disorder after acute response: randomised, placebo-controlled trial with fluoxetine. The Fluoxetine Panic Disorder Study Group. Br J Psychiatry 1999;174: 213–18.
17. Davidson J et al. Efficacy of sertraline in preventing relapse of posttraumatic stress disorder: results of a 28-week double-blind, placebo-controlled study. Am J Psychiatry 2001;158:1974–81.
18. Ballenger JC et al. Consensus statement update on posttraumatic stress disorder from the international consensus group on depression and anxiety. J Clin Psychiatry 2004;65(Suppl 1):55–62.
19. Stein DJ et al. Pharmacotherapy for post traumatic stress disorder (PTSD). Cochrane Database Syst Rev 2006;CD002795.
20. Martenyi F et al. Fluoxetine v. placebo in prevention of relapse in post-traumatic stress disorder. Br J Psychiatry 2002;181:315–20.
21. Ravizza L et al. Long term treatment of obsessive-compulsive disorder. CNS Drugs 1998;10:247–55.
22. The Expert Consensus Panel for obsessive-compulsive disorder. Treatment of obsessive-compulsive disorder. J Clin Psychiatry 1997;58(Suppl 4):2–72.
23. Ravizza L et al. Drug treatment of obsessive-compulsive disorder (OCD): long-term trial with clomipramine and selective serotonin reuptake inhibitors (SSRIs). Psychopharmacol Bull 1996;32: 167–73.
24. National Institute for Clinical Excellence. Obsessive-compulsive disorder: Information for the public. Clinical Guidance 31. http://www.nice.org.uk. 2005.
25. Greist JH et al. Efficacy and tolerability of serotonin transport inhibitors in obsessive-compulsive disorder. A meta-analysis. Arch Gen Psychiatry 1995;52:53–60.
26. Liebowitz MR et al. A randomized, double-blind, fixed-dose comparison of paroxetine and placebo in the treatment of generalized social anxiety disorder. J Clin Psychiatry 2002;63:66–74.
27. Blomhoff S et al. Randomised controlled general practice trial of sertraline, exposure therapy and combined treatment in generalised social phobia. Br J Psychiatry 2001;179:23–30.
28. Hood SD, Nutt DJ. Psychopharmacological treatments: an overview. In Crozier R, Alden E, eds. International Handbook of Social Anxiety. Oxford: John Wiley and Sons, 2001.
29. Department of Health. Treatment choice in psychological therapies and counselling: Evidence based clinical practice guideline. http://www.dh.gov.uk/. 2001.
30. Allgulander C et al. Venlafaxine extended release (ER) in the treatment of generalised anxiety disorder: twenty-four-week placebo-controlled dose-ranging study. Br J Psychiatry 2001;179:15–22.
31. Rickels K et al. Antidepressants for the treatment of generalized anxiety disorder. A placebo-controlled comparison of imipramine, trazodone, and diazepam. Arch Gen Psychiatry 1993;50:884–95.
32. Lader M et al. A multicentre double-blind comparison of hydroxyzine, buspirone and placebo in patients with generalized anxiety disorder. Psychopharmacology 1998;139:402–6.

Depression & anxiety

33. Kapczinski F et al. Antidepressants for generalized anxiety disorder. Cochrane Database Syst Rev 2003;CD003592.
34. Rickels K et al. Paroxetine treatment of generalized anxiety disorder: a double-blind, placebo-controlled study. Am J Psychiatry 2003;160:749–56.
35. Allgulander C et al. Efficacy of sertraline in a 12-week trial for generalized anxiety disorder. Am J Psychiatry 2004;161:1642–9.
36. Lenox-Smith AJ et al. A double-blind, randomised, placebo controlled study of venlafaxine XL in patients with generalised anxiety disorder in primary care. Br J Gen Pract 2003;53:772–7.
37. Rosenthal M. Tiagabine for the treatment of generalized anxiety disorder: a randomized, open-label, clinical trial with paroxetine as a positive control. J Clin Psychiatry 2003;64:1245–9.
38. Baldwin DS et al. Escitalopram and paroxetine in the treatment of generalised anxiety disorder: randomised, placebo-controlled, double-blind study. Br J Psychiatry 2006;189:264–72.
39. Pande AC et al. Pregabalin in generalized anxiety disorder: a placebo-controlled trial. Am J Psychiatry 2003;160:533–40.
40. Rickels K et al. Remission of generalized anxiety disorder: a review of the paroxetine clinical trials database. J Clin Psychiatry 2006;67:41–7.
41. Mathew SJ et al. Open-label trial of riluzole in generalized anxiety disorder. Am J Psychiatry 2005;162:2379–81.
42. Schuurmans J et al. A randomized, controlled trial of the effectiveness of cognitive-behavioral therapy and sertraline versus a waitlist control group for anxiety disorders in older adults. Am J Geriatr Psychiatry 2006;14:255–63.
43. Chessick CA et al. Azapirones for generalized anxiety disorder. Cochrane Database Syst Rev 2006;3:CD006115.
44. Atmaca M et al. Quetiapine augmentation in patients with treatment resistant obsessive-compulsive disorder: a single-blind, placebo-controlled study. Int Clin Psychopharmacol 2002;17:115–19.
45. McDougle CJ et al. A double-blind, placebo-controlled study of fluvoxamine in adults with autistic disorder. Arch Gen Psychiatry 1996;53:1001–8.
46. Koran LM et al. Rapid benefit of intravenous pulse loading of clomipramine in obsessive-compulsive disorder. Am J Psychiatry 1997;154:396–401.
47. Denys D et al. A double-blind, randomized, placebo-controlled trial of quetiapine addition in patients with obsessive-compulsive disorder refractory to serotonin reuptake inhibitors. J Clin Psychiatry 2004;65:1040–8.
48. Shapira NA et al. A double-blind, placebo-controlled trial of olanzapine addition in fluoxetine-refractory obsessive-compulsive disorder. Biol Psychiatry 2004;55:553–5.
49. Maina G et al. Antipsychotic augmentation for treatment resistant obsessive-compulsive disorder: what if antipsychotic is discontinued? Int Clin Psychopharmacol 2003;18:23–8.
50. Hollander E et al. Risperidone augmentation in treatment-resistant obsessive-compulsive disorder: a double-blind, placebo-controlled study. Int J Neuropsychopharmacol 2003;6:397–401.
51. Pallanti S et al. Response acceleration with mirtazapine augmentation of citalopram in obsessive-compulsive disorder patients without comorbid depression: a pilot study. J Clin Psychiatry 2004;65:1394–9.
52. Hollander E et al. Venlafaxine in treatment-resistant obsessive-compulsive disorder. J Clin Psychiatry 2003;64:546–50.
53. Dell'Osso B et al. Serotonin-norepinephrine reuptake inhibitors in the treatment of obsessive-compulsive disorder: a critical review. J Clin Psychiatry 2006;67:600–10.
54. Sousa MB et al. A randomized clinical trial of cognitive-behavioral group therapy and sertraline in the treatment of obsessive-compulsive disorder. J Clin Psychiatry 2006;67:1133–9.
55. Versiani M et al. Reboxetine, a selective norepinephrine reuptake inhibitor, is an effective and well-tolerated treatment for panic disorder. J Clin Psychiatry 2002;63:31–7.
56. Bakker A et al. SSRIs vs. TCAs in the treatment of panic disorder: a meta-analysis. Acta Psychiatr Scand 2002;106:163–7.
57. Benjamin J et al. Double-blind, placebo-controlled, crossover trial of inositol treatment for panic disorder. Am J Psychiatry 1995;152:1084–6.
58. Baetz M et al. Efficacy of divalproex sodium in patients with panic disorder and mood instability who have not responded to conventional therapy. Can J Psychiatry 1998;43:73–7.
59. Otto MW et al. An effect-size analysis of the relative efficacy and tolerability of serotonin selective reuptake inhibitors for panic disorder. Am J Psychiatry 2001;158:1989–92.
60. Bruce SE et al. Are benzodiazepines still the medication of choice for patients with panic disorder with or without agoraphobia? Am J Psychiatry 2003;160:1432–8.
61. Sheehan DV et al. Efficacy and tolerability of controlled-release paroxetine in the treatment of panic disorder. J Clin Psychiatry 2005;66:34–40.
62. Bradwejn J et al. Venlafaxine extended-release capsules in panic disorder: flexible-dose, double-blind, placebo-controlled study. Br J Psychiatry 2005;187:352–9.
63. Connor KM et al. Fluoxetine in post-traumatic stress disorder. Randomised, double-blind study. Br J Psychiatry 1999;175:17–22.
64. Taylor FB. Tiagabine for posttraumatic stress disorder: a case series of 7 women. J Clin Psychiatry 2003;64:1421–5.
65. Pivac N et al. Olanzapine versus fluphenazine in an open trial in patients with psychotic combat-related post-traumatic stress disorder. Psychopharmacology 2004;175:451–6.

Depression & anxiety

66. Filteau MJ et al. Quetiapine reduces flashbacks in chronic posttraumatic stress disorder. Can J Psychiatry 2003;48:282–3.
67. Jakovljevic M et al. Olanzapine in the treatment-resistant, combat-related PTSD – a series of case reports. Acta Psychiatr Scand 2003;107:394–6.
68. Otte C et al. Valproate monotherapy in the treatment of civilian patients with non-combat-related post-traumatic stress disorder: an open-label study. J Clin Psychopharmacol 2004;24:106–8.
69. Davidson JR et al. Mirtazapine vs. placebo in posttraumatic stress disorder: a pilot trial. Biol Psychiatry 2003;53:188–91.
70. Reich DB et al. A preliminary study of risperidone in the treatment of posttraumatic stress disorder related to childhood abuse in women. J Clin Psychiatry 2004;65:1601–6.
71. Bremner DJ et al. Treatment of posttraumatic stress disorder with phenytoin: an open-label pilot study. J Clin Psychiatry 2004;65:1559–64.
72. Schoenfeld FB et al. Current concepts in pharmacotherapy for posttraumatic stress disorder. Psychiatr Serv 2004;55:519–31.
73. Cooper J et al. Pharmacotherapy for posttraumatic stress disorder: empirical review and clinical recommendations. Aust N Z J Psychiatry 2005;39:674–82.
74. Davidson J et al. Treatment of posttraumatic stress disorder with venlafaxine extended release: a 6-month randomized controlled trial. Arch Gen Psychiatry 2006;63:1158–65.
75. Blanco C et al. Pharmacological treatment of social anxiety disorder: a meta-analysis. Depress Anxiety 2003;18:29–40.
76. Stein MB et al. Efficacy of low and higher dose extended-release venlafaxine in generalized social anxiety disorder: a 6-month randomized controlled trial. Psychopharmacology 2005;177:280–8.
77. Aarre TF. Phenelzine efficacy in refractory social anxiety disorder: a case series. Nord J Psychiatry 2003;57:313–15.
78. Simon NM et al. An open-label study of levetiracetam for the treatment of social anxiety disorder. J Clin Psychiatry 2004;65:1219–22.
79. Kinrys G et al. Valproic acid for the treatment of social anxiety disorder. Int Clin Psychopharmacol 2003;18:169–72.

Further reading

Baldwin DS et al. Evidence-based guidelines for the pharmacological treatment of anxiety disorders: recommendations from the British Association for Psychopharmacology. J Psychopharmacol 2005; 19:567–96.
Heyman I et al. Obsessive-compulsive disorder. BMJ 2006;333:424–9.

Depression & anxiety

Benzodiazepines

Benzodiazepines are normally divided into two groups depending on their half-life: hypnotics (short half-life) or anxiolytics (long half-life). Although benzodiazepines have a place in the treatment of some forms of epilepsy and severe muscle spasm, and as premedicants in some surgical procedures, the vast majority of prescriptions are written for their hypnotic and anxiolytic effects. A detailed account of the pharmacology of benzodiazepines, with respect to their anxiolytic and hypnotic properties has been published[1]. Benzodiazepines are also used for rapid tranquillisation (see page 437) and, as adjuncts, in the treatment of depression and schizophrenia.

Anxiolytic effect

Benzodiazepines reduce pathological anxiety, agitation and tension. Although useful in the emergency management of anxiety, benzodiazepines are addictive and, in the majority of patients, use should be restricted to no more than one month[2,3]. In contrast with the commonly held belief that benzodiazepines should be avoided in bereavement as they inhibit psychological adjustment, an RCT[4] found that benzodiazepines had no effect on the course of bereavement.

NICE recommend that benzodiazepines should not be routinely used in patients with panic disorder – the outcome with CBT or SSRIs is superior[3].

Repeat prescriptions should be avoided in those with major personality problems whose difficulties are unlikely ever to resolve. Benzodiazepines should also be avoided, if possible, in those with a history of substance misuse.

Hypnotic effect

Benzodiazepines inhibit REM sleep and a rebound increase is seen when they are discontinued. There is a debate over the significance of this property[4].

Hypnotics are effective drugs, at least in the short term. A high proportion of hospitalised patients are prescribed hypnotics[5]. Care should be taken to avoid using hypnotics regularly or for long periods of time[6]. Physical causes (pain, dyspnoea, etc.) or substance misuse (most commonly high caffeine consumption) should always be excluded before a hypnotic drug is prescribed. Be particularly careful to avoid prescribing hypnotics on discharge from hospital, as this may result in iatrogenic dependence.

Use in depression

Benzodiazepines are not a treatment for major depressive illness. The National Service Framework for Mental Health[7] highlights this point by including a requirement that GPs audit the ratio of benzodiazepines to antidepressants prescribed in their practice. NICE found no evidence to support the use of benzodiazepines alongside antidepressants in the initial treatment of depression[8].

Depression & anxiety

Use in psychosis

Benzodiazepines are commonly used for RT, either alone[9,10], or in combination with an antipsychotic; note that a Cochrane review concludes that there is no convincing evidence that combining an antipsychotic and a benzodiazepine offers any advantage over the benzodiazepine alone[11]. Benzodiazepines have been shown to be effective in treating the prodromal symptoms of psychotic relapse[12]. A significant minority of patients with established psychotic illness fail to respond adequately to antipsychotics alone, and this can result in benzodiazepines being prescribed on a chronic basis[13]. The literature in this area is confusing. There is evidence that some treatment-resistant patients may benefit from a combination of antipsychotics and benzodiazepines, either by showing a very marked antipsychotic response or by allowing the use of lower-dose antipsychotic regimens[14]. Alprazolam and clonazepam are possibly more effective than the other benzodiazepines in this regard[14].

Side-effects

Headaches, confusion, ataxia, dysarthria, blurred vision, gastrointestinal disturbances, jaundice and paradoxical excitement are all possible side-effects. A high incidence of reversible psychiatric side-effects, specifically loss of memory and depression, led to the withdrawal of triazolam[15]. The use of benzodiazepines has been associated with at least a 50% increase in the risk of hip fracture in the elderly[16,17]. The risk is greatest in the first few days and after one month of continuous use. High doses are particularly problematic. This would seem to be a class effect (the risk is not reduced by using short-half-life drugs). Benzodiazepines can cause anterograde amnesia[18] and can adversely affect driving performance[19]. Benzodiazepines can also cause disinhibition.

Respiratory depression is rare with oral therapy but is possible when the IV route is used. A specific benzodiazepine antagonist, flumazenil, is available. Flumazenil has a much shorter half-life than diazepam, making close observation of the patient essential for several hours after administration.

IV injections can be painful and lead to thrombophlebitis due to the low water solubility of benzodiazepines, and therefore it is necessary to use solvents in the preparation of injectable forms. Diazepam is available in emulsion form (Diazemuls) to overcome these problems.

Drug interactions

Benzodiazepines do not induce microsomal enzymes and so do not frequently precipitate pharmacokinetic interactions with any other drugs. Most benzodiazepines are metabolised by CYP3A4, which is inhibited by erythromycin, several SSRIs and ketoconazole. It is theoretically possible that co-administration of these drugs will result in higher serum levels of benzodiazepines. Pharmacodynamic interactions (usually increased sedation) can occur. Benzodiazepines are associated with an important interaction with methadone (see page 324).

References

1. Nutt DJ et al. New insights into the role of the GABA(A)-benzodiazepine receptor in psychiatric disorder. Br J Psychiatry 2001;179:390–6.
2. Committee on Safety of Medicines. Benzodiazepines, dependence and withdrawal symptoms. Current Problems 1988;21:1–2.
3. National Institute for Clinical Excellence. Anxiety: management of anxiety (panic disorder, with or without agoraphobia, and generalised anxiety disorder) in adults in primary, secondary and community care. http://www.nice.org.uk. 2004.
4. Vogel GW et al. Drug effects on REM sleep and on endogenous depression. Neurosci Biobehav Rev 1990;14:49–63.
5. Mahomed R et al. Prescribing hypnotics in a mental health trust: what consultants say and what they do. Pharm J 2002;268:657–9.
6. Royal College of Psychiatrists. Benzodiazepines: risks, benefits and dependence: a re-evaluation. Council Report 59. http://www.rcpsych.ac.uk/ (London). 1997.
7. Department of Health. National Service Framework for Mental Health: Modern Standards and Service Models. http://www.dh.gov.uk/. 1999.
8. National Institute for Clinical Excellence. Depression: management of depression in primary and secondary care – clinical guidance. http://www.nice.org.uk. 2004.
9. TREC Collaborative Group. Rapid tranquillisation for agitated patients in emergency psychiatric rooms: a randomised trial of midazolam versus haloperidol plus promethazine. BMJ 2003;327:708–13.
10. Alexander J et al. Rapid tranquillisation of violent or agitated patients in a psychiatric emergency setting. Pragmatic randomised trial of intramuscular lorazepam v. haloperidol plus promethazine. Br J Psychiatry 2004;185:63–9.
11. Gillies D et al. Benzodiazepines alone or in combination with antipsychotic drugs for acute psychosis. Cochrane Database Syst Rev 2005;CD003079.
12. Carpenter WT Jr et al. Diazepam treatment of early signs of exacerbation in schizophrenia. Am J Psychiatry 1999;156:299–303.
13. Paton C et al. Benzodiazepines in schizophrenia. Is there a trend towards long-term prescribing? Psychiatr Bull 2000;24:113–15.
14. Wolkowitz OM et al. Benzodiazepines in the treatment of schizophrenia: a review and reappraisal. Am J Psychiatry 1991;148:714–26.
15. Anon. The sudden withdrawal of triazolam – reasons and consequences. Drug Ther Bull 1991; 29:89–90.
16. Wang PS et al. Hazardous benzodiazepine regimens in the elderly: effects of half-life, dosage, and duration on risk of hip fracture. Am J Psychiatry 2001;158:892–8.
17. Cumming RG et al. Benzodiazepines and risk of hip fractures in older people: a review of the evidence. CNS Drugs 2003;17:825–37.
18. Verwey B et al. Memory impairment in those who attempted suicide by benzodiazepine overdose. J Clin Psychiatry 2000;61:456–9.
19. Barbone F et al. Association of road-traffic accidents with benzodiazepine use. Lancet 1998; 352: 1331–6.

Depression & anxiety

Further reading

Ashton H. Guidelines for the rational use of benzodiazepines. Drugs 1994;48:25–40.
Chouinard G. Issues in the clinical use of benzodiazepines: potency, withdrawal and rebound. J Clin Psychiatry 2004;65(Suppl. 5):7–12.
Summers J et al. Benzodiazepine prescribing in a psychiatric hospital. Psychiatr Bull 1998;22:480–3.
Williams DDR et al. Benzodiazepines: time for reassessment. Br J Psychiatry 1998;173:361–2.

Benzodiazepines and disinhibition

Unexpected increases in aggressive behaviour secondary to drug treatment are usually called disinhibitory or paradoxical reactions. These reactions may be characterised by acute excitement, hyperactivity, increased anxiety, vivid dreams, sexual disinhibition, hostility and rage. It is possible for a drug to have the potential both to decrease and increase aggressive behaviour. Examples include amfetamines, methylphenidate, benzodiazepines and alcohol (note that all are potential drugs of misuse).

How common are disinhibitory reactions with benzodiazepines?

The incidence of disinhibitory reactions varies widely depending on the population studied (see 'Who is at risk?' below). For example, a meta-analysis of benzodiazepine randomised, controlled trials (RCTs) that included many hundreds of patients with a wide range of diagnoses reported an incidence of less than 1% (similar to placebo)[1]; a Norwegian study that reported on 415 cases of 'driving under the influence', in which flunitrazepam was the sole substance implicated, found that 6% could be described as due to disinhibitory reactions[2]. An RCT that recruited patients with panic disorder reported an incidence of 13%[3]; authors of case series (often reporting on use in high-risk patients) reported rates of 10–20%[1]; and an RCT that included patients with borderline personality disorder reported a rate of 58%[4].

Who is at risk?

Those who have learning disability, neurological disorder or CNS degenerative disease[5], are young (child or adolescent) or elderly[5,6], or have a history of aggression/poor impulse control[4,7] are at increased risk of experiencing a disinhibitory reaction. The risk is further increased if the benzodiazepine is a high-potency drug, has a short half-life, is given in a high dose or is administered intravenously (high and rapidly fluctuating plasma levels)[5,8]. Some people may be genetically predisposed[9].

What is the mechanism?[8,10,11]

Various theories of the mechanism have been proposed: the anxiolytic and amnesic properties of benzodiazepines may lead to a loss of the restraint that governs normal social behaviour, the sedative and amnesic properties of benzodiazepines may lead to a reduced ability to concentrate on the external social cues that guide appropriate behaviour and the benzodiazepine-mediated increases in GABA neurotransmission may lead to a decrease in the restraining influence of the cortex, resulting in untrammelled excitement, anxiety and hostility.

Subjective reports

People who take benzodiazepines rate themselves as being more tolerant and friendly, but respond more to provocation than placebo-treated patients[12].

People with impulse control problems who take benzodiazepines may self-report feelings of power and overwhelming self-esteem[7]. Psychology rating scales demonstrate increased suggestibility, failure to recognise anger in others and reduced ability to recognise social cues.

Clinical implications

Benzodiazepines are frequently used in rapid tranquillisation and the short-term management of disturbed behaviour. It is important to be aware of their propensity to cause disinhibitory reactions.

Paradoxical/disinhibitory/aggressive outbursts in the context of benzodiazepine use:

- usually occur with high doses of high-potency drugs that are administered parenterally
- are rare in the general population but more frequent in people with impulse control problems or CNS damage and in the very young or very old
- usually occur in response to (very mild) provocation, the exact nature of which is not always obvious to others
- are recognised by others but often not by the sufferer, who often believes that he is friendly and tolerant.

Suspected paradoxical reactions should be clearly documented in the clinical notes. In extreme cases, flumazenil can be used to reverse the reaction. If the benzodiazepine was prescribed to control acute behavioural disturbance, future episodes should be managed with antipsychotic drugs[13] or other non-benzodiazepine sedatives.

References

1. Dietch JT et al. Aggressive dyscontrol in patients treated with benzodiazepines. J Clin Psychiatry 1988; 49:184–8.
2. Bramness JG et al. Flunitrazepam: psychomotor impairment, agitation and paradoxical reactions. Forensic Sci Int 2006;159:83–91.
3. O'Sullivan GH et al. Safety and side-effects of alprazolam. Controlled study in agoraphobia with panic disorder. Br J Psychiatry 1994;165:79–86.
4. Gardner DL et al. Alprazolam-induced dyscontrol in borderline personality disorder. Am J Psychiatry 1985;142:98–100.
5. Bond AJ. Drug-induced behavioural disinhibition incidence, mechanisms and therapeutic implications. CNS Drugs 1998;9:41–57.
6. Hawkridge SM et al. A risk–benefit assessment of pharmacotherapy for anxiety disorders in children and adolescents. Drug Saf 1998;19:283–97.
7. Daderman AM et al. Flunitrazepam (Rohypnol) abuse in combination with alcohol causes premeditated, grievous violence in male juvenile offenders. J Am Acad Psychiatry Law 1999;27:83–99.
8. van der BP et al. Disinhibitory reactions to benzodiazepines: a review. J Oral Maxillofac Surg 1991;49: 519–23.
9. Short TG et al. Paradoxical reactions to benzodiazepines – a genetically determined phenomenon? Anaesth Intensive Care 1987;15:330–1.
10. Weisman AM et al. Effects of clorazepate, diazepam, and oxazepam on a laboratory measurement of aggression in men. Int Clin Psychopharmacol 1998;13:183–8.
11. Blair RJ et al. Selective impairment in the recognition of anger induced by diazepam. Psychopharmacology 1999;147:335–8.
12. Bond AJ et al. Behavioural aggression in panic disorder after 8 weeks' treatment with alprazolam. J Affect Disord 1995;35:117–23.
13. Paton C. Benzodiazepines and disinhibition: a review. Psychiatr Bull 2002;26:460–2.

Benzodiazepines: dependence and detoxification

Benzodiazepines are widely acknowledged as addictive and withdrawal symptoms can occur after 4–6 weeks of continuous use. At least a third of long-term users experience problems on dosage reduction or withdrawal[1]. Short-acting drugs such as lorazepam are associated with more problems on withdrawal than longer-acting drugs such as diazepam[1,2]. To avoid or lessen these problems, good practice dictates that benzodiazepines should not be prescribed as hypnotics or anxiolytics for longer than 4 weeks[3,4]. Intermittent use (i.e. not every day) may also help avoid problems of dependence and tolerance.

Problems on withdrawal[5]

Physical	Psychological
• Stiffness	Anxiety/insomnia
• Weakness	Nightmares
• GI disturbance	Depersonalisation
• Paraesthesia	Decreased memory and concentration
• Flu-like symptoms	Delusions and hallucinations
• Visual disturbances	Depression

In the majority, symptoms last no longer than a few weeks, although a minority experience disabling symptoms for much longer[1,3]. Minimal intervention strategies – for example, simply sending the patient a letter advising them to stop taking benzodiazepine – increases the odds of successfully stopping three-fold[6]. Continuing support may be required (e.g. psychological therapies or self-help groups).

If clinically indicated and assuming the patient is in agreement, benzodiazepines should be withdrawn as follows.

Confirming use

If benzodiazepines are not prescribed and patients are obtaining their own supply, use should be confirmed by urine screening (a negative urine screen in combination with no signs of benzodiazepine withdrawal rules out physical dependence). Very short-acting benzodiazepines may not give a positive urine screen despite daily use.

Tolerance test

This will be required if the patient has been obtaining illicit supplies. No benzodiazepines/alcohol should be consumed for 12 hours before the test. A test dose of 10 mg diazepam should be administered (20 mg if consumption of >50 mg daily is claimed or suspected) and the patient observed for 2–3 hours. If there are no signs of sedation, it is generally safe to prescribe the test dose three times a day. Some patients may require much higher doses. Inpatient assessment may be desirable in these cases.

Switching to diazepam

Patients who take short- or intermediate-acting benzodiazepines should be offered an equivalent dose of diazepam (which has a long half-life and therefore provokes less severe withdrawal)[1]. Note that Cochrane are lukewarm about this approach[7]. Approximate 'diazepam equivalent'[1] doses are shown below.

Chlordiazepoxide	25 mg
Clonazepam	1–2 mg
Diazepam	**10 mg**
Lorazepam	1 mg
Lormetazepam	1 mg
Nitrazepam	10 mg
Oxazepam	30 mg
Temazepam	20 mg

The half-lives of benzodiazepines vary greatly. The degree of sedation that they induce also varies, making it difficult to determine exact equivalents. The above is an approximate guide only. Extra precautions apply in patients with hepatic dysfunction as diazepam may accumulate to toxic levels. Diazepam substitution may not be appropriate in this group of patients.

Dosage reduction

Systematic reduction strategies are twice as likely to lead to abstinence than simply advising the patient to stop[6]. Although gradual withdrawal is more acceptable to patients than abrupt withdrawal[7], note that there is no evidence to support the differential efficacy of different tapering schedules, either fixed dose or symptom guided[6]. The following is a suggested taper schedule; some patients may tolerate more rapid reduction and others may require a slower taper.

- Reduce by 10 mg/day every 1–2 weeks, down to a daily dose of 50 mg.
- Reduce by 5 mg/day every 1–2 weeks, down to a daily dose of 30 mg.
- Reduce by 2 mg/day every 1–2 weeks, down to a daily dose of 20 mg.
- Reduce by 1 mg/day every 1–2 weeks until stopped.

Usually, no more than one week's supply (exact number of tablets) should be issued at any one time.

Anticipating problems[1,5,8]

Problematic withdrawal can be anticipated if previous attempts have been unsuccessful, the patient lacks social support, there is a history of alcohol/

polydrug abuse or withdrawal seizures, the patient is elderly, or there is concomitant severe physical/psychiatric disorder or personality disorder. The acceptable rate of withdrawal may inevitably be slower in these patients. Some may never succeed. Risk–benefit analysis may conclude that maintenance treatment with benzodiazepines is appropriate[3]. Some patients may need interventions for underlying disorders masked by benzodiazepine dependence. If the patient is indifferent to withdrawal (i.e. is not motivated to stop), success is unlikely.

Adjunctive treatments

There is some evidence to support the use of antidepressant and mood-stabilising drugs as adjuncts during benzodiazepine withdrawal[1,6,7,9–12]. People with insomnia may benefit from adjunctive treatment with melatonin and those with panic disorder may benefit from CBT during the taper period[6].

References

1. Schweizer E et al. Benzodiazepine dependence and withdrawal: a review of the syndrome and its clinical management. Acta Psychiatr Scand Suppl 1998;393:95–101.
2. Uhlenhuth EH et al. International study of expert judgment on therapeutic use of benzodiazepines and other psychotherapeutic medications: IV. Therapeutic dose dependence and abuse liability of benzodiazepines in the long-term treatment of anxiety disorders. J Clin Psychopharmacol 1999;19:23S–9S.
3. Royal College of Psychiatrists. Benzodiazepines: risks, benefits and dependence: a re-evaluation. Council Report 59. http://www.rcpsych.ac.uk/ (London). 1997.
4. Committee on Safety in Medicines. Benzodiazepines, dependence and withdrawal symptoms. Current Problems 1988;21:1–2.
5. Petursson H. The benzodiazepine withdrawal syndrome. Addiction 1994;89:1455–9.
6. Voshaar RCO et al. Strategies for discontinuing long-term benzodiazepine use: meta-analysis. Br J Psychiatry 2006;189:213–20.
7. Denis C et al. Pharmacological interventions for benzodiazepine mono-dependence management in outpatient settings. Cochrane Database Syst Rev 2006;CD005194.
8. Tyrer P. Risks of dependence on benzodiazepine drugs: the importance of patient selection. BMJ 1989;298:102,104–5.
9. Rickels K et al. Imipramine and buspirone in treatment of patients with generalized anxiety disorder who are discontinuing long-term benzodiazepine therapy. Am J Psychiatry 2000;157:1973–9.
10. Tyrer P et al. A controlled trial of dothiepin and placebo in treating benzodiazepine withdrawal symptoms. Br J Psychiatry 1996;168:457–61.
11. Schweizer E et al. Carbamazepine treatment in patients discontinuing long-term benzodiazepine therapy. Effects on withdrawal severity and outcome. Arch Gen Psychiatry 1991;48:448–52.
12. Zitman FG et al. Chronic benzodiazepine use in general practice patients with depression: an evaluation of controlled treatment and taper-off: report on behalf of the Dutch Chronic Benzodiazepine Working Group. Br J Psychiatry 2001;178:317–24.

Further reading

Department of Health. Drug misuse and dependence – guidelines on clinical management. London: Department of Health, 1999.
Gerada C et al. ABC of mental health: addiction and dependence. Illicit drugs. BMJ 1997;315: 297–300.
Lader M. Withdrawal reactions after stopping hypnotics in patients with insomnia. CNS Drugs 1998;10:425–40.
Mental Health Foundation. Guidelines for the prevention and treatment of benzodiazepine dependence. London: Mental Health Foundation, 1992.
Rickels K et al. Pharmacological strategies for discontinuing benzodiazepine treatment. J Clin Psychopharmacol 1999;19(Suppl 2):12–16.

Depression & anxiety

Insomnia

A patient complaining of insomnia may describe one or more of the following symptoms:

- difficulty in falling asleep
- frequent waking during the night
- early-morning wakening
- daytime sleepiness
- a general loss of well-being through the individual's perception of a bad night's sleep.

Insomnia is a common complaint affecting approximately one-third of the UK population in any one year[1]. It is more common in women, in the elderly (some reports suggest 50% of those over 65 years) and in those with medical or psychiatric disorders[2]. Population studies in the UK have found that the prevalence of symptoms of underlying psychiatric illness, particularly depression and anxiety, increases with the severity and chronicity of insomnia[3]. Insomnia that lasts for 1 year or more is an established risk factor for the development of depression[4]. Chronic insomnia rarely remits spontaneously[5].

Before treating insomnia with drugs, consider:

- Is the underlying cause being treated (depression, mania, breathing difficulties, urinary frequency, pain, etc.)?
- Is substance misuse or diet a problem?
- Are other drugs being given at appropriate times (i.e. stimulating drugs in the morning, sedating drugs at night)?
- Are the patient's expectations of sleep realistic (sleep requirements decrease with age)?
- Have all sleep hygiene approaches (see table below) been tried[1]?

Table Sleep hygiene approaches
• Increase daily exercise (not in the evening) • Reduce daytime napping • Reduce caffeine or alcohol intake, especially before bedtime • Use the bed only for sleeping • Use anxiety management or relaxation techniques • Develop a regular routine of rising and retiring at the same time each day

Table Guidelines for prescribing hypnotics[6]

- Use the lowest effective dose
- Use intermittent dosing (alternate nights or less) where possible
- Prescribe for short-term use (no more than 4 weeks) in the majority of cases
- Discontinue slowly
- Be alert for rebound insomnia/withdrawal symptoms
- Advise patients of the interaction with alcohol and other sedating drugs
- Avoid the use of hypnotics in patients with respiratory disease or severe hepatic impairment and in addiction-prone individuals

Short-acting hypnotics are better for patients who have difficulty dropping off to sleep, but tolerance and dependence may develop more quickly[4]. Long-acting hypnotics are more suitable for patients with frequent or early-morning wakening. These drugs may be less likely to cause rebound insomnia and can have next-day anxiolytic action, but next-day sedation and maybe loss of coordination are more likely to occur[6]. The risks of treating older people (> 60 years) with hypnotics may outweigh the benefits. A meta-analysis has shown the number needed to treat for improved sleep quality was 13 and the number needed to treat for any adverse event was 6[7]. Older patients prescribed hypnotics (especially those with dementia) should be closely monitored to determine if the prescription continues to be justified.

The most widely prescribed hypnotics are the benzodiazepines. Non-benzodiazepine hypnotics such as zopiclone and zolpidem are becoming more widely used but may be just as likely as the benzodiazepines to cause rebound, dependence and neuropsychiatric reactions[8-10]. Zopiclone may impair driving performance more than benzodiazepines[11]. NICE conclude that there is no difference in efficacy between zaleplon, zolpidem and zopiclone and that patients who fail to respond to one drug should not be offered another[12].

A novel antipsychotic, ramelteon, has been approved for use in the USA and may become available in the UK in 2008. It is a highly selective melatonin (MT_1/MT_2) receptor agonist. Ramelteon produced significant reductions in latency to persistent sleep and increases in total sleep in a group of patients with chronic primary insomnia[13], with no apparent next-day residual effects. Over-the-counter remedies for insomnia include valerian–hops combinations and diphenhydramine which may improve sleep to some extent without causing rebound insomnia[14].

Table Drugs used as hypnotics

Drug	Usual therapeutic dose (mg/day)		Time until onset (minutes)	Duration of action
	Adult	Elderly		
Lormetazepam†	0.5–1.5		30–60	Short
Oxazepam†	15–30		20–50	Medium
Nitrazepam†	5–10		20–50	Long
Temazepam*†	10–20	Quarter to	30–60	Short
Zaleplon	10	half the	30	Very short
Zopiclone	3.75–7.5	adult dose	15–30	Medium
Zolpidem	5–10		7–27	Short
Promethazine (not licensed)	25–50		Unclear, but may be 1–2 hours	Long

*Temazepam is a popular drug of misuse. Some of the Controlled Drug regulations apply to its prescription, supply and administration. Nursing paperwork can be simplified considerably by avoiding the use of this drug.

†Changes in Controlled Drug Regulations as of July 2006 mean that benzodiazepines should only be prescribed for a maximum of 28 days at a time.

Although it is commonly believed that tolerance always develops rapidly to the hypnotic effect of benzodiazepines[12] and zopiclone, there are only limited objective data to support this and the magnitude of the problem may have been overestimated[5]. Long-term treatment with hypnotics may be beneficial in a very small number of patients. Case reports, case series and consensus statements support this approach[4–6,15–17]. Long-term users may overestimate the benefits on continuing use: after a period of rebound symptoms immediately after withdrawal, many chronic users will return to the same sleep pattern (drug free) that they previously associated with hypnotic use[18]. As with all prescribing, the potential benefits and risks of hypnotic drugs have to be considered in the context of the clinical circumstances of each case.

Cognitive behavioural therapy (CBT) may be more effective than hypnotics in improving sleep in the long term[19]. CBT has been shown to improve sleep quality, reduce hypnotic drug use and improve health-related quality of life among long-term hypnotic users with chronic sleep difficulties[20].

References

1. Hajak G. A comparative assessment of the risks and benefits of zopiclone: a review of 15 years' clinical experience. Drug Saf 1999;21:457–69.
2. Shapiro CM. ABC of Sleep Disorders. London: BMJ Publishing Group, 1993.
3. Nutt DJ et al. Evaluation of severe insomnia in the general population – implications for the management of insomnia: the UK perspective. J Psychopharmacol 1999;13:S33–S34.
4. Moller HJ. Effectiveness and safety of benzodiazepines. J Clin Psychopharmacol 1999;19:2S–11S.
5. Nowell PD et al. Benzodiazepines and zolpidem for chronic insomnia: a meta-analysis of treatment efficacy. JAMA 1997;278:2170–7.
6. Royal College of Psychiatrists. Benzodiazepines: risks, benefits and dependence: a re-evaluation. Council Report 59. http://www.rcpsych.ac.uk/ (London). 1997.
7. Glass J et al. Sedative hypnotics in older people with insomnia: meta-analysis of risks and benefits. BMJ 2005;331:1169.
8. Sikdar S et al. Zopiclone abuse among polydrug users. Addiction 1996;91:285–6.
9. Gericke CA et al. Chronic abuse of zolpidem. JAMA 1994;272:1721–2.
10. Voshaar RC et al. Zolpidem is not superior to temazepam with respect to rebound insomnia: a controlled study. Eur Neuropsychopharmacol 2004;14:301–6.
11. Barbone F et al. Association of road-traffic accidents with benzodiazepine use. Lancet 1998;352: 1331–6.
12. National Institute for Clinical Excellence. Insomnia – newer hypnotic drugs. Zaleplon, zolpidem and zopiclone for the management of insomnia. Technology Appraisal 77. http://www.nice.org.uk. 2004.
13. Erman M et al. An efficacy, safety, and dose–response study of Ramelteon in patients with chronic primary insomnia. Sleep Med 2006;7:17–24.
14. Morin CM et al. Valerian–hops combination and diphenhydramine for treating insomnia: a randomized placebo-controlled clinical trial. Sleep 2005;28:1465–71.
15. Lader M. Withdrawal reactions after stopping hypnotics in patients with insomnia. CNS Drugs 1998; 10:425–40.
16. Perlis ML et al. Long-term, non-nightly administration of zolpidem in the treatment of patients with primary insomnia. J Clin Psychiatry 2004;65:1128–37.
17. Mahomed R et al. Prescribing hypnotics in a mental health trust: what consultants say and what they do. Pharm J 2002;268:657–9.
18. Poyares D et al. Chronic benzodiazepine usage and withdrawal in insomnia patients. J Psychiatr Res 2004;38:327–34.
19. Jacobs GD et al. Cognitive behavior therapy and pharmacotherapy for insomnia: a randomized controlled trial and direct comparison. Arch Intern Med 2004;164:1888–96.
20. Morgan K et al. Psychological treatment for insomnia in the regulation of long-term hypnotic drug use. Health Technol Assess 2004;8:iii–68.

Further reading

Benca RM. Diagnosis and treatment of chronic insomnia: a review. Psychiatr Serv 2005;56:332–43.
Terzano MG et al. New drugs for insomnia; comparative tolerability of zopiclone, zolpidem and zaleplon. Drug Safety 2003;26:261–82.

chapter 5

Children and adolescents

Children and adolescents suffer from all the illnesses of adulthood. It is common for psychiatric illness to commence more diffusely, present 'atypically', respond less predictably and be associated with cumulative impairment more subtly. Childhood-onset illness is likely to be at least as severe and functionally disabling as adult-onset illness.

Very few psychotropic drugs are licensed for use in children. This should be carefully explained and informed consent sought from patients and their parents/carers (see page 488).

Children

Principles of prescribing practice in childhood and adolescence[1]

- **Target symptoms, not diagnoses.**
  Diagnosis can be difficult in children and co-morbidity is very common. Treatment should target key symptoms. While a working diagnosis is beneficial to frame expectations and help communication with patients and parents, it should be kept in mind that it may take some time for the illness to evolve.

- **Begin with less, go slow and be prepared to end with more.**
  In outpatient care, dosage will usually commence lower in mg/kg per day terms than adults and finish higher in mg/kg per day terms, if titrated to a point of maximal response.

- **Multiple medications are often required in the severely ill.**
  Monotherapy is ideal. However, childhood-onset illness can be severe and may require treatment with psychosocial approaches in combination with more than one medication[2].

- **Allow time for an adequate trial of treatment.**
  Children are generally more ill than their adult counterparts and will often require longer periods of treatment before responding. An adequate trial of treatment for those who have required inpatient care will therefore involve 8–12 weeks for most major conditions.

- **Where possible, change one drug at a time.**

- **Patient and family medication education is essential.**
  For some child and adolescent psychiatric patients the need for medication will be lifelong. The first experiences with medications are therefore crucial to long-term outcomes and adherence. It is important to adhere to the principles of CAAT (see page 515).

References

1. Nunn K et al. The Clinician's Guide to Psychotropic Prescribing in Children and Adolescents. Sydney: Glade Publishing; 2003.
2. Luk E et al. Polypharmacy or pharmacologically rich? In: Nunn KP et al, eds. The Clinician's Guide to Psychotropic Prescribing in Children and Adolescents. Sydney: Glade Publishing; 2003: 8–11.

Depression in children and adolescents

Psychological treatments should always be considered as first-line treatments. If these are inappropriate, have failed or are simply not available, **fluoxetine**[1-3] is the treatment of choice. Note that the placebo response rate is high in younger people[4] and that the benefits of active treatment are likely to be marginal: it is estimated that 1 in 6 may benefit[5]. There is limited evidence to suggest dose increases can improve response[6]. The risk–benefit ratios for the other SSRIs are unfavourable (no proven efficacy, and increased risk of suicidal thoughts or acts). If there is no response to fluoxetine and drug treatment is still considered to be the most favourable option, **an alternative SSRI** may be used cautiously by specialists. Sertraline may be marginally effective[7,8] but is inferior to CBT[9]. Citalopram and escitalopram are probably not effective[2,10,11]. Note that paroxetine and venlafaxine are considered to be unsuitable options[12]. It is important that the dose is increased slowly to minimise the risk of treatment-emergent agitation and that patients are monitored closely for the development of treatment-emergent suicidal thoughts and acts. Patients should be seen at least weekly in the early stages of treatment. There is now no doubt that antidepressants increase the risk of suicide in children[13-18].

Patients and their parents/carers should be well informed about the potential problems associated with SSRI treatment and know how to seek help in an emergency. They should be given a copy of the MHRA leaflet about the use of SSRIs in young people (available via the MHRA website)[2].

Tricyclic antidepressants are not effective in prepubertal children but may have marginal efficacy in adolescents[12]. Amitriptyline (up to 200 mg/day), imipramine (up to 300 mg/day) and nortriptyline have all been studied in RCTs. Note that due to more extensive metabolism, young people require higher mg/kg doses than adults. The side-effect burden associated with TCAs may be considerable. Vertigo, orthostatic hypotension, tremor and dry mouth limit tolerability. Tricyclics are also more cardiotoxic in young people than in adults. Baseline and on-treatment ECGs should be performed. Co-prescribing with other drugs known to prolong the QTc interval should be avoided. There is no evidence that adolescents who fail to respond to SSRIs respond to tricyclics.

Omega-3 fatty acids may be effective in childhood depression but evidence is minimal[19].

Severe depression that is life-threatening or unresponsive to other treatments may respond to ECT[20]. ECT should not be used in children under 12[20]. The effects of ECT on the developing brain are unknown.

There is no good evidence to support the optimum duration of treatment. Adult guidelines are usually followed (see Chapter 4). At the end of treatment, the antidepressant dose should be tapered down slowly to minimise discontinuation symptoms. Ideally this should be done over 6–12 weeks[5].

Note that up to a third of young people who present with an episode of depression will have a diagnosis of bipolar affective disorder within 5 years. When the presentation is of severe depression, associated with psychosis or rapid mood shifts, and worsens on treatment with antidepressants, early bipolar

Children

illness should be suspected. Treatment with antidepressants alone is associated with new or worsening rapid cycling in as many as 23% of bipolar patients[21]. The younger the child, the greater the risk[22]. Early treatment with mood stabilisers should be considered.

References

1. Whittington CJ et al. Selective serotonin reuptake inhibitors in childhood depression: systematic review of published versus unpublished data. Lancet 2004;363:1341–5.
2. Medicines and Healthcare Products Regulatory Agency. Selective serotonin reuptake inhibitors (SSRIs): overview of regulatory status and CSM advice relating to major depressive disorder (MDD) in children and adolescents including a summary of available safety and efficacy data. www.mhra.gov.uk. 2005.
3. Kratochvil CJ et al. Selective serotonin reuptake inhibitors in pediatric depression: is the balance between benefits and risks favorable? J Child Adolesc Psychopharmacol 2006;16:11–24.
4. Jureidini JN et al. Efficacy and safety of antidepressants for children and adolescents. BMJ 2004;328:879–83.
5. National Institute for Clinical Excellence. Depression in children and young people: identification and management in primary, community and secondary care. Clinical Guidance. www.mhra.gov.uk. 2005.
6. Heiligenstein JH et al. Fluoxetine 40–60 mg versus fluoxetine 20 mg in the treatment of children and adolescents with a less-than-complete response to nine-week treatment with fluoxetine 10–20 mg: a pilot study. J Child Adolesc Psychopharmacol 2006;16:207–17.
7. Donnelly CL et al. Sertraline in children and adolescents with major depressive disorder. J Am Acad Child Adolesc Psychiatry 2006;45:1162–70.
8. Rynn M et al. Long-term sertraline treatment of children and adolescents with major depressive disorder. J Child Adolesc Psychopharmacol 2006;16:103–16.
9. Melvin GA et al. A comparison of cognitive-behavioral therapy, sertraline, and their combination for adolescent depression. J Am Acad Child Adolesc Psychiatry 2006;45:1151–61.
10. Wagner KD et al. A double-blind, randomized, placebo-controlled trial of escitalopram in the treatment of pediatric depression. J Am Acad Child Adolesc Psychiatry 2006;45:280–8.
11. von Knorring AL et al. A randomized, double-blind, placebo-controlled study of citalopram in adolescents with major depressive disorder. J Clin Psychopharmacol 2006;26:311–15.
12. Hazell P et al. Tricyclic drugs for depression in children and adolescents. Cochrane Database Syst Rev 2002;CD002317.
13. Martinez C et al. Antidepressant treatment and the risk of fatal and non-fatal self harm in first episode depression: nested case-control study. BMJ 2005;330:389.
14. Kaizar EE et al. Do antidepressants cause suicidality in children? A Bayesian meta-analysis. Clin Trials 2006;3:73–90.
15. Mosholder AD et al. Suicidal adverse events in pediatric randomized, controlled clinical trials of antidepressant drugs are associated with active drug treatment: a meta-analysis. J Child Adolesc Psychopharmacol 2006;16:25–32.
16. Simon GE et al. Suicide risk during antidepressant treatment. Am J Psychiatry 2006;163:41–7.
17. Olfson M et al. Antidepressant drug therapy and suicide in severely depressed children and adults: a case-control study. Arch Gen Psychiatry 2006;63:865–72.
18. Hammad TA et al. Suicidality in pediatric patients treated with antidepressant drugs. Arch Gen Psychiatry 2006;63:332–9.
19. Nemets H et al. Omega-3 treatment of childhood depression: a controlled, double-blind pilot study. Am J Psychiatry 2006;163:1098–100.
20. McKeough G. Electroconvulsive therapy. In: Nunn KP et al, eds. The Clinician's Guide to Psychotropic Prescribing in Children and Adolescents. Sydney: Glade Publishing; 2003:358–65.
21. Ghaemi SN et al. Diagnosing bipolar disorder and the effect of antidepressants: a naturalistic study. J Clin Psychiatry 2000;61:804–8.
22. Martin A et al. Age effects on antidepressant-induced manic conversion. Arch Pediatr Adolesc Med 2004;158:773–80.

Children

Further reading

Bloch Y et al. Electroconvulsive therapy in adolescents: similarities to and differences from adults. J Am Acad Child Adolesc Psychiatry 2001;40:1332–6.
Moreno C et al. Antidepressants in child and adolescent depression: where are the bugs? Acta Psychiatr Scand 2007;115:184–95.

Bipolar illness in children and adolescents

Bipolar illness with an onset in childhood or adolescence has a poorer prognosis than adult-onset illness[1]. The prevalence of co-morbid psychiatric illness is high: anxiety disorders, conduct disorder, obsessive compulsive disorder (OCD) and substance abuse are common. Bipolar onset may precede substance abuse in many cases[2].

Medication	Comment
Valproate[3-12]	Effective in approximately 50% of acute manic or mixed episodes
	More effective when combined with lithium or an SGA
	Marked weight gain can occur (association between weight gain, hyperandrogenism and polycystic ovarian syndrome. Adolescent girls may be more vulnerable than adults)
	Rare reports of serious hepatotoxicity in children
	Very teratogenic (see page 369). Adequate contraception essential in sexually active adolescents. NICE suggest avoiding valproate in adolescent girls
Lithium[3,4,12-21]	Generally better at preventing manic episodes than depression
	Often ineffective in rapid cycling
	May be more effective when combined with risperidone
	Younger children generally have more side-effects than older children (lower serum levels may be appropriate)
	Very toxic in overdose
	Rapid withdrawal may precipitate a manic episode and this may be problematic in poor compliers. May be effective in reducing co-morbid substance abuse and suicide
Carbamazepine[3]	High potential for drug interactions
Lamotrigine[22-26]	Anecdotal reports of success in younger populations, with sometimes dramatic impact on reducing self-harm. Effective in bipolar depression
	Risk of Stevens–Johnson syndrome 1% (greatest in the first 8 weeks). Risk reduced with slow dose titration and special dosing guidelines for concomitant valproate – see manufacturer's guidelines. Safety data available from paediatric epilepsy populations
	Evidence is lacking but, anecdotally, adolescent dosing similar to adults is appropriate (100–125 mg b.d.)
Olanzapine[27-30]	Open-label studies support efficacy in acute mania
	Dietician involvement recommended for weight management

Children

Table (Cont.)	
Medication	**Comment**
Quetiapine[6,11,27,31–33]	Limited data suggest similar efficacy to valproate
Aripiprazole[34,35]	Minimal evidence in the literature. No RCT but seems well tolerated
Antidepressants[36–40]	Should only be used when a combination of mood stabilisers has failed
	Can cause switching and increase rapidity of cycling even in the presence of mood stabilisers
	Avoid in rapid cycling
	If commenced and patient is stabilised, use continuously as discontinuation may cause depressive relapse; i.e. acute treatment only in times of depression may be detrimental

Three or more untreated episodes may lead to cognitive impairment[41]. The more episodes, the more difficult they are to treat[42]. It is important to start treatment early and monitor carefully for the development of suicidal behaviour.

The evidence base supporting the use of mood stabilizers in early-onset illness is poor. There are no adequately powered RCTs.

Valproate is usually the medication of first choice, followed by **lithium** and then **carbamazepine**. Response rates (total clinical global improvement and YMRS improvement) have been estimated to be: valproate 53%, lithium 38% and carbamazepine 38%[3]. **Lamotrigine** is used if treatment-resistant depressive episodes are present. Adolescents often respond poorly to monotherapy and more than one drug may be required to control symptoms[43,44]. **SGA** drugs may be required (see above).

Once symptomatic improvement occurs, treatment should be continued for at least 2 years to prevent relapse. Poor treatment response and recurrence are common[45].

Biochemical and physical monitoring should be carried out as for adults (see page 37).

References

1. Mick E et al. Defining a developmental subtype of bipolar disorder in a sample of nonreferred adults by age at onset. J Child Adolesc Psychopharmacol 2003;13:453–62.
2. Findling RL et al. Rapid, continuous cycling and psychiatric co-morbidity in pediatric bipolar I disorder. Bipolar Disord 2001;3:202–10.
3. Kowatch RA et al. Effect size of lithium, divalproex sodium, and carbamazepine in children and adolescents with bipolar disorder. J Am Acad Child Adolesc Psychiatry 2000;39:713–20.
4. Findling RL et al. Combination lithium and divalproex sodium in pediatric bipolarity. J Am Acad Child Adolesc Psychiatry 2003;42:895–901.
5. Isojarvi JI et al. Polycystic ovaries and hyperandrogenism in women taking valproate for epilepsy. N Engl J Med 1993;329:1383–8.
6. Delbello MP et al. A double-blind, randomized, placebo-controlled study of quetiapine as adjunctive treatment for adolescent mania. J Am Acad Child Adolesc Psychiatry 2002;41:1216–23.
7. Bowden C. The effectiveness of divalproate in all forms of mania and the broader bipolar spectrum: many questions, few answers. J Affect Disord 2004;79(Suppl 1):S9–14.
8. Freeman TW et al. A double-blind comparison of valproate and lithium in the treatment of acute mania. Am J Psychiatry 1992;149:108–11.
9. Bowden CL. Valproate. Bipolar Disord 2003;5:189–202.
10. Pavuluri MN et al. Divalproex sodium for pediatric mixed mania: a 6-month prospective trial. Bipolar Disord 2005;7:266–73.
11. Delbello MP et al. A double-blind randomized pilot study comparing quetiapine and divalproex for adolescent mania. J Am Acad Child Adolesc Psychiatry 2006;45:305–13.
12. Pavuluri MN et al. Open-label prospective trial of risperidone in combination with lithium or divalproex sodium in pediatric mania. J Affect Disord 2004;82(Suppl 1):S103–11.
13. Kafantaris V et al. Lithium treatment of acute mania in adolescents: a placebo-controlled discontinuation study. J Am Acad Child Adolesc Psychiatry 2004;43:984–93.
14. Campbell M et al. Predictors of side effects associated with lithium administration in children. Psychopharmacol Bull 1991;27:373–80.
15. Geller B et al. Double-blind and placebo-controlled study of lithium for adolescent bipolar disorders with secondary substance dependency. J Am Acad Child Adolesc Psychiatry 1998;37:171–8.
16. Faedda GL et al. Outcome after rapid vs gradual discontinuation of lithium treatment in bipolar disorders. Arch Gen Psychiatry 1993;50:448–55.
17. Kafantaris V et al. Are childhood psychiatric histories of bipolar adolescents associated with family history, psychosis, and response to lithium treatment? J Affect Disord 1998;51:153–64.
18. Goodwin FK et al. Suicide risk in bipolar disorder during treatment with lithium and divalproex. JAMA 2003;290:1467–73.
19. Moore GJ et al. Lithium-induced increase in human brain grey matter. Lancet 2000;356:1241–2.
20. Manji HK et al. Lithium at 50: have the neuroprotective effects of this unique cation been overlooked? Biol Psychiatry 1999;46:929–40.
21. Pavuluri MN et al. A one-year open-label trial of risperidone augmentation in lithium nonresponder youth with preschool-onset bipolar disorder. J Child Adolesc Psychopharmacol 2006;16:336–50.
22. Carandang CG et al. Lamotrigine in adolescent mood disorders (Letter to the editor). J Am Acad Child Adolesc Psychiatry 2003;42:750–1.
23. Calabrese JR et al. Latest maintenance data on lamotrigine in bipolar disorder. Eur Neuropsychopharmacol 2003;13(Suppl 2):S57–66.
24. Calabrese JR et al. A double-blind, placebo-controlled, prophylaxis study of lamotrigine in rapid-cycling bipolar disorder. Lamictal 614 Study Group. J Clin Psychiatry 2000;61:841–50.
25. Rzany B et al. Risk of Stevens–Johnson syndrome and toxic epidermal necrolysis during first weeks of antiepileptic therapy: a case-control study. Study Group of the International Case Control Study on Severe Cutaneous Adverse Reactions. Lancet 1999;353:2190–4.
26. Chang K et al. An open-label study of lamotrigine adjunct or monotherapy for the treatment of adolescents with bipolar depression. J Am Acad Child Adolesc Psychiatry 2006;45:298–304.
27. Kafantaris V et al. Adjunctive antipsychotic treatment of adolescents with bipolar psychosis. J Am Acad Child Adolesc Psychiatry 2001;40:1448–56.
28. Frazier JA et al. A prospective open-label treatment trial of olanzapine monotherapy in children and adolescents with bipolar disorder. J Child Adolesc Psychopharmacol 2001;11:239–50.
29. Biederman J et al. Open-label, 8-week trial of olanzapine and risperidone for the treatment of bipolar disorder in preschool-age children. Biol Psychiatry 2005;58:589–94.
30. Fleischhaker C et al. Weight gain associated with clozapine, olanzapine and risperidone in children and adolescents. J Neural Transm 2007;114:273–80.
31. Vieta E et al. Quetiapine in the treatment of rapid cycling bipolar disorder. Bipolar Disord 2002; 4:335–40.
32. Sokolski KN et al. Adjunctive quetiapine in bipolar patients partially responsive to lithium or valproate. Prog Neuropsychopharmacol Biol Psychiatry 2003;27:863–6.
33. Shaw JA et al. A study of quetiapine: efficacy and tolerability in psychotic adolescents. J Child Adolesc Psychopharmacol 2001;11:415–24.
34. Barzman DH et al. The effectiveness and tolerability of aripiprazole for pediatric bipolar disorders: a retrospective chart review. J Child Adolesc Psychopharmacol 2004;14:593–600.

Children

35. Rugino TA et al. Aripiprazole in children and adolescents: clinical experience. J Child Neurol 2005;20: 603–10.
36. American Psychiatric Association. Practice guideline for the treatment of patients with bipolar disorder (revision). Am J Psychiatry 2002;159:1–50.
37. Martin A et al. Age effects on antidepressant-induced manic conversion. Arch Pediatr Adolesc Med 2004;158:773–80.
38. Keck PE, Jr. et al. Advances in the pharmacologic treatment of bipolar depression. Biol Psychiatry 2003; 53:671–9.
39. Bottlender R et al. Mood-stabilisers reduce the risk of developing antidepressant-induced maniform states in acute treatment of bipolar I depressed patients. J Affect Disord 2001;63:79–83.
40. Altshuler L et al. Impact of antidepressant discontinuation after acute bipolar depression remission on rates of depressive relapse at 1-year follow-up. Am J Psychiatry 2003;160:1252–62.
41. Vieta E et al. Brain imaging correlates of cognitive dysfunction in bipolar disorder. Bipolar Disord 2004;6(Suppl 1):19.
42. Kessing LV et al. Predictors of recurrence in affective disorder – analyses accounting for individual heterogeneity. J Affect Disord 2000;57:139–45.
43. Bhangoo RK et al. Medication use in children and adolescents treated in the community for bipolar disorder. J Child Adolesc Psychopharmacol 2003;13:515–22.
44. Tillman R et al. Definitions of rapid, ultrarapid, and ultradian cycling and of episode duration in pediatric and adult bipolar disorders: a proposal to distinguish episodes from cycles. J Child Adolesc Psychopharmacol 2003;13:267–71.
45. Weckerly J. Pediatric bipolar mood disorder. J Dev Behav Pediatr 2002;23:42–56.

Anxiety in children and adolescents

Where a generalised anxiety disorder (GAD) is the primary diagnosis, psychological interventions such as CBT are first-line treatments[1]. Where anxiety is secondary to another psychiatric disorder, treatment should target the primary illness.

If anxiety is severe and disabling and CBT is inappropriate or has failed, the use of medication is likely to be considered. The evidence base is poor. CBT should always be reconsidered if the young person makes a partial response to medication.

The treatment of anxiety in children and adolescents is generally the same as in adults (see page 251). The following additional considerations apply:

- Young people are more likely to develop disinhibition with benzodiazepines than are adults[2]. Extreme care is required.

- Young people treated with SSRIs are more likely to develop treatment-emergent suicidal thoughts and acts than are adults[3]. Venlafaxine is considered to be unsuitable for use in the treatment of depression in this age group[3] but is effective in anxiety in children and adolescents[4]. Fluoxetine is effective[5,6] and is probably the drug of choice.

- Tricyclic antidepressants are generally poorly tolerated in young people[7]. They are more cardiotoxic in children than in adults and should be avoided in childhood GAD.

- Buspirone can cause disinhibitory reactions and worsen aggression in children[8,9]. These risks are reduced in adolescents.

- Benzodiazepines are widely used to alleviate acute anxiety in children (e.g. before dental procedures) but are not recommended for GAD.

References

1. Compton SN et al. Cognitive-behavioral psychotherapy for anxiety and depressive disorders in children and adolescents: an evidence-based medicine review. J Am Acad Child Adolesc Psychiatry 2004;43: 930–59.
2. Paton C. Benzodiazepines and disinhibition: a review. Psychiatr Bull 2002;26:460–2.
3. National Institute for Clinical Excellence et al. Depression in children and young people: identification and management in primary, community and secondary care. Clinical Guidance. www. mhra.gov.uk. 2005.
4. Rynn MA et al. Efficacy and safety of extended-release venlafaxine in the treatment of generalized anxiety disorder in children and adolescents: two placebo-controlled trials. Am J Psychiatry 2007;164: 290–300.
5. Birmaher B et al. Fluoxetine for the treatment of childhood anxiety disorders. J Am Acad Child Adolesc Psychiatry 2003;42:415–23.
6. Clark DB et al. Fluoxetine for the treatment of childhood anxiety disorders: open-label, long-term extension to a controlled trial. J Am Acad Child Adolesc Psychiatry 2005;44:1263–70.
7. Hazell P et al. Tricyclic drugs for depression in children and adolescents. Cochrane Database Syst Rev 2002;CD002317.
8. Kranzler HR. Use of buspirone in an adolescent with overanxious disorder. J Am Acad Child Adolesc Psychiatry 1988;27:789–90.
9. Pfeffer CR et al. Buspirone treatment of psychiatrically hospitalized prepubertal children with symptoms of anxiety and moderately severe aggression. J Child Adolesc Psychopharmacol 1997;7:145–55.

Children

Obsessive compulsive disorder (OCD) in children and adolescents

The treatment of OCD in children follows the same principles as in adults (see page 251). Note that **sertraline**[1-3] (from age 6 years) and **fluvoxamine** (from age 8 years) are the only SSRIs licensed in the UK for the treatment of OCD in young people. Care should be taken when prescribing SSRIs as this group of drugs has been linked with the development of suicidal thoughts and acts in children who are being treated for depression (see page 275). Cognitive behavioural therapy is effective in this patient group and is treatment of first choice[4,5].

Benzodiazepines should be avoided as the risk of disinhibitory reactions is high[6].

Note that Tourette's syndrome is known to be associated with OCD[7] (see page 292).

References

1. Cook EH et al. Long-term sertraline treatment of children and adolescents with obsessive-compulsive disorder. J Am Acad Child Adolesc Psychiatry 2001;40:1175–81.
2. Pediatric OCD Treatment Study Team (POTS). Cognitive-behavior therapy, sertraline, and their combination for children and adolescents with obsessive-compulsive disorder: the Pediatric OCD Treatment Study (POTS) randomized controlled trial. JAMA 2004;292:1969–76.
3. Geller DA et al. Which SSRI? A meta-analysis of pharmacotherapy trials in pediatric obsessive-compulsive disorder. Am J Psychiatry 2003;160:1919–28.
4. O'Kearney RT et al. Behavioural and cognitive behavioural therapy for obsessive compulsive disorder in children and adolescents. Cochrane Database Syst Rev 2006;CD004856.
5. Freeman JB et al. Cognitive behavioral treatment for young children with obsessive-compulsive disorder. Biol Psychiatry 2007;61:337–43.
6. Paton C. Benzodiazepines and disinhibition: a review. Psychiatr Bull 2002;26:460–2.
7. Leonard HL et al. Childhood rituals: normal development or obsessive-compulsive symptoms? J Am Acad Child Adolesc Psychiatry 1990;29:17–23.

Further reading

Lenane MC et al. Psychiatric disorders in first degree relatives of children and adolescents with obsessive compulsive disorders. J Am Acad Child Adolesc Psychiatry 1990;29:407–12.

McDougle C et al. A double-blind, placebo-controlled study of risperidone addition in serotonin reuptake inhibitor-refractory obsessive-compulsive disorder. Arch Gen Psychiatry 2000;57:794–801.

Nunn K et al. Medication table. The Clinician's Guide to Psychotropic Prescribing in Children and Adolescents. Sydney: Glade Publishing; 2004.

Children

Attention deficit hyperactivity disorder (ADHD)

Children

- A diagnosis of ADHD should be made only after a comprehensive assessment by a child psychiatrist or paediatrician with expertise in ADHD[1]. Appropriate psychological, psychosocial and behavioural interventions should be put in place. Drug treatments should only be part of the overall treatment plan.

- Stimulant drugs (**methylphenidate** and **dexamfetamine**) should be used as first-line treatment. Up to 90% of children will respond[2]. Stimulants are more effective in treating hyperactivity than inattention. Dosage regimens and monitoring are outlined below.

- **Atomoxetine**[3-5] is a suitable first-line alternative. It may be useful for children who do not respond to stimulants or whose medication cannot be administered during the day. It may also be suitable where stimulant diversion is a problem or when tics become problematic on stimulants. Monitoring of liver function is advisable.

- Third-line drugs include **clonidine**[6] and **tricyclic antidepressants**[7]. Very few children should receive these drugs for ADHD alone. There is some evidence supporting the efficacy of **carbamazepine**[8]. There is no evidence to support the use of **second-generation antipsychotics (SGAs)**[9], although risperidone may be helpful in those with moderate learning disability[10]. Modafinil appears to be effective[11] but has not been compared with standard treatments.

- Co-morbid psychiatric illness is common in ADHD children. Stimulants are often helpful overall[7] but are unlikely to be appropriate for children who have a psychotic illness or established problem with substance misuse[2].

- Once stimulant treatment has been established, it is appropriate for repeat prescriptions to be supplied through general practitioners[1].

Summary of NICE guidance[12]

- Methylphenidate, dexamfetamine and atomoxetine are recommended within their licensed indications

- Choice of drug should be based on:
  - co-morbid conditions (tics, Tourette's syndrome, epilepsy)
  - tolerability and adverse effects
  - convenience of dosing
  - potential for diversion
  - patient/parent preference

- Where more than one agent is considered suitable, the product with the lowest cost should be prescribed

Adults

- Although adult ADHD is recognised by both ICD-10 and DSM-IV, it remains a controversial diagnosis in the UK.

- Up to 10% of ADHD children may still have symptoms at the age of 30. It is appropriate to **continue treatment started in childhood** in adults whose symptoms remain disabling.

- A new diagnosis of ADHD in an adult should only follow a comprehensive assessment, including interviews with adults who knew the patient as a child.

- The prevalence of substance misuse and antisocial personality disorder are high in adults whose ADHD was not recognised in childhood[13]. Although methylphenidate is very effective in this population[14], most psychiatrists would feel uncomfortable about initiating stimulants in adults.

- **Atomoxetine** is effective[15] but not licensed for initiation in adults. Monitoring of liver function is advisable.

References

1. National Institute for Clinical Excellence. Guidance on the use of methylphenidate (Ritalin/ Equasym) for attention deficit hyperactivity disorder (ADHD) in childhood. Technology Appraisal 13. www.nice.org.uk. 2000.
2. Hutchins P et al. Attention deficit hyperactivity disorder (ADHD). In: Nunn KD et al, eds. The Clinician's Guide to Psychotropic Prescribing in Children and Adolescents. Sydney: Glade Publishing; 2003: 162–71.
3. Michelson D et al. Once-daily atomoxetine treatment for children and adolescents with attention deficit hyperactivity disorder: a randomized, placebo-controlled study. Am J Psychiatry 2002;159:1896–901.
4. Kratochvil CJ et al. Atomoxetine and methylphenidate treatment in children with ADHD: a prospective, randomized, open-label trial. J Am Acad Child Adolesc Psychiatry 2002;41:776–84.
5. Weiss M et al. A randomized, placebo-controlled study of once-daily atomoxetine in the school setting in children with ADHD. J Am Acad Child Adolesc Psychiatry 2005;44:647–55.
6. Connor DF et al. A meta-analysis of clonidine for symptoms of attention-deficit hyperactivity disorder. J Am Acad Child Adolesc Psychiatry 1999;38:1551–9.
7. Hazell P. Tricyclic antidepressants in children: is there a rationale for use? CNS Drugs 1996;5:233–9.
8. Silva RR et al. Carbamazepine use in children and adolescents with features of attention-deficit hyper- activity disorder: a meta-analysis. J Am Acad Child Adolesc Psychiatry 1996;35:352–8.
9. Einarson TR et al. Novel antipsychotics for patients with attention-deficit hyperactivity disorder: a sys- tematic review. Ottawa: Canadian Coordinating Office for Health Technology Assessment (CCOHTA) 2001;Technology Report No 17.
10. Correia Filho AG et al. Comparison of risperidone and methylphenidate for reducing ADHD symptoms in children and adolescents with moderate mental retardation. J Am Acad Child Adolesc Psychiatry 2005;44:748–55.
11. Biederman J et al. A comparison of once-daily and divided doses of modafinil in children with attention- deficit/hyperactivity disorder: a randomized, double-blind, and placebo-controlled study. J Clin Psychiatry 2006;67:727–35.
12. National Institute for Clinical Excellence. Methylphenidate, atomoxetine and dexamfetamine for atten- tion deficit hyperactivity disorder (ADHD) in children and adolescents – guidance. Technology Appraisal 98. www.nice.org.uk. 2006.
13. Cosgrove PVF. Attention deficit hyperactivity disorder. Primary Care Psychiatry 1997;3:101–14.
14. Spencer T et al. A double-blind, crossover comparison of methylphenidate and placebo in adults with childhood-onset attention-deficit hyperactivity disorder. Arch Gen Psychiatry 1995;52:434–43.
15. Spencer T et al. Effectiveness and tolerability of atomoxetine in adults with attention deficit hyperac- tivity disorder. Am J Psychiatry 1998;155:693–5.

Children

Further reading

Kutcher S et al. International consensus statement on attention-deficit/hyperactivity disorder (ADHD) and disruptive behaviour disorders (DBDs): clinical implications and treatment practice suggestions. Eur Neuropsychopharmacol 2004;14:11–28.

Nutt DJ et al. Evidence-based guidelines for management of attention-deficit/hyperactivity disorder in adolescents in transition to adult services and in adults: recommendations from the British Association for Psychopharmacology. J Psychopharmacol 2007;21:10–41.

Taylor E et al. European clinical guidelines for hyperkinetic disorder – first upgrade. Eur Child Adolesc Psychiatry 2004;13(Suppl 1):I7–30.

Children

Table Prescribing in ADHD

Medication	Onset and duration of action	Dose	Comment	Recommended monitoring
Methylphenidate immediate release (Ritalin)[2,3]	Onset: 20–60 min Duration: 2–4 hours	Initially 5–10 mg daily titrated up to a maximum of 60 mg/day in divided doses using weekly increments of 5–10 mg	Usually first-line treatment Generally well tolerated[1] 'Controlled Drug'	BP Pulse Height and weight (risks probably overstated)[4–6] Monitor for insomnia, mood and appetite change and the development of tics[7]
Methylphenidate sustained release (Concerta XL)[2,3,8–10] Also Equasym XL[11,12]	Concerta: Onset: 30 min–2 hours Duration: 12 hours Equasym XL: Onset: 20–60 min Duration: 8 hours	Concerta: Initially 18 mg in the morning, titrated up to a maximum of 54 mg 18 mg Concerta = 15 mg Ritalin Equasym XL: Initially 10 mg increasing as necessary to 60 mg once daily	An afternoon dose of Ritalin may be required in some children to optimise treatment 'Controlled Drug'	Discontinue if no benefits seen in 1 month

Dexamfetamine immediate release (Dexedrine)[1,13]	Onset: 20–60 min Duration: 3–6 hours	2.5–10 mg daily to start, titrated up to a maximum of 20 mg (occasionally 40 mg) in divided doses using weekly increments of 2.5 mg	Considered to be less well tolerated than methylphenidate[1] 'Controlled Drug'	
Atomoxetine[14,15]	Approximately 4–6 weeks (atomoxetine is an NA reuptake inhibitor)	When switching from a stimulant, continue stimulant for first 4 weeks of therapy For children <70 kg: start with 0.5 mg/kg/day and increase after a minimum of 7 days to 1.2 mg/kg (single or divided doses) and increase up to 1.8 mg/kg/day if necessary For children >70 kg: start with 40 mg and increase after a minimum of 7 days to 80 mg	Open, randomized study reports equal efficacy to methylphenidate[16] May be useful where stimulant diversion is a problem[17] Once-daily dosing convenient in schoolchildren Not licensed in adults Not a CD	Pulse BP Height Weight LFTs

References

1. Efron D et al. Side effects of methylphenidate and dexamphetamine in children with attention deficit hyperactivity disorder: a double-blind, crossover trial. Pediatrics 1997;100:662–6.
2. Wolraich ML et al. Pharmacokinetic considerations in the treatment of attention-deficit hyperactivity disorder with methylphenidate. CNS Drugs 2004;18:243–50.
3. British National Formulary. London: British Medical Association and Royal Pharmaceutical Society of Great Britain; 2004.
4. MTA Cooperative Group. A 14-month randomized clinical trial of treatment strategies for attention-deficit/ hyperactivity disorder. Multimodal Treatment Study of Children with ADHD. Arch Gen Psychiatry 1999;56: 1073–86.
5. Kramer JR et al. Predictors of adult height and weight in boys treated with methylphenidate for child-hood behavior problems. J Am Acad Child Adolesc Psychiatry 2000;39:517–24.
6. Poulton A et al. Slowing of growth in height and weight on stimulants: a characteristic pattern. J Paediatr Child Health 2003;39:180–5.
7. Gadow KD et al. Efficacy of methylphenidate for attention-deficit hyperactivity disorder in children with tic disorder. Arch Gen Psychiatry 1995;52:444–55.
8. Hoare P et al. 12-month efficacy and safety of OROS MPH in children and adolescents with attention-deficit/hyperactivity disorder switched from MPH. Eur Child Adolesc Psychiatry 2005;14:305–9.
9. Remschmidt H et al. Symptom control in children and adolescents with attention-deficit/hyperactivity disorder on switching from immediate-release MPH to OROS MPH. Results of a 3-week open-label study. Eur Child Adolesc Psychiatry 2005;14:297–304.
10. Wolraich ML et al. Randomized, controlled trial of oros methylphenidate once a day in children with attention-deficit/hyperactivity disorder. Pediatrics 2001;108:883–92.
11. Findling RL et al. Comparison of the clinical efficacy of twice-daily Ritalin and once-daily Equasym XL with placebo in children with attention deficit/hyperactivity disorder. Eur Child Adolesc Psychiatry 2006; 15:450–9.
12. Anderson VR et al. Spotlight on methylphenidate controlled-delivery capsules (Equasym XL, Metadate CD) in the treatment of children and adolescents with attention-deficit hyperactivity disorder. CNS Drugs 2007;21:173–5.
13. Cyr M et al. Current drug therapy recommendations for the treatment of attention deficit hyperactivity disorder. Drugs 1998;56:215–23.
14. Kelsey DK et al. Once-daily atomoxetine treatment for children with attention-deficit/hyperactivity dis-order, including an assessment of evening and morning behaviour: a double-blind, placebo-controlled trial. Pediatrics 2004;114:e1–e8.
15. Wernicke JF et al. Cardiovascular effects of atomoxetine in children, adolescents, and adults. Drug Saf 2003;26:729–40.
16. Kratochvil CJ et al. Atomoxetine and methylphenidate treatment in children with ADHD: a prospective, randomized, open-label trial. J Am Acad Child Adolesc Psychiatry 2002;41:776–84.
17. Heil SH et al. Comparison of the subjective, physiological, and psychomotor effects of atomoxetine and methylphenidate in light drug users. Drug Alcohol Depend 2002;67:149–56.

Children

Psychosis in children and adolescents

Schizophrenia is rare in children but the incidence increases rapidly in adolescence. Outcome in early-onset illness is generally poor[1]. While drug treatment is undoubtedly indicated, the evidence base underpinning the efficacy and tolerability of antipsychotic drugs in young people is poor.

First-generation drugs, particularly haloperidol, have been subject to small RCTs. While haloperidol is effective, young people are more prone to EPSEs than adults[2]. Treatment-emergent dyskinesias can also be problematic[3]. FGAs should generally be avoided in children.

There have been a handful of randomised controlled trials of antipsychotics in early-onset schizophrenia. Results of these studies suggest that risperidone and olanzapine are equally effective[4,5], with advantages over haloperidol[4]. Clozapine is more effective than halperidol[6] and olanzapine[7]. Data relating to other SGAs are few and far between[8,9]. Ziprasidone should probably be avoided[10,11]. While open studies and case series support a lower risk of treatment-emergent EPSEs with SGAs[1], this has to be balanced against the risk of significant weight gain[1,12,13] and all the physical (and psychological) health consequences thereof.

Clozapine seems to be effective in treatment-resistant psychosis in adolescents, although this population may be more prone to neutropenia and seizures than adults[6].

Overall, algorithms for treating psychosis in young people are the same as those for adult patients (see page 28/29).

References

1. Schulz SC et al. Treatment and outcomes in adolescents with schizophrenia. J Clin Psychiatry 1998; 59(Suppl 1):50–4.
2. Findling RL et al. Atypical antipsychotics in the treatment of children and adolescents: clinical applications. J Clin Psychiatry 2004;65(Suppl 6):30–44.
3. Connor DF et al. Neuroleptic-related dyskinesias in children and adolescents. J Clin Psychiatry 2001; 62:967–74.
4. Sikich L et al. A pilot study of risperidone, olanzapine, and haloperidol in psychotic youth: a double-blind, randomized, 8-week trial. Neuropsychopharmacology 2004;29:133–45.
5. Mozes T et al. An open-label randomized comparison of olanzapine versus risperidone in the treatment of childhood-onset schizophrenia. J Child Adolesc Psychopharmacol 2006;16:393–403.
6. Kumra S et al. Childhood-onset schizophrenia. A double-blind clozapine–haloperidol comparison. Arch Gen Psychiatry 1996;53:1090–7.
7. Shaw P et al. Childhood-onset schizophrenia: a double-blind, randomized clozapine–olanzapine comparison. Arch Gen Psychiatry 2006;63:721–30.
8. Shaw JA et al. A study of quetiapine: efficacy and tolerability in psychotic adolescents. J Child Adolesc Psychopharmacol 2001;11:415–24.
9. Gibson AP et al. Effectiveness and tolerability of aripiprazole in child and adolescent inpatients: a retrospective evaluation. Int Clin Psychopharmacol 2007;22:101–5.
10. Scahill L et al. Sudden death in a patient with Tourette syndrome during a clinical trial of ziprasidone. J Psychopharmacol 2005;19:205–6.
11. Blair J et al. Electrocardiographic changes in children and adolescents treated with ziprasidone: a prospective study. J Am Acad Child Adolesc Psychiatry 2005;44:73–9.

Children

12. Theisen FM et al. Prevalence of obesity in adolescent and young adult patients with and without schizophrenia and in relationship to antipsychotic medication. J Psychiatr Res 2001;35: 339–45.
13. Toren P et al. Benefit–risk assessment of atypical antipsychotics in the treatment of schizophrenia and comorbid disorders in children and adolescents. Drug Saf 2004;27:1135–56.

Further reading

Masi G et al. Children with schizophrenia: clinical picture and pharmacological treatment. CNS Drugs 2006;20:841–66.

Children

Autism

Autism is a chronic and debilitating pervasive developmental disorder involving deficits in language, social interaction and behaviour. Onset is before 3 years of age and the aetiology is unclear. Prevalence is estimated at 6 cases per 1000 children[1], with boys being affected at least three times as frequently as girls[2]. As few as 10% of children with autism may be able to live independently as adults[3].

Deficits in communication make it difficult directly to elicit psychopathology in people with autism. Co-morbid conditions such as mood disorders and ADHD often have to be diagnosed solely from observing behaviour. It therefore follows that case reports and case series should be interpreted with caution. Besides the obvious bias associated with the reporting of open data, the patients included may not be representative of people with autism as a whole.

SSRIs

Case reports and open-case series suggest that SSRIs may be effective in ameliorating repetitive and aggressive behaviours[4]. A double-blind study of fluvoxamine in adults confirmed these findings and also reported improvements in language and social interaction for active drug over placebo[5]. A recent review[6] suggests that SSRIs provide some therapeutic benefit, but further research is required.

Antipsychotics

Small, placebo-controlled studies have found haloperidol to be effective in reducing social withdrawal, stereotypies, overactivity mood dysregulation and irritability, and pimozide to be effective in reducing aggression[4]. There are a great many publications reporting on the efficacy of risperidone in autism[7], three of which are randomised, double-blind, placebo-controlled studies[8–10]. Risperidone is probably effective in the treatment of hyperactivity, aggression and repetitive behaviour and possibly effective in the treatment of depression and irritability[8]: it appears to maintain its efficacy over several months[11,12]. Evidence supporting the efficacy of other SGAs is scant. Note that haloperidol is associated with a high prevalence of EPSEs in young people and all SGAs can cause significant weight gain[13,14].

Anticonvulsants/mood stabilisers

Approximately 30% of people with autism have co-morbid epilepsy[15] and affective illness is also thought to be common[16]. In a review of the literature on the use of anticonvulsant drugs in people with autism and epilepsy, Di Martino and Tuchman[16] report that irritability, aggressiveness and communication improve irrespective of whether or not seizures improve. It is possible that the effect of these drugs in regulating mood is relevant. Caution, however, is required. A case series reported improvements in behaviour with lamotrigine but this finding was not replicated in a double-blind, placebo-controlled trial[17]. Levetiracetam is not effective[18]. There are no randomised, placebo-controlled studies of other anticonvulsant drugs.

Other drugs

Small, controlled studies have reported beneficial effects with clomipramine (for aggression, repetitiveness and irritability), methylphenidate and atomoxetine (for overactivity), clonidine (for overactivity, irritability and aggression), galantamine (for aggression), omega-3 fatty acids (for hyperactivity) and naltrexone (for overactivity),[4,19–21]. Large doses of vitamin B_6 (200 mg/day per 70-kg adult) in combination with magnesium (100 mg/day per 70-kg adult) have been reported to lead to improvements in communication and interpersonal skills. A Cochrane Review concluded that there is insufficient evidence to make any recommendation regarding the use of high doses of vitamin B_6[22]. One positive study has been published since this review[23]. Note that there are unresolved concerns regarding the safety of high doses of vitamin B_6.

The future

There is some evidence that glutamate antagonists (e.g. phencyclidine) and $5HT_{2a}$ agonists (e.g. LSD) can mimic the symptoms of autism[24]. These observations may lead to the development of novel treatments. It may be of note that lamotrigine (a glutamate antagonist) is probably ineffective and risperidone (a $5HT_{2a}$ antagonist) probably effective in ameliorating symptoms of autism.

References

1. Bertrand J et al. Prevalence of autism in a United States population: the Brick Township, New Jersey, investigation. Pediatrics 2001;108:1155–61.
2. Lotter V. Epidemiology of autistic conditions in young children. I. Prevalence. Soc Psychiatry 1966;1:137.
3. Wing L. The diagnosis of autism. In: Gillberg C, ed. Diagnosis and Treatment of Autism. New York: Plenum; 1989:5–22.
4. Palermo MT et al. Pharmacologic treatment of autism. J Child Neurol 2004;19:155–64.
5. McDougle CJ et al. A double-blind, placebo-controlled study of fluvoxamine in adults with autistic disorder. Arch Gen Psychiatry 1996;53:1001–8.
6. Kolevzon A et al. Selective serotonin reuptake inhibitors in autism: a review of efficacy and tolerability. J Clin Psychiatry 2006;67:407–14.
7. Chavez B et al. Role of risperidone in children with autism spectrum disorder. Ann Pharmacother 2006;40:909–16.
8. Barnard L et al. A systematic review of the use of atypical antipsychotics in autism. J Psychopharmacol 2002;16:93–101.
9. Reyes M et al. A randomized, double-blind, placebo-controlled study of risperidone maintenance treatment in children and adolescents with disruptive behavior disorders. Am J Psychiatry 2006;163:402–10.
10. Pandina GJ et al. Risperidone improves behavioral symptoms in children with autism in a randomized, double-blind, placebo-controlled trial. J Autism Dev Disord 2007;37:367–73.
11. Research Units on Pediatric Psychopharmacology Autism Network. Risperidone treatment of autistic disorder: longer-term benefits and blinded discontinuation after 6 months. Am J Psychiatry 2005;162:1361–9.
12. Troost PW et al. Neuropsychological effects of risperidone in children with pervasive developmental disorders: a blinded discontinuation study. J Child Adolesc Psychopharmacol 2006;16:561–73.
13. Hollander E et al. A double-blind placebo-controlled pilot study of olanzapine in childhood/adolescent pervasive developmental disorder. J Child Adolesc Psychopharmacol 2006;16:541–8.
14. Dinca O et al. Systematic review of randomized controlled trials of atypical antipsychotics and selective serotonin reuptake inhibitors for behavioural problems associated with pervasive developmental disorders. J Psychopharmacol 2005;19:521–32.
15. Olsson I et al. Epilepsy in autism and autistic-like conditions. A population-based study. Arch Neurol 1988;45:666–8.
16. Di Martino A et al. Antiepileptic drugs: affective use in autism spectrum disorders. Pediatr Neurol 2001;25:199–207.
17. Belsito KM et al. Lamotrigine therapy for autistic disorder: a randomized, double-blind, placebo-controlled trial. J Autism Dev Disord 2001;31:175–81.
18. Wasserman S et al. Levetiracetam versus placebo in childhood and adolescent autism: a double-blind placebo-controlled study. Int Clin Psychopharmacol 2006;21:363–7.

Children

19. Arnold LE et al. Atomoxetine for hyperactivity in autism spectrum disorders: placebo-controlled crossover pilot trial. J Am Acad Child Adolesc Psychiatry 2006;45:1196–205.
20. Amminger GP et al. Omega-3 fatty acids supplementation in children with autism: a double-blind randomized, placebo-controlled pilot study. Biol Psychiatry 2007;61:551–3.
21. Nicolson R et al. A prospective, open-label trial of galantamine in autistic disorder. J Child Adolesc Psychopharmacol 2006;16:621–9.
22. Nye C et al. Combined vitamin B_6–magnesium treatment in autism spectrum disorder. Cochrane Database Syst Rev 2005;CD003497.
23. Mousain-Bosc M et al. Improvement of neurobehavioral disorders in children supplemented with magnesium–vitamin B_6. II. Pervasive developmental disorder-autism. Magnes Res 2006;19:53–62.
24. Carlsson ML. Hypothesis: is infantile autism a hypoglutamatergic disorder? Relevance of glutamate–serotonin interactions for pharmacotherapy. J Neural Transm 1998;105:525–35.

Children

Tourette's syndrome

Tourette's syndrome is defined by persistent motor and vocal tics. These tics wax and wane over time and are known to be exacerbated by external factors such as stress, anxiety and fatigue. The pathophysiology of Tourette's syndrome is not completely understood. Dopamine, acetylcholine, norepinephrine sex hormones, GABA, serotonin and opiate pathways have all been implicated.

The prevalence of Tourette's syndrome in children and adolescents is estimated to be 1:1000 boys and 1:10,000 girls[1]. Co-morbid depression, anxiety, attention deficit disorder, OCD and behavioural problems are more prevalent than would be expected by chance association alone[2]. These co-morbid conditions are usually treated first before assessing the level of disability caused by the tics. Treatment aimed primarily at reducing tics is warranted if they cause distress to the patient or are functionally disabling.

Studies of pharmacological interventions in Tourette's syndrome are difficult to interpret for several reasons[3]:

- There is a large interindividual variation in tic frequency and severity. Small, randomised studies may include patients that are very different at baseline.
- The severity of tics in a given individual varies markedly over time, making it difficult to separate drug effect from natural variation.
- The placebo effect is large.
- The bulk of the literature consists of case reports, case series, open studies and hugely underpowered, randomised studies. Publication bias is also likely to be an issue.
- A high proportion of patients have co-morbid psychiatric illness. It is difficult to disentangle any direct effect on Tourette's syndrome from an effect on the co-morbid illness. For example, patients with co-morbid OCD would be expected to fare better on a SSRI than placebo or an antipsychotic. This makes it difficult to interpret studies that report improvements in global functioning rather than specific reductions in tics.

The bulk of the published literature concerns children and adolescents. It is commonly believed that younger people are more responsive to treatment than adults but this observation is poorly supported by objective evidence.

Antipsychotics

A 24-week, double-blind, placebo-controlled double crossover study of 22 children and adolescents found pimozide (mean dose 3.4 mg/day) to be statistically superior to placebo in controlling tics[4]. Outcome in the haloperidol arm of this study (mean dose 3.5 mg) was numerically superior to placebo but did not reach statistical significance. Although this study is widely quoted as being positive for pimozide and negative for haloperidol, the absolute difference in response between the two active treatment arms was small. Two children developed severe anxiety and depression during the haloperidol phase that resulted in early termination of treatment. Haloperidol tends to be poorly tolerated by children and adolescents[5]. The high burden of side-effects leads to less than a third being willing to continue treatment in the longer term[6].

Risperidone has been shown to be more effective than placebo in a small ($N = 34$), randomised study[7]. Fatigue and increased appetite were problematic in the risperidone arm and a mean weight gain of 2.8 kg over 8 weeks was reported. Although there is a suggestion that risperidone[8] and olanzapine[9] may be more effective than pimozide, weight gain may be more pronounced in children and adolescents than in adults and this may limit the use of atypicals in young people[8].

Sulpiride has been shown to be effective and relatively well tolerated[10], as has ziprasidone[11]. Open studies support the efficacy of quetiapine[12] and olanzapine[13]. Case series suggest aripiprazole is effective and well tolerated[14-16]. One very small crossover study ($N = 7$) found no effect for clozapine[17].

Other drugs

Clonidine has been shown in open studies to reduce the severity and frequency of tics but this effect does not seem to be convincingly larger that placebo[18]. There may be an age-specific effect, with clonidine being more effective than placebo in adults[19]. Motor tics may be more responsive than vocal tics[19]. Guanfacine (also an adrenergic alpha 2 agonist) has been shown to lead to a 30% reduction in tic-rating-scale scores[20]. Problems with under-powering and the subsequent interpretation of the literature in this area are illustrated by a randomised, controlled trial that found risperidone and clonidine to be equally effective[21].

A small ($N = 10$), double-blind, placebo-controlled, crossover trial of baclofen was suggestive of beneficial effects in overall impairment rather than a specific effect on tics[22]. The numerical benefits shown in this study did not reach statistical significance. Similarly, a double-blind, placebo-controlled trial of nicotine augmentation of haloperidol found beneficial effects in overall impairment rather than a specific effect on tics[23]. These benefits persisted for several weeks after nicotine (in the form of patches) was withdrawn. Nicotine patches were associated with a high prevalence of nausea and vomiting (71% and 40%, respectively). The authors suggest that PRN use may be appropriate. Pergolide (a D1-D2-D3 agonist) given in low dose significantly reduced tics in a double-blind, placebo-controlled, crossover study in children and adolescents[24]. Side-effects included sedation, dizziness, nausea and irritability. Flutamide, an antiandrogen, has been the subject of a small RCT in adults with Tourette's syndrome. Modest, short-lived effects were seen in motor but not phonic tics[3]. A small RCT has shown significant advantages for metoclopramide over placebo[25].

Case reports or case series describing positive effects for ondansetron[26], clomiphene[27], tramadol[28], ketanserin[29], topiramate[30], cyproterone[31], levetiracetam[32] and cannabis[33] have been published. Many other drugs have been reported to be effective in single case reports. Patients in these reports all had co-morbid psychiatric illness, making it difficult to determine the effect of these drugs on Tourette's syndrome alone.

References

1. Awaad Y. Tics in Tourette syndrome: new treatment options. J Child Neurol 1999;14:316–19.
2. Riddle MA et al. Clinical psychopharmacology for Tourette syndrome and associated disorders. Adv Neurol 2001;85:343–54.
3. Peterson BS et al. A double-blind, placebo-controlled, crossover trial of an antiandrogen in the treatment of Tourette's syndrome. J Clin Psychopharmacol 1998;18:324–31.
4. Sallee FR et al. Relative efficacy of haloperidol and pimozide in children and adolescents with Tourette's disorder. Am J Psychiatry 1997;154:1057–62.
5. Richardson MA et al. Neuroleptic use, parkinsonian symptoms, tardive dyskinesia, and associated factors in child and adolescent psychiatric patients. Am J Psychiatry 1991;148:1322–8.
6. Chappell PB et al. The pharmacologic treatment of tic disorders. Child Adolesc Psychiatr Clin N Am 1995;4:197–216.
7. Scahill L et al. A placebo-controlled trial of risperidone in Tourette syndrome. Neurology 2003;60: 1130–5.
8. Bruggeman R et al. Risperidone versus pimozide in Tourette's disorder: a comparative double-blind parallel-group study. J Clin Psychiatry 2001;62:50–6.
9. Onofrj M et al. Olanzapine in severe Gilles de la Tourette syndrome: a 52-week double-blind cross-over study vs. low-dose pimozide. J Neurol 2000;247:443–6.
10. Robertson MM et al. Management of Gilles de la Tourette syndrome using sulpiride. Clin Neuropharmacol 1990;13:229–35.
11. Sallee FR et al. Ziprasidone treatment of children and adolescents with Tourette's syndrome: a pilot study. J Am Acad Child Adolesc Psychiatry 2000;39:292–9.
12. Mukaddes NM et al. Quetiapine treatment of children and adolescents with Tourette's disorder. J Child Adolesc Psychopharmacol 2003;13:295–9.
13. Budman CL et al. An open-label study of the treatment efficacy of olanzapine for Tourette's disorder. J Clin Psychiatry 2001;62:290–4.
14. Bubl E et al. Aripiprazole in patients with Tourette syndrome. World J Biol Psychiatry 2006;7:123–5.
15. Yoo HK et al. A pilot study of aripiprazole in children and adolescents with Tourette's disorder. J Child Adolesc Psychopharmacol 2006;16:505–6.
16. Davies L et al. A case series of patients with Tourette's syndrome in the United Kingdom treated with aripiprazole. Hum Psychopharmacol 2006;21:447–53.
17. Caine ED et al. The trial use of clozapine for abnormal involuntary movement disorders. Am J Psychiatry 1979;136:317–20.
18. Goetz CG et al. Clonidine and Gilles de la Tourette's syndrome: double-blind study using objective rating methods. Ann Neurol 1987;21:307–10.
19. Leckman JF et al. Clonidine treatment of Gilles de la Tourette's syndrome. Arch Gen Psychiatry 1991; 48:324–8.
20. Scahill L et al. A placebo-controlled study of guanfacine in the treatment of children with tic disorders and attention deficit hyperactivity disorder. Am J Psychiatry 2001;158:1067–74.
21. Gaffney GR et al. Risperidone versus clonidine in the treatment of children and adolescents with Tourette's syndrome. J Am Acad Child Adolesc Psychiatry 2002;41:330–6.
22. Singer HS et al. Baclofen treatment in Tourette syndrome: a double-blind, placebo-controlled, crossover trial. Neurology 2001;56:599–604.
23. Silver AA et al. Transdermal nicotine and haloperidol in Tourette's disorder: a double-blind placebo-controlled study. J Clin Psychiatry 2001;62:707–14.
24. Gilbert DL et al. Tourette's syndrome improvement with pergolide in a randomized, double-blind, crossover trial. Neurology 2000;54:1310–15.
25. Nicolson R et al. A randomized, double-blind, placebo-controlled trial of metoclopramide for the treatment of Tourette's disorder. J Am Acad Child Adolesc Psychiatry 2005;44:640–6.
26. Toren P et al. Ondansetron treatment in patients with Tourette's syndrome. Int Clin Psychopharmacol 1999;14:373–6.
27. Sandyk R. Clomiphene citrate in Tourette's syndrome. Int J Neurosci 1988;43:103–6.
28. Shapira NA et al. Novel use of tramadol hydrochloride in the treatment of Tourette's syndrome. J Clin Psychiatry 1997;58:174–5.
29. Bonnier C et al. Ketanserin treatment of Tourette's syndrome in children. Am J Psychiatry 1999;156: 1122–3.
30. Abuzzahab FS et al. Control of Tourette's syndrome with topiramate. Am J Psychiatry 2001;158:968.
31. Izmir M et al. Cyproterone acetate treatment of Tourette's syndrome. Can J Psychiatry 1999;44: 710–11.
32. Awaad Y et al. Use of levetiracetam to treat tics in children and adolescents with Tourette syndrome. Mov Disord 2005;20:714–18.
33. Sandyk R et al. Marijuana and Tourette's syndrome. J Clin Psychopharmacol 1988;8:444–5.

Melatonin in the treatment of insomnia in children and adolescents

Insomnia is a common problem in children with sensory deficits and some learning disability syndromes. It is also a symptom of childhood psychiatric disorders such as depression and ADHD. Approximately 10% of otherwise normal children[1] and up to 80% of children with developmental disorders[2] suffer from delayed sleep phase syndrome.

Melatonin is a hormone that is produced by the pineal gland in a circadian manner. The evening rise in melatonin, enabled by darkness, precedes the onset of natural sleep by about 90 minutes[3]. There is no direct evidence that melatonin is involved in sleep consolidation. Given its association with circadian rhythms and the fact that it is a 'natural' product, melatonin is commonly prescribed to treat insomnia in children and adolescents. Melatonin is not a licensed medicine in the UK.

Efficacy

Five placebo-controlled studies have been published to date. Four studies demonstrated improvements in the time taken to fall asleep[1–6]. The fifth study recruited children with fragmented sleep and melatonin had no effect[7]. In the four positive RCTs there was no consistent effect on total sleep duration or number of awakenings. An open-label study found melatonin to be effective in sleep disorders in people with autism[8].

Side-effects

Many of the children who have received melatonin in RCTs and published case series had developmental problems and/or sensory deficits. The scope for detecting subtle adverse effects in this population is limited. Screening for side-effects was not routine in all studies. Melatonin has been reported to worsen seizures[1,9] and may also exacerbate asthma[10,11] in the short term. Other reported side-effects include headache, depression, restlessness, confusion, nausea, tachycardia and pruritus[12,13]. Long-term side-effects have not been evaluated.

Dose

The cut-off point between physiological and pharmacological doses in children is less than 500 μg. Physiological doses of melatonin result in very high receptor occupancy. The doses used in RCTs and published case series vary hugely, between 500 μg and 5 mg being the most common, although much lower and higher doses have been used. The optimal dose is unknown and there is no evidence to support a direct relationship between dose and response. Pharmacological doses may mediate their effect via GABA receptors[14].

Children

References

1. Smits MG et al. Melatonin for chronic sleep onset insomnia in children: a randomized placebo-controlled trial. J Child Neurol 2001;16:86–92.
2. Jan JE et al. Use of melatonin in the treatment of paediatric sleep disorders. J Pineal Res 1996;21: 193–9.
3. Tzischinsky O et al. Melatonin possesses time-dependent hypnotic effects. Sleep 1994;17:638–45.
4. McArthur AJ et al. Sleep dysfunction in Rett syndrome: a trial of exogenous melatonin treatment. Dev Med Child Neurol 1998;40:186–92.
5. Dodge NN et al. Melatonin for treatment of sleep disorders in children with developmental disabilities. J Child Neurol 2001;16:581–4.
6. Smits MG et al. Melatonin improves health status and sleep in children with idiopathic chronic sleep-onset insomnia: a randomized placebo-controlled trial. J Am Acad Child Adolesc Psychiatry 2003; 42:1286–93.
7. Camfield P et al. Melatonin appears ineffective in children with intellectual deficits and fragmented sleep: six "N of 1" trials. J Child Neurol 1996;11:341–3.
8. Giannotti F et al. An open-label study of controlled-release melatonin in treatment of sleep disorders in children with autism. J Autism Dev Disord 2006;36:741–52.
9. Sheldon SH. Pro-convulsant effects of oral melatonin in neurologically disabled children. Lancet 1998; 351:1254.
10. Maestroni GJ. The immunoneuroendocrine role of melatonin. J Pineal Res 1993;14:1–10.
11. Sutherland ER et al. Elevated serum melatonin is associated with the nocturnal worsening of asthma. J Allergy Clin Immunol 2003;112:513–17.
12. Chase JE et al. Melatonin: therapeutic use in sleep disorders. Ann Pharmacother 1997;31:1218–26.
13. Jan JE et al. Melatonin treatment of sleep–wake cycle disorders in children and adolescents. Dev Med Child Neurol 1999;41:491–500.
14. Sack RL et al. Sleep-promoting effects of melatonin: at what dose, in whom, under what conditions, and by what mechanisms? Sleep 1997;20:908–15.

Children

Rapid tranquillisation (RT) in children and adolescents

As in adults, a comprehensive mental state assessment and appropriately implemented treatment plan along with staff skilled in the use of de-escalation techniques and appropriate placement of the patient are key to minimising the need for enforced parenteral medication.

Oral medication should always be offered before resorting to IM. Monitoring after RT is the same as in adults (see page 439).

Children

Table Recommended drugs for RT

Medication	Dose	Onset of action	Comment
Olanzapine IM[1,2]	2.5–10 mg	15–30 min IM	Possibly increased risk of respiratory depression when administered with benzodiazepines
			Separate administration by at least 1 hour
Haloperidol[3]	0.025–0.075 mg/kg/dose (max 2.5 mg) IM Adolescents >12 years can receive the adult dose (2.5–5 mg)	20–30 min IM	Must have parenteral anticholinergics present in case of laryngeal spasm (young people more vulnerable to severe EPSEs)
			ECG essential
Lorazepam[3,4]	0.05–0.1 mg/kg/dose IM	20–40 min	Slower onset of action than midazolam
			Flumazenil is the reversing agent
			Risk of disinhibitory reactions
Midazolam[4,5]	0.1–0.15 mg/kg	10–20 min IM (1–3 min IV)	Quicker onset and shorter duration of action than lorazepam or diazepam
			Shorter onset and duration of action than haloperidol
			Can be given as buccal liquid (same dose regimen as shown). Onset of action is 15–30 minutes[6]. No published data in mental health but used in epilepsy. Unlicensed product
Diazepam–IV only (not for IM administration)[7]	0.1 mg/kg/dose by slow IV injection. Max 40 mg total daily dose <12 years and 60 mg >12 years	5–10 min	Long half-life that does not correlate with length of sedation. Possibility of accumulation
			Flumazenil is the reversing agent
			Never give as IM injection
Ziprasidone[8,9]	10–20 mg	15–30 min IM	Apparently effective
			QT prolongation is of concern in this patient group

References

1. Breier A et al. A double-blind, placebo-controlled dose–response comparison of intramuscular olanzapine and haloperidol in the treatment of acute agitation in schizophrenia. Arch Gen Psychiatry 2002;59:441–8.
2. Lindborg SR et al. Effects of intramuscular olanzapine vs. haloperidol and placebo on QTc intervals in acutely agitated patients. Psychiatry Res 2003;119:113–23.
3. Sorrentino A. Chemical restraints for the agitated, violent, or psychotic pediatric patient in the emergency department: controversies and recommendations. Curr Opin Pediatr 2004;16:201–5.
4. Nobay F et al. A prospective, double-blind, randomized trial of midazolam versus haloperidol versus lorazepam in the chemical restraint of violent and severely agitated patients. Acad Emerg Med 2004;11: 744–9.
5. Kennedy RM et al. The "ouchless emergency department". Getting closer: advances in decreasing distress during painful procedures in the emergency department. Pediatr Clin North Am 1999;46.
6. Schwagmeier R et al. Midazolam pharmacokinetics following intravenous and buccal administration. Br J Clin Pharmacol 1998;46:203–6.
7. Nunn K et al. Medication table. In: Nunn K et al, eds. The Clinician's Guide to Psychotropic Prescribing in Children and Adolescents. Sydney: Glade Publishing; 2003:383–452.
8. Khan SS et al. A naturalistic evaluation of intramuscular ziprasidone versus intramuscular olanzapine for the management of acute agitation and aggression in children and adolescents. J Child Adolesc Psychopharmacol 2006;16:671–7.
9. Staller JA. Intramuscular ziprasidone in youth: a retrospective chart review. J Child Adolesc Psychopharmacol 2004;14:590–2.

Children

Persistent aggression in children and adolescents

As in adults, persistent aggression may be secondary to a number of under-lying psychiatric illnesses. The most common primary diagnoses in children include conduct disorder, bipolar illness, autism and psychotic illness. It is important to understand what drives the aggressive behaviour and to inter-vene appropriately.

There is most evidence supporting the use of risperidone in aggressive behaviour[1,2]. There are fewer data for olanzapine, quetiapine and clozapine. Risperidone can cause significant EPSEs in young people[1] and all atypicals can cause considerable weight gain.

Lithium may also be effective[3-5].

References

1. Schur SB et al. Treatment recommendations for the use of antipsychotics for aggressive youth (TRAAY). Part I: a review. J Am Acad Child Adolesc Psychiatry 2003;42:132–44.
2. Pappadopulos E et al. Treatment recommendations for the use of antipsychotics for aggressive youth (TRAAY). Part II. J Am Acad Child Adolesc Psychiatry 2003;42:145–61.
3. Campbell M et al. Lithium in hospitalized aggressive children with conduct disorder: a double-blind and placebo-controlled study. J Am Acad Child Adolesc Psychiatry 1995;34:445–53.
4. Malone RP et al. A double-blind placebo-controlled study of lithium in hospitalized aggressive children and adolescents with conduct disorder. Arch Gen Psychiatry 2000;57:649–54.
5. Campbell M et al. Predictors of side effects associated with lithium administration in children. Psycho-pharmacol Bull 1991;27:373–80.

Further reading

Ipser J et al. Systematic review of pharmacotherapy of disruptive behavior disorders in children and adolescents. Psychopharmacology (Berl) 2006.
Kranzler H et al. Clozapine: its impact on aggressive behaviour among children and adolescents with schizophrenia. J Am Acad Child Adolesc Psychiatry 2005;44:55–63.

Children

Doses of commonly used psychotropic drugs in children and adolescents

Suggested approximate oral starting doses (see primary literature for doses in individual indications). Lower dose in suggested range is for children weighing less than 25 kg.

Drug	Dose-range	Comments
Risperidone	0.25–2 mg	Adjust dose according to response and adverse effects
Olanzapine	2.5–5 mg	Use plasma levels to determine maintenance dose
Clozapine	6.25–12.5 mg	Use plasma levels to determine maintenance dose
Fluoxetine	5–10 mg/day	Adjust dose according to response and adverse effects
Lithium	100–200 mg/day lithium carbonate	Use plasma levels to determine maintenance dose
Valproate	10–20 mg/kg/day in divided doses	Use plasma levels to determine maintenance dose
Carbamazepine	5 mg/kg/day in divided doses	Use plasma levels to determine maintenance dose

Children

chapter 6

Substance misuse

Introduction

Mental and behavioural problems due to psychoactive substance use are common. Many psychoactive substances may be problematic, including alcohol, opioids, cannabinoids, sedatives, stimulants, hallucinogens, tobacco and volatile substances. The World Health Organization (WHO) in the International Classification of Diseases-10 (ICD-10)[1] identifies acute intoxication, harmful use, dependence syndrome, withdrawal state, withdrawal state with delirium, psychotic disorder, amnesic syndrome, residual and late-onset psychotic disorder, other mental and behavioural disorders and unspecified mental and behavioural disorders as substance-related disorders. Substance misuse is commonly seen in people with severe mental illness (so-called dual diagnosis) and personality disorder. In many units, dual diagnosis is the norm rather than the exception in adult psychiatry.

According to ICD-10[1], dependence syndrome is 'a cluster of physiological, behavioural, and cognitive phenomena in which the use of a substance or a class of substances takes on a much higher priority for a given individual than other behaviours that once had greater value'. A definite diagnosis of dependence should only be made if at least three of the following have been present together in the last year:

- compulsion to take substance
- difficulties controlling substance-taking behaviour
- physiological withdrawal state
- evidence of tolerance
- neglect of alternative interests
- persistent use despite harm.

Substance use disorders should generally be treated with a combination of psychosocial and pharmacological interventions. This chapter will concentrate on pharmacological interventions for alcohol, opioids and nicotine use. Cocaine, other stimulants and benzodiazepine use will be discussed briefly. Note that NICE guidelines[2], Department of Health Substance Misuse Guidelines[3], and National Treatment Agency for Substance Misuse Guidelines[4] also provide a comprehensive overview of treatment approaches, as does a British Association for Psychopharmacology consensus[5] and a meta-analysis from the Scottish Intercollegiate Guidelines Network[6].

References

1. World Health Organisation. The ICD-10 Classification of Mental and Behavioural Disorders. Switzerland: World Health Organisation, 2003.
2. National Institute for Clinical Excellence. The clinical effectiveness and cost effectiveness of bupropion (Zyban) and Nicotine Replacement Therapy for smoking cessation. Technical Appraisal 39. http://www.nice.org.uk. 2002.
3. Department of Health. Drug misuse and dependence: guidelines on clinical management. Norwich: Department of Health, 1999.
4. Day E. National Treatment Agency for Substance Misuse. Opiate detoxification in an inpatient setting. http://www.nta.nhs.uk/. 2005.
5. Lingford-Hughes AR et al. Evidence-based guidelines for the pharmacological management of substance misuse, addiction and comorbidity: recommendations from the British Association for Psychopharmacology. J Psychopharmacol 2004;18:293–335.
6. Scottish Intercollegiate Guidelines Network. The management of harmful drinking and alcohol dependence in primary care. Guideline No. 74. http://www.sign.ac.uk. 2003.

Alcohol misuse

Pharmacotherapy for alcohol withdrawal

- Alcohol withdrawal is associated with significant morbidity and mortality when improperly managed.
- All patients need general support; a proportion will need pharmacotherapy to modify the course of reversal of alcohol-induced neuro-adaptation.
- Benzodiazepines are recognised as the treatment of choice for alcohol withdrawal. They are cross-tolerant with alcohol and have anticonvulsant properties.
- Parenteral vitamin replacement is an important adjunctive treatment for the prophylaxis and/or treatment of Wernicke–Korsakoff syndrome and other vitamin-related neuropsychiatric conditions.

Management of alcohol withdrawal and detoxification

Most patients undergoing alcohol withdrawal can do so safely at home with regular supervision by their GP and a community team. Some individuals with alcohol dependence will need pharmacological treatment in order to withdraw safely from alcohol. Prior to any managed episode of alcohol withdrawal there should be consideration of the following: Does the client want to undergo detoxification? What are the goals of treatment? Intended goals usually include symptom suppression, prevention of complications of subsequent abstinence. Managed withdrawal should be considered within the wider context of the ongoing care/treatment package. Are plans in place for the post-withdrawal period? In addition, a risk assessment should be carried out to determine the appropriate setting (see guidelines for inpatient treatment below). Care should be ensured with older patients who might be more safely managed as inpatients.

The majority of patients can be detoxified in the community. However, supervised medically assisted inpatient treatment is indicated where there is:

- severe dependence
- a history of delerium tremers (DTs) and alcohol withdrawal seizures
- a history of failed community detoxification(s)
- poor social support
- cognitive impairment
- psychiatric co-morbidity
- poor physical health, e.g. diabetes, liver disease, hypertension.

The alcohol withdrawal syndrome

In alcohol-dependent drinkers, the central nervous system has adjusted to the constant presence of alcohol in the body. When the blood alcohol concentration (BAC) is suddenly lowered (as alcohol is metabolised too quickly for the brain to adjust), the brain remains in a hyperactive and hyperexcited state, causing the withdrawal syndrome.

The alcohol withdrawal syndrome is not a uniform entity. It varies significantly in clinical manifestations and severity. Symptoms can range from mild insomnia to delirium tremens (DTs).

The first symptoms and signs occur within hours of the last drink and peak within 24–48 hours. They include restlessness, tremor, sweating, anxiety, nausea, vomiting, loss of appetite and insomnia. Tachycardia and systolic hypertension are also evident. Generalised seizures occur rarely, usually within 24 hours of cessation. In DTs there is confusion, disorientation, agitation, tachycardia and hypertension. Fever is common. Visual and auditory hallucinations and para-noid ideation are also seen. DTs often present insidiously with night-time con-fusion. The mortality is appoximately 1–2%. Treatment of DTs requires early diagnosis and prompt transfer to the general medical setting where intra-venous diazepam and careful attention to medical disorders, fluid and elec-trolyte replacement, thiamine and other vitamins can be accomplished.

In most alcohol-dependent individuals symptoms of alcohol withdrawal are mild-to-moderate and disappear within 5–7 days after the last drink. In more severe cases (approximately 5% of cases), DTs may develop.

Risk factors for DTs and seizures

- severe alcohol dependence
- past experience of DTs
- long history of alcohol dependence with multiple previous episodes of inpatient treatment
- older age
- concomitant acute illness
- severe withdrawal symptoms when presenting for treatment.

Alcohol withdrawal assessment

- history (including history of previous episodes of alcohol withdrawal)
- physical examination
- time of most recent drink
- concomitant drug (illicit and prescribed) intake
- severity of withdrawal symptoms
- co-existing medical/psychiatric disorders
- laboratory investigations: FBC, U&E, LFTs, INR, prothrombin time and urinary drug screen
- breathalyser: BAC may be estimated by a breathalyser reading.

Withdrawal scales can be helpful. They can be used as a baseline against which withdrawal severity can be measured over time. Use of these scales can minimise over- and under-dosing with benzodiazepines.

The Clinical Institute Withdrawal Assessment of Alcohol Scale, Revised (CIWA-Ar)[1] is a 10-item scale which can be completed in around 5 minutes.

Clinical Institute Withdrawal Assessment of Alcohol Scale, Revised[1]

Patient:_____ **Date:** _____
Time: _____(24 hour clock, midnight = 00:00)

Pulse or heart rate, taken for 1 minute:_____
Blood pressure:_____

NAUSEA AND VOMITING – Ask 'Do you feel sick to your stomach? Have you vomited?' Observation.
0 no nausea and no vomiting
1 mild nausea with no vomiting
2
3
4 intermittent nausea with dry heaves
5
6
7 constant nausea, frequent dry heaves and vomiting

TACTILE DISTURBANCES – Ask 'Have you any itching, pins and needles sensations, any burning, any numbness, or do you feel bugs crawling on or under your skin?' Observation.
0 none
1 very mild itching, pins and needles, burning or numbness
2 mild itching, pins and needles, burning or numbness
3 moderate itching, pins and needles, burning or numbness
4 moderately severe hallucinations
5 severe hallucinations
6 extremely severe hallucinations
7 continuous hallucinations

TREMOR – Arms extended and fingers spread apart. Observation.
0 no tremor
1 not visible, but can be felt fingertip to fingertip
2
3
4 moderate, with patient's arms extended
5
6
7 severe, even with arms not extended

AUDITORY DISTURBANCES – Ask 'Are you more aware of sounds around you? Are they harsh? Do they frighten you? Are you hearing anything that is disturbing to you? Are you hearing things you know are not there?' Observation.
0 not present
1 very mild harshness or ability to frighten
2 mild harshness or ability to frighten
3 moderate harshness or ability to frighten
4 moderately severe hallucinations
5 severe hallucinations
6 extremely severe hallucinations
7 continuous hallucinations

PAROXYSMAL SWEATS – Observation.
0 no sweat visible
1 barely perceptible sweating, palms moist
2
3
4 beads of sweat obvious on forehead
5
6
7 drenching sweats

VISUAL DISTURBANCES – Ask 'Does the light appear to be too bright? Is its colour different? Does it hurt your eyes? Are you seeing anything that is disturbing to you? Are you seeing things you know are not there?' Observation.
0 not present
1 very mild sensitivity
2 mild sensitivity
3 moderate sensitivity
4 moderately severe hallucinations
5 severe hallucinations
6 extremely severe hallucinations
7 continuous hallucinations

ANXIETY – Ask 'Do you feel nervous?' Observation.
0 no anxiety, at ease
1 mildly anxious
2
3
4 moderately anxious, or guarded, so anxiety is inferred
5
6
7 equivalent to acute panic states as seen in severe delirium or acute schizophrenic reactions

HEADACHE, FULLNESS IN HEAD – Ask 'Does your head feel different? Does it feel like there is a band around your head?' Do not rate for dizziness or lightheadedness. Otherwise, rate severity.
0 not present
1 very mild
2 mild
3 moderate
4 moderately severe
5 severe
6 very severe
7 extremely severe

AGITATION – Observation.
0 normal activity
1 somewhat more than normal activity
2
3
4 moderately fidgety and restless
5
6
7 paces back and forth during most of the interview, or constantly thrashes about
Scores
≤10 – mild withdrawal (do not need additional medication)
≤15 – moderate withdrawal
>15 – severe withdrawal

ORIENTATION AND CLOUDING OF SENSORIUM – Ask 'What day is this? Where are you? Who am I?'
0 oriented and can do serial additions
1 cannot do serial additions or is uncertain about date
2 disoriented for date by no more than 2 calendar days
3 disoriented for date by more than 2 calendar days
4 disoriented for place/or person

Total **CIWA-Ar** Score_____
Rater's Initials _____

Maximum Possible Score 67

Withdrawal in the community

- There should be someone at home who is able to monitor and supervise the withdrawal process. This should ideally be over the full 24-hour period. In situations where the supporter cannot be present full-time, there should be a high level of home supervision.
- Discuss treatment plan with the patient and person who will be supporting them. It is helpful to write this out and keep a copy in notes. This should include contingency plans. Give a copy to the patient and send a copy to GP.
- Arrange for medication to be picked up on a daily basis.
- If a patient resumes drinking, stop detoxification.
- Give patient and carer contact details so they can contact you if there are any problems.

Use of benzodiazepines

- Benzodiazepines are typically given for 7 days.
- The choice of benzodiazepine should be contingent upon the circumstances: e.g. shorter-acting benzodiazepines such as lorazepam and oxazepam in patients with alcoholic liver disease.
- Longer-acting benzodiazepines may be more effective in preventing seizures and delirium, but there is a risk of accumulation in elderly patients and those with liver failure[2].
- Additional titration using as-required medication may be used to achieve complete symptom suppression in the first 2 days[3].
- Benzodiazepines can be given in a number of ways: (1) in 'front-loading' a loading dose is given followed by doses every 90 minutes or so, to achieve light sedation; no further doses are needed; (2) symptom-triggered therapy (in patients without a history of complications)[3]; or (3) a tapering dose regimen, described here.

Dose of benzodiazepines

The dose needed will depend on an assessment of:

- severity of alcohol dependence (clinical history, number of units per drinking day and score on Severity of Alcohol Dependence Questionnaire (SADQ)).
- severity of alcohol withdrawal symptoms. CIWA-Ar ($>$10–20 – moderate and $>$20 – severe) or Short Alcohol Withdrawal Scale (SAWS)[4] $>$12.

Table Short Alcohol Withdrawal Scale (SAWS)

	None (0)	Mild (1)	Moderate (2)	Severe (3)
Anxious				
Sleep disturbance				
Problems with memory				
Nausea				
Restless				
Tremor (shakes)				
Feeling confused				
Sweating				
Miserable				
Heart pounding				

The SAWS is a self-completion questionnaire. Symptoms cover the previous 24-hour period. Scores above 12 require pharmacotherapy.

Use of chlordiazepoxide[5]

Mild dependence usually requires very small doses of chlordiazepoxide or else may be managed without medication.

Moderate dependence requires a larger dose of chlordiazepoxide. A typical regimen might be 10–20 mg qds, reducing gradually over 5–7 days. Note that 5–7 days' treatment is adequate *and longer treatment is rarely helpful or necessary*. It is advisable to monitor withdrawal and BAC daily prior to providing the day's medication. This may mean that community pharmacologically assisted alcohol withdrawals need to start on Monday to last 5 days. The protocol below may also be used for an inpatient with moderate dependence.

Chlordiazepoxide – moderate dependence

Day 1.. 20 mg qds
Day 2.. 15 mg qds
Day 3.. 10 mg qds
Day 4.. 5 mg qds
Day 5.. 5 mg bd

Severe dependence requires even larger doses of chlordiazepoxide and will often require specialist/inpatient treatment. Intensive daily monitoring is advised for the first 2–3 days, especially for severe dependence (see below). This may require special arrangements over a weekend. Prescribing should not start if the patient is heavily intoxicated, and in such circumstances the patient should be advised to return when not intoxicated, at an early opportunity.

Inpatient treatment

The approach should be flexible with regard to the number of days pre-scribed, depending on the individual. Severely dependent patients should get 7 days' treatment with the flexibility of as-required medication in the first 2 days. If symptoms are controlled within the first 2 days, then it will be easier to implement the reducing regimen. Patients who have a history of DTs, head injury or cognitive impairment may need lengthier withdrawal regimens, e.g. lasting 10 days.

Chlordiazepoxide should be prescribed according to a flexible regimen over the first 24 (up to 48) hours, with dosage titrated against the rated severity of withdrawal symptoms. This is followed by a fixed 5-day reducing regimen, based upon the dosage requirement estimated during the first 24 (−48) hours. Occasionally (e.g. in DTs) the flexible regimen may need to be prolonged beyond the first 24 hours. However, rarely (if ever) is it necessary to resort to the use of other drugs, such as antipsychotics (associated with reduced seizure threshold) or intravenous diazepam (associated with risk of overdose).

The intention of the flexible protocol for the first 24 hours is to titrate dosage of chlordiazepoxide against severity of alcohol withdrawal symptoms. It is necessary to avoid either under-treatment (associated with patient discomfort and a higher incidence of complications such as seizures or DTs), or over-treatment (associated with excessive sedation and risk of toxicity/interaction with alcohol consumed prior to admission).

In the inpatient setting it is possible to be more responsive, with constant monitoring of the severity of withdrawal symptoms, linked to the adminis-tered dose of chlordiazepoxide.

Prescribing in alcohol withdrawal for severe dependence

First 24 hours (day 1)
On admission, the patient should be assessed by a doctor and prescribed chlordiazepoxide (diazepam is used in some centres). *Observations should be at regular intervals during the first 24 hours.* Three doses of chlordiazepoxide must be specified:

FIRST DOSE (STAT)
This is the first dose of chlordiazepoxide which will be administered by ward staff immediately following admission, as a fixed 'stat' dose. It should be estimated upon:

- clinical signs and symptoms of withdrawal (see below)
- breath alcohol concentration on admission (20 minutes after last drink to avoid falsely high readings from the mouth) and 1 hour later.

The dose prescribed should usually be within the range of 5–50 mg. However, if withdrawal symptoms on admission are mild, or if the breath alcohol is very high, or rising, the initial dose may be 0 mg (i.e. nothing). It is the relative fall in blood alcohol concentration that determines the need for medication not the absolute figure (hence the need to take 2 breathalyser readings at an interval soon after admission). Caution is needed if a patient shows a high BAC reading.

INCREMENTAL DOSE (RANGE)
This is the range within which subsequent doses of chlordiazepoxide should be administered during the first 24 hours (see below). A dose of 5–40 mg will cover almost all circumstances.

MAXIMUM DOSE IN 24 HOURS
This is the maximum cumulative dose that may be given during the first 24 hours. It may be estimated according to clinical judgement, but **250 mg should be adequate for most cases.** Doses above 250 mg should not be prescribed without prior discussion with a consultant or specialist registrar.

The cumulative chlordiazepoxide dose administered during the initial 24-hour period assessment is called the *baseline dose*, and this is used to calculate the subsequent reducing regimen.

Days 2–5
After the initial 24-hour assessment period a standardised reducing regimen is used. Chlordiazepoxide is given in divided doses, 4 times daily. The afternoon and evening doses can be proportionately higher in order to provide night sedation (but note that the effect of chlordiazepoxide and its metabolites is long-lived). The dose should be reduced each day by approximately 20% of the baseline dose, so that no chlordiazepoxide is given on day 6. **However, a longer regimen may be required in the case of patients who have DTs or a history of DTs. This should be discussed with a specialist registrar or consultant, and the dose tailored according to clinical need**.

Note
Chlordiazepoxide should not routinely be prescribed on a PRN basis after the initial assessment (first 2 days) is complete. Patients exhibiting significant further symptoms may have psychiatric (or other) complications and should be seen by the ward or duty doctor.

Observations and administration
After chlordiazepoxide has been prescribed as above, the first 'stat' dose is given immediately. Subsequent doses during the first 24 hours are administered with a frequency and dosage that depend upon the observations of alcohol withdrawal status rated by the ward staff.

Substance misuse

OBSERVATIONS

Each set of observations consists of:

- alcohol withdrawal scale (e.g. CIWA-Ar) and/or clinical observations
- BP
- heart rate
- breathalyser (first and second observations only).

Observations should be recorded:

- on admission procedure immediately after arrival on the ward
- throughout the first 24 hours, approximately every 1–2 hours, at a frequency that depends on:
  - severity of withdrawal
  - whether or not chlordiazepoxide has been administered
- twice-daily from days 2–6.

If patient is asleep (and this is not due to intoxication), they should not be woken up for observations. However, it should be recorded that they were asleep.

During the first 24 hours, chlordiazepoxide should be administered when withdrawal symptoms are considered significant (usually a CIWA-Ar score >15). If a patient suffers hallucinations or agitation, an increased dose should be administered, according to clinical judgement.

Table Alcohol withdrawal treatment interventions – summary

Severity	Supportive care	Medical care	Pharmacotherapy for neuro-adaptation reversal	Setting
Mild CIWA-Ar ≤10	Moderate-to-high level required	Little required	Little to none required – maybe symptomatic treatment only (e.g. paracetamol)	Home
Moderate CIWA-Ar ≤15	Moderate-to-high level required	Little required	Little to none required – maybe symptomatic treatment only	Home or community
Severe CIWA-Ar >15	High level required	Medical monitoring	Usually required – probably symptomatic and substitution treatment (e.g. chlordiazepoxide)	Community or hospital
Complicated CIWA-Ar >10, plus medical problems	High level required	Specialist medical care required	Substitution and symptomatic treatments probably required	Hospital

Example of a chlordiazepoxide regimen for severe dependence		
		Total (mg)
Day 1 (first 24 hours)	40 mg qds + 40 mg PRN	200
Day 2	40 mg qds	160
Day 3	30 mg tds and 40 mg nocte (or 30 mg qds)	120–130
Day 4	30 mg bd and 20 mg bd (or 25 mg qds)	100
Day 5	20 mg qds	80
Day 6	20 mg bd and 10 mg bd	60
Day 7	10 mg qds	40
Day 8	10 mg tds or 10 mg bd and 5 mg bd	30
Day 9	10 mg bd (or 5 mg qds)	20
Day 10	10 mg nocte	10

Also, please see above for first 24-hour dose assessment period.

Vitamin supplementation

All patients undergoing inpatient detoxification should be given **parenteral** thiamine as prophylaxis for Wernicke's encephalopathy (WE). This is probably best given for 5 days and may be followed by oral vitamin B compound. The only parenteral high-potency B-complex vitamin therapy licensed in the UK is Pabrinex. Intravenous Pabrinex remains the treatment of choice in patients in whom a presumptive diagnosis of WE has been made, or for whom the diagnosis is clear. However, IM Pabrinex is also typically given as prophylaxis for inpatients undergoing medically assisted withdrawal. Clients undergoing community detoxification should also be considered for parenteral prophylaxis with Pabrinex because oral thiamine is not adequately absorbed and there is considerable doubt about the usefulness of oral replacement.

IM thiamine preparations have a lower incidence of anaphylactic reactions than IV preparations, at 1 per 5 million pairs of ampoules of Pabrinex, which is far lower than many frequently used drugs that carry no special warning in the *BNF*. However, this risk has resulted in fears about using parenteral preparations, and the inappropriate use of oral thiamine preparations. Given the nature of Wernicke's encephalopathy, the benefit-to-risk ratio favours parenteral thiamine[3,6,7]. One pair of IM high-potency Pabrinex ampoules should be administered once daily for 5 days[7]. *BNF* guidance/CSM advice states that facilities for treating anaphylaxis should be available. This includes the need for staff to be trained in the management of anaphylaxis and administration of epinephrine IM.

Wernicke's encephalopathy

The classical triad of ophthalmoplegia, ataxia and confusion is rarely present in Wernicke's encephalopathy, and the syndrome is much more common than is widely believed[8]. A presumptive diagnosis of Wernicke's encephalopathy should therefore be made in any patient undergoing detoxification who experiences any of the following signs:

- ataxia
- hypothermia and hypotension
- confusion
- ophthalmoplegia/nystagmus
- memory disturbance
- coma/unconsciousness.

Note that alcohol and benzodiazepines can cause ataxia and nystagmus, which may be confused with Wernicke's encephalopathy.

It is advised that parenteral B-complex must be administered before glucose is administered in all patients presenting with altered mental status.

Prophylactic treatment for patients at risk of Wernicke's encephalopathy should be:
One pair IM/IV ampoules high-potency B-complex vitamins (Pabrinex) daily for 3–5 days.
(Thiamine 200–300 mg IM daily may be given if Pabrinex is unavailable.)

Note: All patients should receive this regimen as an absolute minimum.

Therapeutic treatment: Wernicke's encephalopathy (to be undertaken within the general medical hospital setting) consists of:

At least 2 pairs of IV ampoules (i.e. 4 ampoules) of high-potency B-complex vitamins three times daily for 2 days.

- If no response, then discontinue treatment.
- If signs/symptoms respond, continue 1 pair IV or IM ampoules daily for 5 days or for as long as improvement continues.

For outpatient detoxification, the options available are:

- Oral vitamin supplementation with vitamin B Compound Strong, one tablet 3 times daily (but this is unlikely to be absorbed effectively and is therefore of little or no benefit to alcohol-dependent patients).
- Parenteral supplementation, as above, in a clinical setting where appropriate resuscitation facilities are available.

Seizure prophylaxis

A meta-analysis of trials assessing efficacy of drugs preventing alcohol withdrawal seizures has demonstrated that benzodiazepines, particularly long-acting preparations such as diazepam, significantly reduced seizures *de novo*[9].

Most clinicians prefer to use diazepam for medically assisted withdrawal in those with a previous history of seizures. Some units advocate carbamazepine loading in patients with untreated epilepsy; those with a history of more than two seizures during previous withdrawal episodes; or previous seizures despite adequate diazepam loading. Phenytoin does not prevent alcohol-withdrawal seizures and is therefore not indicated. Please note that there is no need to continue an anticonvulsant if it has been used to treat an alcohol-withdrawal-related seizure. A recent Cochrane review evaluated anticonvulsants for alcohol withdrawal and found no definitive evidence on the effectiveness in alcohol withdrawal[10]. Please also see BAP guidelines[3].

Those who have a seizure for the first time should be investigated to rule out an organic disease or structural lesion.

Liver disease

For individuals with impaired liver functioning, oxazepam (a short-acting benzodiazepine) may be preferred to chlordiazepoxide, in order to avoid excessive build-up of metabolites and over-sedation.

Hallucinations

Mild perceptual disturbances usually respond to chlordiazepoxide. However, hallucinations can be treated with oral haloperidol. Haloperidol may also be given intramuscularly (but BP should be monitored for hypotension and ECG for QT prolongation). Caution is needed because haloperidol can reduce seizure threshold. Have parenteral procyclidine available in case of dystonic reactions.

Symptomatic pharmacotherapy

Dehydration:	Ensure adequate fluid intake in order to maintain hydration and electrolyte balance. Dehydration can lead to cardiac arrhythmia and death.
Pain:	Paracetamol.
Nausea and vomiting:	Metoclopramide (Maxolon) 10 mg or prochlorperazine (Stemetil) 5 mg 4–6-hourly.
Diarrhoea:	Diphenoxylate and atropine (Lomotil). Loperamide (Imodium).
Hepatic encephalopathy:	Lactulose (within the general medical hospital)
Skin itching	Occurs commonly and not only in individuals with alcoholic liver disease: Antihistamines.

Relapse prevention

There is no place for the continued use of benzodiazepines beyond treatment of the acute alcohol withdrawal syndrome and they should not be prescribed. Acamprosate and supervised disulfiram are licensed for treatment in the UK and can be considered as adjuncts to psychosocial treatment. These should be initiated by a specialist service. After 12 weeks, transfer of the prescribing to the GP may be appropriate, although specialist care may continue (shared care).

Acamprosate

Acamprosate is a synthetic taurine analogue, which appears to act centrally on glutamate and gamma-aminobutyric acid (GABA) neurotransmitter systems, although the mechanism has not been fully established. It is licensed to prevent relapse to alcohol use and was found in a recent meta-analysis to be associated with a modest treatment effect[11]. Acamprosate should be initiated as soon as possible after abstinence has been achieved and should be maintained if the patient relapses. However continued alcohol use cancels out any benefit. Acamprosate should be prescribed in combination with psychosocial treatment. Contraindications are severe renal or hepatic impairment and therefore liver and kidney function tests should be performed prior to commencing acamprosate. It should be avoided in individuals who are pregnant or breastfeeding.

Please see the *BNF* for current dosages. For adults 18–65 years at 60 kg and over, the starting dose is 666 mg 3 times daily. For adults less than 60 kg, the dose should be reduced to 666 mg (morning), 333 mg (midday) and 333 mg (night).

Disulfiram (Antabuse)

Disulfiram inhibits aldehyde dehydrogenase, leading to acetaldehyde accumulation after drinking alcohol, which can cause extremely unpleasant physical effects. Continued drinking can lead to arrhythmias, hypotension and collapse. Despite being available for many years, the number of controlled clinical trials is limited. Disulfiram appears to reduce the number of drinking days but to not increase abstinence. Supervised disulfiram may improve efficacy[3,12].

Because of the known adverse effects of disulfiram, in order to initiate treatment, the clinician must ensure that no alcohol has been consumed for at least 24 hours before commencing treatment. Contraindications to use include cardiac failure, coronary artery disease, history of cerebrovascular disease, pregnancy and breastfeeding, liver disease and peripheral neuropathy. Please refer to the *BNF* for the full range of contraindications and dosages.

Doses as stated in the *BNF* are 800 mg for the first dose, reducing to 100–200 mg daily. Patients should ideally have supervised consumption of disulfiram by a relative or pharmacist, with regular review, and this should not be continued for longer than 6 months. Halitosis is a common side-effect.

Naltrexone

Naltrexone is an opioid receptor antagonist and does not have marketing authorisation for the treatment of alcohol dependence in the UK. A systematic review of naltrexone treatment concluded that short-term treatment with naltrexone was effective at reducing craving for alcohol; however, there were a number of limitations[13].

Pregnancy and alcohol use

Evidence has suggested that alcohol consumption during pregnancy may cause harm to the fetus. The Royal College of Obstetricians and Gynaecologists

(RCOG) recently released a statement stating that it is safest to avoid alcohol during pregnancy. If a woman continues to drink alcohol, no more than one to two units, once or twice a week should be consumed. RCOG also recommend screening for alcohol use during routine antenatal assessment and easy access to psychosocial interventions, which are the mainstay of treatment[14].

For alcohol-dependent women who have withdrawal symptoms, pharmacological cover for detoxification should be offered, ideally as an inpatient. It is important to carry out a risk–benefit assessment of alcohol withdrawal symptoms versus prescribed benzodiazepines that may carry a risk of fetal abnormalities. This should also be assessed against risk of continued alcohol consumption to the fetus. Chlordiazepoxide has been suggested as being unlikely to pose a substantial risk; however, dose-dependent malformations have been observed[15]. The timing of detoxification in relation to the trimester of pregnancy should be risk-assessed against continued alcohol consumption and risks to the fetus[3]. The Regional Drug & Therapeutics Centre Teratology Information Service[16] provides national advice for healthcare professionals and like to follow-up on pregnancies that require alcohol detoxification. Please refer to the references below. Specialist advice should always be sought. (See also section on pregnancy page 365.)

References

1. Sullivan JT et al. Assessment of alcohol withdrawal: the revised clinical institute withdrawal assessment for alcohol scale (CIWA-Ar). Br J Addict 1989;84:1353–7.
2. Mayo-Smith MF. Pharmacological management of alcohol withdrawal. A meta-analysis and evidence-based practice guideline. American Society of Addiction Medicine Working Group on Pharmacological Management of Alcohol Withdrawal. JAMA 1997;278:144–51.
3. Lingford-Hughes AR et al. Evidence-based guidelines for the pharmacological management of substance misuse, addiction and comorbidity: recommendations from the British Association for Psychopharmacology. J Psychopharmacol 2004;18:293–335.
4. Gossop M et al. A Short Alcohol Withdrawal Scale (SAWS): development and psychometric properties. Addict Biol 2002;7:37–43.
5. Duncan D et al. Chlormethiazole or chlordiazepoxide in alcohol detoxification. Psychiatr Bull 1996;20: 599–601.
6. Thomson AD et al. The Royal College of Physicians report on alcohol: guidelines for managing Wernicke's encephalopathy in the Accident and Emergency Department. Alcohol Alcohol 2002;37: 513–21.
7. Thomson AD et al. The treatment of patients at risk of developing Wernicke's encephalopathy in the community. Alcohol Alcohol 2006;41:159–67.
8. Thomson AD et al. The natural history and pathophysiology of Wernicke's encephalopathy and Korsakoff's psychosis. Alcohol Alcohol 2006;41:151–8.
9. Ntais C et al. Benzodiazepines for alcohol withdrawal. Cochrane Database Syst Rev 2005;CD005063.
10. Polycarpou A et al. Anticonvulsants for alcohol withdrawal. Cochrane Database Syst Rev 2005; CD005064.
11. Boothby LA et al. Acamprosate for the treatment of alcohol dependence. Clin Ther 2005;27:695–714.
12. Hughes JC et al. The efficacy of disulfiram: a review of outcome studies. Addiction 1997;92:381–95.
13. Srisurapanont M et al. Opioid antagonists for alcohol dependence. Cochrane Database Syst Rev 2005;CD001867.
14. Royal College of Obstetricians and Gynaecologists. Alcohol consumption and the outcomes of pregnancy. Statement No. 5. http://www.rcog.org.uk/. 2006.
15. Flannery W, Wolff K. Substance use disorders in pregnancy. In: O'Keane V, Marsh MS, Senevirante T, eds. Psychiatric Disorders and Pregnancy: Obstetric and Psychiatric Care. London: Taylor and Francis, 2005.
16. Regional Drug & Therapeutics Centre. Teratology. http://www.nyrdtc.nhs.uk/. 2007.

Substance misuse

Opioid misuse

Prescribing for opioid dependence

> **Note**: Treatment of opioid dependence usually requires specialist intervention – generalists should always contact substance misuse services (where available) before attempting to treat opioid dependence. It is strongly recommended that general adult psychiatrists do not initiate opioid substitute treatment unless directly advised by specialist services. It cannot be overemphasised that the use of methadone is readily fatal; opioid withdrawal is not.

Treatment aims
- to reduce or prevent withdrawal symptoms
- to reduce or eliminate non-prescribed drug use
- to stabilise drug intake and lifestyle
- to reduce drug-related harm (particularly injecting behaviour)
- to engage and provide an opportunity to work with the patient.

Treatment
This will depend upon:

- patient's medical history
- what pharmacotherapies and/or other interventions are available
- patient's previous history of drug use and treatment
- patient's current drug use and circumstances.

Principles of prescribing[1]
Use licensed medications for heroin dependence treatment (methadone and buprenorphine):

- daily dispensing advised
- supervised consumption in the first 3 months or until stability achieved.

Evidence of opioid dependence
Opioid dependence should be corroborated by positive urine results for opioids and objective signs of withdrawal or general restlessness should be present before considering prescribing any substitute pharmacotherapy. Recent sites of injection may also be present (depending on route of administration of opioid).

Table Objective opioid withdrawal scales

Symptoms	Absent/normal	Mild-moderate	Severe
Lactorrhoea	Absent	Eyes watery	Eyes streaming/ wiping eyes
Rhinorrhoea	Absent	Sniffing	Profuse secretion (wiping nose)
Agitation	Absent	Fidgeting	Can't remain seated
Perspiration	Absent	Clammy skin	Beads of sweat
Piloerection	Absent	Barely palpable hairs standing up	Readily palpable, visible
Pulse rate (BPM)	<80	>80 but <100	>100
Vomiting	Absent	Absent	Present
Shivering	Absent	Absent	Present
Yawning /10 min	<3	3–5	6 or more
Dilated pupils	Normal <4 mm	Dilated 4–6 mm	Widely dilated >6 mm

Opioid withdrawal symptoms can include nausea; stomach cramps; muscular tension; muscle spasms/twitching; aches and pains; insomnia.

> **Note:** Untreated heroin withdrawal symptoms typically reach their peak 32–72 hours after the last dose and symptoms will have subsided substantially after 5 days. Untreated methadone withdrawal typically reaches its peak at 4–6 days after last dose and symptoms do not substantially subside for 10–12 days[1].

Induction and stabilisation of substitute prescribing
It is usually preferable to use a longer-acting opioid agonist or partial agonist (e.g. methadone or buprenorphine, respectively) in opioid dependence, as it is generally easier to maintain stability[1]. However, patients with a less severe opioid dependency (e.g. history of using codeine or dihydrocodeine-containing preparations only) may in some cases be better managed by maintaining/ detoxifying them using that preparation or equivalent.

Choosing between buprenorphine and methadone for substitute treatment
Current evidence has not identified particular groups of patients who routinely do better on buprenorphine or methadone. Hence, the decision should

be made after discussion with the patient and taking the following into consideration:

- Buprenorphine appears to have a milder withdrawal syndrome than methadone and therefore may be preferred for detoxification programmes[2,3].
- Side-effects: differences in side-effect profiles (e.g. buprenorphine is often described as less sedating) may affect patient preference.
- Buprenorphine appears to provide greater 'blockade' effects than doses of methadone <60 mg[4–7]. This may be considered an advantage or disadvantage by patients. In particular, patients with chronic pain conditions that frequently require additional opioid analgesia may have difficulties being treated with buprenorphine.
- Buprenorphine is more effective than placebo for reducing opioid use and retaining patients. Buprenorphine is comparable to methadone at lower doses (30–60 mg). Higher-dose methadone maintenance treatment (>60 mg) appears more effective than buprenorphine. However, there are no adequate trials of high-dose buprenorphine (16–32 mg) compared with high-dose methadone maintenance treatment[8].
- Methadone levels may alter with drugs that inhibit/induce CYP3A4 such as erythromycin, several SSRIs, ribovarin and some anticonvulsants. This may make dose assessment difficult, if a person is not consistent in their use of these CYP3A4-inhibiting drugs. Buprenorphine is less affected by such medications, and may be preferable for such patients.
- Women who are pregnant or planning a pregnancy should consider methadone treatment, as there is a risk of buprenoprhine-precipitated withdrawal or risk associated with awaiting spontaneous withdrawal before initiation of buprenorphine in pregnant women.
- Methadone clients unable to reduce to doses of methadone <60 mg without becoming 'unstable' cannot easily be transferred to buprenorphine.
- Patients with a history of diversion of medication may be better served with methadone treatment, as sublingual buprenorphine tablets can be more easily diverted (with the risk of injecting tablets).

Methadone

Clinical effectiveness

Methadone, a long-acting opioid agonist, has been shown to be an effective maintenance therapy intervention for the treatment of heroin dependence by retaining patients in treatment and decreasing heroin use more than non-opioid-based replacement therapy[8]. In addition, higher doses of methadone (60–100 mg/day) have been shown to be more effective than lower dosages in retaining patients and in reducing illicit heroin and cocaine use during treatment[9]. Methadone is also effective at reducing withdrawal severity when used for detoxification from heroin; however, there is a high relapse following termination of treatment[10].

Prescribing information

Methadone is a Controlled Drug with a high dependency potential and a low lethal dose. The initial 2 weeks of treatment with methadone are associated with a substantially increased risk of overdose mortality[1,11–14]. It is important that appropriate assessment, titration of doses and monitoring is performed during this period.

Prescribing should only commence if:

- opioid drugs are being taken on a regular basis (typically daily)
- there is convincing evidence of dependence (see above)
- consumption of methadone can be supervised.

Supervised daily consumption is recommended for new prescriptions, for a minimum of 3 months[1]. If not possible, instalment prescriptions for daily dispensing and collection should be used. Certainly no more than 1 week's supply should be dispensed at one time, except in very exceptional circumstances[1].

Methadone should be prescribed in the oral liquid formulation (mixture or linctus). Tablets can potentially be crushed and inappropriately injected and therefore should not be prescribed[1,15].

Important: All patients starting a methadone treatment programme must be informed of the risks of toxicity and overdose, and the necessity for safe storage[1,13,14,16].

METHADONE DOSE

For patients who are *currently prescribed* methadone and if *all* the criteria listed below are met, then it is safe to prescribe the same dose:

- Dose confirmed by prescriber.
- Last consumption confirmed and supervised (e.g. pharmacy contacted) and is within last 3 days.
- Prescriptions are not being issued elsewhere.
- Patient is comfortable on dose (no signs of intoxication/withdrawal).
- No other contraindications or cautions are present.

Otherwise the following recommendations should be followed.

STARTING DOSE

Consideration must be given to the potential for opioid toxicity, taking into account:

- Tolerance to opioids can be affected by a number of factors and it obviously significantly influences an individual's risk of toxicity[17]. Tolerance should be assessed on the history of quantity, frequency and route of administration (be aware of the likelihood of over-reporting). An individual's tolerance to methadone can be significantly reduced within 3–4 days of not using, so that caution must be exercised when re-instating their dose.
- Use of other drugs, particularly CNS depressants (e.g. alcohol and benzodiazepines).
- Long half-life of methadone, as cumulative toxicity may develop[18,19].
- Inappropriate dosing can result in fatal overdose, particularly in the first few days[11–14]. Deaths have occurred following the commencement of a daily dose of 40 mg methadone[1]. It is safer to keep to a low dose that can subsequently be increased at intervals if this dose later proves to be insufficient.

Substance misuse

> *Note:* **Opioid withdrawal is not a life-threatening condition. Opioid toxicity is.**

Direct conversion tables for opioids and methadone should be viewed cautiously, as there are a number of factors influencing the values at any given time. It is much safer to titrate the dose against presenting withdrawal symptoms.

The **initial total** daily dose for most cases will be in the range of 10–40 mg methadone, depending on the level of tolerance (low: 10–20 mg, moderate: 25–40 mg). Starting doses >30 mg should be prescribed with caution because of the risk of overdose and death. It is safer to use a starting dose of 10–20 mg and reassess the patient after a period of 2–4 hours. Further incremental doses of 5–10 mg can be given, depending on the severity of the withdrawal symptoms. *Note:* onset of action should be evident within half an hour, with peak plasma levels being achieved after approximately 2–4 hours of dosing.

Heavily dependent users with high tolerance may require larger doses. A starting dose, not exceeding 30 mg can be given, followed by a second dose after a minimum interval of 2–4 hours. The second dose can be up to 30 mg, depending on the persisting severity of withdrawal symptoms. High doses should only be prescribed by experienced specialist medical practitioners.

Table Methadone dose after initial dose

Severity of withdrawal after initial dose	*Additional dosage*
Mild	Nil
Moderate (muscle aches and pains, pupil dilation, nausea, yawning, clammy skin)	5–10 mg
Severe (vomiting, profuse sweating, piloerection, tachycardia, elevated BP)	20–30 mg

METHADONE STABILISATION DOSE
- **First week**
  Outpatients should attend daily for the first few days to enable assessment by the prescriber and any dose titration against withdrawal symptoms. Dose increases should not exceed 5–10 mg/day and 30 mg/week above the initial starting dose. Note that steady-state plasma levels are only achieved approximately 5 days after the last dose increase. Once the patient has been stabilised on an adequate dose, methadone should be prescribed as a single daily dose. It should not be prescribed on a PRN basis.

- **Subsequent period**
  Subsequent increases should not exceed 10 mg/week beyond the induction period[1], up to a total daily dose of 60–120 mg. Stabilisation is usually

achieved within 6 weeks but may take longer. However, it is important to consider that some patients may require a quicker stabilisation. This would need to be balanced by a high level of supervision, thereby allowing the ability to increase doses more rapidly.

METHADONE CAUTIONS

- **Intoxication.** Methadone should not be given to any patient showing signs of intoxication, especially due to alcohol or other CNS depressant drugs (e.g. benzodiazepines)[17,20]. Risk of fatal overdose is greatly enhanced when methadone is taken concomitantly with alcohol and other respiratory depressant drugs. Concurrent alcohol and illicit drug consumption must be borne in mind when considering subsequent prescribing of methadone due to the increased risk of overdose associated with poly-substance misuse[11,14,20,21].

- **Severe hepatic/renal dysfunction**. Metabolism and elimination of methadone may be affected, in which case the dose or dosing interval should be adjusted accordingly against clinical presentation. Because of extended plasma half-life, the interval between assessments during initial dosing may need to be extended.

METHADONE OVERDOSE
In the event of methadone overdose, naloxone should be administered following the *BNF* guidelines. Naloxone can be given by the intravenous, intramuscular or subcutaneous route.

Dose: 0.4–2 mg repeated at intervals of 2–3 minutes to a maximum of 10 mg if respiratory function does not improve. If no response, consider alternative causes for overdose.

Although the onset of action will be slower with the intramuscular route, this is the preferred route within the psychiatric setting or addiction service, where the intravenous route may be difficult and actually take longer to administer.

In the medical setting, a continuous intravenous infusion (2 mg/500 ml) at a rate adjusted according to response may be used.

Since naloxone is a short-acting agent and the effect may reverse within 20 minutes to 1 hour, an individual can revert back to an overdose state. Medical monitoring should therefore be provided after naloxone administration.

Substance misuse

Always Call Emergency Services

Analgesia for methadone-prescribed patients
Non-opioid analgesics should be used in preference (e.g. paracetamol, NSAIDs). If opioid analgesia is indicated (e.g. codeine, dihydrocodeine, MST), the drug should be titrated accordingly against pain relief, with the methadone dose remaining constant to alleviate withdrawal symptoms. Titrating the methadone dose to provide analgesia may be used in certain circumstances but should only be carried out by experienced specialists.

Methadone and risk of torsade de pointes/QT interval prolongation

Methadone may be a risk factor for developing QT interval prolongation on the electrocardiogram[22–24]. This is associated with torsade de pointes, which is often fatal. Limitations to the evidence may be confounding variables. However, it is possible that methadone combined with other QT-prolonging agents may increase the likelihood of QT prolongation.

MHRA guidance is that increased monitoring should occur with patients on high-dose methadone (>100 mg/day) and/or with other QT interval prolongation risk factors including heart or liver disease, electrolyte abnormalities, concomitant treatment with CYP3A4 inhibitors, or medicines/illicit drugs with the potential to cause QT interval prolongation[25].

Recommended ECG monitoring

Consider an ECG at baseline before commencing methadone if a patient has QT interval prolongation risk factors as described above. This should be repeated after a period of stabilisation (approximately 4 weeks). For existing clients on methadone, an ECG should be considered if the patient fulfils the MHRA criteria above. ECG monitoring should occur at 6–12-month intervals depending on clinical circumstances.

Remember that QT should be corrected for heart rate to produce a corrected QT (QTc) in milliseconds (ms). This is normally documented on the ECG recording. Refer to the earlier sections (page 116) on QT prolongation for actions depending on the ECG results. Brief guidelines as to actions to take are documented below. Always seek specialist advice if unsure.

Table Guidelines for ECG monitoring

	Borderline prolonged QTc	Action	Prolonged QTc	Action	Very prolonged QTc	Action
Females Males	≥470 ms ≥440 ms	Repeat ECG Electrolytes Try to modify QT risk factors Regular ECG until normal	≥500 ms	Repeat ECG Electrolytes Try to modify QT risk factors Seek specialist help Consider stopping methadone/ switching to buprenorphine Regular ECGs until normal	≥550 ms	Urgent specialist referral Repeat ECG Electrolytes Try to modify QT risk factors Stop methadone

Substance misuse

325

Injectable opioid maintenance treatment
Injectable medications and diamorphine prescriptions for opioid addiction should only be started and maintained by addictions specialists. Please also note that a home office licence is required to prescribe diamorphine for addictions treatment. At present there is insufficient evidence supporting the use of injectable opioid drugs for maintenance treatment[26]. However, it may be considered in some patients as a 'second-line' treatment option for whom an adequate trial (e.g. at least 6 months) of optimised methadone maintenance treatment (e.g. doses > 80 mg, regular supervised dosing, regular attendance at key worker and medical reviews, and appropriate management of medical or psychiatric co-morbidity) is proving ineffective in controlling illicit injecting drug use. A substance misuse specialist should initiate injectable methadone or diamorphine treatment. National Treatment Agency (NTA) guidelines advocate that all clients currently on injectable opioids should be supervised whilst taking their prescribed drug on a regular basis, enabling assessment of a patient's tolerance and injecting techniques.

There appears to be considerable individual variation in appropriate dose conversions between oral and injectable methadone. It appears that oral methadone has a bioavailability of approximately 80% (ranging from 40 to 99%)[27]. Hence it is suggested that the injectable methadone dose = 80% x oral methadone dose, and that clients are regularly monitored in subsequent days and the dose titrated (up or down) as clinically indicated.

Dose conversions between oral methadone and injectable diamorphine vary from between 3:1 and 6:1 according to the dose. Readers are referred to NTA guidance regarding injectable opioid prescribing[27].

Buprenorphine

Clinical effectiveness

Buprenorphine (Subutex) is a synthetic partial opioid agonist with a low intrinsic activity and high affinity at μ-opioid receptors. It is an effective treatment for use in maintenance treatment for heroin addiction, although not more effective than methadone at adequate dosages[8]. There is no significant difference between buprenorphine and methadone in terms of completion of detoxification treatment, but withdrawal symptoms may resolve more quickly with buprenorphine[28].

Prescribing information
Buprenorphine is absorbed via the sublingual route, which takes approximately 5–10 minutes to complete. It is effective in treating opioid dependence because:

- It alleviates/prevents opioid withdrawal and craving.
- It reduces the effects of additional opioid use because of its high receptor affinity[4–6].
- It is long-acting, allowing daily (or less-frequent) dosing. The duration of action is related to the buprenorphine dose administered: low doses (e.g. 2 mg) exert effects for up to 12 hours; higher doses (e.g. 16–32 mg) exert effects for as long as 48–72 hours.

BUPRENORPHINE STARTING DOSE

The same principles as for methadone apply when starting treatment with buprenorphine. However, of particular interest with buprenorphine is the phenomenon of precipitated withdrawal. Patient education is an important factor in reducing the problems during induction.

INDUCTING HEROIN USERS

The first dose of buprenorphine should be administered when the patient is experiencing opioid withdrawal symptoms to reduce the risk of precipitated withdrawal. The initial dose recommendations are as follows:

Patient in withdrawal and no risk factors	8 mg buprenorphine
Patient not experiencing withdrawal and no risk factors	4 mg buprenorphine
Patient has concomitant risk factors (e.g. medical condition, polydrug misuse, low or uncertain severity of dependence)	2–4 mg buprenorphine

BUPRENORPHINE TRANSFERRING FROM METHADONE

Patients transferring from methadone are at risk of experiencing precipitated withdrawal symptoms that may continue at a milder level for 1–2 weeks. Factors affecting precipitated withdrawal are listed in the following table.

Table Factors affecting risk of precipitated withdrawal with buprenorphine

Factor	Discussion	Recommended strategy
Dose of methadone	More likely with doses of methadone above 30 mg. Generally – the higher the dose the more severe the precipitated withdrawal[29]	Attempt transfer from doses of methadone <40 mg (preferably ≤30 mg). Transfer from >60 mg should not be attempted
Time between last methadone dose and first buprenorphine dose	Interval should be at least 24 hours. Increasing the interval reduces the incidence and severity of withdrawal[30,31]	Cease methadone and delay first dose until patient experiencing withdrawal from methadone
Dose of buprenorphine	Very low doses of buprenorphine (e.g. 2 mg) are generally inadequate to substitute for methadone. High first doses of buprenorphine (e.g. 8 mg) are more likely to precipitate withdrawal	First dose should generally be 4 mg; review patient 2–3 hours later
Patient expectancy	Patients not prepared for precipitated withdrawal are more likely to become distressed and confused by the effect	Inform patients in advance. Have contingency plan for severe symptoms
Use of other medications	Symptomatic medication (e.g. lofexidine) can be useful to relieve symptoms	Prescribe in accordance to management plan

TRANSFERRING FROM METHADONE DOSE <40 MG (IDEALLY <30 MG)
Methadone should be ceased abruptly, and the first dose of buprenorphine given at least 24 hours after the last methadone dose. The following conversion rates are recommended:

Last methadone dose	Day 1 – initial buprenorphine dose	Day 2 buprenorphine dose
20–40 mg	4 mg	6–8 mg
10–20 mg	4 mg	4–8 mg
1–10 mg	2 mg	2–4 mg

TRANSFERRING FROM METHADONE DOSE 40–60 MG

- The methadone dose should be reduced as far as possible without the patient becoming unstable or chaotic, and then abruptly stopped.
- The first buprenorphine dose should be delayed until the patient displays clear signs of withdrawal, generally 48–96 hours after the last dose of methadone. Symptomatic medication (lofexidine) may be useful to provide transitory relief.
- An initial dose of 2–4 mg should be given. The patient should then be reviewed 2–3 hours later.
- If withdrawal has been precipitated, further symptomatic medication can be prescribed.
- If there has been no precipitation or worsening of withdrawal, an additional 2–4 mg of buprenorphine can be dispensed and administered on the same day.
- The patient should be reviewed the following day, at which point the dose should be increased to 8–12 mg.

TRANSFERRING FROM METHADONE DOSES >60 MG
Such transfers should not be attempted in an outpatient setting. Consider referral to inpatient unit if required.

BUPRENORPHINE TRANSFERRING FROM OTHER PRESCRIBED OPIOIDS
There is little experience in transferring patients from other prescribed opioids (e.g. codeine, dihydrocodeine, morphine). Basic principles suggest that transferring from opioids with short half-lives should be similar to inducting heroin users, whereas transferring from opioids with longer half-lives will be similar to transferring from methadone.

STABILISATION DOSE OF BUPRENORPHINE
Outpatients should attend regularly for the first few days to enable assessment by the prescriber and any dose titration. Dose increases should be made in increments of 2–4 mg at a time, daily if necessary, up to a maximum daily dose of 32 mg. Effective maintenance doses are usually in the range of 12–24 mg daily[32] and patients should generally be able to achieve maintenance levels within 1–2 weeks of starting buprenorphine.

BUPHRENORPHINE LESS THAN DAILY DOSING
Buprenorphine is licensed in the UK as a medication to be taken daily. International evidence and experience indicate that many clients can be comfortably maintained on one dose every 2–3 days[33–36]. This may be pertinent for patients in buprenorphine treatment who are considered unsuitable for take-away medication because of the risk of diversion. The following conversion rate is recommended:

2-day buprenorphine dose = 2 × daily dose of buprenorphine (to a maximum 32 mg)
3-day buprenorphine dose = 3 × daily dose of buprenorphine (to a maximum 32 mg)

Note: In the event of patients being unable to stabilise comfortably on buprenorphine (often those transferring from methadone), the option of transferring to methadone should be available. Methadone can be commenced 24 hours after the last buprenorphine dose. Doses should be titrated according to clinical response, being mindful of the residual 'blockade' effect of buprenorphine, which may last for several days.

Cautions with buprenorphine

- **Liver function:** There is some evidence suggesting that high-dose buprenorphine can cause changes in liver function in individuals with a history of liver disease[37]. Such patients should have LFTs measured before commencing with follow-up investigations conducted 6–12 weeks after commencing buprenorphine. More frequent testing should be considered in patients of particular concern, e.g. severe liver disease. Elevated liver enzymes in the absence of clinically significant liver disease, however, does not necessarily contraindicate treatment with buprenorphine.
- **Intoxication:** Buprenorphine should not be given to any patient showing signs of intoxication, especially when due to alcohol or other depressant drugs (e.g. benzodiazepines). Buprenorphine in combination with other sedative drugs can result in respiratory depression, sedation, coma and death. Concurrent alcohol and illicit drug consumption must be borne in mind when considering subsequent prescribing of buprenorphine due to the increased risk of overdose associated with polysubstance misuse.

OVERDOSE WITH BUPRENORPHINE

Buprenorphine as a single drug in overdose is generally regarded as safer than methadone and heroin because it causes less respiratory depression. However, in combination with other respiratory depressant drugs the effects may be harder to manage. Very high doses of naloxone (e.g. 10–15 mg) may be needed to reverse buprenorphine effects (although lower doses such as 0.8–2 mg may be sufficient); hence, ventilator support is often required in cases where buprenorphine is contributing to respiratory depression (e.g. in polydrug overdose).

Always Call Emergency Services

ANALGESIA FOR BUPRENORPHINE-PRESCRIBED PATIENTS

Non-opioid analgesics should be used in preference (e.g. paracetamol, NSAIDs). Buprenorphine reduces or blocks the effect of full opioid agonists, complicating their use as analgesics in patients on buprenorphine. If adequate pain control cannot be achieved, it may be necessary to transfer the patient to a stable methadone dose so that an opioid analgesic can be effectively used for pain control (see note on analgesia for methadone-prescribed patients).

Opioid detoxification and reduction regimens

Opioid maintenance can be continued in the long term, however if a person wants to withdraw from maintenance treatment, detoxification will be required.

Community setting

- **Methadone**
  Following a period of stabilisation with methadone, a contract may be negotiated between the patient and prescriber to reduce the daily methadone dose by 5–10 mg weekly or fortnightly. However, this should be reviewed regularly and remain flexible to adjustments and changes in the patient's readiness for total abstinence. Factors such as an increase in heroin or other drug use, or worsening of the patient's physical, psychological or social well-being, may warrant a temporary increase or stabilisation of the dose or a slowing-down of the reduction rate. Towards the end of the detoxification, the dose reduction may be slower, at 1–2 mg per week.
- **Buprenorphine**
  The same principles as for methadone apply when planning a buprenorphine detoxification regimen. Dose reduction should be gradual to minimise withdrawal discomfort. Suggested reduction regimen:

Daily buprenorphine dose	Reduction rate
Above 16 mg	4 mg every 1–2 weeks
8–16 mg	2–4 mg every 1–2 weeks
2–8 mg	2 mg per week or fortnight
Below 2 mg	Reduce by 0.4–0.8 mg per week

- **Lofexidine**
  Lofexidine is licensed for the management of symptoms of opioid withdrawal. It is non-opioid and therefore less liable to misuse and diversion. Its use in community detoxification is more likely to be successful for patients with a low level of heroin use, for non-polydrug users and for those with shorter drug and treatment histories, or for those at an end stage of methadone detoxification (patients taking not more than 20 mg daily).
  - *Precautions:* severe coronary insufficiency, recent MI, bradycardia, cerebrovascular disease, chronic renal failure, pregnancy and breastfeeding. QT prolongation has been reported[38]. Consider ECG monitoring during treatment based on other cardiac risk factors.
  - *Interactions:* alcohol and other CNS depressants – lofexidine may enhance the effects. Tricyclic antidepressants – concomitant use may reduce the efficacy of lofexidine.
  - *Side-effects:* drowsiness, dryness of mouth, throat and nose, hypotension, bradycardia and rebound hypertension on withdrawal.
  Before commencing treatment with lofexidine, baseline blood pressure should be measured. Once lofexidine has been commenced, BP should be monitored over the first few days. If there is a significant drop in BP (systolic less than 90 mmHg or 30 mmHg below baseline), or pulse is

below 55, lofexidine should be withheld. Treatment should be reviewed with the option to either continue at a reduced dose or discontinue.

- *Dose*: Initially, 0.4–0.6 mg twice daily, increased as necessary, to control withdrawal symptoms, in increments of 0.2–0.4 mg daily, to a maximum total daily dose of 2.4 mg. The total daily dose should be given in 2–4 divided doses, with one dose at bedtime to offset insomnia associated with opioid withdrawal. Treatment course should be 7–10 days, followed by a gradual withdrawal over 2–4 days. For patients currently taking methadone before detoxification, low, reducing doses of methadone (e.g. 15 mg/10 mg/5 mg daily) may be given over the initial days of treatment with lofexidine as a cross-over period, to minimise withdrawal symptoms. Additional short-term medication may be required for nausea, stomach cramps, diarrhoea and insomnia.

Inpatient setting

- **Methadone**
  Patients should have a starting dose assessment of methadone, over 48 hours following the same guidelines listed above. The dose may then be reduced following a linear regimen over 10 days.
- **Buprenorphine**
  Buprenorphine can be used effectively for short-term inpatient detoxifications following the same principles as for methadone.
- **Lofexidine** (see community detoxification regimens above for more information)
  Higher doses of lofexidine (up to the maximum daily dose of 2.4 mg) may be given initially, particularly for patients with moderately severe heroin dependence). This is provided there is adequate monitoring of BP, pulse and adverse effects, and appropriate action can be taken in any such event. If there is a significant drop in BP or pulse (systolic less than 90 mmHg or 30 mmHg below baseline, or pulse below 55), lofexidine should be withheld until normal measurements are obtained and then reintroduced cautiously at a lower dose. In certain cases lofexidine may need to be discontinued and alternative detoxification treatment regimens considered.

  The total daily dose should be given in four divided doses over the first 2–3 days with the full treatment course continuing for 7–10 days. This should then be followed by a gradual withdrawal over 2–4 days.

  Additional short-term medication may be required for nausea, stomach cramps, diarrhoea and insomnia.

Relapse prevention – naltrexone

Evidence for the effectiveness of naltrexone as a treatment for relapse prevention in opioid misusers is inconclusive[39]. Combined use of naltrexone and psychosocial therapy has proved to be more effective than either therapy alone in improving post-treatment outcomes[40]. The available trials do not provide a final evaluation of naltrexone maintenance treatment. A trend in favour of treatment with naltrexone has been observed with highly motivated client groups only[39]. There is a risk of adverse events such as fatal overdose in those who relapse to opioid use due to lowering of opioid tolerance induced by prior naltrexone maintenance. Therefore this intervention should be used cautiously in highly selected patients.

Naltrexone-initiating treatment

Naltrexone has the propensity to cause a severe withdrawal reaction in patients who are either currently taking opioid drugs or who were previously taking opioid drugs and have not allowed a sufficient wash-out period prior to administering naltrexone.

The minimum recommended interval between stopping the opioid and starting naltrexone depends on the opioid used, duration of use and the amount taken as a last dose. Opioid agonists with long half-lives such as methadone will require a wash-out period of up to 10 days, whereas shorter-acting opioids such as heroin may only require up to 7 days.

Experience with buprenorphine indicates that a wash-out period of up to 7 days is sufficient (final buprenorphine dose >2 mg; duration of use >2 weeks) and in some cases naltrexone may be started within 2–3 days of a patient stopping (final buprenorphine dose <2 mg; duration of use <2 weeks).

A test dose of naloxone (0.2–0.8 mg), which has a much shorter half-life than naltrexone, may be given to the patient prior to starting naltrexone treatment. Any withdrawal symptoms precipitated will be of shorter duration than if precipitated by naltrexone.

Patients *must* be advised of the risk of withdrawal prior to giving the dose. It is worth thoroughly questioning the patient as to whether they have taken any opioid-containing preparation unknowingly (e.g. over-the-counter analgesic).

Patients must also be warned of the risk of acute opioid toxicity occurring in an attempt to overcome the blockade effect of naltrexone. Changes in the individual's opioid tolerance level are likely to be very significant, particularly following a detoxification programme and any period of abstinence.

Dose of naltrexone

An initial dose of 25 mg naltrexone should be administered after a suitable opioid-free interval (and naloxone challenge if appropriate). The patient should be monitored for 4 hours after the first dose, for symptoms of opioid withdrawal. Symptomatic medication for withdrawal (lofexidine) should be available for use, if necessary, on the first day of naltrexone dosing (withdrawal symptoms may last up to 4–8 hours). Once the patient has tolerated this low naltrexone dose, subsequent doses can be increased to 50 mg daily as a maintenance dose.

Pregnancy and opioid use

Detoxification should be avoided in the first trimester, ideally undertaken in the second trimester and undertaken with caution in the third trimester.

It is useful to anticipate potential problems for women prescribed opioids during pregnancy with regard to opioid pain relief.

Pregnancy and breastfeeding – methadone

There is no evidence of an increase in congenital defects with methadone; however, the newborn may experience a withdrawal syndrome[41]. It is important to prevent the pregnant woman going into a withdrawal state, since this is dangerous for both mother and fetus. Specialist advice should be obtained before initiating opioid substitution treatment or detoxification, particularly with regards to management and treatment plan during pregnancy. Maternal metabolism of methadone may increase towards the third trimester of pregnancy. At this time an increased methadone dose may be required or occasionally split dosing on the medication to prevent withdrawal. Maternal methadone dose does not appear to correlate with severity of neonatal withdrawal for doses above 20 mg. Continued use of heroin during pregnancy and rate of clearance of methadone may also be predictors of neonatal withdrawal severity[42].

Methadone is considered compatible with breastfeeding, with no adverse effects to nursing infant associated with maternal doses of 20 mg or less[41].

Pregnancy and breastfeeding – buprenorphine
Currently there is insufficient evidence regarding the use of buprenorphine as an opioid substitute treatment during pregnancy or breastfeeding to be able to define its safety profile[41]. More evidence is available on the safety of methadone, which for that reason makes it the preferred choice. However, women well maintained on buprenorphine prior to pregnancy refusing alternative pharmacotherapy may remain on buprenorphine following full informed consent and advice that safety of buprenorphine in pregnancy has not been demonstrated at their own risk[42]. Please note that buprenorphine is not licensed in pregnancy.

Opioid overdose and use of naloxone

All addiction services and psychiatric units should have naloxone available.

If pregnant, breastfeeding or <18 years old, please call the emergency services and get specialist help.

Opioid overdose with heroin or other opioids
Can be recognised by:
* pin-point pupils
* respiratory depression (<8 breaths per minute)
* cold to touch/blue lips
* unconscious.

Actions to be taken on discovering an opioid overdose
* Check area safe, then try to rouse overdose victim.
* If unrousable – call for help/ambulance.
* Check airway and breathing:
  * if not breathing, give 2 rescue breaths (optional)
  * if breathing, place in recovery position.
* Administer 0.4 mg naloxone IM.
* Consider use of high-flow oxygen (where available).
* Await emergency team/ambulance.
* Patient to have medical monitoring for several hours after naloxone, as the effects of naloxone are short-acting (between 30 minutes to 1 hour) and the effects of an opioid overdose may re-emerge. Patients may need additional doses of naloxone.

'Take-home naloxone'

Research trials have assessed the impact of providing take-home naloxone and overdose management training to opioid-using patients. Although no randomised controlled trials have been carried out the available evidence is promising for reducing heroin-related overdose deaths[43,44]. Some services are providing one dose of take-home naloxone (400 µg) in combination opioid overdose management training (as above) to opioid-using clients in treatment.

References

1. Department of Health. Drug misuse and dependence: guidelines on clinical management. Norwich: Department of Health, 1999.
2. Seifert J et al. Detoxification of opiate addicts with multiple drug abuse: a comparison of buprenorphine vs. methadone. Pharmacopsychiatry 2002;35:159–64.
3. Jasinski DR et al. Human pharmacology and abuse potential of the analgesic buprenorphine: a potential agent for treating narcotic addiction. Arch Gen Psychiatry 1978;35:501–16.
4. Bickel WK et al. Buprenorphine: dose-related blockade of opioid challenge effects in opioid dependent humans. J Pharmacol Exp Ther 1988;247:47–53.
5. Walsh SL et al. Acute administration of buprenorphine in humans: partial agonist and blockade effects. J Pharmacol Exp Ther 1995;274:361–72.
6. Comer SD et al. Buprenorphine sublingual tablets: effects on IV heroin self-administration by humans. Psychopharmacology 2001;154:28–37.
7. Donny EC et al. High-dose methadone produces superior opioid blockade and comparable withdrawal suppression to lower doses in opioid-dependent humans. Psychopharmacology 2002;161:202–12.
8. Mattick RP et al. Buprenorphine maintenance versus placebo or methadone maintenance for opioid dependence. Cochrane Database Syst Rev 2003;CD002207.
9. Faggiano F et al. Methadone maintenance at different dosages for opioid dependence. Cochrane Database Syst Rev 2003;CD002208.
10. Amato L et al. Methadone at tapered doses for the management of opioid withdrawal. Cochrane Database Syst Rev 2005;CD003409.
11. Harding-Pink D. Methadone: one person's maintenance dose is another's poison. Lancet 1993; 341: 665–6.
12. Drummer OH et al. Methadone toxicity causing death in ten subjects starting on a methadone maintenance program. Am J Forensic Med Pathol 1992;13:346–50.
13. Caplehorn JR. Deaths in the first two weeks of maintenance treatment in NSW in 1994: identifying cases of iatrogenic methadone toxicity. Drug Alcohol Rev 1998;17:9–17.
14. Zador D et al. Deaths in methadone maintenance treatment in New South Wales, Australia 1990–1995. Addiction 2000;95:77–84.
15. Department of Health, Task Force to Review Services for Drug Misusers. Report of an independent review of drug treatment services in England. http://www.dh.gov.uk/. 1996.
16. Hall W. Reducing the toll of opioid overdose deaths in Australia. Drug Alcohol Rev 1999;18:213–20.
17. White JM et al. Mechanisms of fatal opioid overdose. Addiction 1999;94:961–72.
18. Wolff K et al. The pharmacokinetics of methadone in healthy subjects and opiate users. Br J Clin Pharmacol 1997;44:325–34.
19. Rostami-Hodjegan A et al. Population pharmacokinetics of methadone in opiate users: characterization of time-dependent changes. Br J Clin Pharmacol 1999;48:43–52.
20. Farrell M et al. Suicide and overdose among opiate addicts. Addiction 1996;91:321–3.
21. Neale J. Methadone, methadone treatment and non-fatal overdose. Drug Alcohol Depend 2000;58: 117–24.
22. Krantz MJ et al. Torsade de pointes associated with very-high-dose methadone. Ann Intern Med 2002; 137:501–4.
23. Kornick CA et al. QTc interval prolongation associated with intravenous methadone. Pain 2003;105: 499–506.
24. Martell BA et al. The impact of methadone induction on cardiac conduction in opiate users. Ann Intern Med 2003;139:154–5.
25. Medicines and Healthcare Products Regulatory Agency. Risk of QT interval prolongation with methadone. Curr Probl Pharmacovigilance 2006;31:6.
26. Lingford-Hughes AR et al. Evidence-based guidelines for the pharmacological management of substance misuse, addiction and comorbidity: recommendations from the British Association for Psychopharmacology. J Psychopharmacol 2004;18:293–335.
27. National Treatment Agency for Substance Misuse. Injectable heroin and injectable methadone in the treatment of opioid dependence: dosing guidance for pilot sites (Draft). http://www.nta.nhs.uk/. 2004.
28. Gowing L et al. Buprenorphine for the management of opioid withdrawal. Cochrane Database Syst Rev 2006;CD002025.
29. Walsh SL et al. Effects of buprenorphine and methadone in methadone-maintained subjects. Psychopharmacology 1995;119:268–76.

30. Strain EC et al. Acute effects of buprenorphine, hydromorphone and naloxone in methadone-maintained volunteers. J Pharmacol Exp Ther 1992;261:985–93.
31. Strain EC et al. Buprenorphine effects in methadone-maintained volunteers: effects at two hours after methadone. J Pharmacol Exp Ther 1995;272:628–38.
32. Ling W et al. Buprenorphine maintenance treatment of opiate dependence: a multicenter, randomized clinical trial. Addiction 1998;93:475–86.
33. Amass L et al. Alternate-day dosing during buprenorphine treatment of opioid dependence. Life Sci 1994;54:1215–28.
34. Amass L et al. Alternate-day buprenorphine dosing is preferred to daily dosing by opioid-dependent humans. Psychopharmacology 1998;136:217–25.
35. Johnson RE et al. Buprenorphine treatment of opioid dependence: clinical trial of daily versus alternate-day dosing. Drug Alcohol Depend 1995;40:27–35.
36. Eissenberg T et al. Controlled opioid withdrawal evaluation during 72 h dose omission in buprenorphine-maintained patients. Drug Alcohol Depend 1997;45:81–91.
37. Berson A et al. Hepatitis after intravenous buprenorphine misuse in heroin addicts. J Hepatol 2001; 34:346–50.
38. Schmittner J et al. QT interval increased after single dose of lofexidine. BMJ 2004;329:1075.
39. Kirchmayer U et al. Naltrexone maintenance treatment for opioid dependence. Cochrane Database Syst Rev 2003;CD001333.
40. Tucker TK et al. Naltrexone in the treatment of heroin dependence: a literature review. Drug Alcohol Rev 2000;19:73–82.
41. Briggs GG, Freeman RK, Yaffe SJ. Drugs in Pregnancy and Lactation. A Reference Guide to Fetal and Neonatal Risk. Philadelphia: Lippincott, Williams & Wilkins, 2001.
42. New South Wales Department of Health. National clinical guidelines for the management of drug use during pregnancy, birth and the early development years of the newborn. http://www.health.nsw.gov. au/. 2006.
43. Baca CT et al. Take-home naloxone to reduce heroin death. Addiction 2005;100:1823–31.
44. Strang J et al. Emergency naloxone for heroin overdose. BMJ 2006;333:614–5.

Further reading

National Institute for Clinical Excellence. Methadone and buprenorphine for the management of opioid dependence. NICE technology appraisal guidance 114, 2007.
National Institute for Clinical Excellence Naltrexone for the management of opioid dependence. NICE technology appraisal guidance 115, 2007.

Substance
misuse

NICE Guidance – Summary
Methadone and buprenorphine for the management of opioid dependence

- Methadone and buprenorphine (oral formulations), using flexible dosing regimens, are recommended as options for maintenance therapy in the management of opioid dependence.
- The decision about which drug to use should be made on a case by case basis, taking into account a number of factors, including the person's history of opioid dependence, their commitment to a particular long-term management strategy, and an estimate of the risks and benefits of each treatment made by the responsible clinician in consultation with the person. If both drugs are equally suitable, methadone should be prescribed as the first choice.
- Methadone and buprenorphine should be administered daily, under supervision, for at least the first 3 months. Supervision should be relaxed only when the patient's compliance is assured. Both drugs should be given as part of a programme of supportive care.

NICE Guidance – Summary
Naltrexone for the management of opioid dependence

- Naltrexone is recommended as a treatment option in detoxified formerly opioid-dependent people who are highly motivated to remain in an abstinence programme.
- Naltrexone should only be administered under adequate supervision to people who have been fully informed of the potential adverse effects of treatment. It should be given as part of a programme of supportive care.
- The effectiveness of naltrexone in preventing opioid misuse in people being treated should be reviewed regularly. Discontinuation of naltrexone treatment should be considered if there is evidence of such misuse.

Substance misuse

Nicotine and smoking cessation

NICE guidance on smoking cessation

Harmful effects from nicotine dependence are related only to the harm caused by smoking cigarettes and therefore the primary goal of treatment is complete cessation of smoking. The three main treatments licensed in the UK for smoking cessation are nicotine replacement (all formulations are available over the counter), the antidepressant bupropion prolonged-release, and since December 2006, varenicline tartrate. Nicotine replacement therapy (NRT) and bupropion have been investigated in a large number of well-conducted RCTs and varenicline in four similar trials. NICE have developed treatment guidance for nicotine dependence and smoking cessation.

NICE guidance also made recommendations on brief interventions and referral to NHS smoking cessation services, some of which are outlined below[1]:

- Everyone who smokes should be advised to stop.
- All smokers should be asked how interested they are in quitting.
- Healthcare workers (including GPs and hospital doctors) should offer referral to smoking cessation services and if the person does not want to attend these services, can initate pharmacotherpy as per NICE guidance[2] if sufficiently experienced.

The original NICE guidance assessed bupropion and NRT and new guidance is expected to include varenicline. NICE have made several recommendations for treatment.

- NRT and bupropion are recommended for those who want to quit smoking.
- NRT and bupropion should only be prescribed as part of an 'abstinent-contingent treatment' model in which smokers make a committment to stop smoking on a particular date and medication is only continued if the user remains abstinent from smoking at follow-ups. To increase cost-efficacy, the total treatment course is dispensed in divided prescriptions. NRT should initially be prescribed to last for 2 weeks after the quit date and bupropion for 3–4 weeks after the quit date. Subsequent prescriptions should be given if the smoker is making good progress.
- Bupropion should not be used in the under-18s or pregnant and breastfeeding women.
- NHS-funded smoking cessation treatments should not usually be offered within 6 months of an unsuccessful attempt at smoking cessastion with either NRT or bupropion, unless there are external cicrumstances which led to relapse.
- The evidence is insufficient to recommend NRT combined with bupropion.
- Factors to consider when deciding which treatment to initiate include:
  - motivation to quit
  - availability of counselling
  - previous experience with smoking cessation aids
  - contraindications to use (particularly for bupropion)
  - personal preference of smoker.

Nicotine replacement therapy

Clinical effectiveness

A Cochrane review of 23 RCTs of NRT compared with placebo or non-NRT for smoking cessation with at least 6 months follow-up[3] concluded that all six commercially available forms of NRT are effective. NRT increases the odds of quitting by approximately 1.5- to 2-fold, regardless of clinical setting. NRT significantly reduces the severity of nicotine withdrawal symptoms and urge to smoke and should be given as per recommended doses in the *BNF* and as outlined below. The dosages may vary according to the degree of nicotine dependence, as indicated by markers such as daily cigarette consumption, latency to first cigarette in the morning, severity of withdrawal symptoms on previous quit attempts.

Notes: The MHRA recently issued new advice on the use of NRT to widen access in at-risk patient groups. NRT may now be used by:

- Adolescents aged 12–18, but as there are limited data on the safety and efficacy, duration should be restricted to 12 weeks. Treatment should only be continued longer than 12 weeks on the advice of a healthcare professional.

- Pregnant women – ideally they should stop smoking without using NRT but, if this is not possible, NRT may be recommended to assist a quit attempt as it is considered that the risk to the fetus of continued smoking by the mother outweighs any potential adverse effects of NRT. The decision to use NRT should be made following a risk–benefit assessment as early in pregnancy as possible. The aim should be to discontinue NRT use after 2–3 months. Intermittent (oral) forms of NRT are preferable during pregnancy, although a patch may be appropriate if nausea and/or vomiting are a problem. If patches are used, they should be removed before going to bed at night.

- Breastfeeding – NRT can be used by women who are breastfeeding. The amount of nicotine the infant is exposed to from breast milk is relatively small and less hazardous than the second-hand smoke they would otherwise be exposed to if the mother continued to smoke. If possible, patches should be avoided. NRT products taken intermittently (oral forms) are preferred, as their use can be adjusted to allow the maximum time between their administration and feeding of the baby, to minimise the amount of nicotine in the milk.

- Cardiovascular disease – dependent smokers with a myocardial infarction (MI), severe dysrhythmia or recent cerebrovascular accident (CVA) who are in hospital should be encouraged to stop smoking with non-pharmacological interventions. If this fails, NRT may be considered, but as data on safety in these patient groups are limited, initiation of NRT should only be done under medical supervision. For patients with stable cardiovascular disease, NRT is a lesser risk than continuing to smoke.

- Diabetes – nicotine releases catecholamines, which can affect carbohydrate metabolism. Diabetic patients should be advised to monitor their blood sugar levels more closely than usual when starting NRT.

- Renal or hepatic impairment – NRT should be used with caution in patients with moderate to severe hepatic impairment and/or severe renal impairment, as the clearance of nicotine or its metabolites may be decreased, with the potential for increased adverse effects.

- Drug interactions with NRT – drug interactions may occur as a *result of quitting smoking* rather from NRT *per se*. The only interaction that is possibly directly attributable to NRT is with adenosine (adverse haemodynamic effects).

Preparations and dose
All NRTs should be used for about 8–12 weeks but may be continued beyond this time if needed to prevent relapse. They can also be used in combination if required; usually the patch plus a faster-acting oral NRT for relief of situational urges to smoke. Cochrane report an odds ratio of 1.42 for combination NRT versus patch alone for long-term abstinence[3].

1. Sublingual tablets (2 mg): recommended dose of one tablet per hour or, for heavy smokers (smoking more than 20 cigarettes per day), two tablets per hour, maximum 40 × 2 mg daily.

2. Gum (2 mg or 4 mg chewed slowly when urge to smoke occurs) up to maximum of 15 pieces daily. Gum needs to be rested against the gums or buccal mucosa for absorption to occur.

3. Patch: two different types are available (24-hour or 16-hour patches). There is no difference in efficacy. Both types come in three strengths to allow gradual weaning:
   - 16-hour patches deliver nicotine over a 16-hour period and are removed at bedtime (dose 15 mg, 10 mg, 5 mg).
   - 24-hour patches are worn throughout the night and taken off and replaced in the morning (21 mg, 14 mg, 7 mg).

4. Nasal spray (each metered spray delivers 0.5 mg nicotine. A dose = 1 spray to each nostril, up to maximum of 2 doses per hour or 32 doses per day). Most suitable for highly dependent smokers.

5. Inhalator (10 mg/cartridge) used with a plastic mouthpiece. Dose initially up to 12 cartridges per day – puffed for 20 minutes every hour.

6. Lozenges (1 mg, 2 mg and 4 mg), up to maximum of 15 per day.

Side-effects
Mainly mild local irritant effects such as skin irritation or stinging in the mouth/throat/nose, depending on formulation. Side effects usually disappear with continued use as tolerance develops rapidly.

Bupropion (amfebutamone)

Clinical effectiveness
Bupropion (Zyban) is an atypical antidepressant, with dopaminergic and noradrenergic actions, and has been advocated by NICE for smoking cessation. A systematic review of 19 RCTs of bupropion revealed a doubling of smoking cessation compared with the placebo control. Trials show it significantly reduces

the severity of nicotine withdrawal symptoms and urges to smoke and in some patients will make smoking less pleasurable and rewarding.

There is a risk of seizures of about 1 in 1000 associated with bupropion use and therefore this must be considered before initiation of treatment.

Bupropion is contraindicated in patients with a history of seizures, eating disorders, a CNS tumour, bipolar disorder, pregnancy, breastfeeding or those experiencing acute benzodiazepine or alcohol withdrawal. As many drugs reduce seizure threshold, including other antidepressants, a risk–benefit assessment must be made in such cases, and if bupropion is prescribed it should be at half dose.

Side-effects
Insomnia, dry mouth, headache are common (~30%). Seizure, hypersensitivity reaction or rash are rare (~0.1%).

Dose
Refer to the BNF for current dose ranges. Start 1–2 weeks before the planned 'quit date' at 150 mg daily for 6 days, then 150 mg twice daily for a maximum of 7–9 weeks. The dose will need to be reduced in the elderly or in those experiencing side-effects. Not recommended for individuals <18 years old.

Varenicline

Varenicline tartrate is a new drug for smoking cessation that was recently licensed by the European Medicines Agency (under the brand name Champix) and was launched in the UK in December 2006. It is a partial agonist binding with high affinity to the $\alpha_4\beta_2$ nicotinic acetylcholine receptor. Two large-scale randomised placebo-controlled trials comparing it directly with bupropion suggest it is nearly 80% more effective[4,5]. Trials comparing it with NRT are underway. Like NRT and bupropion, varenicline significantly reduces nicotine withdrawal symptoms, but there is also evidence it makes smoking less rewarding, so may help prevent 'slips' developing into full relapse.

Dose
Days 1–3, 0.5 mg once daily; days 4–7, 0.5 mg twice daily; and from day 8 to end of week 12, 1 mg twice daily. Smokers should set a 'quit date' between day 8–14. For patients who have successfully stopped smoking at the end of 12 weeks, an additional course of 12 weeks treatment at 1 mg twice daily may be considered. The only contraindication is hypersensitivity to the drug or excipients. There are no known drug interactions.

Warnings and precautions
Smoking cessation, with or without pharmacotherapy, has been associated with exacerbation of underlying psychiatric illness (e.g. depression). There is no clinical experience with varenicline in patients with epilepsy or psychiatric illness. It should not be used in the under-18s, pregnant or breastfeeding women, or in those with end-stage renal disease. Those with severe renal impairment may require a dosage reduction.

Substance misuse

Side-effects
The main side-effect is nausea (30%). No serious adverse events have been reported to date.

Note. Stopping smoking may alter the pharmacokinetics or pharmacodynamics of other drugs, including several used in psychiatry, for which dosage adjustment may be necessary (examples include alprazolam, theophylline, chlorpromazine, diazepam, warfarin, insulin, clomipramine, clozapine, desipramine, doxepin, fluphenazine, haloperidol, imipramine and oxazepam). Stopping smoking is not thought to alter blood levels of chlordiazepoxide, ethanol, lorazepam, midazolam or trizolam. It is unclear if quitting affects blood levels of amitriptyline and nortriptyline[6]. Smoking cessation usually results in an increase of plasma levels of CYP1A2 substrates (smoking induces CYP1A2) (see page 502).

Pregnancy and nicotine use

As stated earlier ideally women should stop smoking without using NRT but, if this is not possible, NRT may be recommended to assist a quit attempt. Please see above.

References

1. National Institute for Clinical Excellence. Brief interventions and referral for smoking cessation in primary care and other settings. Public Health Intervention Guidance No 1. http://www.nice. org.uk. 2006.
2. National Institute for Clinical Excellence. The clinical effectiveness and cost effectiveness of bupropion (Zyban) and Nicotine Replacement Therapy for smoking cessation. Technical Appraisal 39. http://www. nice.org.uk. 2002.
3. Silagy C et al. Nicotine replacement therapy for smoking cessation. Cochrane Database Syst Rev 2004;CD000146.
4. Gonzales D et al. Varenicline, an alpha4beta2 nicotinic acetylcholine receptor partial agonist, vs sustained-release bupropion and placebo for smoking cessation: a randomized controlled trial. JAMA 2006;296: 47–55.
5. Jorenby DE et al. Efficacy of varenicline, an alpha4beta2 nicotinic acetylcholine receptor partial agonist, vs placebo or sustained-release bupropion for smoking cessation: a randomized controlled trial. JAMA 2006;296:56–63.
6. Desai HD et al. Smoking in patients receiving psychotropic medications: a pharmacokinetic perspective. CNS Drugs 2001;15:469–94.

Cocaine and other stimulant use

Cocaine and other stimulant use has increased in the last 10 years and is a growing public health problem. **There is no effective pharmacotherapy for the treatment of cocaine dependence and other stimulant dependence.** Psychosocial interventions may be more effective.

Pharmacological treatments for cocaine dependence have been investigated. Systematic reviews found no evidence supporting the clinical use of carbamazepine, antidepressants or dopamine agonists for the treatment of cocaine dependence[1-3]. There is limited evidence for pharmacological treatment of amfetamine dependence but no pharmacological treatment is advocated[4]. There is no evidence to support amfetamine substitute prescribing for the treatment of cocaine or amfetamine dependence. If a patient has been prescribed long-term amfetamines for an addiction problem, this should be slowly withdrawn unless there are exceptional circumstances.

Stimulants should not be prescribed to patients who have a history of heart disease. Cocaine and other stimulants cause coronary artery constriction, can contribute to heart disease and have been implicated in causing QT prolongation. An ECG would be recommended for patients using these substances also presenting with cardiac symptoms.

Pregnancy and stimulant use

Current recommendations are to stop using stimulants before planned pregnancy. If a woman is found to be pregnant and using stimulants, she should be advised to stop using those substances.

References

1. Lima AR et al. Carbamazepine for cocaine dependence. Cochrane Database Syst Rev 2002;CD002023.
2. Lima MS et al. Antidepressants for cocaine dependence. Cochrane Database Syst Rev 2003;CD002950.
3. Soares BG et al. Dopamine agonists for cocaine dependence. Cochrane Database Syst Rev 2003; CD003352.
4. Srisurapanont M et al. Treatment for amphetamine psychosis. Cochrane Database Syst Rev 2001; CD003026.

Substance misuse

Benzodiazepine use (see page 264)

Benzodiazepine prescription has increased since the seventies, mainly due to the discontinuation of barbiturates and perceived safety profile. However benzodiazepines have a high potential for causing dependence. Prescriptions originally started for other disorders may have been continued long term and developed into dependence. A review evaluated the evidence for pharmacological interventions for benzodiazepine mono-dependence. This concluded that a gradual reduction of benzodiazepines was preferable to an abrupt discontinuation[1].

A large number of patients presenting to addictions services may be using illicit benzodiazepines on top of their primary substance of abuse. Athough some services provide prescriptions of benzodiazepines, there is no evidence that substitute prescribing of benzodiazepines reduces benzodiazepine use. In exceptional circumstances, if benzodiazepines are prescribed, this should be for a short–term time limited (2–3 weeks) prescription.

If patients have been prescribed benzodiazepines for a substantial period of time, it may be preferable to convert to eqivalents of diazepam as this is long acting. Benzodiazepine dependence as part of polysubstance dependence should also be treated by a gradual withdrawal of the medication. Benzodiazepines prescribed at greater than 30mg diazepam equivalent may cause harm[2] and so this should be avoided. Psychosocial interventions including contingency management have had some some success at reducing benzodiazepine use.

Pregnancy and benzodiazepine use

There is a risk of teratogencity with benzodiazepine use, so ideally benzodiazepine prescriptions should be gradually discontinued before a planned pregancy. If a woman is prescribed benzodiazepines and found to be pregnant, the prescription should be gradually withdrawn. A risk benefit analysis should be undertaken and specialist advice sought at the time.

References

1. Denis C et al. Pharmacological interventions for benzodiazepine mono-dependence management in outpatient settings. Cochrane Database Syst Rev 2006;CD005194.
2. Department of Health. Drug misuse and dependence: guidelines on clinical management. Norwich: Department of Health, 1999.

Substance misuse

Drugs of misuse – a summary

One in ten adults uses illicit drugs in any one year[1], and at least a third of those with mental illness can be classified as having a 'dual diagnosis'[2,3]. It is therefore important to be aware of the main mental state changes associated with drugs of abuse. Urine-testing for illicit drugs is routine on many psychiatric wards. It is important to be aware of the duration of detection of drugs in urine and of other commonly used substances and drugs that can give a false-positive result.

The following table provides a summary of the characteristics of major substances of misuse.

Drug	Physical signs/ symptoms of intoxication	Most common mental state changes[4]	Withdrawal symptoms
Amfetamine[8]	Tachycardia; increased BP anorexia; tremor; restlessness	Visual/tactille/ olfactory auditory hallucinations; paranoia; decreased concentration; elation	Extreme fatigue; hunger; depression;
Benzodiazepines	Sedation (possible); dizziness; respiratory depression	Relaxation; visual hallucinations; disorientation; sleep disturbance	Seizures; psychosis; paraesthesia
Barbiturates	Headache; hypotension; respiratory depression	Restlessness/ataxia; confusion/excitement; drowsiness	Similar to alcohol: tremor; vomiting; seizures; delirium tremens
Cannabis[5,9]	Tachycardia; lack of coordination; red eyes; postural hypotension	Elation; psychosis; perceptual distortions; disturbance of memory/judgement; twofold increase in risk of developing schizophrenia[10]	Restlessness; irritability; insomnia; anxiety[6]
Cocaine	Tachycardia/ tachypnoea; increased BP/ headache; respiratory; depression; chest pain	Euphoria; paranoid psychosis; panic attacks/anxiety; insomnia/excitement	Profound lethargy; decreased consciousness
Heroin	Pinpoint pupils; clammy skin; respiratory depression	Drowsiness; euphoria; hallucinations	Nausea pains/ gooseflesh; general aches and runny nose/eyes; diarrhoea
Methadone	Respiratory depression; pulmonary oedema	As above	As above but milder and longer lasting

Duration of withdrawal	Duration of detection in the urine[5-7]	Other substances which give a positive result[7]
Peaks 7–34 hours; lasts maximum of 5 days	Up to 72 hours	Cough and decongestant preparations, selegiline, large quantities of tyramine, tranylcypromine, chloroquine, ranitidine
Usually short-lived but may last weeks to months	Up to 28 days: depending on half-life of drug taken	Zopiclone Nefopam
Depends on half-life – likely to be at least several days	Up to 21 days, depending on half-life	None known
Uncertain Probably less than 1 month[5] (longer in heavy users[6])	Single use: 3 days; chronic heavy use: up to 21 days	Passive 'smoking' of cannabis Efavirenz
12–18 hours	Up to 96 hours	Food/tea containing coco leaves Codeine Ephedrine Pseudoephedrine
Peaks after 36–72 hours	Up to 72 hours	Food/tea containing poppy seed Procaine Any opiate analgesic Diphenoxylate, naltrexone
Peaks after 4–6 days; can last 3 weeks	Up to 7 days with chronic use	Imipramine Pethidine Chlorpheniramine (high doses) Diphenydramine Cetirizine Doxylamine

Substance misuse

347

References

1. Ramsay M, Spiller J. Drug Misuse Declared in 1996: Latest Results from the British Crime Survey. London: Home Office, 1996.
2. Menezes PR et al. Drug and alcohol problems among individuals with severe mental illness in south London. Br J Psychiatry 1996;168:612–19.
3. Phillips P et al. Drug and alcohol misuse among in-patients with psychotic illnesses in three inner-London psychiatric units. Psychiatr Bull 2003;27:217–20.
4. Micromedex® Healthcare Series. CD-ROM, version 5.1. http://www.micromedex.com/. 2004. Thomson Micromedex.
5. Johns A. Psychiatric effects of cannabis. Br J Psychiatry 2001;178:116–22.
6. Budney AJ et al. Review of the validity and significance of cannabis withdrawal syndrome. Am J Psychiatry 2004;161:1967–77.
7. Euromed. Technical Bulletin – January 2006. www.euromedltd.com. 2006.
8. Srisurapanont M et al. Treatment for amphetamine psychosis. Cochrane Database Syst Rev 2001;CD003026.
9. Hall W et al. Long-term cannabis use and mental health. Br J Psychiatry 1997;171:107–8.
10. Arseneault L et al. Causal association between cannabis and psychosis: examination of the evidence. Br J Psychiatry 2004;184:110–17.

Substance misuse

Interactions between 'street drugs' and prescribed psychotropic drugs

There are some significant interactions between 'street drugs' and drugs that are prescribed for the treatment of mental illness. Information comes from case reports or theoretical assumptions, rarely from systematic investigation. A summary can be found in the table, but remember that the knowledge base is poor. Always be cautious.

In all patients who misuse street drugs:
- Infection with hepatitis B and C is common. This may lead to a reduced ability to metabolise other drugs and increased sensitivity to side-effects.
- Infection with HIV is common[1,2]. Antiretroviral drugs are involved in pharmacokinetic interactions with a number of prescribed drugs; see page 454 for a summary. Interactions with street drugs are likely.
- Prescribed drugs may be used in the same way as illicit drugs (i.e. erratically and not as intended). Large quantities of prescribed drugs should not be given to outpatients.

Acute behavioural disturbance

Acute intoxication with street drugs may result in behavioural disturbance. Non-drug management is preferable. If at all possible, a urine drug screen should be done to determine the drugs that have been taken, before prescribing any psychotropic. A physical examination should be done if possible (BP, TPR and ECG).

If intervention with a psychotropic is unavoidable, olanzapine 10 mg po/IM is probably the safest option. Temperature, pulse, respiration and blood pressure *must* be monitored afterwards. Benzodiazepines are commonly misused with other street drugs and so standard doses may be ineffective in tolerant users. Interactions are also possible (see table). Try to avoid.

Table Interactions between 'street drugs' and psychotropics (for references, see page 352)

	Cannabis	Heroin/methadone[3]	Cocaine, amfetamines, ecstasy	Alcohol
General considerations	• Usually smoked in cigarettes (induces CYP1A2) • Can be sedative[4] • Dose-related tachycardia[5]	• Can produce sedation/respiratory depression • QTc prolongation also reported with methadone (see page XXX)	• Stimulants (cocaine can be sedative in higher doses) • Arrhythmia possible • Cerebral/cardiac ischaemia with cocaine[6] • Hyperthermia/dehydration with Ecstasy[7]	• Sedative • Liver damage possible
Older antipsychotics (FGAs)	• Antipsychotics reduce the psychotropic effects of almost all drugs of abuse by blocking dopamine receptors (dopamine is the neurotransmitter responsible for 'reward') • Patients prescribed antipsychotics may increase their consumption of illicit substances to compensate • Patients who have taken ecstasy may be more prone to EPSEs • Cardiotoxic or very sedative antipsychotics are best avoided, at least initially. Sulpiride is a reasonably safe first choice			
SGAs	• Risk of additive sedation • Cannabis smoking can reduce serum levels of olanzapine and clozapine via induction of CYP1A2[8]	• Risk of additive sedation • Case report of methadone withdrawal being precipitated by risperidone[9]	• Antipsychotics may reduce craving and cocaine-induced euphoria[10-12]	• Increased risk of hypotension with olanzapine (and possibly other blockers)
Antidepressants	• Tachycardia has been reported (monitor pulse and take care with TCAs[13])	• Avoid very sedative antidepressants • Some SSRIs can increase methadone plasma levels[14] (citalopram is SSRI of choice)	• Avoid TCAs (arrhythmia) • MAOIs contraindicated (hypertension) • Moclobemide and SSRIs may increase stimulant toxicity[15-17] and SSRIs may	• Avoid very sedative antidepressants • Avoid antidepressants that are toxic in OD

Drug				
(antidepressants, continued)			attenuate psychological effects[18] • Antidepressants have been used in 'crack' withdrawal. They are ineffective for cocaine dependence[19]. One small study suggests no interaction between cocaine and trazodone[20]. Deaths have been reported with combinations of Ecstasy and SSRIs	• Impaired psychomotor skills (*not* SSRIs)
Anticholinergics	• Misuse is likely. Try to avoid if at all possible (by using an SGA if an antipsychotic is required) • Can cause hallucinations, elation and cognitive impairment			
Lithium	• Very toxic if taken erratically • Always consider the effects of dehydration (particularly problematic with alcohol or ecstasy)			
Carbamazepine/ valproate		• Carbamazepine (CBZ) decreases methadone levels[6] (danger if CBZ stopped suddenly) • Valproate seems less likely to interact	• Carbamazepine induces CYP3A4, which leads to increased formation of norcocaine (hepatotoxic and more cardiotoxic than cocaine)[21]	• Monitor LFTs
Benzodiazepines (Always remember that benzodiazepines are liable to misuse)	• Monitor level of sedation	• Oversedation (and respiratory depression possible) • Concomitant use can lead to accidental overdose • Possible pharmacokinetic interaction (increased methadone levels)	• Oversedation (if high doses of cocaine have been taken) • Widely used after cocaine intoxication • Future misuse possible • Widely used in alcohol detoxification	• Oversedation (and respiratory depression) possible

References

1. Vocci FJ et al. Medication development for addictive disorders: the state of the science. Am J Psychiatry 2005;162:1432–40.
2. Tsuang J et al. Pharmacological treatment of patients with schizophrenia and substance abuse disorders. Addict Disord Treat 2005;4:127–37.
3. Department of Health. Annex 14. Drug interactions – methadone drug interactions. Drug Misuse and Dependence – Guidelines on Clinical Management, Norwich: Department of Health, 1999.
4. Johns A. Psychiatric effects of cannabis. Br J Psychiatry 2001;178:116–22.
5. Ashton CH. Pharmacology and effects of cannabis: a brief review. Br J Psychiatry 2001;178:101–6.
6. Miller BL, Mena I, Giombetti R, Villanueva-Meyer J, Djenderedjian AH. Neuropsychiatric effects of cocaine: SPECT measurements. In Paredes A, Gorelick DA, eds. Cocaine: Physiological and Physiopathological Effects. New York: Haworth Press, 1993; 47–58.
7. Gowing LR et al. The health effects of ecstasy: a literature review. Drug Alcohol Rev 2002;21:53–63.
8. Zullino DF et al. Tobacco and cannabis smoking cessation can lead to intoxication with clozapine or olanzapine. Int Clin Psychopharmacol 2002;17:141–3.
9. Wines JD Jr et al. Opioid withdrawal during risperidone treatment. J Clin Psychopharmacol 1999; 19:265–7.
10. Poling J et al. Risperidone for substance dependent psychotic patients. Addict Disord Treat 2005;4:1–3.
11. Newton TF et al. Risperidone pre-treatment reduces the euphoric effects of experimentally administered cocaine. Psychiatry Res 2001;102:227–33.
12. Albanese MJ et al. Risperidone in cocaine-dependent patients with comorbid psychiatric disorders. J Psychiatr Pract 2006;12:306–11.
13. Benowitz NL et al. Effects of delta-9-tetrahydrocannabinol on drug distribution and metabolism. Antipyrine, pentobarbital, and ethanol. Clin Pharmacol Ther 1977;22:259–68.
14. Ketter TA et al. Principles of clinically important drug interactions with carbamazepine. Part I. J Clin Psychopharmacol 1991;11:198–203.
15. Vuori E et al. Death following ingestion of MDMA (ecstasy) and moclobemide. Addiction 2003;98: 365–8.
16. O'Dell LE et al. Antidepressant drugs appear to enhance cocaine-induced toxicity. Exp Clin Psychopharmacol 2000;8:133–41.
17. Macedo DS et al. Effect of anxiolytic, antidepressant, and antipsychotic drugs on cocaine-induced seizures and mortality. Epilepsy Behav 2004;5:852–6.
18. Liechti ME et al. Acute psychological effects of 3,4-methylenedioxymethamphetamine (MDMA, "Ecstasy") are attenuated by the serotonin uptake inhibitor citalopram. Neuropsychopharmacology 2000;22:513–21.
19. Lima MS et al. Antidepressants for cocaine dependence. Cochrane Database Syst Rev 2001;CD002950.
20. Rowbotham MC et al. Trazodone–oral cocaine interactions. Arch Gen Psychiatry 1984;41:895–9.
21. Roldan CJ et al. Toxicity, cocaine. http://www.emedicine.com/. 2004.

Further reading

Howard LA et al. The role of pharmacogenetically-variable cytochrome P450 enzyme in drug abuse and dependence. Pharmacogenomics 2002;3:185–199.

Ley A et al. Treatment programmes for people with both severe mental illness and substance misuse. Cochrane Database Syst Rev Update Software, Oxford, 2002.

Williams R et al. Substance use and misuse in psychiatric wards. Psychiatr Bull 2000;24:43–6.

chapter 7

Use of psychotropics in special patient groups

Depression and psychosis in epilepsy

The prevalence of clinical depression in people with epilepsy varies from 9% to 22%[1,2], and depressive symptoms may occur in up to 60% of people with intractable epilepsy[3]. Suicide rates have been estimated to be 4–5 times that of the general population[1,2]. The prevalence of psychotic illness in people with epilepsy is at least 4%[4]. Peri-ictal depression or psychosis (that is, symptoms temporally related to seizure activity) should initially be treated by optimising anticonvulsant therapy[4]. Interictal depression or psychosis (symptoms occurring independently of seizures) are likely to require treatment with antidepressants or antipsychotics[2,4].

Use of antidepressants and antipsychotics in epilepsy

The prevalence of active epilepsy in adults under the age of 65 is 0.6% and the annual incidence 0.03%[5]; reports of seizures apparently associated with drug treatment should be interpreted in this context, particularly if no control group data are available. Note also that almost all antidepressants and antipsychotics have been associated with hyponatraemia (see page 137); seizures may occur if this is severe[6]. The majority of antipsychotics and antidepressants can reduce the seizure threshold[1,2,7,8] and the risk is dose-related. Although it has been stated that treatment with an antidepressant or antipsychotic drug increases the risk of *de novo* seizures in non-epileptic subjects 10-fold[7], it has been suggested that most antidepressant drugs in standard doses actually have anticonvulsant properties and that proconvulsant effects only become apparent at very high doses[9].

There are few systematic studies of antipsychotics or antidepressants in people with epilepsy. Data are mainly derived from animal studies, clinical trials, case reports and CSM reports. The table below gives some general guidance. Treatment should be commenced at the lowest dose and this should be gradually increased until a therapeutic dose is achieved[2,8,10]. As a general rule, the more sedating a drug is, the more likely it is to induce seizures[8].

Electroconvulsive therapy (ECT) has anticonvulsive properties and is worth considering in the treatment of depression in patients with unstable epilepsy[1,2].

Table Psychotropics in epilepsy*		
Antidepressant	**Safety in epilepsy**	**Special considerations**
Moclobemide[15]	Good choice	Not known to be proconvulsive
SSRIs[16]	Good choice	Low proconvulsive effect[2,17]; there is no clear difference in risk between the available SSRIs[5]. Seizure risk is dose-related
Mirtazapine/reboxetine/venlafaxine[18,19]	Care required	Less data and clinical experience than with SSRIs. Venlafaxine proconvulsive in OD. Use with care
Duloxetine[6,11]	Care required	Very limited data and clinical experience Seizures have been reported rarely
Amitriptyline Dosulepin (dothiepin)[20] Clomipramine[21] Bupropion	Avoid	Most are epileptogenic Ideally, should be avoided completely
Lithium[2]	Care required	Low proconvulsive effect at therapeutic doses Marked proconvulsive activity in overdose
Antipsychotic		
Trifluoperazine/haloperidol[2,8,22,23]	Good choice	Low proconvulsive effect Carbamazepine increases the metabolism of some antipsychotics and larger doses of an antipsychotic may be required
Sulpiride	Good choice	Low proconvulsive effect (less clinical experience) No known interactions with anticonvulsants

Table Psychotropics in epilepsy* (Cont.)

Antidepressant	Safety in epilepsy	Special considerations
Risperidone[19] Olanzapine[24,25] Quetiapine[26,27] Amisulpride	Care required	Limited clinical experience but probably safe Olanzapine may affect EEG[28]. Myoclonic seizures have been reported[29] Seizures rarely reported with quetiapine
Aripiprazole	Care required	Very limited data and clinical experience Seizures have been reported rarely[30]
Clozapine[4,7,31]	Avoid if possible	Very epileptogenic. Approximately 4–5% who receive more than 600 mg/ day develop seizures Sodium valproate is the anticonvulsant of choice as it has a lower incidence of leucopenia than carbamazepine
Chlorpromazine[4,32,33] Loxapine[34]	Avoid	Most epileptogenic of the older drugs. Ideally best avoided completely
Zotepine[35]	Avoid	Has established dose-related proconvulsive effect Best avoided completely
Depot antipsychotics	Avoid	None of the depot preparations currently available are thought to be epileptogenic, however: • the kinetics of depots are complex (seizures may be delayed) • if seizures do occur, the offending drug may not be easily withdrawn Depots should be used with extreme care

*This table contains information about the proconvulsive effects of antidepressants and antipsychotics when used in therapeutic doses. See page 473 for information about overdose.

Special groups

355

Depression and psychosis associated with anticonvulsant drugs

Anticonvulsant drugs have been associated with new-onset depression and psychosis[1]. If anticonvulsants have recently been changed, this should always be considered as a potential cause of a new/worsening depressive or psychotic illness. Lowering of folate levels by some anticonvulsants may also influence the expression of depression[1]. Folate levels should be checked.

Psychosis[11]

Summaries of Product Characteristics and case reports associate the following anticonvulsants with the onset of psychotic symptoms: carbamazepine, ethosuximide, tiagabine, topiramate, valproate and vigabatrin. There are case reports in the literature describing psychosis related to topiramate[12], zonisamide[13] and levetiracetam[14]. Some of these reports may relate to the process of 'forced normalisation' in which a diminished frequency of seizures allows psychotic symptoms to emerge.

Depression[11,36]

Manufacturer's data and case reports associate the following anticonvulsants with the onset of depressive symptoms: acetazolamide, barbiturates, carbamazepine, ethosuximide, gabapentin, phenytoin, piracetam, tiagabine, topiramate and vigabatrin.

Interactions

Pharmacokinetic interactions between anticonvulsants and antidepressants/antipsychotics are common. These interactions are primarily mediated through cytochrome P450 enzymes[1,2]. Fluoxetine and paroxetine are potent inhibitors of several hepatic CYP enzyme systems (CYP2D6, CYP3A4). Sertraline is a less potent inhibitor, but this effect is dose-related and higher doses of sertraline are commonly used. Citalopram is a weak inhibitor. Carbamazepine and phenytoin have a narrow therapeutic index and plasma levels can be increased by enzyme inhibitors. This is particularly dangerous with phenytoin. Plasma levels should be monitored and dosage adjustment may be required.

Carbamazepine is an enzyme inducer (mainly CYP3A4) and can lower plasma levels of some antipsychotic drugs[37]. Many other medicines can cause problems in people with epilepsy by raising or reducing the seizure threshold or interacting with anticonvulsant drugs. Check Appendix 1 (Interactions) of the *BNF* or contact pharmacy for advice (see also page 359 for a summary).

Epilepsy and driving

People with epilepsy may not drive a car if they have had a seizure while awake in the previous year or, if seizures occur only during sleep, this has been an established nocturnal pattern for at least 3 years. The consequences of inducing seizure with antidepressants or antipsychotics can therefore be significant. For further information see www.dvla.gov.uk.

References

1. Harden CL et al. Mood disorders in patients with epilepsy: epidemiology and management. CNS Drugs 2002;16:291–302.
2. Curran S et al. Selecting an antidepressant for use in a patient with epilepsy. Safety considerations. Drug Saf 1998;18:125–33.
3. Lambert MV et al. Depression in epilepsy: etiology, phenomenology, and treatment. Epilepsia 1999; 40(Suppl 10):S21–S47.
4. Blumer D et al. Treatment of the interictal psychoses. J Clin Psychiatry 2000;61:110–22.
5. Montgomery SA. Antidepressants and seizures: emphasis on newer agents and clinical implications. Int J Clin Pract 2005;59:1435–40.
6. Maramattom BV. Duloxetine-induced syndrome of inappropriate antidiuretic hormone secretion and seizures. Neurology 2006;66:773–4.
7. Pisani F et al. Effects of psychotropic drugs on seizure threshold. Drug Saf 2002;25:91–110.
8. Marks RC et al. Antipsychotic medications and seizures. Psychiatr Med 1991;9:37–52.
9. Jobe PC et al. The serotonergic and noradrenergic effects of antidepressant drugs are anticonvulsant, not proconvulsant. Epilepsy Behav 2005;7:602–19.
10. Rosenstein DL et al. Seizures associated with antidepressants: a review. J Clin Psychiatry 1993;54: 289–99.
11. Datapharm Communications Ltd. Electronic Medicines Compendium. http://medguides.medicines.org. uk/. 2006.
12. Hofer A et al. Worsening of psychosis after replacement of adjunctive valproate with topiramate in a schizophrenia patient. J Clin Psychiatry 2003;64:1267–8.
13. Miyamoto T et al. Psychotic episodes during zonisamide treatment. Seizure 2000;9:65–70.
14. Youroukos S et al. Acute psychosis associated with levetiracetam. Epileptic Disord 2003;5:117–19.
15. Schiwy W et al. Therapeutic and side-effect profile of a selective and reversible MAO-A inhibitor, bro-faromine. Results of dose-finding trials in depressed patients. J Neural Transm Suppl 1989;28:33–44.
16. Wedin GP et al. Relative toxicity of cyclic antidepressants. Ann Emerg Med 1986;15:797–804.
17. Duncan D et al. Which is the safest antidepressant to use in epilepsy? Psychiatr Bull 1995;19:355.
18. Juckel G et al. Epileptiform EEG patterns induced by mirtazapine in both psychiatric patients and healthy volunteers. J Clin Psychopharmacol 2003;23:421–2.
19. Alldredge BK. Seizure risk associated with psychotropic drugs: clinical and pharmacokinetic consider-ations. Neurology 1999;53:S68–S75.
20. Buckley NA et al. Greater toxicity in overdose of dothiepin than of other tricyclic antidepressants. Lancet 1994;343:159–62.
21. Stimmel GL et al. Psychotrophic drug-induced reductions in seizure threshold: incidence and conse-quences. CNS Drugs 1996;5:3750.
22. Markowitz JC et al. Seizures with neuroleptics and antidepressants. Gen Hosp Psychiatry 1987;9: 135–41.
23. Darby JK et al. Haloperidol dose and blood level variability: toxicity and interindividual and intraindi-vidual variability in the nonresponder patient in the clinical practice setting. J Clin Psychopharmacol 1995;15:334–40.
24. Beasley CM Jr. et al. Safety of olanzapine. J Clin Psychiatry 1997;58(Suppl 10):13–17.
25. Lee JW et al. Seizure associated with olanzapine. Ann Pharmacother 1999;33:554–6.
26. Dogu O et al. Seizures associated with quetiapine treatment. Ann Pharmacother 2003;37:1224–7.
27. Hedges DW et al. New-onset seizure associated with quetiapine and olanzapine. Ann Pharmacother 2002;36:437–9.
28. Amann BL et al. EEG abnormalities associated with antipsychotics: a comparison of quetiapine, olan-zapine, haloperidol and healthy subjects. Hum Psychopharmacol 2003;18:641–6.
29. Camacho A et al. Olanzapine-induced myoclonic seizure. Clin Neuropharmacol 2005;28:145–7.
30. Tsai JF. Aripiprazole-associated seizure. J Clin Psychiatry 2006;67:995–6.
31. Toth P et al. Clozapine and seizures: a review. Can J Psychiatry 1994;39:236–8.
32. Itil TM et al. Epileptogenic side effects of psychotropic drugs. Practical recommendations. JAMA 1980; 244:1460–3.
33. Logothetis J. Spontaneous epileptic seizures and electroencephalographic changes in the course of phenothiazine therapy. Neurology 1967;17:869–77.
34. Peterson CD. Seizures induced by acute loxapine overdose. Am J Psychiatry 1981;138:1089–91.
35. Tsuchiya H et al. Generalized seizures during treatment of schizophrenia with zotepine. Yonago Acta Med 1986;29:103–11.
36. Besag FM. Behavioural effects of the newer antiepileptic drugs: an update. Expert Opin Drug Saf 2004;3:1–8.
37. Tiihonen J et al. Carbamazepine-induced changes in plasma levels of neuroleptics. Pharmacopsychiatry 1995;28:26–8.

Special groups

357

Further reading

Centorrino F et al. EEG abnormalities during treatment with typical and atypical antipsychotics. Am J Psychiatry 2002;159:109–15.

Farooq S. Interventions for psychotic symptoms concomitant with epilepsy (Protocol). Cochrane Database Syst Rev 2006;CD006118.

Schmitz B. Antidepressant drugs: indications and guidelines for use in epilepsy. Epilepsia 2002; 43(Suppl 2):14–18.

Van der Feltz-Cornelis CM. Treatment of interictal psychiatric disorder in epilepsy. I. Affective and anxiety disorders. Acta Neuropsychiatr 2002;14:39–43.

Van der Feltz-Cornelis CM. Treatment of interictal psychiatric disorder in epilepsy. II. Chronic psychosis. Acta Neuropsychiatr 2002;14:44–8.

Van der Feltz-Cornelis CM. Treatment of interictal psychiatric disorder in epilepsy. III. Personality disorder, aggression and mental retardation. Acta Neuropsychiatr 2002;14:49–54.

Special groups

Pharmacokinetic drug interactions between antiepileptic drugs and other psychotropic drugs

Antiepileptic drug	Increases level of	Decreases level of	Level increased by	Level decreased by
Carbamazepine	Phenytoin	Clobazam Clonazepam Ethosuximide Lamotrigine Midazolam Phenytoin Primidone Tiagabine Topiramate Valproic acid Zonisamide Aripiprazole Clozapine Haloperidol Olanzapine Quetiapine Risperidone Sertindole Zotepine Mianserin Mirtazepine Paroxetine ?Sertraline TCAs Trazodone Benzodiazepines Bupropion Donepezil Methadone Methylphenidate Modafinil Thyroxine	Valproic acid and primidone increase levels of 10,11-epoxide (metabolite of carbamazepine) Clobazam Lamotrigine Oxcarbazepine Fluoxetine Fluvoxamine Sertraline	Oxcarbazepine Phenobarbital Phenytoin Primidone St John's Wort Valproate
Phenytoin	Carbamazepine Phenobarbital Valproate	Carbamazepine Ethosuximide Lamotrigine Phenobarbital Primidone Tiagabine Topiramate Valproate Zonisamide	Carbamazepine Ethosuximide Oxcarbazepine Phenobarbital Primidone Topiramate Valproate Phenothiazines ?Zotepine	Carbamazepine Clonazepam Diazepam Phenobarbital Primidone Valproate Vigabatrin Alcohol (chronic)

Table Pharmacokinetic drug interactions between antiepileptic drugs and other psychotropic drugs (Cont.)

Antiepileptic drug	Increases level of	Decreases level of	Level increased by	Level decreased by
Phenytoin		Clonazepam Oxazepam Aripiprazole Clozapine Haloperidol Phenothiazines Quetiapine Risperidone Sertindole Mianserin Mirtazepine Paroxetine TCAs Bupropion Donepezil Methadone Thyroxine	Fluoxetine Fluvoxamine Paroxetine Sertraline TCAs Trazodone Clobazam Chlordiazepoxide Diazepam Disulfiram Modafanil Thyroxine	Phenothiazines St John's Wort
Lamotrigine	Oxcarbazepine Risperidone	None known	Sertraline Valproate	Carbamazepine Oxcarbazepine Phenobarbital Phenytoin Primidone
Valproate	Ethosuximide Free phenytoin Lamotrigine Oxcarbazepine Phenobarbital Primidone Benzodiazepines Bupropion TCAs	Topiramate 10-monohydroxy metabolite of oxcarbazepine Total phenytoin	Risperidone	Carbamazepine Phenobarbital Phenytoin Primidone Topiramate ?Fluoxetine
Gabapentin	None known	None known	None known	None known
Levetiracetam	None known	None known	None known	None known
Vigabatrin	Carbamazepine	?Phenobarbital Phenytoin Primidone	None known	None known
Oxcarbazepine	10,11-epoxide, metabolite of carbamazepine Phenobarbital Phenytoin	Carbamazepine Lamotrigine	None known	Carbamazepine Phenobarbital Phenytoin Valproate

Table Pharmacokinetic drug interactions between antiepileptic drugs and other psychotropic drugs (Cont.)

Antiepileptic drug	Increases level of	Decreases level of	Level increased by	Level decreased by
Phenobarbital	Phenytoin	Carbamazepine Clonazepam Ethosuximide Lamotrigine Oxcarbazepine Phenytoin Tiagabine Topiramate Valproate Zotepine Aripiprazole ?Chlorpromazine Clozapine Haloperidol Promethazine Quetiapine Mianserin TCAs Paroxetine Bupropion Mondafanil Thyroxine Zonisamide	Carbamazepine Oxcarbazepine Phenytoin Valproate Alcohol (acute) Methylphenidate	Vigabatrin Alcohol (chronic) St John's Wort
Tiagabine	None known	Valproate	None known	Carbamazepine Phenobarbital Phenytoin Primidone
Topiramate	Phenytoin	?Valproate	None known	Carbamazepine Phenobarbital Phenytoin Valproate
Ethosuximide	?Phenytoin	None known	Valproate	Carbamazepine Phenobarbital Phenytoin Primidone

For pharmacodynamic interactions, see page 353.
For interactions with lithium, see page 146.
For interactions in the elderly, see page 412.

Further reading

British Medical Association and Royal Pharmaceutical Society. British National Formulary, Issue 52, Appendix 1, 2006.

Micromedex® Healthcare Series. CD-ROM, version 5.1. http://www.micromedex.com/. 2004. Thomson Micromedex.

Patsalos PN et al. The importance of drug interactions in epilepsy therapy. Epilepsia 2002;43:365–85.

Schmitz B. Antidepressant drugs: indications and guidelines for use in epilepsy. Epilepsia 2002; 43(Suppl 2):14–18.

www.medicines.org.uk

Special
groups

Withdrawing anticonvulsant drugs

Patients with epilepsy

Optimal treatment with anticonvulsant drugs will render two-thirds of people with epilepsy seizure-free[1,2]. Many patients ask about drug withdrawal. It should be noted that this is a specialist area of practice, and it is strongly recommended that patients are referred for a neurological opinion.

The withdrawal of anticonvulsants in people with epilepsy has been associated with relapse rates of 12–63%[2]. This wide variation probably reflects the heterogeneous nature of the patients studied. It should be noted that patients who remain on anticonvulsant drugs also relapse[3].

The following factors are associated with unsuccessful withdrawal[2,4,5].

Onset of epilepsy during or after adolescence.

Family history of epilepsy.

Epilepsy of proven or suspected organic origin.

Mental retardation.

Abnormal neurological examination.

Poor initial response to treatment.

Ongoing seizures during treatment.

Prescription of two or more anticonvulsant drugs.

Ongoing abnormal EEG.

Abnormal EEG developing during withdrawal period.

The dose of anticonvulsant drugs should be gradually tapered over a period of 6 months. If the patient is taking more than one anticonvulsant (note that such a patient is at increased risk of relapse), they should be withdrawn sequentially. The risk of seizure recurrence is greatest during the period of anticonvulsant withdrawal and steadily decreases over the first year; 70–80% of relapses occur within a year[3]. For those patients who discontinue their anticonvulsant medication because they are seizure-free and whose seizures return, approximately 1 in 4 may continue to have seizures after anticonvulsants are reinstated[6].

Recommendation

Patients with epilepsy should be referred to a neurologist for advice about withdrawing anticonvulsant drugs.

Special groups

Patients with affective disorders

There is no systematic research that addresses the risk of relapse after withdrawal in patients who take anticonvulsant drugs for their mood-stabilising properties. There are three possibilities:

1. The natural course of the illness is improved by a period of treatment with mood-stabilising drugs. There is no evidence to suggest that this is true. Patients with bipolar illness tend to have more episodes and shorter periods of stability as they get older.

2. The illness resumes its natural course. It then follows that the more effective the mood-stabilising medication has been, the greater the chance of relapse when it is stopped.

3. Prognosis may be worsened in some way that is poorly understood. This has been demonstrated for lithium. Treatment with lithium for at least 3 years followed by gradual taper over at least 1 month minimises this risk. It is unknown if these observations hold true for anticonvulsant drugs. There is some evidence to suggest that the risk of completed suicide is high in the month after (presumably abrupt) discontinuation of either lithium or valproate[7].

Recommendation

When used as mood stabilisers, it would be prudent to withdraw anticonvulsant drugs slowly. The optimum duration of taper is unknown. A period of at least 1 month is suggested.

References

1. Cockerell OC et al. Remission of epilepsy: results from the National General Practice Study of Epilepsy. Lancet 1995;346:140–4.
2. Cockerell OC et al. Prognosis of epilepsy: a review and further analysis of the first nine years of the British National General Practice Study of Epilepsy, a prospective population-based study. Epilepsia 1997;38:31–46.
3. Britton JW. Antiepileptic drug withdrawal: literature review. Mayo Clin Proc 2002;77:1378–88.
4. Medical Research Council Antiepileptic Drug Withdrawal Study Group. Randomised study of antiepileptic drug withdrawal in patients in remission. Lancet 1991;337:1175–80.
5. Schmidt D et al. A practical guide to when (and how) to withdraw antiepileptic drugs in seizure-free patients. Drugs 1996;52:870–4.
6. Sillanpaa M et al. Prognosis of seizure recurrence after stopping antiepileptic drugs in seizure-free patients: a long-term population-based study of childhood-onset epilepsy. Epilepsy Behav 2006;8: 713–9.
7. Goodwin FK et al. Suicide risk in bipolar disorder during treatment with lithium and divalproex. JAMA 2003;290:1467–73.

Special groups

Drug choice in pregnancy

A 'normal' outcome to pregnancy can never be guaranteed. The spontaneous abortion rate in confirmed early pregnancy is 10–20% and the risk of spontaneous major malformation is 2–3% (approx. 1 in 40 pregnancies)[1]. Drugs account for a very small proportion of abnormalities (approximately 5% of the total). Potential risks of drugs include major malformation (first-trimester exposure), neonatal toxicity (third-trimester exposure) and long-term neurobehavioural effects.

The safety of psychotropics in pregnancy cannot be clearly established because robust, prospective trials are obviously unethical. Individual decisions on psychotropic use in pregnancy are therefore dependent upon an imperfect retrospective database and a 'best guess' assessment of the risks and benefits associated with withdrawal or continuation of drug treatment. Pregnancy does not protect against mental illness and may even elevate overall risk. The patient's view of risks and benefits will have paramount importance. This section provides a brief summary of knowledge to date.

General principles of prescribing in pregnancy

- Always discuss the possibility of pregnancy with women of child-bearing potential – many pregnancies are unplanned.
- Try to avoid using drugs that are contraindicated during pregnancy in women of reproductive age, especially sodium valproate and carbamazepine. If these drugs are prescribed, women should be made fully aware of their teratogenic properties even if not planning pregnancy.
- Treatment should be discussed with each woman individually in relation to risk–benefit. The general guidelines should be that discontinuation of treatment abruptly post-conception for women with SMI and at a high risk of relapse is unwise. On the other hand, treatment should be discontinued if a woman is well and at low risk of relapse. Ensure that the prospective parents are fully involved in all discussions. Refer to specialist perinatal services, where available.
- Always take into account the risk of relapse when considering discontinuing psychotropics – relapse may ultimately be more harmful to the mother and child than continued, effective drug therapy.
- Try to avoid all drugs in the first trimester (when major organs are being formed). If this is not possible, use the lowest effective dose.
- Use an established drug at the lowest effective dose.
- Avoid polypharmacy whenever possible.
- Be prepared to adjust doses as pregnancy progresses and drug handling is altered. Dose increases are frequently required in the third trimester when blood volume expands by around 30%. Plasma level monitoring is helpful, where available.
- Ensure adequate foetal screening during pregnancy.
- Be aware of potential problems with individual drugs around the time of delivery.
- Inform obstetric team of psychotropic use and possible complications.
- Monitor the neonate for withdrawal effects after birth.
- Document all decisions.

Special groups

365

Risk of psychosis during pregnancy and postpartum[2-5]

- Pregnancy does not protect against relapse.
- The risk of perinatal psychosis is 0.1–0.25% in the general population, but is about 50% in women with a history of bipolar disorder.
- During the month after childbirth there is a 20-fold increase in the relative risk of psychosis.
- The risk of postpartum psychosis in patients with a history of postpartum psychosis is 50–90%.

The risks of not treating psychosis include:

- harm to the mother through poor self-care, lack of obstetric care, poor judgement or impulsive acts
- harm to the foetus or neonate (ranging from neglect to infanticide).

The mental health of the mother in the perinatal period influences foetal well-being, obstetric outcome and child development.

Treatment with antipsychotics

It has long been established that people with schizophrenia are more likely to have minor physical anomalies than the general population[6]. Some of these anomalies may be apparent at birth, while others are more subtle and may not be obvious until later in life. This background risk complicates the assessment of antipsychotic drug risk. Data relating to antipsychotics and pregnancy are poor: Cochrane suggests that the risk of harm remains unknown[7].

Older, first-generation antipsychotics are generally considered to have minimal risk of teratogenicity[8,9], although data are less than convincing, as might be expected[10,11]. It remains uncertain whether first-generation antipsychotics are entirely without risk to the fetus or to later development – an association with malformation has been suggested[10] and neonatal dyskinesia reported[12]. However, this continued uncertainty and the wide use of these drugs over several decades suggest that any risk is small – an assumption borne out by most studies[8,13].

Data relating to second-generation antipsychotics are growing in number. The use of clozapine appears to present no increased risk of malformation, although gestational diabetes and neonatal seizures may be more likely to occur[14] and stillbirth has been reported[15]. Similarly, limited data suggest that olanzapine is not associated with teratogenicity, but may increase the risk of gestational diabetes[10,14,16,17]. Not all authorities agree that olanzapine is free of risk of teratogenicity[18-20]. Limited data suggest that neither risperidone[17,21,22] nor quetiapine[17,23,24] is teratogenic in humans. Data relating to aripiprazole are scarce[25]. There are virtually no published data relating to other SGAs.

Overall, these data do not allow an assessment of relative risks associated with different agents and certainly do not confirm absolutely the safety of any particular drug. Older drugs may still be preferred in pregnancy, but, considering data available on some atypical drugs, it may not now be appropriate always to switch to these first-generation drugs, should continued treatment be necessary. As with other drugs, decisions must be based on the latest available information and an individualised assessment of probable risks and benefits. If possible, specialist advice should be sought and primary reference sources consulted.

Recommendations – psychosis in pregnancy

- Patients with a history of psychosis who are maintained on antipsychotic medication should be advised to discuss a planned pregnancy as early as possible.
- Such patients, particularly if they have suffered repeated relapses, are best maintained on antipsychotics during and after pregnancy. This may minimise fetal exposure by avoiding the need for higher doses should relapse occur.
- There is most experience with **chlorpromazine** (constipation and sedation can be a problem), **trifluoperazine, haloperidol, olanzapine** and **clozapine** (gestational diabetes may be a problem with both SGAs). If the patient is established on another antipsychotic, the most up-to-date advice should always be obtained. Experience with other drugs is growing and a change in treatment may not be necessary or wise. Olanzapine is widely used by perinatal services in the UK.
- A few authorities recommend discontinuation of antipsychotics 5–10 days before anticipated delivery to minimise the chances of neonatal effects. This may, however, put mother and infant at risk and needs to be considered carefully. Antipsychotic discontinuation symptoms can occur in the neonate (e.g. crying, agitation, increased suckling). Some centres used mixed (breast/bottle) feeding to minimise withdrawal. With SGAs, discontinuation may not be necessary or desirable. Consult specialist services for the latest advice on pre-delivery prescribing.

Risk of depression during pregnancy and postpartum[4,24,26,27]

- Approximately 10% of pregnant women develop a depressive illness and a further 16% a self-limiting depressive reaction. Much postpartum depression begins before birth.
- There is a significant increase in new psychiatric episodes in the first 3 months after delivery. At least 80% are mood disorders, primarily depression.
- Women who have had a previous episode of depressive illness (postpartum or not) are at higher risk of further episodes during pregnancy and postpartum.
- The risk is highest in women with bipolar illness.

- Pregnancy does not protect against depression; relapse rates are high in those with a history of depression who discontinue medication.

The risks of not treating depression include:

- harm to the mother through poor self-care, lack of obstetric care or self-harm
- harm to the foetus or neonate (ranging from neglect to infanticide).

The mental health of the mother influences foetal well-being, obstetric outcome and child development.

Treatment with antidepressants

Tricyclic antidepressants have been widely used throughout pregnancy without apparent detriment to the foetus[11,28] and have for many years been agents of choice in pregnancy. Some authorities recommend the use of nortriptyline and desipramine (not available in the UK) because these drugs are less anticholinergic and hypotensive than amitriptyline and imipramine (respectively, their tertiary amine parent molecules). Note that use of tricyclics in the third trimester is well known to produce neonatal withdrawal effects (agitation, irritability, seizures)[29]. Fetal exposure to tricyclics (via umbilicus and amniotic fluid) is high[30,31]. In addition, little is known of the developmental effects of prenatal exposure to tricyclics, although one small study detected no adverse consequences[32].

With the possible exception of paroxetine, SSRIs also appear not to be teratogenic, with most data supporting the safety of fluoxetine[28,29,32–36]. One study[37] revealed a slight increase in rate of malformation with SSRIs, and paroxetine is more clearly linked to cardiac malformations,[38] particularly after high-dose (>25 mg/day), first-trimester exposure[39]. SSRIs have also been associated with decreased gestational age (mean 1 week), spontaneous abortion[40] and decreased birth weight (mean 175 g)[33,34,41,42]. (Note that depression itself carries an increased risk of early birth and of obstetric complications, so evaluating these findings is difficult.) Sertraline appears to result in the least placental exposure[43]. Third-trimester exposure has been associated with reduced early APGAR scores[33]. Third-trimester use of paroxetine may give rise to neonatal complications, presumably related to abrupt withdrawal[44–46]. Other SSRIs have similar, possibly less severe effects[46,47]. Exposure to SSRIs in late pregnancy may increase the risk of persistent pulmonary hypertension of the newborn (PPHN)[48], although the absolute risk is small. Numerous data relating to neurodevelopmental outcome of fetal exposure to SSRIs suggest that these drugs are safe, although data are less than conclusive[49].

Rather more scarce data suggest the absence of teratogenic potential with moclobemide[50], reboxetine[51] and venlafaxine (although neonatal withdrawal may occur)[34,52,53], but none of these drugs can be specifically recommended at the time of writing. Similarly, trazodone, bupropion (amfebutamone) and mirtazapine cannot be recommended because there are few data supporting their safety[11,28,34,54,55]. Recent data suggest that both bupropion and mirtazapine are not associated with malformations but, like SSRIs, may be linked to an increased rate of spontaneous abortion[56,57].

MAOIs should be avoided in pregnancy because of a suspected increased risk of congenital malformation and because of the risk of hypertensive crisis[58].

There is no evidence to suggest that ECT causes harm to either the mother or fetus during pregnancy[59] although general anaesthesia is of course not without risks. Omega-3 fatty acids may also be a treatment option[60], although efficacy and safety data are scant.

Recommendations – depression in pregnancy

- Patients who are already receiving antidepressants and are at high risk of relapse are best maintained on antidepressants during and after pregnancy.
- Those who develop a moderate or severe depressive illness during pregnancy should be treated with antidepressant drugs if psychological management has failed or is not available.
- There is most experience with **amitriptyline, imipramine** (constipation and sedation can be a problem with both; withdrawal symptoms may occur) and **fluoxetine** (increased chance of earlier delivery and reduced birth weight). If the patient is established on another antidepressant, always obtain the most up-to-date advice. Experience with other drugs is growing and a change in treatment may not be necessary or wise. **Avoid paroxetine**.
- The neonate may experience discontinuation symptoms such as agitation and irritability, or even convulsions (with SSRIs). The risk is assumed to be particularly high with short half-life drugs such as paroxetine and venlafaxine. Continuing to breast-feed and then 'weaning' by switching to mixed (breast/bottle) feeding may help reduce the severity of reactions.
- Note the probable increased risk of persistent pulmonary hypertension of the newborn when SSRIs are taken in late pregnancy.

Risks in patients with bipolar illness during pregnancy and postpartum

- The risk of relapse after delivery is hugely increased: up to eight-fold in the first month postpartum.

The risks of not treating bipolar disorder include:

- harm to the mother through poor self-care, lack of obstetric care or self-harm
- harm to the fetus or neonate (ranging from neglect to infanticide).

The mental health of the mother influences fetal well-being, obstetric outcome and child development.

Special groups

Treatment with mood stabilisers

Lithium use during pregnancy has a well-known association with the cardiac malformation Ebstein's anomaly[11] (relative risk is 10–20 times more than control, but the absolute risk is low at 1:1000)[61]. The period of maximum risk to the fetus is 2–6 weeks after conception[62], before many women know that they are pregnant. Although the risk of major malformations in the infant has probably been overestimated, lithium should be avoided in pregnancy if possible. Slow discontinuation before conception is the preferred course of action[14,63] because abrupt discontinuation is suspected of worsening the risk of relapse. The relapse rate postpartum may be as high as 70% in women who discontinued lithium before conception[64]. If discontinuation is unsuccessful during pregnancy – restart and continue. If lithium is continued during pregnancy, high-resolution ultrasound and echocardiography should be performed at 6 and 18 weeks of gestation. In the third trimester, the use of lithium may be problematic because of changing pharmacokinetics: an increasing dose of lithium is required to maintain the lithium level during pregnancy as total body water increases, but the requirements return abruptly to pre-pregnancy levels immediately after delivery. Lithium completely equilibrates across the placenta[65]. Neonatal goitre, hypotonia, lethargy and cardiac arrhythmia can occur.

Most data relating to carbamazepine and valproate come from studies in epilepsy, a condition associated with increased neonatal malformation. These data may not be precisely relevant to use in mental illness. Nonetheless, both carbamazepine and valproate have a clear causal link with increased risk of a variety of fetal abnormalities, particularly spina bifida[11,28,66]. Both drugs should be avoided, if possible. Valproate is more dangerous than carbamazapine[67,68] and should be avoided (see page 377). Where continued use is deemed essential, low-dose monotherapy is strongly recommended, as the teratogenic effect is probably dose-related[69,70]. Ideally, all patients should take folic acid (5 mg daily) for at least a month before conception (this may reduce the risk of neonatal neural tube defects). Note, however, that some authorities recommend a lower dose[71], presumably because of a risk of twin births[72]. Use of carbamazepine in the third trimester may necessitate maternal vitamin K. Early data for lamotrigine suggest a low risk of fetal malformations when used as monotherapy[71,73,74], although a substantially increased risk of cleft palate has recently been reported[75]. Clearance of lamotrigine seems to increase radically during pregnancy[76].

Recommendations – bipolar disorder in pregnancy

- For women who have had a long period without relapse, the possibility of withdrawing treatment before conception and for at least the first trimester should be considered.
- The risk of relapse both pre- and postpartum is very high if medication is discontinued abruptly.
- Women with severe illness or who are known to relapse quickly after discontinuation of a mood stabiliser should be advised to continue their medication following discussion of the risks.
- No mood stabiliser is clearly safe. Women prescribed lithium should undergo level 2 ultrasound of the fetus at 6 and 18 weeks' gestation to screen for Ebstein's anomaly. Those prescribed valproate or carbamazepine (both teratogenic) should receive prophylactic folic acid to reduce the incidence of neural tube defects. Prophylactic vitamin K should be administered to the mother and neonate after delivery.
- Valproate (the most teratogenic) and combinations of mood stabilisers should be avoided.
- Lamotrigine may be associated with cleft palate.

Risks in patients with epilepsy during pregnancy and postpartum[77,78]

- There is an increased risk of maternal complications such as severe morning sickness, eclampsia, vaginal bleeding and premature labour. Women should get as much sleep and rest as possible and comply with medication (if prescribed) in order to minimise the risk of seizures.
- The risk of having a child with minor malformations may be increased regardless of treatment with antiepileptic drugs (AEDs).
- The risks of not treating epilepsy are as follows:
  - If seizures are inadequately controlled, there is an increased risk of accidents resulting in fetal injury. Postpartum the mother may be less able to look after herself and her child.
  - The risk of seizures during delivery is 1–2%, potentially worsening maternal and neonatal mortality.

Treatment with anticonvulsant drugs[79-82]

It is established that treatment with anticonvulsant drugs increases the risk of having a child with major congenital malformation to two- to three-fold that seen in the general population. Congenital heart defects (1.8%) and facial clefts (1.7%) are the most common congenital malformations. Both carbamazepine and valproate are associated with a hugely increased incidence of spina bifida at 0.5–1% and 1–2%, respectively. The risk of other neural tube defects is also increased. In women with epilepsy, the risk of fetal malformations with carbamazepine is 2.3%; with lamotrigine, 3%; and with valproate,

Special groups

371

7.2%[83], possibly even higher[68,70]. Higher doses (particularly doses of valproate exceeding 1000 mg/day) and anticonvulsant polypharmacy are particularly problematic[70]. Cognitive deficits have been reported in older children who have been exposed to valproate in utero. Those exposed to carbamazepine may not be similarly disadvantaged[84]. Early data with lamotrigine[73,85] and oxcarbazepine[86] suggest a relatively lower risk of malformation, but confirmation is required (and note risk of cleft palate with lamotrigine[75]).

Pharmacokinetics change during pregnancy. Dosage adjustment may be required to keep the patient seizure-free[87]. Serum levels usually return to pre-pregnancy levels within a month of delivery – often much more rapidly. Doses may need to be reduced at this point.

Best practice guidelines recommend that a woman should receive the lowest possible dose of a single anticonvulsant.

Recommendations – epilepsy in pregnancy

- For women who have been seizure-free for a long period, the possibility of withdrawing treatment before conception and for at least the first trimester should be considered.
- No anticonvulsant is clearly safer. Valproate should be avoided if possible. Women prescribed valproate or carbamazepine should receive prophylactic folic acid to reduce the risk of neural tube defects. Prophylactic vitamin K should be administered to the mother and neonate after delivery.
- Valproate and combinations of anticonvulsants should be avoided if possible.
- All women with epilepsy should have a full discussion with their neurologist to quantify the risks and benefits of continuing anticonvulsant drugs.

Sedatives

Anxiety disorders and insomnia are commonly seen in pregnancy[88]. First-trimester exposure to benzodiazepines appears to be associated with an increased risk of oral clefts in newborns, although there is debate about the magnitude of this risk[89]. Third-trimester use is commonly associated with neonatal difficulties (floppy baby syndrome)[90]. Benzodiazepines are best avoided in pregnancy.

Promethazine has been used in hyperemesis gravidarum and appears not to be teratogenic, although data are limited.

Recommendations – psychotropics in pregnancy

Psychotropic group	Recommendations
Antidepressants	Nortriptyline Amitriptyline Imipramine Fluoxetine
Antipsychotics	**Conventional drugs** have been widely used, although safety is not fully established. Most experience with **chlorpromazine, haloperidol** and **trifluoperazine**. No clear evidence that **clozapine** and **olanzapine** have teratogenic potential but data are limited
Benzodiazepines	Best avoided
Mood stabilisers	Avoid unless risks and consequences of relapse outweigh known risk of teratogenesis. Women of childbearing potential taking carbamazepine or valproate should receive prophylactic folic acid. Avoid valproate and combinations where possible
Sedatives	Promethazine is widely used but supporting data are scarce

References

1. McElhatton PR. General principles of drug use in pregnancy. Pharm J 2003;270:232–4.
2. Oates M. Patients as parents: the risk to children. Br J Psychiatry Suppl 1997;(32):22–7.
3. Terp IM et al. Post-partum psychoses. Clinical diagnoses and relative risk of admission after parturition. Br J Psychiatry 1998;172:521–6.
4. Stein G. Postpartum and related disorders. In Stein G, Wilkinson G, eds. Seminars in General Adult Psychiatry. London: Royal College of Psychiatrists, 1998:903–58.
5. Spinelli MG. A systematic investigation of 16 cases of neonaticide. Am J Psychiatry 2001;158:811–13.
6. Ismail B et al. Minor physical anomalies in schizophrenic patients and their siblings. Am J Psychiatry 1998;155:1695–702.
7. Webb RT et al. Antipsychotic drugs for non-affective psychosis during pregnancy and postpartum. Cochrane Database Syst Rev 2004;CD004411.
8. Trixler M et al. Use of antipsychotics in the management of schizophrenia during pregnancy. Drugs 2005;65:1193–206.
9. Diav-Citrin O et al. Safety of haloperidol and penfluridol in pregnancy: a multicenter, prospective, controlled study. J Clin Psychiatry 2005;66:317–22.
10. Patton SW et al. Antipsychotic medication during pregnancy and lactation in women with schizophrenia: evaluating the risk. Can J Psychiatry 2002;47:959–65.
11. Cohen LS et al. Psychotropic drug use during pregnancy: weighing the risks. J Clin Psychiatry 1998; 59(Suppl 2):18–28.
12. Collins KO et al. Maternal haloperidol therapy associated with dyskinesia in a newborn. Am J Health Syst Pharm 2003;60:2253–5.
13. Trixler M et al. Antipsychotic use in pregnancy. What are the best treatment options? Drug Saf 1997; 16:403–10.
14. Ernst CL et al. The reproductive safety profile of mood stabilizers, atypical antipsychotics, and broad-spectrum psychotropics. J Clin Psychiatry 2002;63(Suppl 4):42–55.
15. Mendhekar DN et al. Clozapine and pregnancy (Letter). J Clin Psychiatry 2003;64:850.
16. Eli Lilly and Company Limited. Zyprexa – use in pregnancy. Personal communication. 2003.

Special groups

17. McKenna K et al. Pregnancy outcome of women using atypical antipsychotic drugs: a prospective comparative study. J Clin Psychiatry 2005;66:444–9.
18. Howard L et al. Safety of antipsychotic drugs for pregnant and breastfeeding women with non-affective psychosis. BMJ 2004;329:933–4.
19. Spyropoulou AC et al. Hip dysplasia following a case of olanzapine exposed pregnancy: a questionable association. Arch Womens Ment Health 2006;9:219–22.
20. Arora M et al. Meningocele and ankyloblepharon following in utero exposure to olanzapine. Eur Psychiatry 2006;21:345–6.
21. Ratnayake T et al. No complications with risperidone treatment before and throughout pregnancy and during the nursing period. J Clin Psychiatry 2002;63:76–7.
22. Dabbert D et al. Follow-up of a pregnancy with risperidone microspheres. Pharmacopsychiatry 2006;39:235.
23. Tenyi T et al. Quetiapine and pregnancy. Am J Psychiatry 2002;159:674.
24. Taylor TM et al. Safety of quetiapine during pregnancy (Letter). Am J Psychiatry 2003;160:588–9.
25. Mendhekar DN et al. Aripiprazole use in a pregnant schizoaffective woman. Bipolar Disord 2006;8:299–300.
26. Llewellyn AM et al. Depression during pregnancy and the puerperium. J Clin Psychiatry 1997;58(Suppl 15):26–32.
27. Cohen LS et al. Relapse of major depression during pregnancy in women who maintain or discontinue antidepressant treatment. JAMA 2006;295:499–507.
28. Altshuler LL et al. Pharmacologic management of psychiatric illness during pregnancy: dilemmas and guidelines. Am J Psychiatry 1996;153:592–606.
29. Wisner KL et al. Pharmacologic treatment of depression during pregnancy. JAMA 1999;282:1264–9.
30. Loughhead AM et al. Placental passage of tricyclic antidepressants. Biol Psychiatry 2006;59:287–90.
31. Loughhead AM et al. Antidepressants in amniotic fluid: another route of fetal exposure. Am J Psychiatry 2006;163:145–7.
32. Nulman I et al. Child development following exposure to tricyclic antidepressants or fluoxetine throughout fetal life: a prospective, controlled study. Am J Psychiatry 2002;159:1889–95.
33. Hallberg P et al. The use of selective serotonin reuptake inhibitors during pregnancy and breast-feeding: a review and clinical aspects. J Clin Psychopharmacol 2005;25:59–73.
34. Gentile S. The safety of newer antidepressants in pregnancy and breastfeeding. Drug Saf 2005;28:137–52.
35. Kallen BA et al. Maternal use of selective serotonin re-uptake inhibitors in early pregnancy and infant congenital malformations. Birth Defects Res A Clin Mol Teratol 2007 [Epub ahead of print].
36. Einarson TR et al. Newer antidepressants in pregnancy and rates of major malformations: a meta-analysis of prospective comparative studies. Pharmacoepidemiol Drug Saf 2005;14:823–7.
37. Wogelius P et al. Maternal use of selective serotonin reuptake inhibitors and risk of congenital malformations. Epidemiology 2006;17:701–4.
38. Thormahlen GM. Paroxetine use during pregnancy: is it safe? Ann Pharmacother 2006;40:1834–7.
39. Berard A et al. First trimester exposure to paroxetine and risk of cardiac malformations in infants: the importance of dosage. Birth Defects Res B Dev Reprod Toxicol 2007;80:18–27.
40. Hemels ME et al. Antidepressant use during pregnancy and the rates of spontaneous abortions: a meta-analysis. Ann Pharmacother 2005;39:803–9.
41. Simon GE et al. Outcomes of prenatal antidepressant exposure. Am J Psychiatry 2002;159:2055–61.
42. Oberlander TF et al. Neonatal outcomes after prenatal exposure to selective serotonin reuptake inhibitor antidepressants and maternal depression using population-based linked health data. Arch Gen Psychiatry 2006;63:898–906.
43. Hendrick V et al. Placental passage of antidepressant medications. Am J Psychiatry 2003;160:993–6.
44. Costei AM et al. Perinatal outcome following third trimester exposure to paroxetine. Arch Pediatr Adolesc Med 2002;156:1129–32.
45. Haddad PM et al. Neonatal symptoms following maternal paroxetine treatment: serotonin toxicity or paroxetine discontinuation syndrome? J Psychopharmacol 2005;19:554–7.
46. Sanz EJ et al. Selective serotonin reuptake inhibitors in pregnant women and neonatal withdrawal syndrome: a database analysis. Lancet 2005;365:482–7.
47. Koren G. Discontinuation syndrome following late pregnancy exposure to antidepressants. Arch Pediatr Adolesc Med 2004;158:307–8.
48. Chambers CD et al. Selective serotonin-reuptake inhibitors and risk of persistent pulmonary hypertension of the newborn. N Engl J Med 2006;354:579–87.
49. Gentile S. SSRIs in pregnancy and lactation: emphasis on neurodevelopmental outcome. CNS Drugs 2005;19:623–33.
50. Rybakowski JK. Moclobemide in pregnancy. Pharmacopsychiatry 2001;34:82–3.
51. Pharmacia Ltd. Erdronax: use on pregnancy, renally and hepatically impaired patients. Personal communication. 2003.
52. Einarson A et al. Pregnancy outcome following gestational exposure to venlafaxine: a multicenter prospective controlled study. Am J Psychiatry 2001;158:1728–30.
53. Ferreira E et al. Effects of selective serotonin reuptake inhibitors and venlafaxine during pregnancy in term and preterm neonates. Pediatrics 2007;119:52–9.

54. Einarson A et al. A multicentre prospective controlled study to determine the safety of trazodone and nefazodone use during pregnancy. Can J Psychiatry 2003;48:106–10.
55. Rohde A et al. Mirtazapine (Remergil) for treatment resistant hyperemesis gravidarum: rescue of a twin pregnancy. Arch Gynecol Obstet 2003;268:219–21.
56. Chun-Fai-Chan B et al. Pregnancy outcome of women exposed to bupropion during pregnancy: a prospective comparative study. Am J Obstet Gynecol 2005;192:932–6.
57. Djulus J et al. Exposure to mirtazapine during pregnancy: a prospective, comparative study of birth outcomes. J Clin Psychiatry 2006;67:1280–4.
58. Hendrick V et al. Management of major depression during pregnancy. Am J Psychiatry 2002;159: 1667–73.
59. Miller LJ. Use of electroconvulsive therapy during pregnancy. Hosp Community Psychiatry 1994;45: 444–50.
60. Freeman MP et al. An open trial of Omega-3 fatty acids for depression in pregnancy. Acta Neuro-psychiatr 2006;18:21–4.
61. Cohen LS et al. A reevaluation of risk of in utero exposure to lithium. JAMA 1994;271:146–50.
62. Yonkers KA et al. Lithium during pregnancy: drug effects and therapeutic implications. CNS Drugs 1998;4:269.
63. Dodd S et al. The pharmacology of bipolar disorder during pregnancy and breastfeeding. Expert Opin Drug Saf 2004;3:221–9.
64. Viguera AC et al. Risk of recurrence of bipolar disorder in pregnant and nonpregnant women after discontinuing lithium maintenance. Am J Psychiatry 2000;157:179–84.
65. Newport DJ et al. Lithium placental passage and obstetrical outcome: implications for clinical manage-ment during late pregnancy. Am J Psychiatry 2005;162:2162–70.
66. Holmes LB et al. The teratogenicity of anticonvulsant drugs. N Engl J Med 2001;344:1132–8.
67. Wide K et al. Major malformations in infants exposed to antiepileptic drugs in utero, with emphasis on carbamazepine and valproic acid: a nation-wide, population-based register study. Acta Paediatr 2004; 93:174–6.
68. Wyszynski DF et al. Increased rate of major malformations in offspring exposed to valproate during pregnancy. Neurology 2005;64:961–5.
69. Vajda FJ et al. Critical relationship between sodium valproate dose and human teratogenicity: results of the Australian register of anti-epileptic drugs in pregnancy. J Clin Neurosci 2004;11:854–8.
70. Vajda FJ et al. Maternal valproate dosage and fetal malformations. Acta Neurol Scand 2005;112: 137–43.
71. Yonkers KA et al. Management of bipolar disorder during pregnancy and the postpartum period. Am J Psychiatry 2004;161:608–20.
72. Czeizel AE. Folic acid and the prevention of neural-tube defects. N Engl J Med 2004;350:2209–11.
73. Sabers A et al. Epilepsy and pregnancy: lamotrigine as main drug used. Acta Neurol Scand 2004;109:9–13.
74. Cunnington M et al. Lamotrigine and the risk of malformations in pregnancy. Neurology 2005;64: 955–60.
75. Holmes LB et al. Increased risk for non-syndromic cleft palate among infants exposed to lamotrigine during pregnancy. Birth Defects Research 2006;76:318.
76. de Haan GJ et al. Gestation-induced changes in lamotrigine pharmacokinetics: a monotherapy study. Neurology 2004;63:571–3.
77. Shorvon S. Antiepileptic drug therapy during pregnancy: the neurologist's perspective. J Med Genet 2002;39:248–50.
78. Cleland PG. Risk–benefit assessment of anticonvulsants in women of child-bearing potential. Drug Saf 1991;6:70–81.
79. Dolk H et al. Assessing epidemiological evidence for the teratogenic effects of anticonvulsant medica-tions. J Med Genet 2002;39:243–4.
80. Holmes LB. The teratogenicity of anticonvulsant drugs: a progress report. J Med Genet 2002;39: 245–7.
81. Adab N et al. Common antiepileptic drugs in pregnancy in women with epilepsy. Cochrane Database Syst Rev 2004;CD004848.
82. Iqbal MM et al. The effects of lithium, valproic acid, and carbamazepine during pregnancy and lactation. J Toxicol Clin Toxicol 2001;39:381–92.
83. National Institute for Clinical Excellence. The clinical effectiveness and cost effectiveness of newer drugs for epilepsy in adults. Technology Appraisal 76. http://www.nice.org.uk. 2004.
84. Gaily E et al. Normal intelligence in children with prenatal exposure to carbamazepine. Neurology 2004;62:28–32.
85. Vajda FJ et al. The Australian registry of anti-epileptic drugs in pregnancy: experience after 30 months. J Clin Neurosci 2003;10:543–9.
86. Meischenguiser R et al. Oxcarbazepine in pregnancy: clinical experience in Argentina. Epilepsy Behav 2004;5:163–7.
87. Adab N. Therapeutic monitoring of antiepileptic drugs during pregnancy and in the postpartum period: is it useful? CNS Drugs 2006;20:791–800.
88. Ross LE et al. Anxiety disorders during pregnancy and the postpartum period: a systematic review. J Clin Psychiatry 2006;67:1285–98.

375

89. Dolovich LR et al. Benzodiazepine use in pregnancy and major malformations or oral cleft: meta-analysis of cohort and case-control studies. BMJ 1998;317:839–43.
90. McElhatton PR. The effects of benzodiazepine use during pregnancy and lactation. Reprod Toxicol 1994;8:461–75.

Further reading

Einarson A et al. Abrupt discontinuation of psychotropic drugs during pregnancy: fear of teratogenic risk and impact of counselling. J Psychiatry Neurosci 2001;26:44–8.

Gentile S. Clinical utilization of atypical antipsychotics in pregnancy and lactation. Ann Pharmacother 2004;38:1265–71.

Hallberg P et al. The use of selective serotonin reuptake inhibitors during pregnancy and breast-feeding: a review and clinical aspects. J Clin Psychopharmacol 2005;25:59–73.

National Institute for Health and Clinical Excellence. Clinical guideline 45, Antenatal and postnatal mental health. February 2007.

Ruchkin V et al. SSRIs and the developing brain. Lancet 2005;365:451–3.

Sanz EJ et al. Selective serotonin reuptake inhibitors in pregnant women and neonatal withdrawal syndrome: a database analysis. Lancet 2005;365:482–7.

Special groups

Psychotropics in breast feeding

Data on the safety of psychotropic medication in breast-feeding are largely derived from small studies or case reports and case series. With the majority of data, only acute adverse effects (or their absence) are reported. Long-term safety cannot therefore be guaranteed for the psychotropics mentioned. The information presented must be interpreted with caution with respect to the limited data from which it is derived and the need for such information to be regularly updated.

General principles of prescribing psychotropics in breast-feeding

- In each case, the benefits of breast-feeding to the mother and infant must be weighed against the risk of drug exposure in the infant.
- Premature infants and infants with renal, hepatic, cardiac or neurological impairment are at a greater risk from exposure to drugs.
- The infants should be monitored for any specific adverse effects of the drugs as well as for feeding patterns and growth and development.
- It is usually inappropriate to withhold treatment to allow breast-feeding. Treatment of maternal illness is the highest priority.

Wherever possible:

- use the lowest effective dose
- avoid polypharmacy
- time the feeds to avoid peak drug levels in the milk or express milk to give later.

Summary of recommendations (see full review below for details)

Drug group	Recommended drugs
Antidepressants	Paroxetine or sertraline (others may be used – see table)
Antipsychotics	Sulpiride; olanzapine (others may be used – see table)
Mood stabilisers	Avoid if possible; valproate if essential
Sedatives	Lorazepam for anxiety; zolpidem for sleep (others may be used – see table)

377

Antidepressants in breast-feeding

Drug	Comment
Tricyclic antidepressants (TCAs)[1-8]	All TCAs are excreted in human breast milk. Infant serum levels range from undetectable to low. Adverse effects have not been reported in infants exposed to amitriptyline, nortriptyline, clomipramine, imipramine, dosulepin (dothiepin) and desipramine. There are two case reports of doxepin exposure during breast-feeding leading to adverse effects in the infant. In one, an 8-week-old infant experienced respiratory depression, which resolved 24 hours after stopping nursing. In the other, poor suckling, muscle hypotonia and drowsiness were observed in a newborn, again resolving 24 hours after removing doxepin exposure. A study of 15 children did not show a negative outcome on cognitive development in children 3–5 years postpartum, following breast milk exposure to dosulepin. Data on TCAs not mentioned in this section were not available and their use can therefore not be recommended unless used during pregnancy.
Citalopram[1,9-15]	Citalopram is excreted in breast milk. Infant serum levels appear to be low or undetectable, although higher than reported with fluvoxamine, sertraline and paroxetine. Breast milk peak levels have been observed 3–9 hours after maternal dose. There is one case report of uneasy sleep in an infant exposed to citalopram while breast-feeding. This resolved on halving the mother's dose. Irregular breathing, sleep disorder, hypo- and hypertonia were observed up to 3 weeks after delivery in another breast-feeding infant exposed to citalopram in utero. The symptoms were attributed to withdrawal syndrome from citalopram despite the mother continuing citalopram postpartum. In a study of 31 infants exposed to citalopram via breast milk, one case each of colic, decreased feeding, and irritability/restlessness was reported.
Escitalopram[16-18]	Escitalopram is excreted in breast milk but adverse effects were not seen in two separate case reports. In a study of 8 women, breast milk peak levels of escitalopram were observed 2–11 hours post maternal dose. No adverse effects were noted in the infants. Serum levels were found to be low or undetectable in all five of the infants from whom blood could be taken.

378

Fluvoxamine[1,19-24]	Fluvoxamine is excreted in breast milk. The levels detected in infants exposed to fluvoxamine while breast-feeding vary from undetectable to up to half the maternal serum level. No adverse effects were noted in these infants. Peak drug levels in breast milk have been observed 4 hours after maternal dose.
Fluoxetine[1,25-30]	Of the SSRIs, most data relate to fluoxetine. Fluoxetine is excreted in breast milk. Infant serum levels appear to be low, although higher than reported with paroxetine, fluvoxamine and sertraline, and close to those reported for citalopram. Adverse effects have not been reported for the majority of fluoxetine-exposed infants. However, in two infants, reported adverse effects included excessive crying, decreased sleep, diarrhoea and vomiting in one and somnolence, decreased feeding, hypotonia, moaning, grunting and fever in the other. In another, seizure activity at 3 weeks, 4 months and then 5 months was reported. The mother was taking a combination of fluoxetine and carbamazepine. A retrospective study found the growth curves of breast-fed infants of mothers taking fluoxetine to be significantly below those of infants receiving breast milk free of fluoxetine. However, in another study of 11 infants exposed to fluoxetine during pregnancy and lactation, neurological developments and weight gain were found to be normal. No developmental abnormalities were noted in another four infants exposed to fluoxetine during breast-feeding.
Paroxetine[1,19,29,31-37]	Paroxetine is excreted in breast milk. Infant serum levels vary from low to undetectable. There is a single case of adverse consequences arising from maternal paroxetine consumption. Vomiting and irritability were reported in a breast-feeding baby of 18 months. The symptoms were attributed to severe hyponatraemia in the infant. The maternal paroxetine dose was 40 mg. Paroxetine levels were not determined in the breast milk or infant serum. Adverse effects were not noted in the other cases cited. Breast-fed infants of 27 women taking paroxetine reached the usual developmental milestones at 3, 6 and 12 months, similar to a control group.
Sertraline[29,35,38]	Sertraline is excreted in breast milk. Infant serum levels appear to be low. Peak drug levels in breast milk have been observed 7–10 hours after the maternal dose. No adverse effects were noted in these infants.

Special groups

Table Antidepressants in breast-feeding (Cont.)

Drug	Comment
Sertraline (cont.)	Withdrawal symptoms (agitation, restlessness, insomnia and an enhanced startle reaction) developed in a breast-fed neonate after abrupt withdrawal of maternal sertraline. The neonate was exposed to sertraline in utero.
Nefazodone[39,40]	From the three published case reports available, it appears that nefazodone is excreted in breast milk. Recorded infant serum levels are low. In one infant, drowsiness and poor feeding were reported. These symptoms resolved over a 72-hour period after breast-feeding ceased. Peak breast milk levels were seen 1–3 hours after the maternal dose.
Reboxetine[41]	Reboxetine is excreted in breast milk. Infant serum levels ranged from low to undetectable and no adverse effects were noted in four infants. In addition, normal developmental milestones were reached by three of the infants. The fourth infant had developmental problems thought not to be related to maternal reboxetine therapy. Breast milk peak levels were observed 1–9 hours after maternal dose.
Venlafaxine[29,35,42,43]	Venlafaxine is excreted in breast milk. Infant serum levels were found to be low. Although not directly compared, these levels appear to be higher than those seen with fluvoxamine, sertraline and paroxetine. No adverse effects have been observed. Symptoms of lethargy, jitteriness, rapid breathing, poor suckling and dehydration seen 2 days after delivery of an infant exposed to venlafaxine in utero subsided over a week on exposure to venlafaxine via breast milk. It was suggested in this case that breast-feeding may have helped manage the withdrawal symptoms experienced postpartum.
MAOIs	There are no published data available.
Moclobemide[44,45]	Moclobemide is excreted in breast milk. Infant serum levels appear to be low. No adverse effects were detected in these infants. Peak drug levels in breast milk were seen at 3 hours.
Mianserin[46]	Mianserin is excreted in breast milk. Adverse effects were not seen in two infants studied.

Special groups

Mirtazapine[47]	Psychomotor development in an infant exposed to mirtazapine in breast milk was found to be normal after 6 weeks of exposure. No sedation or abnormal weight gain was noted in the infant.
Trazodone[48]	Trazodone is excreted in breast milk in small quantities (based on assessments after a single maternal dose).

Antipsychotics in breast-feeding

Drug	Comment
Butyrophenones[1,2,29,49,50]	Haloperidol is excreted in breast milk. The extent appears variable. Normal development was noted in one infant. However, delayed development was noted in three infants exposed to a combination of haloperidol and chlorpromazine in breast milk. Data on butyrophenones not mentioned in this section were not available.
Phenothiazines[1,2,49,50]	Most of the data relate to chlorpromazine. Chlorpromazine is excreted in breast milk. There is a wide variation in the breast milk concentrations quoted. Similarly, infant serum levels vary greatly. Lethargy was reported in one infant whose mother was taking chlorpromazine while breast-feeding. In another case, however, an infant exposed to much higher levels showed no signs of lethargy. There is a report of delayed development in three infants exposed to a combination of chlorpromazine and haloperidol while breast-feeding. In the one case of perphenazine exposure and two cases of trifluoperazine exposure, no adverse effects were noted in the infants. Data on phenothiazines not mentioned in this section were not available.
Thioxanthenes[1,51,52]	There are two cases of infant exposure to flupentixol and one to zuclopenthixol. The amount excreted in breast milk of both drugs is low. No adverse effects or developmental abnormalities were noted in the infant exposed to flupentixol. The clinical status of the other infant was not reported.

Table   Antipsychotics in breast-feeding (Cont.)

Drug	Comment
Sulpiride[53–57]	There are a number of small studies in which sulpiride has been shown to improve lactation in nursing mothers. The amounts excreted in breast milk were low. No adverse effects were noted in the nursing infants.
Amisulpride	There are no published data available.
Aripiprazole	There are no published data available.
Clozapine[1,2,29,50]	Clozapine is excreted in breast milk. In a study of four infants exposed to clozapine in breast milk, sedation was noted in one and another developed agranulocytosis, which resolved on stopping clozapine. No adverse effects were noted in the other two. Decreased sucking reflex, irritability, seizures and cardiovascular instability have also been reported in nursing infants exposed to clozapine. Because of the risk of neutropenia and seizures, it is advisable to avoid breast-feeding while on clozapine until more data become available.
Olanzapine[1,29,58–61]	Olanzapine is excreted in breast milk. Estimates of infant serum levels are low. There is one case of an infant developing jaundice and sedation on exposure to olanzapine during breast-feeding. This continued on cessation of breast-feeding. This infant was exposed to olanzapine in utero and had cardiomegaly. No adverse effects were reported in four of seven breast-fed infants of mothers taking olanzapine. Of the rest, one was not assessed, one had a lower developmental age than chronological age (but the mother had also been taking additional psychotropic medication), and drowsiness was noted in another, which resolved on halving the maternal dose. The median maximum concentration in the milk was found at around 5 hours after maternal ingestion.
Quetiapine[62–65]	Quetiapine is excreted in breast milk. From a single case report the levels were found to be low although the maternal dose was only 200 mg/day. No adverse effects were noted in the infant. In a separate case, no adverse effects were noted in an infant when quetiapine (up to 400 mg/day) was added to maternal paroxetine therapy. In addition, no adverse effects were noted in an infant exposed via breast milk to a combination of quetiapine and fluvoxamine. The baby reached developmental milestones.

Quetiapine (cont.)	In a small study of quetiapine augmentation of maternal antidepressant therapy, two out of six babies showed mild developmental delays not thought to be related to quetiapine treatment. The doses in this study ranged from 25 to 400 mg/day.
Risperidone[66–69]	Risperidone is excreted in breast milk. In five cases reported in the literature, no adverse effects were noted. In two cases where development was assessed, no abnormalities were observed.
Sertindole	There are no published data available.
Ziprasidone	There are no published data available.

Mood stabilisers in breast-feeding

Drug	Comment
Carbamazepine[1,70–72]	Carbamazepine is excreted in breast milk. Infant serum levels range from 6% to 65% of maternal serum levels. Adverse effects have been reported in a number of infants exposed to carbamazepine during breast-feeding. These include one case of cholestatic hepatitis, and one of transient hepatic dysfunction with hyperbilirubinaemia and elevated GGT. The adverse effects in the first case resolved after discontinuation of breast-feeding and the second resolved despite continued feeding. Other adverse effects reported include seizure-like activity, drowsiness, irritability and high-pitched crying in one infant whose mother was on multiple agents, hyperexcitability in two infants and poor feeding in another three. In contrast, in a number of infants, no adverse effects were noted.
Lamotrigine[73–78]	Lamotrigine is excreted in breast milk. Infant serum levels range between 18% and 50% of maternal serum levels. No adverse effects have been reported in exposed infants. However, because of the risk of life-threatening rashes, it is advisable to avoid lamotrigine while breast-feeding until more data on its effects become available.
Lithium[70,72,79]	Lithium is excreted in breast milk. Infant serum levels range from 5% to 200% of maternal serum concentrations. Adverse effects have been reported in infants exposed to lithium while breast-feeding. One infant developed cyanosis, lethargy, hypothermia, hypotonia and a heart murmur, all of which resolved within 3 days of stopping breast-feeding. The infant was exposed

Special groups

Table	Mood stabilisers in breast-feeding (Cont.)
Drug	**Comment**
Lithium (cont.)	to lithium in utero. Non-specific signs of toxicity have been reported in others. There are also reports of no adverse effects in some infants exposed to lithium while breast-feeding. Opinions on the use of lithium while breast-feeding vary from absolute contraindication to mother's informed choice. Conditions which may alter the infant's electrolyte balance and state of hydration must be borne in mind. If it is used, the infant must be carefully monitored for signs of toxicity.
Valproate[1,70–72,80]	Valproate is excreted in breast milk. Infant serum levels vary from undetectable to 40% of maternal serum levels. Thrombocytopenia and anaemia were reported in a 3-month-old infant exposed to valproate in utero and while breast-feeding. This reversed on stopping breast-feeding.

Sedatives in breast-feeding

Drug	**Comment**
Benzodiazepines[1,29,81–85]	Diazepam is excreted in breast milk. Infant serum levels vary from undetectable to nearly 14% of the maternal serum levels. In some infants, no adverse effects were noted. In others, reported adverse effects included sedation, lethargy and weight loss. Lorazepam, temazepam and clonazepam are excreted in breast milk in small amounts. Apart from one case report of persistent apnoea in one infant exposed to clonazepam in utero and during breast-feeding, no adverse effects were reported. Any infant exposed to benzodiazepines in breast milk should be monitored for CNS depression and apnoea.
Promethazine	There are no published data available.
Zopiclone, zolpidem and zaleplon[86–88]	All three are excreted in breast milk in small amounts. No adverse effects were noted in exposed infants. Peak concentrations of zolpidem in breast milk were found 4 hours after ingestion of a single 20 mg dose. Zaleplon peak breast milk levels were found 1 hour after the dose and breast milk concentrations were approximately 50% of plasma concentrations.

References

1. Burt VK et al. The use of psychotropic medications during breast-feeding. Am J Psychiatry 2001;158: 1001–9.
2. Yoshida K et al. Psychotropic drugs in mothers' milk: a comprehensive review of assay methods, pharmacokinetics and of safety of breast-feeding. J Psychopharmacol 1999;13:64–80.
3. Misri S et al. Benefits and risks to mother and infant of drug treatment for postnatal depression. Drug Saf 2002;25:903–11.
4. Yoshida K et al. Investigation of pharmacokinetics and of possible adverse effects in infants exposed to tricyclic antidepressants in breast-milk. J Affect Disord 1997;43:225–37.
5. Frey OR et al. Adverse effects in a newborn infant breast-fed by a mother treated with doxepin. Ann Pharmacother 1999;33:690–3.
6. Ilett KF et al. The excretion of dothiepin and its primary metabolites in breast milk. Br J Clin Pharmacol 1992;33:635–9.
7. Kemp J et al. Excretion of doxepin and N-desmethyldoxepin in human milk. Br J Clin Pharmacol 1985;20:497–9.
8. Buist A et al. Effect of exposure to dothiepin and northiaden in breast milk on child development. Br J Psychiatry 1995;167:370–3.
9. Lee A et al. Frequency of infant adverse events that are associated with citalopram use during breast-feeding. Am J Obstet Gynecol 2004;190:218–21.
10. Heikkinen T et al. Citalopram in pregnancy and lactation. Clin Pharmacol Ther 2002;72:184–91.
11. Jensen PN et al. Citalopram and desmethylcitalopram concentrations in breast milk and in serum of mother and infant. Ther Drug Monit 1997;19:236–9.
12. Spigset O et al. Excretion of citalopram in breast milk. Br J Clin Pharmacol 1997;44:295–8.
13. Rampono J et al. Citalopram and demethylcitalopram in human milk; distribution, excretion and effects in breast fed infants. Br J Clin Pharmacol 2000;50:263–8.
14. Schmidt K et al. Citalopram and breast-feeding: serum concentration and side effects in the infant. Biol Psychiatry 2000;47:164–5.
15. Franssen EJ et al. Citalopram serum and milk levels in mother and infant during lactation. Ther Drug Monit 2006;28:2–4.
16. Gentile S. Escitalopram late in pregnancy and while breast-feeding (Letter). Ann Pharmacother 2006; 40:1696–7.
17. Castberg I et al. Excretion of escitalopram in breast milk. J Clin Psychopharmacol 2006;26:536–8.
18. Rampono J et al. Transfer of escitalopram and its metabolite demethylescitalopram into breastmilk. Br J Clin Pharmacol 2006;62:316–22.
19. Hendrick V et al. Use of sertraline, paroxetine and fluvoxamine by nursing women. Br J Psychiatry 2001; 179:163–6.
20. Piontek CM et al. Serum fluvoxamine levels in breastfed infants. J Clin Psychiatry 2001;62:111–13.
21. Yoshida K et al. Fluvoxamine in breast-milk and infant development. Br J Clin Pharmacol 1997;44:210–11.
22. Hagg S et al. Excretion of fluvoxamine into breast milk. Br J Clin Pharmacol 2000;49:286–8.
23. Arnold LM et al. Fluvoxamine concentrations in breast milk and in maternal and infant sera. J Clin Psychopharmacol 2000;20:491–2.
24. Kristensen JH et al. The amount of fluvoxamine in milk is unlikely to be a cause of adverse effects in breastfed infants. J Hum Lact 2002;18:139–43.
25. Yoshida K et al. Fluoxetine in breast-milk and developmental outcome of breast-fed infants. Br J Psychiatry 1998;172:175–8.
26. Lester BM et al. Possible association between fluoxetine hydrochloride and colic in an infant. J Am Acad Child Adolesc Psychiatry 1993;32:1253–5.
27. Hendrick V et al. Fluoxetine and norfluoxetine concentrations in nursing infants and breast milk. Biol Psychiatry 2001;50:775–82.
28. Hale TW et al. Fluoxetine toxicity in a breastfed infant. Clin Pediatr 2001;40:681–4.
29. Malone K et al. Antidepressants, antipsychotics, benzodiazepines, and the breastfeeding dyad. Perspect Psychiatr Care 2004;40:73–85.
30. Heikkinen T et al. Pharmacokinetics of fluoxetine and norfluoxetine in pregnancy and lactation. Clin Pharmacol Ther 2003;73:330–7.
31. Begg EJ et al. Paroxetine in human milk. Br J Clin Pharmacol 1999;48:142–7.
32. Stowe ZN et al. Paroxetine in human breast milk and nursing infants. Am J Psychiatry 2000; 157:185–9.
33. Misri S et al. Paroxetine levels in postpartum depressed women, breast milk, and infant serum. J Clin Psychiatry 2000;61:828–32.
34. Ohman R et al. Excretion of paroxetine into breast milk. J Clin Psychiatry 1999;60:519–23.
35. Berle JO et al. Breastfeeding during maternal antidepressant treatment with serotonin reuptake inhibitors: infant exposure, clinical symptoms, and cytochrome p450 genotypes. J Clin Psychiatry 2004;65:1228–34.
36. Merlob P et al. Paroxetine during breast-feeding: infant weight gain and maternal adherence to counsel. Eur J Pediatr 2004;163:135–9.
37. Abdul Aziz A et al. Severe paroxetine induced hyponatremia in a breast fed infant. J Bahrain Med Soc 2004;16:195–8.

385

38. Llewellyn A et al. Psychotropic medications in lactation. J Clin Psychiatry 1998;59(Suppl 2):41–52.
39. Yapp P et al. Drowsiness and poor feeding in a breast-fed infant: association with nefazodone and its metabolites. Ann Pharmacother 2000;34:1269–72.
40. Dodd S et al. Nefazodone in the breast milk of nursing mothers: a report of two patients. J Clin Psychopharmacol 2000;20:717–18.
41. Hackett LP et al. Transfer of reboxetine into breastmilk, its plasma concentrations and lack of adverse effects in the breastfed infant. Eur J Clin Pharmacol 2006;62:633–8.
42. Koren G et al. Can venlafaxine in breast milk attenuate the norepinephrine and serotonin reuptake neonatal withdrawal syndrome? J Obstet Gynaecol Can 2006;28:299–302.
43. Ilett KF et al. Distribution of venlafaxine and its O-desmethyl metabolite in human milk and their effects in breastfed infants. Br J Clin Pharmacol 2002;53:17–22.
44. Pons G et al. Moclobemide excretion in human breast milk. Br J Clin Pharmacol 1990;29:27–31.
45. Buist A et al. Plasma and human milk concentrations of moclobemide in nursing mothers. Hum Psychopharmacol 1998;13:579–82.
46. Buist A et al. Mianserin in breast milk (Letter). Br J Clin Pharmacol 1993;36:133–4.
47. Aichhorn W et al. Mirtazapine and breast-feeding. Am J Psychiatry 2004;161:2325.
48. Verbeeck RK et al. Excretion of trazodone in breast milk. Br J Clin Pharmacol 1986;22:367–70.
49. Yoshida K et al. Breast-feeding and psychotropic drugs. Int Rev Psychiatry 1996;8:117–24.
50. Patton SW et al. Antipsychotic medication during pregnancy and lactation in women with schizophrenia: evaluating the risk. Can J Psychiatry 2002;47:959–65.
51. Matheson I et al. Milk concentrations of flupenthixol, nortriptyline and zuclopenthixol and between-breast differences in two patients. Eur J Clin Pharmacol 1988;35:217–20.
52. Kirk L et al. Concentrations of Cis(Z)-flupentixol in maternal serum, amniotic fluid, umbilical cord serum, and milk. Psychopharmacology 1980;72:107–8.
53. Ylikorkala O et al. Treatment of inadequate lactation with oral sulpiride and buccal oxytocin. Obstet Gynecol 1984;63:57–60.
54. Aono T et al. Augmentation of puerperal lactation by oral administration of sulpiride. J Clin Endocrinol Metab 1970;48:478–82.
55. Ylikorkala O et al. Sulpiride improves inadequate lactation. Br Med J 1982;285:249–51.
56. Aono T et al. Effect of sulpiride on poor puerperal lactation. Am J Obstet Gynecol 1982;143:927–32.
57. Polatti F. Sulpiride isomers and milk secretion in puerperium. Clin Exp Obstet Gynecol 1982;9:144–7.
58. Goldstein DJ et al. Olanzapine-exposed pregnancies and lactation: early experience. J Clin Psychopharmacol 2000;20:399–403.
59. Croke S et al. Olanzapine excretion in human breast milk: estimation of infant exposure. Int J Neuropsychopharmacol 2002;5:243–7.
60. Gardiner SJ et al. Transfer of olanzapine into breast milk, calculation of infant drug dose, and effect on breast-fed infants. Am J Psychiatry 2003;160:1428–31.
61. Ambresin G et al. Olanzapine excretion into breast milk: a case report. J Clin Psychopharmacol 2004;24:93–5.
62. Lee A et al. Excretion of quetiapine in breast milk. Am J Psychiatry 2004;161:1715–16.
63. Gentile S. Quetiapine–fluvoxamine combination during pregnancy and while breastfeeding (Letter). Arch Womens Ment Health 2006;9:158–9.
64. Misri S et al. Quetiapine augmentation in lactation: a series of case reports. J Clin Psychopharmacol 2006;26:508–11.
65. Ritz S. Quetiapine monotherapy in post-partum onset bipolar disorder with a mixed affective state. Eur Neuropsychopharmacol 2005;15(Suppl 3):S407.
66. Ratnayake T et al. No complications with risperidone treatment before and throughout pregnancy and during the nursing period. J Clin Psychiatry 2002;63:76–7.
67. Hill RC et al. Risperidone distribution and excretion into human milk: case report and estimated infant exposure during breast-feeding. J Clin Psychopharmacol 2000;20:285–6.
68. Aichhorn W et al. Risperidone and breast-feeding. J Psychopharmacol 2005;19:211–13.
69. Ilett KF et al. Transfer of risperidone and 9-hydroxyrisperidone into human milk. Ann Pharmacother 2004;38:273–6.
70. Chaudron LH et al. Mood stabilizers during breastfeeding: a review. J Clin Psychiatry 2000;61:79–90.
71. Wisner KL et al. Serum levels of valproate and carbamazepine in breastfeeding mother–infant pairs. J Clin Psychopharmacol 1998;18:167–9.
72. Ernst CL et al. The reproductive safety profile of mood stabilizers, atypical antipsychotics, and broad-spectrum psychotropics. J Clin Psychiatry 2002;63(Suppl 4):42–55.
73. Ohman I et al. Lamotrigine in pregnancy: pharmacokinetics during delivery, in the neonate, and during lactation. Epilepsia 2000;41:709–13.
74. Liporace J et al. Concerns regarding lamotrigine and breast-feeding. Epilepsy Behav 2004;5:102–5.
75. Gentile S. Lamotrigine in pregnancy and lactation (Letter). Arch Womens Ment Health 2005; 8:57–8.
76. Page-Sharp M et al. Transfer of lamotrigine into breast milk (Letter). Ann Pharmacother 2006;40:1470–1.
77. Rambeck B et al. Concentrations of lamotrigine in a mother on lamotrigine treatment and her newborn child. Eur J Clin Pharmacol 1997;51:481–4.
78. Tomson T et al. Lamotrigine in pregnancy and lactation: a case report. Epilepsia 1997;38:1039–41.
79. Moretti ME et al. Monitoring lithium in breast milk: an individualized approach for breast-feeding mothers. Ther Drug Monit 2003;25:364–6.

386

80. Piontek CM et al. Serum valproate levels in 6 breastfeeding mother–infant pairs. J Clin Psychiatry 2000;61:170–2.
81. Spigset O et al. Excretion of psychotropic drugs into breast milk: pharmacokinetic overview and therapeutic implications. CNS Drugs 1998;9:111–34.
82. Hagg S et al. Anticonvulsant use during lactation. Drug Saf 2000;22:425–40.
83. Iqbal MM et al. Effects of commonly used benzodiazepines on the fetus, the neonate, and the nursing infant. Psychiatr Serv 2002;53:39–49.
84. Buist A et al. Breastfeeding and the use of psychotropic medication: a review. J Affect Disord 1990;19: 197–206.
85. Fisher JB et al. Neonatal apnea associated with maternal clonazepam therapy: a case report. Obstet Gynecol 1985;66:34S-5S.
86. Darwish M et al. Rapid disappearance of zaleplon from breast milk after oral administration to lactating women. J Clin Pharmacol 1999;39:670–4.
87. Pons G et al. Excretion of psychoactive drugs into breast milk. Pharmacokinetic principles and recommendations. Clin Pharmacokinet 1994;27:270–89.
88. Matheson I et al. The excretion of zopiclone into breast milk. Br J Clin Pharmacol 1990;30:267–71.

Special
groups

Renal impairment

- Using drugs in patients with renal impairment can be difficult. This is because some drugs are nephrotoxic and also because pharmacokinetics (absorption, distribution, metabolism, excretion) of drugs is altered in renal impairment.
- Essentially, **patients with renal impairment have a reduced capacity to excrete drugs** and their metabolites.

Prescribing in renal impairment – general principles

1. **Estimate the excretory capacity of the kidney** by calculating the glomerular filtration rate (GFR). GFR can be directly measured by collection of urine over 24 hours or estimated in *adults* in one of 2 ways[1]: i.e. creatinine clearance (CrCl) using the Cockroft and Gault equation or estimated GFR (eGFR) using the modification of diet in renal disease (MDRD) below.

(a) Cockroft and Gault equation*

$$CrCl \text{ (ml/min)} = \frac{F(140 - \text{age (in years)}) \times \text{ideal body weight (kg)}}{\text{Serum creatinine } (\mu\text{mol/l})}$$

$F = 1.23$ (men) and 1.04 (women)
Ideal body weight should be used for patients at extremes of body weight or else the calculation is inaccurate:
For men, ideal body weight (kg) = 50 kg + 2.3 kg per inch over 5 feet
For women, ideal body weight (kg) = 45.5 kg + 2.3 kg per inch over 5 feet

*This equation is not accurate if plasma creatinine is unstable, in pregnant women, children or in diseases causing production of abnormal amounts of creatinine, and has only been validated in Caucasian patients. Creatinine clearance is less representative of GFR in severe renal failure.

When calculating drug doses, use estimated CrCl from the Cockroft and Gault equation. Do not use MDRD formula (below) for dose calculation because most current dose recommendations are based on the creatinine clearance estimations from Cockroft and Gault.

(b) Modification of diet in renal disease (MDRD) formula

- This gives an estimated GFR (eGFR) for a 1.73 m^2 body surface area. If the body surface area is greater than or less than 1.73 m^2 then eGFR is incorrect.
- Body surface area can be calculated as follows:

$$m^2 = \frac{\text{height (cm)} \times \text{weight (kg)}}{3600}$$

- The equation below is what Pathology departments use to report eGFR.
  eGFR (ml/min/1.73 m^2) = 175 × {[serum creatinine (μmol/l)/88.4]$^{-1.154}$} × {age (years)$^{-0.203}$}
  × 0.742 if female
  × 1.21 if African-American or African-Caribbean
  An online calculator is available at www.renal.org/eGFRcalc/GFR.pl
- **Use Cockroft and Gault for drug dose calculation.**

2. Classify the stage of renal impairment as below:

Stage	Description
1	Normal GFR ≥90 ml/min/1.73 m^2 **with** other evidence of chronic kidney disease*
2	Mild impairment; GFR=60–89 ml/min/1.73 m^2 **with** other evidence of kidney damage*
3	Moderate impairment, GFR=30–59 ml/min/1.73 m^2
4	Severe impairment, GFR=15–29 ml/min/1.73 m^2
5	Established renal failure, GFR < 15 ml/min/1.73 m^2 **or** on dialysis

*Other evidence of chronic kidney damage is one or more of the following; persistent microalbuminuria; persistent proteinuria; persistent haematuria; structural kidney abnormalities; biopsy-proven chronic glomerulonephritis.

3. **Elderly patients are assumed to have mild renal impairment.** Their creatinine may not be raised because they have a smaller muscle mass.
4. **Avoid drugs that are nephrotoxic** (e.g. lithium) in moderate or severe renal failure.
5. **Choose a drug that is safer to use in renal impairment** (see tables below).
6. **Be cautious when using drugs that are extensively renally cleared** (e.g. sulpiride, amisulpride, lithium).
7. **Start at a low dose and increase slowly** because, in renal impairment, the half-life of a drug and the time for it to reach steady state are often prolonged. Plasma level monitoring may be useful for some drugs.
8. **Avoid long-acting drugs** (e.g. depot preparations). Their dose and frequency cannot be easily adjusted should renal function change.

9. **Prescribe as few drugs as possible.** Patients with renal failure take many medications requiring regular review. Interactions and side-effects can be avoided if fewer drugs are used.
10. **Monitor patient for adverse effects.** Patients with renal impairment are more likely to experience side-effects and they may take longer to develop than in healthy patients. Adverse effects such as sedation, confusion and postural hypotension can be more common.
11. **Be cautious when using drugs with anticholinergic effects**, since they may cause urinary retention.
12. There are **few clinical studies** of the use of psychotropic drugs in people with renal impairment. Advice about drug use in renal impairment is often based on knowledge of the drug's pharmacokinetics in healthy patients.
13. **The effect of renal replacement therapies on drugs is difficult to predict.** Dosing advice is available from tables and data on each drug's volume of distribution and protein binding affinity. Seek specialist advice.
14. **Avoid drugs known to prolong QTc.** In established renal failure, electrolyte changes are common so best to avoid drugs with the greatest risk of QTc prolongation (see page 115).
15. **Monitor weight carefully.** Weight gain predisposes to diabetes, which can cause rhabdomyolysis[2] and renal failure. Psychotropic medication commonly causes weight gain.
16. **Be vigilant for dystonias and neuroleptic malignant syndrome (NMS),** as the resulting rhabdomyolysis can cause NMS and there are case reports of rhabdomyolysis occurring with antipsychotics without other symptoms of NMS[3-5].

Table Antipsychotics in renal impairment

Drug	Comments
Amisulpride[6-9]	Primarily renally excreted. 50% excreted unchanged in urine. Limited experience in renal disease. Manufacturer states no data with doses of >50 mg, but recommends following dosing: 50% of dose if GFR 30–60 ml/min; 33% of dose if GFR is 10–30 ml/min; no recommendations for GFR <10 ml/min so best avoided in established renal failure.
Aripiprazole[6,7]	Less than 1% of unchanged aripiprazole renally excreted. Manufacturer states no dose adjustment required in renal failure as pharmacokinetics are similar in healthy and severely renally impaired patients. However, no published studies in patients with renal disease.
Chlorpromazine[6,7,9-11]	Less than 1% excreted unchanged in urine. Manufacturer advises avoiding in renal dysfunction. Dosing: GFR 10–50 ml/min, dose as in normal renal function; GFR <10 ml/min, start with a small dose because of an increased risk of anticholinergic, sedative and hypotensive side-effects. Monitor carefully.

Clozapine[7,11–14]	Only trace amounts of unchanged clozapine excreted in urine; however, there are rare case reports of interstitial nephritis and acute renal failure. Nocturnal enuresis and urinary retention are common side-effects. Contraindicated by manufacturer in severe renal disease. Anticholinergic, sedative and hypotensive side-effects occur more frequently in patients with renal disease. Levels are useful to guide dosing. May cause and aggravate diabetes, a common cause of renal disease.
Flupentixol[6,7]	Negligible renal excretion of unchanged flupentixol. Dose adjustment may not be necessary in renal impairment. Manufacturer recommends caution in renal failure.
Fluphenazine[7]	Little information available; manufacturer contraindicates in renal insufficiency and renal failure.
Haloperidol[4,6,7,9,11,15,16]	Less than 1% excreted unchanged in the urine. Manufacturer advises caution in renal failure. Dosing: GFR 10–50 ml/min, dose as in normal renal function; GFR <10 ml/min start with a lower dose. A case report of haloperidol use in renal failure suggests starting at a low dose and increasing slowly.
Olanzapine[3,6,7,9,16]	57% of an oral dose of olanzapine is excreted, mainly as metabolites. Manufacturer recommends a starting dose of 5 mg, so start at this dose and increase with caution. May cause and aggravate diabetes, a common cause of renal disease.
Pimozide[6,7,9]	Less than 1% of pimozide is excreted unchanged in the urine; dose reductions not usually needed in renal impairment. Dosing; GFR 10–50 ml/min, dose as in normal renal function; GFR <10 ml/min start with 50% of normal dose. Manufacturer advises caution in renal dysfunction.
Quetiapine[5–7,9,17,18]	Less than 5% of quetiapine is excreted unchanged in the urine. Plasma clearance is reduced by an average of 25% in patients with a GFR <30 ml/min. In patients with GFR of <50 ml/min start at 25 mg/day and increase in daily increments of 25–50 mg to an effective dose. Two separate case reports – one of thrombotic thrombocytopenic purpura and another of non-NMS rhabdomyolyisis, both resulting in acute renal failure with quetiapine – have been described.

Table Antipsychotics in renal impairment (Cont.)

Drug	Comments
Risperidone[6,7,9,16,19,20]	Clearance of risperidone and the active metabolite of risperidone is reduced by 60% in patients with moderate to severe renal disease. Dosing: GFR<50 ml/min, 0.5 mg twice daily for at least 1 week, then increasing by 0.5 mg twice daily to 1–2 mg bd. The manufacturer advises caution when using risperidone in renal impairment. The long-acting injection should only be used after titration with oral risperidone as described above. If 2 mg orally is tolerated, 25 mg intramuscularly every 2 weeks can be administered. A case report of the successful use of risperidone in a child with steroid-induced psychosis and nephrotic syndrome has been described.
Sertindole[6,7,21]	Less than 1% of sertindole is excreted into urine. A single-dose study of sertindole found no dose adjustment needed in mild, moderate or severe renal impairment. The manufacturers state no dose adjustment needed in renal impairment.
Sulpiride[2,6,7,9,22]	Almost totally renally excreted, with 95% excreted in urine and faeces as unchanged sulpiride. Dosing regimen: GFR 30–60 ml/min, give 70% of normal dose; GFR 10–30 ml/min, give 50% of normal dose; GFR <10 ml/min, give 30% of normal dose. There is a case report of renal failure with sulpiride due to diabetic coma and rhabdomyolysis. Manufacturer contraindicates in severe renal disease. Probably best avoided in renal impairment.
Trifluoperazine[9]	Less than 1% excreted unchanged in the urine; dose as for normal renal function.
Ziprasidone[6,16,23]	<1% is renally excreted unchanged. No dose adjustment needed for GFR >10 ml/min but care needed with using the injection as it contains a renally eliminated excipient (cyclodextrin sodium).
Zotepine[6,9,24]	<0.1% is excreted as unchanged zotepine in urine. Patients with renal dysfunction have higher plasma levels than healthy patients, so start low, gradually titrate and reduce the maximum daily dose. The manufacturer suggests a starting dose of 25 mg twice daily, gradually titrating to a maximum of 75 mg twice daily in patients with established renal impairment.

Special groups

Table Antidepressants in renal impairment

Drug	Comments
Amitriptyline[6,7,9,11,16,25–27]	<10% excreted unchanged in urine; no dose adjustment needed in renal failure. Dose as in normal renal function but start at a low dose and increase slowly. Monitor patient for urinary retention, confusion, sedation and postural hypotension. Has been used to treat pain in those with renal disease. Plasma level monitoring may be useful.
Bupropion[6,7,9,11,16,28] (amfebutamone)	0.5% excreted unchanged in the urine. Dosing: GFR <50 ml/min, 150 mg once daily. A single-dose study in haemodialysis patients (stage 5 disease) recommended a dose of 150 mg every 3 days. Metabolites may accumulate in renal impairment. Elevated levels increase risk of seizures.
Citalopram[6,7,9,16,29–31]	<13% of citalopram is excreted unchanged in the urine. Single-dose studies in mild and moderate renal impairment show no change in the pharmacokinetics of citalopram. Dosing is as for normal renal function; however, use with caution if GFR <10 ml/min due to reduced clearance. The manufacturer does not advise use if GFR <20 ml/min. Renal failure has been reported with citalopram overdose.
Clomipramine[6,7,9,11]	2% of unchanged clomipramine is excreted in the urine. Dosing: GFR 20–50 ml/min, dose as for normal renal function; GFR <20 ml/min, effects unknown, start at a low dose and monitor patient for urinary retention, confusion, sedation and postural hypotension
Dosulepin[6,9,32] (dothiepin)	56% of mainly active metabolites renally excreted. They have a long half-life and may accumulate, resulting in excessive sedation. Dosing: GFR 20–50 ml/min, dose as for normal renal function; GFR <20 ml/min, start with 25 mg at night and monitor patient for urinary retention, confusion, sedation and postural hypotension.
Doxepin[6,7,9]	<1% excreted unchanged in urine. Dose as in normal renal function but monitor patient for urinary retention, confusion, sedation and postural hypotension. Manufacturer advises using with caution. Haemolytic anaemia with renal failure has been reported with doxepin.

393

Table	Antidepressants in renal impairment (Cont.)
Drug	*Comments*
Duloxetine[6,7]	Manufacturer states no dose adjustment is necessary for GFR >30 ml/min; however, starting at a low dose and increasing slowly is advised. Duloxetine is contraindicated in patients with a GFR <30 ml/min. Licensed to treat diabetic neuropathic pain. Diabetes is a common cause of renal impairment.
Escitalopram[6,7,33]	8% excreted unchanged in urine. The manufacturer states dosage adjustment is not necessary in patients with mild or moderate renal impairment but caution is advised if GFR <30 ml/min. A case study of reversible renal tubular defects has been reported with escitalopram.
Fluvoxamine[6,7,16]	Little information on its use in renal impairment. Dose as for normal renal function but start on a low dose and monitor carefully.
Fluoxetine[6,7,9,11,16,34–36]	2.5–5% of fluoxetine and 10% of the active metabolite norfluoxetine are excreted unchanged in the urine. Dosing: GFR 20–50 ml/min, dose as normal renal function; GFR <20 ml/min, dose as normal renal function or on alternate days. One small placebo-controlled study of fluoxetine in patients on chronic dialysis found no significant differences in depression scores between the two groups.
Imipramine[6,7,9,11,25]	<5% excreted unchanged in the urine. No specific dose adjustment necessary in renal impairment. Monitor patient for urinary retention, confusion, sedation and postural hypotension. Renal impairment with imipramine has been reported and manufacturer advises caution in severe renal impairment. Renal damage reported rarely.
Lofepramine[6,7,37]	There is little information about the use of lofepramine in renal impairment. Most lofepramine is excreted in the urine along with some as the active metabolite desipramine. Desipramine has a long half-life (12–24 hours) and can accumulate, so avoid in renal impairment. Manufacturer contraindicates in severe renal disease and cautions in non-severe renal impairment.
Mirtazapine[6,7,9,38]	75% excreted unchanged in the urine. Clearance is reduced by 30% in patients with a GFR of 11–39 ml/min and by 50% in patients with a GFR <10 ml/min. Dosing advice: GFR 20–50 ml/min, dose as for normal renal function; GFR <10 ml/min, start at a low dose and monitor closely. Mirtazapine has been used to treat pruritus

	caused by renal failure and is associated with kidney calculus formation.
Moclobemide[6,7,39,40]	<1% of parent drug excreted unchanged in the urine. However, an active metabolite was found to be raised in patients with renal impairment but was not thought to affect dosing. The manufacturer advises that dose adjustments are not required in renal impairment.
Nortriptyline[6,9,16,25,41]	If GFR 10–50 ml/min, dose as in normal renal function; if GFR <10 ml/min, start at a low dose. Plasma level monitoring recommended at doses of >100 mg/day, as plasma concentrations of active metabolites are raised in renal impairment. Worsening of GFR in elderly patients has also been reported. Plasma level monitoring can be useful.
Paroxetine[6,7,9,11,42–45]	Less than 2% of oral dose is excreted unchanged in the urine. Single-dose studies show increased plasma concentrations of paroxetine when GFR <30 ml/min. Start at 10 mg/day if GFR <30 ml/min and increase dose according to response. Paroxetine 10 mg daily and psychotherapy have been used successfully to treat depression in patients on chronic haemodialysis. Rarely associated with Fanconi syndrome.
Phenelzine[6,9]	Approximately 1% excreted unchanged in the urine. No dose adjustment required in renal failure.
Reboxetine[6,7,9,46,47]	Approximately 10% of unchanged drug is excreted unchanged in the urine. Dosing: GFR <20 ml/min, 2 mg twice daily, adjusting dose according to response. Half-life is prolonged as renal function decreases.
Sertraline[6,7,9,11,48]	<0.2% of unchanged sertraline excreted in urine. Pharmacokinetics in renal impairment unchanged in single-dose studies but no published data on multiple dosing. Dosing is as for normal renal function. Sertraline has been used to treat dialysis-associated hypotension; however, acute renal failure has been reported so it should be used with caution.
Trazodone[6,7,9,11,49]	<5% excreted unchanged in urine but care needed as approximately 70% of active metabolite also excreted. Dosing: GFR 20–50 ml/min, dose as normal renal function; GFR 10–20 ml/min, dose as normal renal function but start with small dose and increase gradually; GFR 10 ml/min, avoid or use half the dose or halve frequency.

Table Antidepressants in renal impairment (Cont.)

Drug	Comments
Trimipramine[6,11,25,50,51]	No dose reduction required in renal impairment; however, elevated urea and interstitial nephritis have been reported. As with all tricyclic antidepressants, monitor patient for urinary retention, confusion, sedation and postural hypotension as patients with renal impairment are at increased risk of having these side-effects.
Venlafaxine[6,7,11,52–54]	1–10% is excreted unchanged in the urine (30% as the active metabolite). Clearance is decreased and half-life prolonged in renal impairment. Dosing advice differs: GFR 30–50 ml/min, dose as in normal renal function or reduce by 50%; GFR 10–30 ml/min, reduce dose by 50% and give once daily; GFR <10 ml/min, reduce dose by 50% and give once daily; however, manufacturer advises avoiding use in these patients. Avoid using the XL preparation if GFR <30 ml/min. Rhabdomyolysis and renal failure have been reported rarely with venlafaxine

Table Mood stabilisers in renal impairment

Drug	Comments
Carbamazepine[6,7,9,55–60]	2–3% of the dose is excreted unchanged in urine. Dose reduction is not necessary in renal disease, although cases of renal failure, tubular necrosis and tubulointerstitial nephritis have been reported rarely.
Lamotrigine[6,7,9,61–64]	<10% of lamotrigine is excreted unchanged in the urine. Single-dose studies in renal failure show pharmacokinetics are little affected; however, inactive metabolites can accumulate (effects unknown) and half-life can be prolonged. Renal failure and interstitial nephritis have also been reported. Dosing: GFR <10–50 ml/min, use cautiously, start with a low dose, increase slowly and monitor closely.
Lithium[6,7,9,11,65,66]	Lithium is nephrotoxic and contraindicated in severe renal impairment; 95% is excreted unchanged in the urine. Long-term treatment may result in impaired renal function ('creeping creatinine') and both reversible and irreversible kidney damage. If lithium is used in renal impairment, toxicity is more likely. The maufacturer

Table	Mood stabilisers in renal impairment (Cont.)
Drug	**Comments**
	contraindicates lithium in renal impairment. Dosing: GFR 10–50 ml/min, avoid or reduce dose (50–75% of normal dose) and monitor levels; GFR <10 ml/min, avoid if possible; however, if used, it is essential to reduce dose (25–50% of normal dose). Renal damage is more likely with chronic toxicity than acute.
Valproate[6,7,9,67–73]	Approximately 2% excreted unchanged. Dose adjustment is usually not required in renal impairment; however, free valproate levels may be increased. Renal impairment, interstitial nephritis, Fanconi syndrome, renal tubular acidosis and renal failure have been reported. Dose as in normal renal function; however, in severe impairment it may be necessary to alter doses according to free (unbound) valproate levels.

Table	Anxiolytics and hypnotics in renal impairment
Drug	**Comments**
Buspirone[6,7,9,11]	Less than 1% is excreted unchanged; however, active metabolite is renally excreted. Dosing advice contradictory; suggest: GFR 10–50 ml/min, dose as normal; GFR <10 ml/min, avoid if possible due to accumulation of active metabolites; if essential, reduce dose by 25–50% if patient is anuric.
Clomethiazole[6,7,9,74] (chlormethiazole)	0.1–5% of unchanged drug excreted unchanged in urine. Dose as in normal renal function but monitor for excessive sedation. Manufacturer recommends caution in renal disease.
Chlordiazepoxide[7,9,11]	<5% excreted unchanged but chlordiazepoxide has a long-acting active metabolite that can accumulate. Dosing: GFR 10–50 ml/min, dose as normal renal function; GFR <10 ml/min, reduce dose by 50%. Monitor for excessive sedation.
Clonazepam[6,7,9,11]	<1% of clonazepam excreted unchanged in urine. Dose adjustment not required in impaired renal function; however, with long-term administration, active metabolites may accumulate so lower doses may be needed. Monitor for excessive sedation.

Table Anxiolytics and hypnotics in renal impairment (Cont.)

Drug	Comments
Diazepam[6,9,11,75]	Less than 1% is excreted unchanged. Dosing: GFR 20–50 ml/min, dose as in normal renal function; GFR <20 ml/min, use small doses and titrate to response. Long-acting, active metabolites accumulate in renal impairment; monitor patients for excessive sedation and encephalopathy. One case of interstitial nephritis with diazepam has been reported in a patient with chronic renal failure.
Lorazepam[6,7,9,11,76–79]	<5% excreted unchanged in urine, dose as in normal renal function but carefully according to response as some may need lower doses. Monitor for excessive sedation. Impaired elimination reported in two patients with severe renal impairment and also reports of propylene glycol in lorazepam injection causing renal impairment and acute tubular necrosis.
Nitrazepam[7,9]	Less than 5% excreted unchanged in the urine. Dosing: GFR 10–50 ml/min, as in normal renal function; GFR <10 ml/min, start with small dose and increase slowly. Manufacturer advises halving dose in renal impairment. Monitor patient for sedation.
Oxazepam[6,9,11,80]	Less than 1% excreted unchanged in the urine. Dose adjustment needed in severe renal impairment. Oxazepam may take longer to reach steady state in patients with renal impairment. Dosing: GFR 10–50 ml/min, dose as in normal renal function; GFR <10 ml/min, 10–20 mg three or four times a day. Monitor for excessive sedation.
Promethazine[6,7,9,11]	Dose reduction usually not necessary; however, promethazine has a long half-life so monitor for excessive sedative effects in patients with renal impairment. Manufacturer advises caution in renal impairment.
Temazepam[6,7,9,11]	<2% excreted unchanged in urine. In renal impairment the inactive metabolite can accumulate. Monitor for excessive sedative effects. Dosing: GFR 20–50 ml/min, dose as normal renal function; GFR 10–20 ml/min, start with small doses, maximum 20 mg/day; GFR <10 ml/min, start with small doses, maximum 10 mg daily.
Zaleplon[6,7,81,82]	<0.1% excreted unchanged in the urine. In renal impairment inactive metabolites accumulate. No dose adjustment appears to be necessary in patients with a GFR >20 ml/min. Zaleplon is not recommended if GFR <20 ml/min; however, it has been used in patients on haemodialysis.

Table Anxiolytics and hypnotics in renal impairment (Cont.)

Drug	Comments
Zolpidem[6,7,9,81]	Clearance moderately reduced in renal impairment. No dose adjustment required in renal impairment; however, there are no published studies of zolpidem in severe renal impairment.
Zopiclone[6,7,9,83,84]	5–11% excreted unchanged in urine. Manufacturer states no accumulation of zopiclone in renal impairment but suggests starting at 3.75 mg in those with GFR <10 ml/min. Can cause interstitial nephritis rarely.

Summary – psychotropics in renal impairment

Drug group	Recommended drugs
Antipsychotics	No agent clearly preferred, however: • avoid sulpiride and amisulpride • avoid highly anticholinergic agents because they may cause urinary retention • First-generation antipsychotic – suggest **haloperidol** 2–6 mg/day • Second-generation antipsychotic – suggest **olanzapine** 5 mg/day
Antidepressants	No agent clearly preferred, however: • **citalopram** and **sertraline** are suggested as reasonable choices
Mood stabilisers	No agent clearly preferred to another, however: • avoid lithium • suggest start one of the following at a low dose and increase slowly, monitoring for adverse effects: **valproate**, **carbamazepine** or **lamotrigine**
Anxiolytics and hypnotics	No agent clearly preferred to another, however: • excessive sedation is more likely to occur in patients with renal impairment, so monitor all patients carefully • **lorazepam** and **zopiclone** are suggested as reasonable choices

Special groups

References

1. Devaney A et al. Chronic kidney disease – new approaches to classification. Hospital Pharmacist 2006; 13:410.
2. Toprak O et al. New-onset type II diabetes mellitus, hyperosmolar non-ketotic coma, rhabdomyolysis and acute renal failure in a patient treated with sulpiride. Nephrol Dial Transplant 2005;20:662–3.
3. Baumgart U et al. Olanzapine-induced acute rhabdomyolysis – a case report. Pharmacopsychiatry 2005; 38:36–7.
4. Marsh SJ et al. Rhabdomyolysis and acute renal failure during high-dose haloperidol therapy. Ren Fail 1995;17:475–8.
5. Smith RP et al. Quetiapine overdose and severe rhabdomyolysis. J Clin Psychopharmacol 2004;24:343.
6. Micromedex Inc. DRUGDEX® System. Englewood, Colorado, Fourth quarter: 2006.
7. Datapharm Communications Ltd. Electronic Medicines Compendium. http://medguides.medicines.org.uk/. 2006.
8. Noble S et al. Amisulpride: a review of its clinical potential in dysthymia. CNS Drugs 1999;12:471–83.
9. Ashley C, Currie A. The Renal Drug Handbook, 2nd edn. Oxford: Radcliffe Publishing, 2003.
10. Fabre J et al. Influence of renal insufficiency on the excretion of chloroquine, phenobarbital, phenothiazines and methacycline. Helv Med Acta 1967;33:307–16.
11. Aronoff GR et al. Drug Prescribing in Renal Failure: Dosing Guidelines for Adults. Philadelphia: American College of Physicians, 1999.
12. Fraser D et al. An unexpected and serious complication of treatment with the atypical antipsychotic drug clozapine. Clin Nephrol 2000;54:78–80.
13. Elias TJ et al. Clozapine-induced acute interstitial nephritis. Lancet 1999;354:1180–1.
14. Au AF et al. Clozapine-induced acute interstitial nephritis. Am J Psychiatry 2004;161:1501.
15. Lobeck F et al. Haloperidol concentrations in an elderly patient with moderate chronic renal failure. J Geriatr Drug Ther 1986;1:91–7.
16. Cohen LM et al. Update on psychotropic medication use in renal disease. Psychosomatics 2004; 45:34–48.
17. Thyrum PT et al. Single-dose pharmacokinetics of quetiapine in subjects with renal or hepatic impairment. Prog Neuropsychopharmacol Biol Psychiatry 2000;24:521–33.
18. Huynh M et al. Thrombotic thrombocytopenic purpura associated with quetiapine. Ann Pharmacother 2005;39:1346–8.
19. Snoeck E et al. Influence of age, renal and liver impairment on the pharmacokinetics of risperidone in man. Psychopharmacology 1995;122:223–9.
20. Herguner S et al. Steroid-induced psychosis in an adolescent: treatment and prophylaxis with risperidone. Turk J Pediatr 2006;48:244–7.
21. Wong SL et al. Pharmacokinetics of sertindole and dehydrosertindole in volunteers with normal or impaired renal function. Eur J Clin Pharmacol 1997;52:223–7.
22. Bressolle F et al. Pharmacokinetics of sulpiride after intravenous administration in patients with impaired renal function. Clin Pharmacokinet 1989;17:367–73.
23. Aweeka F et al. The pharmacokinetics of ziprasidone in subjects with normal and impaired renal function. Br J Clin Pharmacol 2000;49:27S–33S.
24. Healthcare Logistics. Zoleptil – Combined summary of product characteristics. 2003.
25. Lieberman JA et al. Tricyclic antidepressant and metabolite levels in chronic renal failure. Clin Pharmacol Ther 1985;37:301–7.
26. Murphy EJ. Acute pain management pharmacology for the patient with concurrent renal or hepatic disease. Anaesth Intensive Care 2005;33:311–22.
27. Mitas JA et al. Diabetic neuropathic pain: control by amitriptyline and fluphenazine in renal insufficiency. South Med J 1983;76:462–3,467.
28. Worrall SP et al. Pharmacokinetics of bupropion and its metabolites in haemodialysis patients who smoke. A single dose study. Nephron Clin Pract 2004;97:c83–c89.
29. Spigset O et al. Citalopram pharmacokinetics in patients with chronic renal failure and the effect of haemodialysis. Eur J Clin Pharmacol 2000;56:699–703.
30. Joffe P et al. Single-dose pharmacokinetics of citalopram in patients with moderate renal insufficiency or hepatic cirrhosis compared with healthy subjects. Eur J Clin Pharmacol 1998;54:237–42.
31. Kelly CA et al. Adult respiratory distress syndrome and renal failure associated with citalopram overdose. Hum Exp Toxicol 2003;22:103–5.
32. Rees JA. Clinical interpretation of pharmacokinetic data on dothiepin hydrochloride (Dosulepin, Prothiaden). J Int Med Res 1981;9:98–102.
33. Adiga GU et al. Renal tubular defects from antidepressant use in an older adult: an uncommon but reversible adverse drug effect. Clin Drug Investig 2006;26:607–10.
34. Blumenfield M et al. Fluoxetine in depressed patients on dialysis. Int J Psychiatry Med 1997;27:71–80.
35. Bergstrom RF et al. The effects of renal and hepatic disease on the pharmacokinetics, renal tolerance, and risk–benefit profile of fluoxetine. Int Clin Psychopharmacol 1993;8:261–6.
36. Rabindranath KS et al. Physical measures for treating depression in dialysis patients. Cochrane Database Syst Rev 2005;CD004541.
37. Lancaster SG et al. Lofepramine. A review of its pharmacodynamic and pharmacokinetic properties, and therapeutic efficacy in depressive illness. Drugs 1989;37:123–40.
38. Davis MP et al. Mirtazapine for pruritus. J Pain Symptom Manage 2003;25:288–91.

39. Schoerlin MP et al. Disposition kinetics of moclobemide, a new MAO-A inhibitor, in subjects with impaired renal function. J Clin Pharmacol 1990;30:272–84.
40. Stoeckel K et al. Absorption and disposition of moclobemide in patients with advanced age or reduced liver or kidney function. Acta Psychiatr Scand Suppl 1990;360:94–7.
41. Pollock BG et al. Metabolic and physiologic consequences of nortriptyline treatment in the elderly. Psychopharmacol Bull 1994;30:145–50.
42. Doyle GD et al. The pharmacokinetics of paroxetine in renal impairment. Acta Psychiatr Scand Suppl 1989;350:89–90.
43. Kaye CM et al. A review of the metabolism and pharmacokinetics of paroxetine in man. Acta Psychiatr Scand Suppl 1989;350:60–75.
44. Koo JR et al. Treatment of depression and effect of antidepression treatment on nutritional status in chronic hemodialysis patients. Am J Med Sci 2005;329:1–5.
45. Ishii T et al. A rare case of combined syndrome of inappropriate antidiuretic hormone secretion and Fanconi syndrome in an elderly woman. Am J Kidney Dis 2006;48:155–8.
46. Coulomb F et al. Pharmacokinetics of single-dose reboxetine in volunteers with renal insufficiency. J Clin Pharmacol 2000;40:482–7.
47. Dostert P et al. Review of the pharmacokinetics and metabolism of reboxetine, a selective noradrenaline reuptake inhibitor. Eur Neuropsychopharmacol 1997;7(Suppl 1):S23–S35.
48. Brewster UC et al. Addition of sertraline to other therapies to reduce dialysis-associated hypotension. Nephrology (Carlton) 2003;8:296–301.
49. Catanese B et al. A comparative study of trazodone serum concentrations in patients with normal or impaired renal function. Boll Chim Farm 1978;117:424–7.
50. Simpson GM et al. A preliminary study of trimipramine in chronic schizophrenia. Curr Ther Res Clin Exp 1966;99:248.
51. Leighton JD et al. Trimipramine-induced acute renal failure (Letter). N Z Med J 1986;99:248.
52. Troy SM et al. The effect of renal disease on the disposition of venlafaxine. Clin Pharmacol Ther 1994;56:14–21.
53. Pascale P et al. Severe rhabdomyolysis following venlafaxine overdose. Ther Drug Monit 2005;27:562–4.
54. Guldiken S et al. Complete relief of pain in acute painful diabetic neuropathy of rapid glycaemic control (insulin neuritis) with venlafaxine HCl. Diabetes Nutr Metab 2004;17:247–9.
55. Verrotti A et al. Renal tubular function in patients receiving anticonvulsant therapy: a long-term study. Epilepsia 2000;41:1432–5.
56. Hogg RJ et al. Carbamazepine-induced acute tubulointerstitial nephritis. J Pediatr 1981;98:830–2.
57. Hegarty J et al. Carbamazepine-induced acute granulomatous interstitial nephritis. Clin Nephrol 2002;57:310–13.
58. Nicholls DP et al. Acute renal failure from carbamazepine (Letter). Br Med J 1972;4:490.
59. Jubert P et al. Carbamazepine-induced acute renal failure. Nephron 1994;66:121.
60. Imai H et al. Carbamazepine-induced granulomatous necrotizing angiitis with acute renal failure. Nephron 1989;51:405–8.
61. Fillastre JP et al. Pharmacokinetics of lamotrigine in patients with renal impairment: influence of haemodialysis. Drugs Exp Clin Res 1993;19:25–32.
62. Wootton R et al. Comparison of the pharmacokinetics of lamotrigine in patients with chronic renal failure and healthy volunteers. Br J Clin Pharmacol 1997;43:23–7.
63. Schaub JE et al. Multisystem adverse reaction to lamotrigine. Lancet 1994;344:481.
64. Fervenza FC et al. Acute granulomatous interstitial nephritis and colitis in anticonvulsant hypersensitivity syndrome associated with lamotrigine treatment. Am J Kidney Dis 2000;36:1034–40.
65. Gitlin M. Lithium and the kidney: an updated review. Drug Saf 1999;20:231–43.
66. Lepkifker E et al. Renal insufficiency in long-term lithium treatment. J Clin Psychiatry 2004;65:850–6.
67. Smith GC et al. Anticonvulsants as a cause of Fanconi syndrome. Nephrol Dial Transplant 1995;10:543–5.
68. Fukuda Y et al. Immunologically mediated chronic tubulo-interstitial nephritis caused by valproate therapy. Nephron 1996;72:328–9.
69. Zaki EL et al. Renal injury from valproic acid: case report and literature review. Pediatr Neurol 2002;27:318–19.
70. Tanaka H et al. Distal type of renal tubular acidosis after anti-epileptic therapy in a girl with infantile spasms. Clin Exp Nephrol 1999;3:311–13.
71. Knorr M et al. Fanconi syndrome caused by antiepileptic therapy with valproic acid. Epilepsia 2004;45:868–71.
72. Watanabe T et al. Secondary renal Fanconi syndrome caused by valproate therapy. Pediatr Nephrol 2005;20:814–17.
73. Rahman MH et al. Acute hemolysis with acute renal failure in a patient with valproic acid poisoning treated with charcoal hemoperfusion. Hemodial Int 2006;10:256–9.
74. Pentikainen PJ et al. Pharmacokinetics of chlormethiazole in healthy volunteers and patients with cirrhosis of the liver. Eur J Clin Pharmacol 1980;17:275–84.
75. Sadjadi SA et al. Allergic interstitial nephritis due to diazepam. Arch Intern Med 1987;147:579.
76. Verbeeck RK et al. Impaired elimination of lorazepam following subchronic administration in two patients with renal failure. Br J Clin Pharmacol 1981;12:749–51.

77. Reynolds HN et al. Hyperlactatemia, increased osmolar gap, and renal dysfunction during continuous lorazepam infusion. Crit Care Med 2000;28:1631–4.
78. Yaucher NE et al. Propylene glycol-associated renal toxicity from lorazepam infusion. Pharmacotherapy 2003;23:1094–9.
79. Hayman M et al. Acute tubular necrosis associated with propylene glycol from concomitant administration of intravenous lorazepam and trimethoprim–sulfamethoxazole. Pharmacotherapy 2003;23:1190–4.
80. Murray TG et al. Renal disease, age, and oxazepam kinetics. Clin Pharmacol Ther 1981;30:805–9.
81. Drover DR. Comparative pharmacokinetics and pharmacodynamics of short-acting hypnosedatives: zaleplon, zolpidem and zopiclone. Clin Pharmacokinet 2004;43:227–38.
82. Sabbatini M et al. Zaleplon improves sleep quality in maintenance hemodialysis patients. Nephron Clin Pract 2003;94:c99–103.
83. Goa KL et al. Zopiclone. A review of its pharmacodynamic and pharmacokinetic properties and therapeutic efficacy as an hypnotic. Drugs 1986;32:48–65.
84. Hussain N et al. Zopiclone-induced acute interstitial nephritis. Am J Kidney Dis 2003;41:E17.

Hepatic impairment

Patients with hepatic impairment may have:

- **reduced capacity to metabolise** biological waste products, dietary proteins and foreign substances such as drugs. Clinical consequences include hepatic encephalopathy and increased dose-related side-effects from drugs.

- **reduced ability to synthesise** plasma proteins and vitamin K-dependent clotting factors. Clinical consequences include hypoalbuminaemia, leading in extreme cases to ascites. Increased toxicity from highly protein-bound drugs should be anticipated. There is also an increased risk of bleeding from GI irritant drugs and perhaps with SSRIs.

- **reduced hepatic blood flow.** Clinical consequences include oesophageal varices and elevated plasma levels of drugs subject to first-pass metabolism.

General principles

Liver function tests (LFTs) are a poor marker of hepatic metabolising capacity, as the hepatic reserve is large. Note that many patients with chronic liver disease are asymptomatic or have fluctuating clinical symptoms. Always consider the clinical presentation rather than adhere to rigid rules involving LFTs.

There are few clinical studies relating to the use of psychotropic drugs in people with hepatic disease. The following principles should be adhered to:

1. Prescribe as **few drugs** as possible.
2. Use **lower starting doses**, particularly of drugs that are highly protein bound. TCAs, SSRIs (except citalopram), trazodone and antipsychotics may have increased free plasma levels, at least initially. This will not be reflected in measured (total) plasma levels. Use lower doses of drugs known to be subject to extensive first-pass metabolism. Examples include TCAs and haloperidol.
3. Be **cautious with drugs that are extensively hepatically metabolised** (most psychotropic drugs). Lower doses may be required. Exceptions are sulpiride, amisulpride, lithium and gabapentin, which all undergo no or minimal hepatic metabolism.
4. **Leave longer intervals between dosage increases.** Remember that the half-life of most drugs is prolonged in hepatic impairment, so it will take longer for plasma levels to reach steady state.
5. Always **monitor carefully for side-effects**, which may be delayed.
6. **Avoid drugs that are very sedative** because of the risk of precipitating hepatic encephalopathy.
7. **Avoid drugs that are very constipating** because of the risk of precipitating hepatic encephalopathy.
8. **Avoid drugs that are known to be hepatotoxic** in their own right (e.g. MAOIs, chlorpromazine).
9. **Choose a low-risk drug** (see tables below) and monitor LFTs weekly, at least initially. If LFTs deteriorate after a new drug is introduced, consider switching to another drug.

These rules should always be observed in severe liver disease (low albumin, increased clotting time, ascites, jaundice, encephalopathy, etc.). The information above and on the following pages should be interpreted in the context of the patient's clinical presentation.

Table Antipsychotics in hepatic impairment

Drug	Comments
Amisulpride[1,2]	Predominantly renally excreted, so dosage reduction should not be necessary as long as renal function is normal but there are no clinical studies in people with hepatic impairment and little clinical experience. Caution required
Aripiprazole[1]	Extensively hepatically metabolised. Limited data that hepatic impairment has minimal effect on pharmacokinetics. SPC states no dosage reduction required in mild–moderate hepatic impairment, but caution required in severe impairment. Limited clinical experience. Caution required
Clozapine[1–5]	Very sedative and constipating. Contraindicated in active liver disease associated with nausea, anorexia or jaundice, progressive liver disease or hepatic failure. In less severe disease, start with 12.5 mg and increase slowly, using plasma levels to gauge metabolising capacity and guide dosage adjustment. Transient elevations in AST, ALT and GGT to over twice the normal range occur in over 10% of physically healthy people. Clozapine-induced hepatitis, jaundice, cholestasis and liver failure have been reported
Flupentixol/ zuclopenthixol[1,2,6,7]	Both are extensively hepatically metabolised. Small, transient elevations in transaminases have been reported in some patients treated with zuclopenthixol. No other literature reports of use or harm. Both drugs have been in use for many years. Depot preparations are best avoided, as altered pharmacokinetics will make dosage adjustment difficult and side-effects from dosage accumulation more likely
Haloperidol[1,8]	Drug of choice in clinical practice and no problems reported although UK SPC states 'caution in liver disease'. Isolated reports of cholestatic hepatitis
Olanzapine[1,2,9–12]	Although extensively hepatically metabolised, the pharmacokinetics of olanzapine seem to change little in severe hepatic impairment. It is sedative and anticholinergic (can cause constipation) so caution is advised. Start with 5 mg/day and consider using plasma levels to guide dosage (aim for 20–40 μg/l).

Special groups

Table	Antipsychotics in hepatic impairment (Cont.)
	Dose-related, transient, asymptomatic elevations in ALT and AST reported in physically healthy adults. People with liver disease may be at increased risk. Rare cases of hepatitis in the literature
Phenothiazines[1,2,13–15]	All cause sedation and constipation. Associated with cholestasis and some reports of fulminant hepatic cirrhosis. Best avoided completely in hepatic impairment. Chlorpromazine is particularly hepato-toxic
Quetiapine[1,2,16–19]	Extensively hepatically metabolised but short half-life. One single-dose, kinetic study suggests that no change in starting dose is required. Clearance reduced by a mean of 30% in hepatic impairment so small dosage adjustments may be required. Can cause sedation and constipation. Little clinical experience in hepatic impairment so caution recom-mended. One case of fatal hepatic failure reported in the literature
Risperidone[1,2,20–25]	Highly protein bound. Manufacturers recommend a maximum dose of 4 mg in hepatic impairment. Transient, asymptomatic elevations in LFTs, cholestatic hepatitis and rare cases of hepatic failure have been reported. Steatohepatitis may arise as a result of weight gain. Clinical experience limited in hepatic impairment so caution recommended
Sulpiride[1,2,26,27]	Almost completely renally excreted with a low potential to cause sedation or constipation. Dosage reduction should not be required. Some clinical experience in hepatic impairment with few problems. Fairly old established drug. Isolated case reports of cholestatic jaundice and primary biliary cirrhosis. SPC states contraindicated in severe hepatic disease

Special groups

Table Antidepressants in hepatic impairment

Drug	Comments
Fluoxetine[1,2,28–32]	Extensively hepatically metabolised with a long half-life. Kinetic studies demonstrate accumulation in compensated cirrhosis. Although dosage reduction (of at least 50%) or alternate day dosing could be used, it would take many weeks to reach steady-state serum levels, making fluoxetine complex to use. Asymptomatic increases in LFTs found in 0.5% of healthy adults. Rare cases of hepatitis reported
Other SSRIs[1,2,32–41]	All are hepatically metabolised and accumulate on chronic dosing. Dosage reduction may be required. Raised LFTs and rare cases of hepatitis, including chronic active hepatitis, have been reported with paroxetine. Sertraline and fluvoxamine have also been associated with hepatitis. Citalopram has minimal effects on hepatic enzymes and may be the SSRI of choice although clinical experience is limited and occasional hepatotoxicity has been reported. Paroxetine is used by some specialised liver units with few apparent problems
Tricyclics[1,2,42]	All are hepatically metabolised, highly protein bound and will accumulate. They vary in their propensity to cause sedation and constipation. All are associated with raised LFTs and rare cases of hepatitis. There is most clinical experience with imipramine. Sedative TCAs such as trimipramine, (dosulepin) dothiepin and amitriptyline are best avoided. Lofepramine is possibly the most hepatotoxic and should be avoided completely
Venlafaxine[1,2,43,44]	Dosage reduction of 50% advised in moderate hepatic impairment. Little clinical experience. Rare cases of hepatitis reported. Caution advised
MAOIs[1,2,45,46]	People with hepatic impairment reported to be more sensitive to the side-effects of MAOIs. MAOIs are also more hepatotoxic than other antidepressants, so best avoided completely
Moclobemide[1,2,47,48]	Clinical experience limited but probably safer than the irreversible MAOIs. 50% reduction in dose advised by manufacturers. Rare cases of hepatotoxicity reported. Caution advised
Reboxetine[1,2,49]	50% reduction in starting dose recommended. Clinical experience limited. Does not seem to be associated with hepatotoxicity. Caution advised
Mirtazapine[1,2]	Hepatically metabolised and sedative. 50% dose reduction recommended based on kinetic data, but clinical experience limited. Mild, asymptomatic increases in LFTs seen in healthy adults. Caution advised

Special groups

406

Table	Antidepressants in hepatic impairment (Cont.)
Duloxetine[1,2,50]	Hepatically metabolised. Clearance markedly reduced even in mild impairment. Reports of hepatocellular injury and, less commonly, jaundice. Isolated case report of fulminant hepatic failure. Limited experience. Best avoided

Table Mood stabilisers in hepatic impairment

Drug	Comments
Carbamazepine[1,2,51-54]	Extensively hepatically metabolised and potent inducer of CYP450 enzymes. Contraindicated in acute liver disease. In chronic stable disease, caution advised. Reduce starting dose by 50%, and titrate up slowly, using plasma levels to guide dosage. Stop if LFTs deteriorate. Associated with hepatitis, cholangitis, cholestatic and hepatocellular jaundice, and hepatic failure (rare). Adverse hepatic effects are most common in the first month of treatment
Lamotrigine[1,2,54,55]	Manufacturers recommend 50% reduction in initial dose, dose escalation and maintenance dose in moderate hepatic impairment and 75% in severe lamotrigine-induced rash (which can be serious). Extreme caution advised, particularly if co-prescribed with valproate. Elevated LFTs and hepatitis reported
Lithium[1,2,56,57]	Not metabolised, so dosage reduction not required as long as renal function is normal. Use serum levels to guide dosage and monitor more frequently if ascites status changes (volume of distribution will change). One case of ascites and one of hyperbilirubinaemia reported over many decades of lithium use worldwide
Valproate[1,2,54,58-60]	Highly protein bound and hepatically metabolised. Dosage reduction with close monitoring of LFTs in moderate hepatic impairment. Use plasma levels (free levels if possible) to guide dosage. Caution advised. Contraindicated in severe and/or active hepatic impairment; impairment of usual metabolic pathway can lead to generation of hepatotoxic metabolites via alternative pathway. Associated with elevated LFTs and serious hepatotoxicity including fulminant hepatic failure. Mitochondrial disease, learning disability, polypharmacy, metabolic disorders and underlying hepatic disease may be risk factors. Particularly hepatotoxic in very young children. The greatest risk is in the first 3 months of treatment

Summary – psychotropics in hepatic impairment	
Drug group	**Recommended drugs**
Antipsychotics	**Haloperidol**: low dose *or* **Sulpiride/amisulpride**: no dosage reduction required if renal function is normal
Antidepressants	**Imipramine**: start with 25 mg/day and titrate slowly (weekly at most) if required *or* **Paroxetine** or **citalopram**: start at 10 mg if severe hepatic impairment. Titrate slowly (if required) as above
Mood stabilisers	**Lithium**: use plasma levels to guide dosage. Care needed if ascites status changes
Sedatives	**Lorazepam**, **oxazepam**, **temazepam**: as short half-life with no active metabolites Use low doses with caution, as sedative drugs can precipitate hepatic encephalopathy **Zopiclone**: 3.75 mg with care in moderate hepatic impairment

Drug-induced hepatic damage

This can be due to:

- Direct dose-related hepatotoxicity (Type 1 Adverse drug reaction (ADR)). A small number of drugs fall into this category, e.g. paracetamol; alcohol.
- Hypersensitivity reactions (Type 2 ADR). These can present with rash, fever and eosinophilia. Almost all drugs have been associated with cases of heptatoxicity; frequency varies.

Almost any type of liver damage can occur, ranging from mild transient asymptomatic increases in LFTs to fulminant hepatic failure. (See tables on pages 402–408 for details of the hepatotoxic potential of individual drugs.)

Risk factors for drug-induced hepatotoxicity include[61]:

- increasing age
- female gender
- alcohol consumption
- co-prescription of enzyme-inducing drugs
- genetic predisposition
- obesity
- pre-existing liver disease (small effect).

When interpreting LFTs, remember that[61]:

- 12% of the healthy adult population have one LFT outside (above or below) the normal reference range.
- Up to 10% of patients with clinically significant hepatic disease have normal LFTs.
- Individual LFTs lack specificity for the liver, but >1 abnormal test greatly increases the likelihood of liver pathology.
- The absolute values of LFTs are a poor indicator of disease severity.

When monitoring LFTs:

- Ideally, LFTs should be measured before treatment starts so that 'baseline' values are available.
- LFT elevations of <2 times the upper limit of the normal reference range are rarely clinically significant.
- Most drug-related LFT elevations occur early in treatment (first month) and are transient. They may indicate adaptation of the liver to the drug rather than damaged per se.
- If LFTs are persistently elevated >threefold, continuing to rise or accompanied by clinical symptoms, the suspected drugs should be withdrawn.
- When tracking change, >20% change in liver enzymes is required to exclude biological or analytical variation.

References

1. Datapharm Communications Ltd. Electronic Medicines Compendium: http://medguides.medicines.org.uk/. 2006.
2. DRUGDEX® System [database on CD-ROM]. Version 5.1. Greenwood Village, Colorado: Thomson Micromedex, 2005.
3. Hummer M et al. Hepatotoxicity of clozapine. J Clin Psychopharmacol 1997;17:314–17.
4. Kellner M et al. Toxic hepatitis by clozapine treatment. Am J Psychiatry 1993;150:985–6.
5. Thatcher GW et al. Clozapine-induced toxic hepatitis. Am J Psychiatry 1995;152:296–7.
6. Amdisen A et al. Zuclopenthixol acetate in Viscoleo – a new drug formulation. An open Nordic multi-centre study of zuclopenthixol acetate in Viscoleo in patients with acute psychoses including mania and exacerbation of chronic psychoses. Acta Psychiatr Scand 1987;75:99–107.
7. Wistedt B et al. Zuclopenthixol decanoate and haloperidol decanoate in chronic schizophrenia: a double-blind multicentre study. Acta Psychiatr Scand 1991;84:14–21.
8. Ozcanli T et al. Severe liver enzyme elevations after three years of olanzapine treatment: a case report and review of olanzapine associated hepatotoxicity. Prog Neuropsychopharmacol Biol Psychiatry 2006;30:1163–6.
9. Beasley CM Jr. et al. Safety of olanzapine. J Clin Psychiatry 1997;58(Suppl 10):13–17.
10. Kolpe M et al. Effect of olanzapine on the liver transaminases. Can J Psychiatry 2003;48:210.
11. Jadallah KA et al. Acute hepatocellular-cholestatic liver injury after olanzapine therapy (Letter). Ann Intern Med 2003;138:357–8.
12. Tchernichovsky E et al. Hepatotoxicity, leucopenia and neutropenia associated with olanzapine therapy. Int J Psychiatry Clin Pract 2004;8:173–7.
13. Regal RE et al. Phenothiazine-induced cholestatic jaundice. Clin Pharm 1987;6:787–94.
14. Zimmerman HJ et al. Drug-induced cholestasis. Med Toxicol 1987;2:112–60.
15. de Abajo FJ et al. Acute and clinically relevant drug-induced liver injury: a population based case-control study. Br J Clin Pharmacol 2004;58:71–80.
16. Thyrum PT et al. Single-dose pharmacokinetics of quetiapine in subjects with renal or hepatic impairment. Prog Neuropsychopharmacol Biol Psychiatry 2000;24:521–33.
17. Nemeroff CB et al. Quetiapine: preclinical studies, pharmacokinetics, drug interactions, and dosing. J Clin Psychiatry 2002;63(Suppl 13):5–11.
18. Green B. Focus on quetiapine. Curr Med Res Opin 1999;15:145–51.
19. El H et al. Subfulminant liver failure associated with quetiapine. Eur J Gastroenterol Hepatol 2004;16:1415–18.
20. Cordeiro Q Jr et al. Pancreatitis and cholestatic hepatitis induced by risperidone. J Clin Psychopharmacol 2001;21:529–30.

21. Phillips EJ et al. Rapid onset of risperidone-induced hepatotoxicity. Ann Pharmacother 1998;32:843.
22. Whitworth AB et al. Transient increase of liver enzymes induced by risperidone: two case reports. J Clin Psychopharmacol 1999;19:475–6.
23. Holtmann M et al. Risperidone-associated steatohepatitis and excessive weight-gain. Pharmacopsychiatry 2003;36:206–7.
24. Ginsberg DL. Risperidone-induced hepatotoxicity. Prim Psychiatry 2005;12:29.
25. Llinares TF et al. Acute cholestatic hepatitis probably associated with risperidone. Int J Psychiatry Med 2005;35:199–205.
26. Melzer E et al. Severe cholestatic jaundice due to sulpiride. Isr J Med Sci 1987;23:1259-60.
27. Ohmoto K et al. Symptomatic primary biliary cirrhosis triggered by administration of sulpiride. Am J Gastroenterol 1999;94:3660–1.
28. Schenker S et al. Fluoxetine disposition and elimination in cirrhosis. Clin Pharmacol Ther 1988;44:353–9.
29. Cai Q et al. Acute hepatitis due to fluoxetine therapy. Mayo Clin Proc 1999;74:692-4.
30. Friedenberg FK et al. Hepatitis secondary to fluoxetine treatment. Am J Psychiatry 1996;153:580.
31. Johnston DE et al. Chronic hepatitis related to use of fluoxetine. Am J Gastroenterol 1997;92:1225–6.
32. Hale AS. New antidepressants: use in high-risk patients. J Clin Psychiatry 1993;54(Suppl):61–70.
33. Benbow SJ et al. Paroxetine and hepatotoxicity. BMJ 1997;314:1387.
34. Odeh M et al. Severe hepatotoxicity with jaundice associated with paroxetine. Am J Gastroenterol 2001;96:2494–6.
35. Dunbar GC. An interim overview of the safety and tolerability of paroxetine. Acta Psychiatr Scand Suppl 1989;350:135–7.
36. Kuhs H et al. A double-blind study of the comparative antidepressant effect of paroxetine and amitriptyline. Acta Psychiatr Scand Suppl 1989;350:145–6.
37. De Bree H et al. Fluvoxamine maleate: disposition in men. Eur J Drug Metab Pharmacokinet 1983;8:175–9.
38. Green BH. Fluvoxamine and hepatic function. Br J Psychiatry 1988;153:130–1.
39. Milne RJ et al. Citalopram. A review of its pharmacodynamic and pharmacokinetic properties, and therapeutic potential in depressive illness. Drugs 1991;41:450–77.
40. Lopez-Torres E et al. Hepatotoxicity related to citalopram (Letter). Am J Psychiatry 2004;161:923–4.
41. Colakoglu O et al. Toxic hepatitis associated with paroxetine. Int J Clin Pract 2005;59:861–2.
42. Committee on Safety in Medicines. Lofepramine (Gamanil) and abnormal blood tests of liver function. Current Problems 1988;23:2.
43. Cardona X et al. Venlafaxine-associated hepatitis. Ann Intern Med 2000;132:417.
44. Phillips BB et al. Hepatitis associated with low-dose venlafaxine for postmenopausal vasomotor symptoms. Ann Pharmacother 2006;40:323–7.
45. Gomez-Gil E et al. Phenelzine-induced fulminant hepatic failure. Ann Intern Med 1996;124:692–3.
46. Bonkovsky HL et al. Severe liver injury due to phenelzine with unique hepatic deposition of extracellular material. Am J Med 1986;80:689–92.
47. Stoeckel K et al. Absorption and disposition of moclobemide in patients with advanced age or reduced liver or kidney function. Acta Psychiatr Scand Suppl 1990;360:94–7.
48. Timmings P et al. Intrahepatic cholestasis associated with moclobemide leading to death. Lancet 1996;347:762–3.
49. Tran A et al. Pharmacokinetics of reboxetine in volunteers with hepatic impairment. Clin Drug Invest 2000;19:473–7.
50. Hanje AJ et al. Case report: fulminant hepatic failure involving duloxetine hydrochloride. Clin Gastroenterol Hepatol 2006;4:912–17.
51. El Serag HB et al. Carbamazepine-associated severe bile duct injury. Am J Gastroenterol 1999;94:526–7.
52. Forbes GM et al. Carbamazepine hepatotoxicity: another cause of the vanishing bile duct syndrome. Gastroenterology 1992;102:1385–8.
53. Morales-Diaz M et al. Suspected carbamazepine-induced hepatotoxicity. Pharmacotherapy 1999;19:252–5.
54. Ahmed SN et al. Antiepileptic drugs and liver disease. Seizure 2006;15:156–64.
55. Sauve G et al. Acute hepatitis after lamotrigine administration. Dig Dis Sci 2000;45:1874–7.
56. Cohen LS et al. Lithium-induced hyperbilirubinemia in an adolescent. J Clin Psychopharmacol 1991;11:274–5.
57. Hazelwood RE. Ascites: a side effect of lithium? Am J Psychiatry 1981;138:257.
58. Krahenbuhl S et al. Mitochondrial diseases represent a risk factor for valproate-induced fulminant liver failure. Liver 2000;20:346–8.
59. Klotz U et al. Disposition of valproic acid in patients with liver disease. Eur J Clin Pharmacol 1978;13:55–60.
60. Pinkston R et al. Multiorgan system failure caused by valproic acid toxicity. Am J Emerg Med 1997;15:504–6.
61. Rosalki SB et al. Liver function profiles and their interpretation. Br J Hosp Med 1994;51:181–6.

Prescribing in the elderly

General principles

The pharmacokinetics and pharmacodynamics of most drugs are altered to an important extent in the elderly. These changes in drug handling and action must be taken into account if treatment is to be effective and adverse effects minimised. The elderly often have a number of concurrent illnesses and may require treatment with several drugs. This leads to a greater chance of problems arising because of drug interactions and to a higher rate of drug-induced problems in general[1]. It is reasonable to assume that all drugs are more likely to cause adverse effects in the elderly than in younger patients.

How drugs affect the ageing body (altered pharmacodynamics)

As we age, control over reflex actions such as blood pressure and temperature regulation is reduced. Receptors may become more sensitive. This results in an increased incidence and severity of side-effects. For example, drugs that decrease gut motility are more likely to cause constipation (e.g. TCAs and opioids) and drugs that affect blood pressure are more likely to cause falls (e.g. TCAs and diuretics). The elderly are more sensitive to the effects of benzodiazepines than younger adults. Therapeutic response can also be delayed; the elderly may take longer to respond to antidepressants than younger adults[2].

The elderly may be more prone to develop serious side-effects from some drugs: for example, agranulocytosis with clozapine[3] and stroke with antipsychotic drugs[4,5].

How ageing affects drug therapy (altered pharmacokinetics)[6]

ABSORPTION
Gut motility decreases with age, as does secretion of gastric acid. This leads to drugs being absorbed more slowly, resulting in a slower onset of action. The same *amount* of drug is absorbed as in a younger adult, but the rate of absorption is slower.

DISTRIBUTION
The elderly have more body fat, less body water and less albumin than younger adults. This leads to an increased volume of distribution and a longer duration of action for some fat-soluble drugs (e.g. diazepam), higher concentrations of some drugs at the site of action (e.g. digoxin) and a reduction in the amount of drug bound to albumin (increased amounts of active 'free drug'; e.g. warfarin, phenytoin).

METABOLISM
The majority of drugs are hepatically metabolised. Liver size is reduced in the elderly, but in the absence of hepatic disease or significantly reduced hepatic blood flow, there is no significant reduction in metabolic capacity. The magnitude of pharmacokinetic interactions is unlikely to be altered but the pharmacodynamic consequences of these interactions may be amplified.

EXCRETION
Renal function declines with age: 35% of function is lost by the age of 65 years and 50% by the age of 80.

More function is lost if there are concurrent medical problems such as heart disease, diabetes or hypertension. Measurement of serum creatinine or urea can be misleading in the elderly because muscle mass is reduced, so less creatinine is produced. Creatinine clearance is the only accurate measure of renal function in this age group. It is best to assume that all elderly patients have at most two-thirds of normal renal function.

Most drugs are eventually (after metabolism) excreted by the kidney. A few do not undergo biotransformation first. Lithium and sulpiride are important examples. Drugs primarily excreted via the kidney will accumulate in the elderly, leading to toxicity and side-effects. Dosage reduction is likely to be required (see page 389 *et seq*. for full review of renal effects of psychotropics).

Drug interactions

Some drugs have a narrow therapeutic index (a small increase in dose can cause toxicity and a small reduction in dose can cause a loss of therapeutic action). The most commonly prescribed ones are: digoxin, warfarin, theophylline, phenytoin and lithium. Changes in the way these drugs are handled in the elderly and the greater chance of interaction with other drugs mean that toxicity and therapeutic failure are more likely. These drugs can be used safely but extra care must be taken and blood levels should be measured where possible.

Some drugs inhibit or induce hepatic metabolising enzymes. Important examples include the SSRIs, erythromycin and carbamazepine (see page 247 for further information). This may lead to the metabolism of another drug being altered. Many drug interactions occur through this mechanism. Details of individual interactions and their consequences can be found in Appendix 1 of the *BNF*. Most can be predicted by a sound knowledge of pharmacology.

Reducing drug-related risk

Adherence to the following principles will reduce drug-related morbidity and mortality:

- Use drugs only when absolutely necessary.
- Avoid, if possible, drugs that block α_1 adrenoceptors, have anticholinergic side-effects, are very sedative, have a long half-life or are potent inhibitors of hepatic metabolising enzymes.
- Start with a low dose and increase slowly but do not undertreat. Some drugs still require the full adult dose.
- Try not to treat the side-effects of one drug with another drug. Find a better-tolerated alternative.
- Keep therapy simple; that is, once daily administration whenever possible.

Administering medicines in foodstuffs[7,8]

Sometimes patients may refuse treatment with medicines, even when such treatment is thought to be in their best interests. Where the patient has a mental illness or has capacity, the Mental Health Act should be used, but if the patient lacks capacity, this option may not be desirable. Medicines should never be administered covertly to elderly patients with dementia without a full discussion with the MDT and the patient's relatives. The outcome of this discussion should be clearly documented in the patient's clinical notes. Medicine should be administered covertly only after such discussion and if the clear and express purpose is to reduce suffering for the patient.

References

1. Royal College of Physicians. Medication for older people. Summary and recommendations of a report of a working party of the Royal College of Physicians. J R Coll Physicians Lond 1997;31:254–7.
2. Paykel ES et al. Residual symptoms after partial remission: an important outcome in depression. Psychol Med 1995;25:1171–80.
3. Munro J et al. Active monitoring of 12,760 clozapine recipients in the UK and Ireland. Beyond pharma-covigilance. Br J Psychiatry 1999;175:576–80.
4. Schneider LS et al. Atypical antipsychotic drug treatment for dementia. Meta-analysis of randomized placebo-controlled trials. JAMA 2005;294:1934–43.
5. Gill SS et al. Atypical antipsychotic drugs and risk of ischaemic stroke: population based retrospective cohort study. BMJ 2005;330:445.
6. Mayersohn M. Special pharmacokinetic considerations in the elderly. In Evans WE, Schentag JJ, Jusko WJ, eds. Applied Pharmacokinetics: Principles of Therapeutic Drug Monitoring. Spokane, WA: Applied Therapeutics Inc, 1986; 229–93.
7. Treloar A et al. Concealing medication in patients' food. Lancet 2001;357:62–4.
8. Treloar A et al. Administering medicines to patients with dementia and other organic cognitive syndromes. Adv Psychiatr Treat 2001;7:444–50.

Further reading

National Service Framework for Older People. London: Department of Health, 2001.

Alzheimer's disease

Acetylcholinesterase (AChE) inhibitors

Three inhibitors of AChE are currently licensed in the UK for the treatment of Alzheimer's disease: donepezil, rivastigmine and galantamine. In addition, rivastigmine is licensed in the treatment of mild to moderate dementia associated with Parkinson's disease. Cholinesterase inhibitors differ in pharmacological action: donepezil and galantamine are selective inhibitors of AChE; rivastigmine affects both AChE and butyrylcholinesterase (BuChE); donepezil and rivastigmine are relatively selective for AChE in the brain; and galantamine also affects nicotinic receptors[1]. To date, these differences have not been shown to result in differences in efficacy or tolerability.

All three drugs seem to have broadly similar clinical effects, as measured with the Mini Mental State Examination (MMSE), a 30-point basic evaluation of cognitive function and the Alzheimer's Disease Assessment Scale – cognitive subscale (ADAS-cog), a 70-point evaluation largely of cognitive dysfunction. Major trials of donepezil[2–4] suggest an advantage over placebo of 2.5–3.1 points on the ADAS-cog scale. For rivastigmine[5,6] the advantage is 2.6–4.9 points and for galantamine[7–9] 2.9–3.9. Estimates of the number needed to treat (NNT) (improvement of >4 points ADAS-cog) range from 4 to 12. Direct comparisons of anticholinesterases have given equivocal results – a Pfizer-sponsored study suggested the superiority of donepezil over galantamine[10]; a Janssen-sponsored study suggested the converse[11].

All the above results need to be interpreted with caution, especially as so few head-to-head studies have been published. Alzheimer's disease is usually characterised by inexorable cognitive decline, which is generally well quantified by tests such as ADAS-cog and MMSE. The average rate of decline is 4–6 points on the ADAS-cog over 1 year, but the range is large. It is therefore difficult to accurately assess treatment effect in individual patients. The effect of anticholinesterases is, on average, to improve modestly cognitive function for several months (scores return to baseline after about 9–12 months)[4,8].

This average incorporates and to some extent conceals three groups of patients: 'non-responders', who continue to decline at the anticipated rate; 'non-decliners', who neither improve significantly nor decline; and 'improvers', who improve to a clinically relevant extent. This last group is usually defined as those who show a >4 point improvement on ADAS-cog. In trials of around 6 months, approximately 25–35% of those on anticholinesterases will be classified as 'improvers' compared with around 15–25% on placebo. Around 55–70% of patients treated with anticholinesterases will show no cognitive decline during a 5–6-month trial[6,8] – about 20% more patients in absolute terms than those on placebo. Note that, for the most part, results of trials so far conducted relate only to patients with mild-to-moderate Alzheimer's disease (those giving a score of 10–26 on MMSE), although data on those with more severe illness are encouraging[12].

Taking into account trial differences and all assessments made, available anticholinesterases can be said to have broadly similar efficacy against cognitive symptoms in clinical trials. Any minor differences observed may be accounted for by differences in trial design or patient characteristics. In the absence of sufficient 'head-to-head' studies, the available drugs should be assumed to have equal efficacy. Overall, in a cohort of patients given anti-cholinesterases at optimal doses under clinical trial conditions, approximately one-third would be expected to improve over 6 months and around another third would be expected not to deteriorate. These observations appear to be broadly reflected in practice.

Other effects
Anticholinesterases may also affect non-cognitive aspects of Alzheimer's disease. For example, they seem to have useful psychotropic activity against neuropsychiatric symptoms[13–15]. These drugs may also lower caregiver burden[16] and improve patients' abilities with daily activities[17]. Differential effects for different drugs have yet to be demonstrated. However, anticholinesterases appear to have minimal effects on time to institutionalisation or progression of disability[18].

Tolerability
Drug tolerability may differ between anticholinesterases, but, again, in the absence of sufficient direct comparisons, it is difficult to draw cogent conclusions. Overall tolerability can be broadly evaluated by reference to the numbers withdrawing from clinical trials. Withdrawal rates in trials of donepezil[2,3] ranged from 4% to 16% (placebo 1–7%). With rivastigmine[5,6], rates ranged from 7% to 29% (placebo 7%) and with galantamine[7–9] from 7% to 23% (placebo 7–9%). (All figures relate to withdrawals specifically associated with adverse effects.)

Tolerability seems to be affected by speed of titration and, perhaps less clearly, by dose. Most adverse effects occurred in trials during titration, and slower titration schedules are recommended in clinical use. This may mean that these drugs are equally well tolerated in practice.

Dosing
Different titration schedules do, to some extent, differentiate anticholin-esterases. **Donepezil** is perhaps easiest to use, starting at 5 mg/day and increasing 'if necessary' (however this might be determined) to 10 mg after a month. **Rivastigmine** is taken twice daily, starting at 1.5 mg b.d. and increasing to 3 mg b.d. after 2 weeks or more and then to 4.5 mg b.d. after a further 2 weeks (maximum 6 mg b.d.). With **galantamine**, the starting dose is 4 mg twice daily, increasing to 8 mg twice daily after 4 weeks and then to 12 mg b.d., if necessary, 4 weeks later (a once daily preparation is now available). Thus, both rivastigmine and galantamine need to be given twice daily and have prolonged titration schedules. These factors may be important to prescribers, patients and carers. This was demonstrated in a retrospective analysis of the patterns of use of AChE, where it was demonstrated that donepezil was significantly more likely to be prescribed at an effective dose than either rivastigmine or galantamine[19].

Interactions
Potential for interaction may also differentiate currently available cholinesterase inhibitors. Donepezil[20] and galantamine[21] are metabolised by cytochromes 2D6 and 3A4 and so drug levels may be altered by other drugs affecting the function of these enzymes. Anticholinesterases themselves may also interfere with the metabolism of other drugs, although this is perhaps a theoretical consideration. Rivastigmine has almost no potential for interaction since it

is metabolised at the site of action and does not affect hepatic cytochromes. Overall, rivastigmine appears to be least likely to cause problematic drug interactions, a factor that may be important in an elderly population subject to polypharmacy.

Adverse effects

When adverse effects occur, they are largely predictable: excess cholinergic stimulation leads to nausea, vomiting, dizziness, insomnia and diarrhoea[22]. Urinary incontinence has also been reported[23]. There appear to be no important differences between drugs in respect to type or frequency of adverse events, although clinical trials do suggest a relatively lower frequency of adverse events for donepezil. This may simply be a reflection of the aggressive titration schedules used in trials of other drugs.

NICE recommendations

Using a protocol like that originally suggested by NICE[24] may mean that, of a cohort of patients referred for treatment, only three-quarters may be considered suitable for treatment, and only one-third of these may continue treatment for a year or more[25]. In contrast, in the artificial environment of a clinical trial, nearly half of patients continued for 2 years or more[26]. (Note that long-term, double-blind trials may underestimate real-life benefits of treatment because non-responders or poor responders are continued on drug treatment[18].) While NICE guidance has now changed (below) a similar (or lower) rate of take-up and persistence with treatment should be anticipated.

Summary of NICE guidance on anticholinesterases[27]

- The three acetylcholinesterase inhibitors (donepezil, galantamine and rivastigmine) are recommended as options in the management of people with Alzheimer's disease of moderate severity (MMSE score of between 10 and 20). Corresponding NICE guidelines on dementia suggest a less rigid adherence to MMSE scores in determining whether or not to treat. Those with MMSEs >20 may start treatment if functionally impaired, for example.
- Only specialists in dementia should initiate treatment.
- A carer's view on the patient's condition at baseline and follow-up should be sought.
- Patients who continue on the drug should be reviewed every 6 months by MMSE score and global, functional and behavioural assessment. The drug should only be continued if the MMSE remains at or above 10 and the drug effect is considered to be worthwhile. (Note, however, that abrupt discontinuation of AChE inhibitors in patients whose MMSE score drops below this level is not advised – a careful trial of graduated discontinuation is preferred.)
- Therapy with AChE inhibitor should be initiated with a drug with the lowest acquisition cost. An alternative may be considered on the basis of adverse effects profile, concordance, medical co-morbidity and possibility of drug interactions.
- People with mild Alzheimer's disease currently receiving AChE inhibitors may be continued on therapy until they, their carers and/or specialist consider it appropriate to stop.

Memantine

Memantine is licensed in the UK for the treatment of moderately severe to severe Alzheimer's disease. It acts as an antagonist at N-methyl-D-aspartate (NMDA) receptors, an action which, in theory, may be neuroprotective and thus disease modifying[28]. Memantine appears to be well tolerated[29,30] and clinical experience is encouraging. Trials in severe dementia[31] and vascular dementia[32] suggest an advantage over placebo of around 2 points on the ADAS-cog scale and NNTs (improvement) of 3–8[33]. Improvement was also seen in other domains of functioning.

Other data suggest memantine is effective in mild to moderate Alzheimer's disease with an advantage over placebo of 1.9 points on ADAS-cog[34].

Ginkgo biloba

Ginkgo biloba has been widely touted as a cognitive enhancer and there are some experimental data to suggest that it has neuroprotective effects[35]. There are also well-controlled human trial data which suggest that *G. biloba* is effective in mild to moderate Alzheimer's disease with an advantage over placebo of around 1.4 points on ADAS-cog[36]. Several reports have noted that *G. biloba* may increase the risk of bleeding[37]. The drug is widely used in Germany but less so elsewhere.

Combination treatment

A wide range of drug combinations have been evaluated but few have involved more modern treatments such as anticholinesterases and memantine[38], perhaps the most obvious combination to use. Nonetheless, a combination of memantine and donepezil has been shown to be more effective than donepezil in patients with moderate to severe Alzheimer's disease[39]. The combination appears to be well tolerated[39,40]. Similarly, the combination of rivastigmine and memantine has also been investigated in a prospective open-label study in patients who failed to respond to donepezil or galantamine. The combination was found to be beneficial without increased side-effects[41].

Vascular dementia

None of the currently available drugs are formally licensed in the UK for vascular dementia. There is growing evidence that donepezil[42,43], rivastigmine[44], galantamine[45,46] and memantine[47] are effective in vascular dementia. Overall effect seems to be similar or slightly less than that seen in Alzheimer's disease. Note, however, that it is impossible to diagnose with certainty vascular or Alzheimer's dementia and much dementia has mixed causation.

Table Summary – anticholinesterases in Alzheimer's disease

Drug	Starting dose	Usual treatment dose	Adverse effects	Costs (1-month treatment) at usual dose
Donepezil	5 mg daily	10 mg daily	Nausea Vomiting Insomnia Diarrhoea	£95.42
Rivastigmine	1.5 mg b.d.	6 mg b.d.	Nausea Vomiting Insomnia Diarrhoea	£83.94
Galantamine	4 mg b.d.	12 mg b.d.	Nausea Vomiting Insomnia Diarrhoea	£90
Galantamine XL	8 mg XL daily	24 mg XL daily	Nausea Vomiting Insomnia Diarrhoea	£90
Memantine	5 mg daily	20 mg daily	Hallucinations Dizziness Confusion	£73.94

Special groups

References

1. Weinstock M. Selectivity of cholinesterase inhibition: clinical implications for the treatment of Alzheimer's disease. CNS Drugs 1999;12:307–23.
2. Rogers SL et al. Donepezil improves cognition and global function in Alzheimer disease: a 15-week, double-blind, placebo-controlled study. Donepezil Study Group. Arch Intern Med 1998;158:1021–31.
3. Rogers SL et al. A 24-week, double-blind, placebo-controlled trial of donepezil in patients with Alzheimer's disease. Donepezil Study Group. Neurology 1998;50:136–45.
4. Rogers SL et al. Long-term efficacy and safety of donepezil in the treatment of Alzheimer's disease: final analysis of a US multicentre open-label study. Eur Neuropsychopharmacol 2000;10:195–203.
5. Corey-Bloom J et al. A randomized trial evaluating the efficacy and safety of ENA 713 (rivastigmine tartrate), a new acetylcholinesterase inhibitor, in patients with mild to moderately severe Alzheimer's disease. Int J Geriatr Psychopharmacol 1998;1:55–64.
6. Rosler M et al. Efficacy and safety of rivastigmine in patients with Alzheimer's disease: international randomised controlled trial. BMJ 1999;318:633–8.
7. Tariot PN et al. A 5-month, randomized, placebo-controlled trial of galantamine in AD. The Galantamine USA-10 Study Group. Neurology 2000;54:2269–76.
8. Raskind MA et al. Galantamine in AD: A 6-month randomized, placebo-controlled trial with a 6-month extension. The Galantamine USA-1 Study Group. Neurology 2000;54:2261–8.
9. Wilcock GK et al. Efficacy and safety of galantamine in patients with mild to moderate Alzheimer's disease: multicentre randomised controlled trial. Galantamine International-1 Study Group. BMJ 2000; 321:1445–9.
10. Jones RW et al. A multinational, randomised, 12-week study comparing the effects of donepezil and galantamine in patients with mild to moderate Alzheimer's disease. Int J Geriatr Psychiatry 2004; 19:58–67.
11. Wilcock G et al. A long-term comparison of galantamine and donepezil in the treatment of Alzheimer's disease. Drugs Aging 2003;20:777–89.
12. Birks JS et al. Donepezil for dementia due to Alzheimer's disease. Cochrane Database Syst Rev 2003; CD001190.
13. Cummings JL et al. Evidence for psychotropic effects of acetylcholinesterase inhibitors. CNS Drugs 2000;13:385–95.
14. Weiner MF et al. Effects of donepezil on emotional/behavioral symptoms in Alzheimer's disease patients. J Clin Psychiatry 2000;61:487–92.
15. Blesa R. Galantamine: therapeutic effects beyond cognition. Dement Geriatr Cogn Disord 2000; 11(Suppl 1):28–34.
16. Feldman H et al. Efficacy of donepezil on maintenance of activities of daily living in patients with moderate to severe Alzheimer's disease and the effect on caregiver burden. J Am Geriatr Soc 2003; 51:737–44.
17. Winblad B et al. A 1-year, randomized, placebo-controlled study of donepezil in patients with mild to moderate AD. Neurology 2001;57:489–95.
18. AD2000 Collaborative Group. Long-term donepezil treatment in 565 patients with Alzheimer's disease (AD2000): randomised double-blind trial. Lancet 2004;363:2105–15.
19. Dybicz SB et al. Patterns of cholinesterase-inhibitor use in the nursing home setting: a retrospective analysis. Am J Geriatr Pharmacother 2006;4:154–60.
20. Dooley M et al. Donepezil: a review of its use in Alzheimer's disease. Drugs Aging 2000;16:199–226.
21. Scott LJ et al. Galantamine: a review of its use in Alzheimer's disease. Drugs 2000;60:1095–122.
22. Dunn NR et al. Adverse effects associated with the use of donepezil in general practice in England. J Psychopharmacol 2000;14:406–8.
23. Hashimoto M et al. Urinary incontinence: an unrecognised adverse effect with donepezil. Lancet 2000;356:568.
24. National Institute for Clinical Excellence. Guidance on the use of donepezil, rivastigmine and galantamine for the treatment of Alzheimer's disease. Technology Appraisal 19. http://www.nice.org. uk. 2001.
25. Matthews HP et al. Donepezil in Alzheimer's disease: eighteen month results from Southampton Memory Clinic. Int J Geriatr Psychiatry 2000;15:713–20.
26. Ieni JR et al. Safety of donepezil in extended treatment of Alzheimer's disease. Eur Neuropsychopharmacol 1999;9(Suppl 5):328–9.
27. National Institute for Clinical Excellence. Donepezil, galantamine, rivastigmine (review) and memantine for the treatment of Alzheimer's disease. Technology Appraisal No. 111. http://www.nice.org.uk. 2006.
28. Danysz W et al. Neuroprotective and symptomatological action of memantine relevant for Alzheimer's disease – a unified glutamatergic hypothesis on the mechanism of action. Neurotox Res 2000;2:85–97.
29. Parsons CG et al. Memantine is a clinically well tolerated N-methyl-D-aspartate (NMDA) receptor antagonist – a review of preclinical data. Neuropharmacology 1999;38:735–67.
30. Reisberg B et al. Memantine in moderate-to-severe Alzheimer's disease. N Engl J Med 2003;348: 1333–41.
31. Winblad B et al. Memantine in severe dementia: results of the 9M-Best Study (Benefit and efficacy in severely demented patients during treatment with memantine). Int J Geriatr Psychiatry 1999;14: 135–46.

32. Orgogozo JM et al. Efficacy and safety of memantine in patients with mild to moderate vascular dementia: a randomized, placebo-controlled trial (MMM 300). Stroke 2002;33:1834–9.
33. Livingston G et al. The place of memantine in the treatment of Alzheimer's disease: a number needed to treat analysis. Int J Geriatr Psychiatry 2004;19:919–25.
34. Peskind ER et al. Memantine treatment in mild to moderate Alzheimer disease: a 24-week randomized, controlled trial. Am J Geriatr Psychiatry 2006;14:704–15.
35. Ahlemeyer B et al. Pharmacological studies supporting the therapeutic use of Ginkgo biloba extract for Alzheimer's disease. Pharmacopsychiatry 2003;36(Suppl 1):S8–14.
36. Kanowski S et al. Ginkgo biloba extract EGb 761 in dementia: intent-to-treat analyses of a 24-week, multi-center, double-blind, placebo-controlled, randomized trial. Pharmacopsychiatry 2003;36:297–303.
37. Bent S et al. Spontaneous bleeding associated with Ginkgo biloba: a case report and systematic review of the literature. J Gen Intern Med 2005;20:657–61.
38. Schmitt B et al. Combination therapy in Alzheimer's disease: a review of current evidence. CNS Drugs 2004;18:827–44.
39. Tariot PN et al. Memantine treatment in patients with moderate to severe Alzheimer disease already receiving donepezil: a randomized controlled trial. JAMA 2004;291:317–24.
40. Hartmann S et al. Tolerability of memantine in combination with cholinesterase inhibitors in dementia therapy. Int Clin Psychopharmacol 2003;18:81–5.
41. Dantoine T et al. Rivastigmine monotherapy and combination therapy with memantine in patients with moderately severe Alzheimer's disease who failed to benefit from previous cholinesterase inhibitor treatment. Int J Clin Pract 2006;60:110–18.
42. Black S et al. Efficacy and tolerability of donepezil in vascular dementia: positive results of a 24-week, multicenter, international, randomized, placebo-controlled clinical trial. Stroke 2003;34:2323–30.
43. Wilkinson D et al. Donepezil in vascular dementia: a randomized, placebo-controlled study. Neurology 2003;61:479–86.
44. Moretti R et al. Rivastigmine superior to aspirin plus nimodipine in subcortical vascular dementia: an open, 16-month, comparative study. Int J Clin Pract 2004;58:346–53.
45. Small G et al. Galantamine in the treatment of cognitive decline in patients with vascular dementia or Alzheimer's disease with cerebrovascular disease. CNS Drugs 2003;17:905–14.
46. Kurz AF et al. Long-term safety and cognitive effects of galantamine in the treatment of probable vascular dementia or Alzheimer's disease with cerebrovascular disease. Eur J Neurol 2003;10:633–40.
47. Wilcock G et al. A double-blind, placebo-controlled multicentre study of memantine in mild to moderate vascular dementia (MMM500). Int Clin Psychopharmacol 2002;17:297–305.

Further reading

Areosa Sastre A et al. Memantine for dementia. In: The Cochrane Library, Issue 1. Oxford: Update Software, 2003.
Burns A et al. Clinical practice with anti-dementia drugs: a consensus statement from British Association for Psychopharmacology. J Psychopharmacol 2006;20:732–55.
Loy C et al. Galantamine for Alzheimer's disease. Cochrane Database Syst Rev 2004;4: CD001747. DOI: 10.1002/14651858.CD001747.pub2.

Special groups

Behavioural disturbance in dementia

Behavioural symptoms are common in patients with dementia but, for a variety of reasons, treatment is not well informed by properly conducted studies.

Antipsychotics
First-generation antipsychotics (FGAs) have been widely used for decades in behavioural disturbance associated with dementia. They are probably effective[1] but, because of extrapyramidal and other adverse effects, are less well tolerated than second-generation antipsychotics (SGAs) while being, if anything, less effective[2–4]. FGAs may also hasten cognitive decline in dementia[5] although there is recent evidence to refute this[6].

Various reviews and trials support the efficacy of olanzapine[2,7], risperidone[8], quetiapine[4,9] and aripiprazole[10,11]. These drugs are not thought to affect cognitive decline[6]. SGAs were once widely recommended in dementia-related behaviour disturbance[12] but their use is now highly controversial. There are three reasons for this: effect size is small; tolerability is poor; and there is a tentative association with increased mortality. The recent CATIE-AD study[13] showed very minor effectiveness advantages for olanzapine and risperidone (but not for quetiapine) over placebo but all drugs were poorly tolerated because of sedation, confusion and EPSEs (the last of these not a problem with quetiapine). Other studies and meta-analyses have detected only minor advantages for olanzapine, risperidone and aripiprazole[12,14,15].

In the UK[16] and USA[17] warnings have been issued regarding increased mortality with olanzapine, risperidone, quetiapine and aripiprazole when used in dementia. Several published analyses support these warnings[18–20], suggesting an association between some SGAs and stroke. Other studies have detected no clear adverse outcome[21–23] and one suggested relatively higher mortality with haloperidol than with risperidone or olanzapine[24]. The relative safety of FGAs cannot be assumed.

In the UK, concerns about a link to stroke and increased mortality have led to a reduction in the use of those SGAs identified as potentially causative. Some centres use amisulpride but its use is only minimally supported[25] and its safety in this group of patients unknown.

Others
Donepezil[26,27], rivastigmine[28–30] and galantamine[31] all seem to be effective in reducing behavioural disturbance in dementia. Their effect seems apparent only after several weeks of treatment. RCT evidence suggests memantine has a similar effect[32].

Benzodiazepines[33] and trazodone[34] are widely used but poorly supported. SSRIs are of doubtful efficacy[35,36]. Mood stabilisers have also been used[37,38]. One RCT of valproate that included an open-label extension found valproate to be ineffective in controlling symptoms. Seven of the 39 patients enrolled died during the 12-week extension phase[39].

Non-drug measures
A variety of non-pharmacological methods have been developed and some are reasonably well supported by cogent research[40,41]. Given concerns over

almost all drug therapies, non-pharmacological measures should always be considered.

Summary

The evidence base available to guide treatment in this area is insufficient to allow specific recommendations on drug choice. Whichever drug is chosen, the '3T' approach should be followed:

> Target symptoms requiring treatment.
> Titrate drug dose from a low starting dose.
> Time-limit prescriptions so that ineffective treatment is not unnecessarily continued.

References

1. Devanand DP et al. A randomized, placebo-controlled dose-comparison trial of haloperidol for psychosis and disruptive behaviors in Alzheimer's disease. Am J Psychiatry 1998;155:1512–20.
2. Verhey FR et al. Olanzapine versus haloperidol in the treatment of agitation in elderly patients with dementia: results of a randomized controlled double-blind trial. Dement Geriatr Cogn Disord 2006;21:1–8.
3. Suh GH et al. Comparative efficacy of risperidone versus haloperidol on behavioural and psychological symptoms of dementia. Int J Geriatr Psychiatry 2006;21:654–60.
4. Savaskan E et al. Treatment of behavioural, cognitive and circadian rest–activity cycle disturbances in Alzheimer's disease: haloperidol vs. quetiapine. Int J Neuropsychopharmacol 2006;9:507–16.
5. McShane R et al. Do neuroleptic drugs hasten cognitive decline in dementia? Prospective study with necropsy follow up. BMJ 1997;314:266–70.
6. Livingston G et al. Antipsychotics and cognitive decline in Alzheimer's disease: the LASER-Alzheimer's disease longitudinal study. J Neurol Neurosurg Psychiatry 2007;78:25–9.
7. Street JS et al. Olanzapine treatment of psychotic and behavioral symptoms in patients with Alzheimer disease in nursing care facilities: a double-blind, randomized, placebo-controlled trial. The HGEU Study Group. Arch Gen Psychiatry 2000;57:968–76.
8. Bhana N et al. Risperidone: a review of its use in the management of the behavioural and psychological symptoms of dementia. Drugs Aging 2000;16:451–71.
9. McManus DQ et al. Quetiapine, a novel antipsychotic: experience in elderly patients with psychotic disorders. Seroquel Trial 48 Study Group. J Clin Psychiatry 1999;60:292–8.
10. Laks J et al. Use of aripiprazole for psychosis and agitation in dementia. Int Psychogeriatr 2006;18:335–40.
11. De Deyn P et al. Aripiprazole for the treatment of psychosis in patients with Alzheimer's disease: a randomized, placebo-controlled study. J Clin Psychopharmacol 2005;25:463–7.
12. Lee PE et al. Atypical antipsychotic drugs in the treatment of behavioural and psychological symptoms of dementia: systematic review. BMJ 2004;329:75.
13. Schneider LS et al. Effectiveness of atypical antipsychotic drugs in patients with Alzheimer's disease. N Engl J Med 2006;355:1525–38.
14. Deberdt WG et al. Comparison of olanzapine and risperidone in the treatment of psychosis and associated behavioral disturbances in patients with dementia. Am J Geriatr Psychiatry 2005;13:722–30.
15. Schneider LS et al. Efficacy and adverse effects of atypical antipsychotics for dementia: meta-analysis of randomized, placebo-controlled trials. Am J Geriatr Psychiatry 2006;14:191–210.
16. Duff G. Atypical antipsychotic drugs and stroke. http://www.mhra.gov.uk. 2004.
17. US Food and Drug Administration. FDA Public Health Advisory. Deaths with antipsychotics in elderly patients with behavioural disturbances. http://www.fda.gov/. 2005.
18. Herrmann N et al. Do atypical antipsychotics cause stroke? CNS Drugs 2005;19:91–103.
19. Kryzhanovskaya LA et al. A review of treatment-emergent adverse events during olanzapine clinical trials in elderly patients with dementia. J Clin Psychiatry 2006;67:933–45.
20. Schneider LS et al. Risk of death with atypical antipsychotic drug treatment for dementia: meta-analysis of randomized placebo-controlled trials. JAMA 2005;294:1934–43.
21. Herrmann N et al. Atypical antipsychotics and risk of cerebrovascular accidents. Am J Psychiatry 2004;161:1113–15.

Special groups

22. Gill SS et al. Atypical antipsychotic drugs and risk of ischaemic stroke: population based retrospective cohort study. BMJ 2005;330:445.
23. Finkel S et al. Risperidone treatment in elderly patients with dementia: relative risk of cerebrovascular events versus other antipsychotics. Int Psychogeriatr 2005;17:617–29.
24. Nasrallah HA et al. Lower mortality in geriatric patients receiving risperidone and olanzapine versus haloperidol: preliminary analysis of retrospective data. Am J Geriatr Psychiatry 2004;12:437–9.
25. Mauri M et al. Amisulpride in the treatment of behavioural disturbances among patients with moderate to severe Alzheimer's disease. Acta Neurol Scand 2006;114:97–101.
26. Terao T et al. Can donepezil be considered a mild antipsychotic in dementia treatment? A report of donepezil use in 6 patients. J Clin Psychiatry 2003;64:1392–3.
27. Weiner MF et al. Effects of donepezil on emotional/behavioral symptoms in Alzheimer's disease patients. J Clin Psychiatry 2000;61:487–92.
28. Finkel SI. Effects of rivastigmine on behavioral and psychological symptoms of dementia in Alzheimer's disease. Clin Ther 2004;26:980–90.
29. Rosler M et al. Effects of two-year treatment with the cholinesterase inhibitor rivastigmine on behavioural symptoms in Alzheimer's disease. Behav Neurol 1998;11:211–16.
30. Cummings JL et al. Effects of rivastigmine treatment on the neuropsychiatric and behavioral disturbances of nursing home residents with moderate to severe probable Alzheimer's disease: a 26-week, multicenter, open-label study. Am J Geriatr Pharmacother 2005;3:137–48.
31. Cummings JL et al. Reduction of behavioral disturbances and caregiver distress by galantamine in patients with Alzheimer's disease. Am J Psychiatry 2004;161:532–8.
32. Cummings JL et al. Behavioral effects of memantine in Alzheimer disease patients receiving donepezil treatment. Neurology 2006;67:57–63.
33. Verdoux H et al. Is benzodiazepine use a risk factor for cognitive decline and dementia? A literature review of epidemiological studies. Psychol Med 2005;35:307–15.
34. Martinon-Torres G et al. Trazodone for agitation in dementia. Cochrane Database Syst Rev 2004; CD004990.
35. Deakin JB et al. Paroxetine does not improve symptoms and impairs cognition in frontotemporal dementia: a double-blind randomized controlled trial. Psychopharmacology 2004;172:400–8.
36. Finkel SI et al. A randomized, placebo-controlled study of the efficacy and safety of sertraline in the treatment of the behavioral manifestations of Alzheimer's disease in outpatients treated with donepezil. Int J Geriatr Psychiatry 2004;19:9–18.
37. Lonergan ET et al. Valproic acid for agitation in dementia. Cochrane Database Syst Rev 2004;CD003945.
38. Tariot PN et al. Efficacy and tolerability of carbamazepine for agitation and aggression in dementia. Am J Psychiatry 1998;155:54–61.
39. Sival RC et al. Sodium valproate in aggressive behaviour in dementia: a twelve-week open label follow-up study. Int J Geriatr Psychiatry 2004;19:305–12.
40. Ayalon L et al. Effectiveness of nonpharmacological interventions for the management of neuropsychiatric symptoms in patients with dementia: a systematic review. Arch Intern Med 2006;166:2182–8.
41. Livingston G et al. Systematic review of psychological approaches to the management of neuropsychiatric symptoms of dementia. Am J Psychiatry 2005;162:1996–2021.

Further reading

Ballard C et al. Quetiapine and rivastigmine and cognitive decline in Alzheimer's disease: randomised double blind placebo controlled trial. BMJ 2005;330:874.
Medicines and Healthcare Products Regulatory Agency. PhVWP Assessment report. Antipsychotics and cerebrovascular accident. http://www.mhra.gov.uk. 2005.
Royal College of Psychiatrists. Atypical antipsychotics and BPSD. Prescribing update v4c. http://www.rcpsych.ac.uk/. 2004.

Special groups

Parkinson's disease

Parkinson's disease (PD) is a progressive, degenerative neurological disorder characterised by resting tremor, cogwheel rigidity, bradykinesia and postural instability. The prevalence of co-morbid psychiatric disorders is high. Approximately 25% will suffer from major depression at some point during the course of their illness, a further 25% from milder forms of depression, 25% from anxiety spectrum disorders, 25% from psychosis and 25–40% will develop dementia[1]. While depression and anxiety can occur at any time, psychosis, dementia and also delirium are more prevalent in the later stages of the illness. Close co-operation between the psychiatrist and neurologist is required to optimise treatment for this group of patients.

Depression in Parkinson's disease

Depression in Parkinson's disease predicts greater cognitive decline, deterioration in functioning and progression of motor symptoms[2]. Pre-existing dementia is an established risk factor for the development of depression.

Recommendations for treatment – depression in Parkinson's disease

Step	Intervention
1	Exclude/treat organic causes such as hypothyroidism (the prevalence of which is higher in Parkinson's disease[2]).
2	**SSRIs** are considered to be first-line treatment. Some patients may experience a worsening of motor symptoms, although the absolute risk is low[3]. Care must be taken when combining SSRIs with selegiline, as the risk of serotonin syndrome is increased[2]. TCAs are generally poorly tolerated because of their anticholinergic (can worsen cognitive problems; constipation) and alpha-blocking effects (can worsen symptoms of autonomic dysfunction). Note that, in the only RCT of the treatment of severe depression in patients with Parkinson's disease, amitriptyline was found to be more effective than fluoxetine[4].
3	Consider **ECT**. Depression and motor symptoms generally respond well[2] but the risk of inducing delirium is high[5], particularly in patients with pre-existing cognitive impairment.
4	Consider augmentation with dopamine agonists/releasers such as amantadine[6] or pramipexole[2].
5	Follow the algorithm for treatment-resistant depression (see page 193) from this point. Be aware of the increased propensity for side-effects and drug interactions in this patient group.

Psychosis in Parkinson's disease

Psychosis in Parkinson's disease is often characterised by visual hallucinations. Auditory hallucinations and delusions occur far less frequently[7]. Psychosis and dementia frequently co-exist. Having one predicts the development of the other[8]. Sleep disorders are also an established risk factor for the development of psychosis[1].

Abnormalities in dopamine, serotonin and acetylcholine neurotransmission have all been implicated, but the exact aetiology of Parkinson's disease psychosis is poorly understood. In the majority of patients, psychotic symptoms are thought to be secondary to dopaminergic medication rather than part of Parkinson's disease itself. From the limited data available, anticholinergics and dopamine agonists seem to be associated with a higher risk of inducing psychosis than levodopa or COMT inhibitors[7,9]. Psychosis is a major contributor to caregiver distress and a risk factor for institutionalisation and early death[8].

Step	Intervention
	**Recommendations for treatment – Psychosis in Parkinson's disease**
1	Exclude organic causes (delirium).
2	Optimise the environment to maximise orientation and minimise problems due to poor caregiver–patient interactions.
3	If the patient has insight and hallucinations are infrequent and not troubling, do not treat.
4	Consider reducing or stopping anticholinergics and dopamine agonists. Monitor for signs of motor deterioration. Be prepared to restart/increase the dose of these drugs again to achieve the best balance between psychosis and mobility.
5	Try a SGA. Low-dose quetiapine is the best tolerated[10], although EPSEs[11] and stereotypical movements[12] can occur. Note that recent studies have cast doubt on the efficacy of quetiapine[13,14] and olanzapine[15,16]. Olanzapine[17–19], risperidone[20–22], aripiprazole[19,20] and ziprasidone[23] probably all have greater adverse effects on motor function than quetiapine. FGAs should be avoided completely. Severe rebound psychosis has been described when antipsychotic drugs (quetiapine or clozapine) are discontinued[24]. Note that atypical antipsychotics have been associated with an increased risk of vascular events in the elderly. See page 422.
6	Consider a **cholinesterase inhibitor**, particularly if the patient has co-morbid dementia[25–27].
7	Try **clozapine**. Start at 6.25 mg – usual dose 25 mg/day[28–30]. Monitor as for clozapine (see page 60). The elderly are more prone to develop serious blood dyscrasia. A case of aplastic anaemia has been reported[31].
8	Consider **ECT**[32]. Psychotic and motor symptoms usually respond well[33] but the risk of inducing delirium is high[5], particularly in patients with pre-existing cognitive impairment.

Dementia in Parkinson's disease

Cholinesterase inhibitors have been shown to improve cognition, delusions and hallucinations in patients with Lewy body dementia (which has some similarities to Parkinson's disease). Motor function may deteriorate[26,34]. Improvements in cognitive functioning are modest[35,36]. A Cochrane review concluded that there was most evidence for rivastigmine; 15% of patients experience clinically meaningful improvements in cognition and activities of daily living[37].

References

1. Reich SG et al. Ten most commonly asked questions about the psychiatric aspects of Parkinson's disease. Neurologist 2003;9:50–6.
2. McDonald WM et al. Prevalence, etiology, and treatment of depression in Parkinson's disease. Biol Psychiatry 2003;54:363–75.
3. Gony M et al. Risk of serious extrapyramidal symptoms in patients with Parkinson's disease receiving antidepressant drugs: a pharmacoepidemiologic study comparing serotonin reuptake inhibitors and other antidepressant drugs. Clin Neuropharmacol 2003;26:142–5.
4. Serrano-Duenas M. A comparison between low doses of amitriptyline and low doses of fluoxetine used in the control of depression in patients suffering from Parkinson's disease (Spanish). Rev Neurol 2002;35: 1010–14.
5. Figiel GS et al. ECT-induced delirium in depressed patients with Parkinson's disease. J Neuropsychiatry Clin Neurosci 1991;3:405–11.
6. Huber TJ et al. Possible use of amantadine in depression. Pharmacopsychiatry 1999;32:47–55.
7. Ismail MS et al. A reality test: How well do we understand psychosis in Parkinson's disease? J Neuropsychiatry Clin Neurosci 2004;16:8–18.
8. Factor SA et al. Longitudinal outcome of Parkinson's disease patients with psychosis. Neurology 2003;60:1756–61.
9. Ives NJ et al. Dopamine agonist therapy in early Parkinson's disease: a systematic review of randomised controlled trials. Mov Disord 2004;19(Suppl 9):S209.
10. Fernandez HH et al. Long-term outcome of quetiapine use for psychosis among Parkinsonian patients. Mov Disord 2003;18:510–14.
11. Prueter C et al. Akathisia as a side effect of antipsychotic treatment with quetiapine in a patient with Parkinson's disease. Mov Disord 2003;18:712–13.
12. Miwa H et al. Stereotyped behaviors or punding after quetiapine administration in Parkinson's disease. Parkinsonism Relat Disord 2004;10:177–80.
13. Prohorov T et al. The effect of quetiapine in psychotic Parkinsonian patients with and without dementia. An open-labeled study utilizing a structured interview. J Neurol 2006;253:171–5.
14. Ondo WG et al. Double-blind, placebo-controlled, unforced titration parallel trial of quetiapine for dopaminergic-induced hallucinations in Parkinson's disease. Mov Disord 2005;20:958–63.
15. Breier A et al. Olanzapine in the treatment of dopamimetic-induced psychosis in patients with Parkinson's disease. Biol Psychiatry 2002;52:438–45.
16. Ondo WG et al. Olanzapine treatment for dopaminergic-induced hallucinations. Mov Disord 2002;17: 1031–5.
17. Friedman J. Olanzapine in the treatment of dopaminomimetic psychosis in patients with Parkinson's disease. Neurology 1998;50:1195–6.
18. Friedman JH et al. Substituting clozapine for olanzapine in psychiatrically stable Parkinson's disease patients: results of an open label pilot study. Clin Neuropharmacol 1998;21:285–8.
19. Goetz CG et al. Olanzapine and clozapine: comparative effects on motor function in hallucinating PD patients. Neurology 2000;55:789–94.
20. Ford B et al. Risperidone in Parkinson's disease. Lancet 1994;344:681.
21. Rich SS et al. Risperidone versus clozapine in the treatment of psychosis in six patients with Parkinson's disease and other akinetic-rigid syndromes. J Clin Psychiatry 1995;56:556–9.
22. Factor SA et al. Risperidone and Parkinson's disease. Mov Disord 2002;17:221–2.
23. Gomez-Esteban JC et al. Use of ziprasidone in parkinsonian patients with psychosis. Clin Neuropharmacol 2005;28:111–14.
24. Fernandez HH et al. Rebound psychosis: effect of discontinuation of antipsychotics in Parkinson's disease. Mov Disord 2005;20:104–5.
25. Shea C et al. Donepezil for treatment of dementia with Lewy bodies: a case series of nine patients. Int Psychogeriatr 1998;10:229–38.
26. McKeith I et al. Efficacy of rivastigmine in dementia with Lewy bodies: a randomised, double-blind, placebo-controlled international study. Lancet 2000;356:2031–6.
27. Fernandez HH et al. Treatment of psychosis in Parkinson's disease: safety considerations. Drug Saf 2003;26:643–59.
28. Parkinson Study Group. Low-dose clozapine for the treatment of drug-induced psychosis in Parkinson's disease. N Engl J Med 1999;340:757–63.
29. Factor SA et al. Clozapine for the treatment of drug-induced psychosis in Parkinson's disease: results of the 12 week open label extension in the PSYCLOPS trial. Mov Disord 2001;16:135–9.

Special groups

30. Pollak P et al. Clozapine in drug induced psychosis in Parkinson's disease: a randomised, placebo controlled study with open follow up. J Neurol Neurosurg Psychiatry 2004;75:689–95.
31. Ziegenbein M et al. Clozapine-induced aplastic anemia in a patient with Parkinson's disease. Can J Psychiatry 2003;48:352.
32. Factor SA et al. Combined clozapine and electroconvulsive therapy for the treatment of drug-induced psychosis in Parkinson's disease. J Neuropsychiatry Clin Neurosci 1995;7:304–7.
33. Martin BA. ECT for Parkinson's? CMAJ 2003;168:1391–2.
34. Richard IH et al. Rivastigmine-induced worsening of motor function and mood in a patient with Parkinson's disease. Mov Disord 2001;16:33–4.
35. Emre M et al. Rivastigmine for dementia associated with Parkinson's disease. N Engl J Med 2004; 351:2509–18.
36. Aarsland D et al. Donepezil for cognitive impairment in Parkinson's disease: a randomised controlled study. J Neurol Neurosurg Psychiatry 2002;72:708–12.
37. Maidment I et al. Cholinesterase inhibitors for Parkinson's disease dementia. Cochrane Database Syst Rev 2006;CD004747.

Further reading

Miyasaki JM et al. Practice parameter: evaluation and treatment of depression, psychosis, and dementia in Parkinson disease (an evidence-based review): report of the Quality Standards Subcommittee of the American Academy of Neurology. Neurology 2006;66:996–1002.
National Institute for Clinical Excellence. Parkinson's disease: diagnosis and management in primary and secondary care. Clinical Guidance 35. http://www.nice.org.uk. 2006.

Special
groups

428

Multiple sclerosis

Multiple sclerosis (MS) is a common cause of neurological disability affecting approximately 85,000 people in the UK, with the onset of the condition usually occurring between 20 and 50 years of age. Individuals with MS may experience a variety of psychiatric disorders such as depression, anxiety, pathological laughter and crying, mania and euphoria, psychosis/bipolar disorder and cognitive impairment. Psychiatric disorders may result from the psychological impact of MS diagnosis and prognosis, perceived lack of social support and dysfunctional coping styles[1], treatment with corticosteroids or beta interferon[2], or damage to neuronal pathways[2].

Depression in multiple sclerosis

Depression is common in MS, with a point prevalence of 14–27%[3,4] and lifetime prevalence of up to 50%[4]. Suicide rates are 7.5 times higher than the general population[5]. Depression in MS may be associated with fatigue and pain, though it is unclear whether depression causes fatigue and worsens pain or whether the experience of fatigue or pain leads to depression. Overlapping symptoms of depression and MS can complicate diagnosis; therefore, cooperation between neurologists and psychiatrists is essential to ensure optimal treatment for individuals with MS.

The role of beta interferon in the aetiology of MS depression is unclear; however, some suggest that concerns are undue[6]. Standard care for initiation of beta interferon should include frequent assessment for depression and, for those with a past history of depressive illness, prophylactic treatment with an antidepressant[2].

Recommendations for treatment – depression in multiple sclerosis	
Step	**Intervention**
1	Screen for depression, utilising HADS/BDI[7]/CES-D[8]. Exclude and treat any organic causes. Consider iatrogenic effects of medications as potential cause of depression. Ensure there is no past history of mania. If mild depression is evident, patients should not be prescribed antidepressants but should be provided with self-help materials based on cognitive behavioural therapy (CBT)
2	SSRIs should be first-line treatment[2,9–11] because of their benign side-effect profile. Due to reduced tolerability of side-effects in this patient group, medications should be titrated from an initial half dose. Many MS patients are prescribed low-dose TCAs for pain/bladder disturbance; therefore, SSRIs should be used with caution and patients should be observed for serotonin syndrome. For those with co-morbid pain and/or depression consideration should be given to treating with an SNRI such as duloxetine or venlafaxine[12]. Tricyclics are often poorly tolerated[13]
3	If SSRIs are not tolerated or there is no response, there are limited data that moclobemide is effective and well tolerated[14,15]. There are no

Table Recommendations for treatment – depression in multiple sclerosis (Cont.)		
Step	**Intervention**	
	published trials focusing on venlafaxine and mirtazapine but these agents are used widely	
4	ECT could be considered for people who are actively suicidal or severely depressed and at high risk, but it may trigger an exacerbation of MS symptoms[16], although some studies suggest no neurological disturbance occurs[17]	
5	CBT is the most appropriate psychological intervention with best efficacy in comparison to supportive therapy or usual care, and should be used in conjunction with medication for those who are moderately–severely depressed[9,18]	

Anxiety in multiple sclerosis

Anxiety affects many people with MS, with point prevalence of 14–25%[19,20] and lifetime incidence of 35–37%[17]. Elevated rates appear attributed to generalised anxiety disorder, panic disorder and obsessive compulsive disorder[17]. Anxiety appears reactive in nature and is linked to perceived lack of support with anxious patients more likely to be depressed, drink excessively and become suicidal. SSRIs such as paroxetine or sertraline should be used and, in non-responsive cases, venlafaxine could be used. Pregabalin is also licensed for anxiety and may be useful in this population group, although control effects can be problematic.

Pathological laughter and crying (PLC)

Up to 10% of individuals with MS experience PLC. It is more common in the advanced stages of the disease and is associated with cognitive impairment[21]. There have been a few open-label trials recommending the use of small doses of TCAs (e.g. amitriptyline) or SSRIs (e.g. fluoxetine)[22,23] with reasonable efficacy and rapid response.

Mania/euphoria/bipolar disorder in multiple sclerosis

Prevalence of bipolar disorder can be as high as 13% in the MS population[2] compared with 1–6% in the general population. Anecdotal evidence suggests that patients presenting with mania should be treated with valproate, as this is better tolerated than lithium[24]. Lithium can cause polyuria and thus lead to difficulties with tolerability. Mania accompanied by psychosis could be treated with low-dose second generation antipsychotics such as risperidone, olanzapine[2] and ziprasidone[25].

Patients requiring psychiatric treatment for steroid-induced mania with psychosis have been known to respond well to olanzapine[26]; further case reports suggest risperidone is also useful. There have been no trials in this area.

Psychosis in multiple sclerosis

Psychosis occurs in 1.1% of the MS population[27]. There have been few published trials in this area, but risperidone[2], olanzapine[2] and ziprasidone[25] all appear to have reasonable efficacy. Psychosis may rarely be the presentation of an MS relapse, in which case steroids may be beneficial but would need to be given under close supervision.

Cognitive impairment

Cognitive impairment occurs in at least 40–65% of people with MS. Some of the iatrogenic effects of medications commonly prescribed can worsen cognition: e.g. pregabalin, tizanidine, diazepam and gabapentin[28]. Although there are no published trials, evidence from clinical case studies suggests that the treatment of sleep difficulties, depression and fatigue can enhance cognitive function[28]. There have been two favourable small trials with donepezil for people with mild–moderate cognitive impairment showing moderate efficacy[29,30].

References

1. Ron MA. Do neurologists provide adequate care for depression in patients with multiple sclerosis? Nat Clin Pract Neurol 2006;2:534–5.
2. Servis ME. Psychiatric comorbidity in Parkinson's disease, multiple sclerosis, and seizure disorder. Continuum 2006;12:72–86.
3. Gottberg K et al. A population-based study of depressive symptoms in multiple sclerosis in Stockholm county: association with functioning and sense of coherence. J Neurol Neurosurg Psychiatry 2007; 78:60–5.
4. Patten SB et al. Major depression in multiple sclerosis: a population-based perspective. Neurology 2003;61:1524–7.
5. Sadovnick AD et al. Cause of death in patients attending multiple sclerosis clinics. Neurology 1991;41:1193–6.
6. Zephir H et al. Multiple sclerosis and depression: influence of interferon beta therapy. Mult Scler 2003; 9:284–8.
7. Moran PJ et al. The validity of Beck Depression Inventory and Hamilton Rating Scale for Depression items in the assessment of depression among patients with multiple sclerosis. J Behav Med 2005;28:35–41.
8. Pandya R et al. Predictive value of the CES-D in detecting depression among candidates for disease-modifying multiple sclerosis treatment. Psychosomatics 2005;46:131–4.
9. Siegert RJ et al. Depression in multiple sclerosis: a review. J Neurol Neurosurg Psychiatry 2005; 76:469–75.
10. Mohr DC et al. Comparative outcomes for individual cognitive-behavior therapy, supportive-expressive group psychotherapy, and sertraline for the treatment of depression in multiple sclerosis. J Consult Clin Psychol 2001;69:942–9.
11. Barak Y et al. Treatment of depression in patients with multiple sclerosis. Neurologist 1998; 4:99–104.
12. Hilty DM et al. Psychopharmacology for neurologists: principles, algorithms, and other resources. Continuum 2006;12:33–46.
13. Schiffer RB et al. Antidepressant pharmacotherapy of depression associated with multiple sclerosis. Am J Psychiatry 1990;147:1493–7.
14. Barak Y et al. Moclobemide treatment in multiple sclerosis patients with comorbid depression: an open-label safety trial. J Neuropsychiatry Clin Neurosci 1999;11:271–3.
15. Then BF et al. Combined treatment with corticosteroids and moclobemide favors normalization of hypothalamo–pituitary–adrenal axis dysregulation in relapsing-remitting multiple sclerosis: a randomized, double blind trial. J Clin Endocrinol Metab 2001;86:1610–15.
16. Feinstein A. Multiple sclerosis, depression, and suicide. BMJ 1997;315:691–2.
17. Corruble E et al. ECT in delusional depression with multiple sclerosis. Am J Psychiatry 2004;161:1715.
18. Larcombe NA et al. An evaluation of cognitive-behaviour therapy for depression in patients with multiple sclerosis. Br J Psychiatry 1984;145:366–71.
19. Korostil M et al. Anxiety disorders and their clinical correlates in multiple sclerosis patients. Mult Scler 2007;13:67–72.
20. Feinstein A et al. The effects of anxiety on psychiatric morbidity in patients with multiple sclerosis. Mult Scler 1999;5:323–6.
21. Feinstein A et al. Prevalence and neurobehavioral correlates of pathological laughing and crying in multiple sclerosis. Arch Neurol 1997;54:1116–21.
22. Schiffer RB et al. Treatment of pathologic laughing and weeping with amitriptyline. N Engl J Med 1985;312:1480–2.
23. Seliger GM et al. Fluoxetine improves emotional incontinence. Brain Inj 1992;6:267–70.
24. Stip E et al. Valproate in the treatment of mood disorder due to multiple sclerosis. Can J Psychiatry 1995;40:219–20.
25. Davids E et al. Antipsychotic treatment of psychosis associated with multiple sclerosis. Prog Neuropsychopharmacol Biol Psychiatry 2004;28:743–4.
26. Budur K et al. Olanzapine for corticosteroid-induced mood disorders. Psychosomatics 2003;44:353.
27. Schifferdecker M et al. Psychoses in multiple sclerosis – a reevaluation (in German). Fortschr Neurol Psychiatr 1995;63:310–19.
28. Pierson SH et al. Treatment of cognitive impairment in multiple sclerosis. Behav Neurol 2006;17: 53–67.
29. Krupp LB et al. Donepezil improved memory in multiple sclerosis in a randomized clinical trial. Neurology 2004;63:1579–85.
30. Greene YM et al. A 12-week, open trial of donepezil hydrochloride in patients with multiple sclerosis and associated cognitive impairments. J Clin Psychopharmacol 2000;20:350–6.

Special groups

432

Eating disorders

Prevalence rates in young females are 0.3% for anorexia nervosa and 1% for bulimia nervosa. In men the rate is about a 10th of that seen in women[1]. There are many similarities between the different types of eating disorders and patients often traverse diagnoses, which can complicate treatment[2].

Other psychiatric conditions (particularly anxiety, depression and obsessive compulsive disorder) often coexist with eating disorders and may in part explain the benefit of medication.

Anorexia nervosa carries considerable risk of mortality or serious physical morbidity. Patients may present with multiple physical conditions including amenorrhoea, muscle wasting, electrolyte abnormalities, cardiovascular complications and osteoporosis. Patients who purge through vomiting are at high risk of loss of tooth enamel, gastro-oesophageal erosion and dehydration[2]. Other modes of purging include laxative and diuretic misuse. Any medication prescribed should accompany close observations of physical state and possible adverse reactions.

Anorexia nervosa

General guidance
There are few controlled trials to guide treatment in anorexia nervosa. Prompt weight restoration, family therapy and structured psychotherapy are the main choices of treatment[3,4]. The aim of (physical) treatment is to improve nutritional health through re-feeding with very limited evidence base for pharmacological treatment. Drugs may be used to treat co-morbid conditions[3].

Healthcare professionals should be aware of the risk of drugs that prolong the QTc interval. All patients with a diagnosis of anorexia nervosa should have an alert placed in their prescribing record concerning the risk of side effects. ECG monitoring should be undertaken if the prescription of medication that may compromise cardiac functioning is essential[3].

Physical aspects
Vitamins & minerals: Treatment with a multivitamin/multimineral supplement in oral form is recommended during both inpatient and outpatient weight restoration[3] (in the UK, Forceval or Sanatogen Gold one capsule daily may be used).

Electrolytes: Electrolyte disturbances (e.g. hypokalaemia) may develop slowly over time and may be asymptomatic and resolve with re-feeding. Hypophosphataemia may be precipitated by re-feeding. Rapid correction may be hazardous. Oral supplementation is therefore used to prevent serious sequelae rather than simply to restore normal levels. If supplements are used urea and electrolytes, HCO_3, Ca, P & Mg need to be monitored and ECG needs to be performed[5].

Osteoporosis: Bone loss is a serious complication of anorexia with serious consequences. Hormonal treatment using oestrogen or dehydroepiandrosterone

433

(DHEA) does not have a positive impact on bone density and oestrogen is not recommended in children and adolescence due to the risk of premature fusion of the bones[3].

Psychiatric aspects
Acute illness: *Antidepressants* - A Cochrane review found no evidence from four placebo-controlled trials that antidepressants improved weight gain, eating disorder or associated psychopathology[6]. It has been suggested that neurochemical abnormalities in starvation may partially explain this non-response[6]. Co-prescribing nutritional supplementation (including tryptophan) with fluoxetine has not been shown to increase efficacy[7].

Other psychotropic drugs - Antipsychotic drugs (e.g. olanzapine), minor tranquilisers or antihistamines (e.g. promethazine) are often used to reduce the high levels of anxiety associated with anorexia nervosa but they are not recommended for the promotion of weight gain[3]. Case reports and retrospective studies have suggested that olanzapine may reduce agitation (and possibly improve weight gain)[8,9]. Many other medications have been investigated in small placebo-controlled trials of varying quality and success, these include zinc[10], naltrexone[11] and cyproheptadine[12].

Relapse prevention: There is evidence from one small trial that fluoxetine may be useful in improving outcome and preventing relapse of patients with anorexia nervosa after weight restoration[13]. Other studies have found no benefit[6,14].

Co-morbid disorders: Antidepressants are often used to treat co-morbid major depressive disorder and obsessive compulsive disorder. However, caution should be used as these conditions may resolve with weight gain alone[3].

Bulimia Nervosa & Binge Eating Disorder

Adults with bulimia nervosa and binge eating disorder (BED) may be offered a trial of an antidepressant. SSRIs (specifically fluoxetine[15–17]) are the drugs of first choice. The effective dose of fluoxetine is 60mg daily[18]. Patients should be informed that this can reduce the frequency of binge eating and purging but long-term effects are unknown[3].

Antidepressant drugs may be used for the treatment of bulimia nervosa in adolescents but they are not licensed for this age group and there is no evidence for this practice. They should not be considered as a first line treatment in adolescent bulimia nervosa[3].

Other atypical eating disorders

There have been no studies of the use of drugs to treat atypical eating disorders other than BED[3,19].

In the absence of evidence to guide the management of atypical eating disorders (also known as eating disorders not otherwise specified) other than binge eating disorder, it is recommended that the clinician considers following the guidance of the eating disorder that mostly resembles the individual patient's eating disorder[3].

Summary of NICE guidance in eating disorders[3]

Anorexia Nervosa
- Psychological interventions are the treatments of choice and should be accompanied by monitoring of the patient's physical state
- No particular medication is recommended. A range of drugs may be used in the treatment of co-morbid conditions.

Bulimia nervosa
- An evidence based self-help programme or cognitive behaviour therapy for bulimia nervosa should be the first choice of treatment
- A trial of fluoxetine may be offered as an alternative or additional first step

Binge eating disorder
- An evidence based self-help programme of cognitive behavioural therapy for binge eating disorder should be the first choice of treatment
- A trial of an SSRI can be considered as an alternative or additional first step

---

References

1. Hoek HW et al. Review of the prevalence and incidence of eating disorders. Int J Eat Disord 2003;34:383–96.
2. Steffen KJ et al. Emerging drugs for eating disorder treatment. Expert Opin Emerg Drugs 2006;11:315–36.
3. National Institute for Clinical Excellence. Eating disorders: Core interventions in the treatment and management of anorexia nervosa, bulimia nervosa and related eating disorders. Clinical Guidance 9. http://www.nice.org.uk. 2004.
4. American Psychiatric Association. Treatment of patients with eating disorders, third edition. Am J Psychiatry 2006;163:4–54.
5. Connan F et al. Biochemical and endocrine complications. Eur Eat Disord Rev 2007;8:144–57.
6. Claudino AM et al. Antidepressants for anorexia nervosa. Cochrane Database Syst Rev 2006;CD004365.
7. Barbarich NC et al. Use of nutritional supplements to increase the efficacy of fluoxetine in the treatment of anorexia nervosa. Int J Eat Disord 2004;35:10–5.
8. Malina A et al. Olanzapine treatment of anorexia nervosa: a retrospective study. Int J Eat Disord 2003;33:234–7.
9. La Via MC et al. Case reports of olanzapine treatment of anorexia nervosa. Int J Eat Disord 2000; 27:363–6.
10. Su JC et al. Zinc supplementation in the treatment of anorexia nervosa. Eat Weight Disord 2002; 7:20–2.
11. Marrazzi MA et al. Naltrexone use in the treatment of anorexia nervosa and bulimia nervosa. Int Clin Psychopharmacol 1995;10:163–72.
12. Halmi KA et al. Anorexia nervosa. Treatment efficacy of cyproheptadine and amitriptyline. Arch Gen Psychiatry 1986;43:177–81.
13. Kaye WH et al. Double-blind placebo-controlled administration of fluoxetine in restricting- and restricting-purging-type anorexia nervosa. Biol Psychiatry 2001;49:644–52.
14. Walsh BT et al. Fluoxetine after weight restoration in anorexia nervosa: a randomized controlled trial. JAMA 2006;295:2605–12.
15. Fluoxetine Bulimia Nervosa Collaborative Study Group. Fluoxetine in the treatment of bulimia nervosa. A multicenter, placebo-controlled, double-blind trial. Arch Gen Psychiatry 1992;49: 139–47.
16. Goldstein DJ et al. Long-term fluoxetine treatment of bulimia nervosa. Fluoxetine Bulimia Nervosa Research Group. Br J Psychiatry 1995;166:660–6.
17. Romano SJ et al. A placebo-controlled study of fluoxetine in continued treatment of bulimia nervosa after successful acute fluoxetine treatment. Am J Psychiatry 2002;159:96–102.
18. Bacaltchuk J et al. Antidepressants versus placebo for people with bulimia nervosa. Cochrane Database Syst Rev 2003;CD003391.
19. Leombruni P et al. A 12 to 24 weeks pilot study of sertraline treatment in obese women binge eaters. Hum Psychopharmacol 2006;21:181–8.

Acutely disturbed or violent behaviour

Acute behavioural disturbance may occur in the context of psychiatric illness, physical illness, substance abuse or personality disorder. Psychotic symptoms are common and the patient may be aggressive towards others secondary to persecutory delusions or auditory, visual or tactile hallucinations.

The clinical practice of rapid tranquillisation (RT) is used when appropriate psychological and behavioural approaches have failed to de-escalate acutely disturbed behaviour. It is, essentially, a treatment of last resort. RT is not underpinned by a strong evidence base. Patients who require RT are often too disturbed to give informed consent and therefore cannot participate in randomised controlled trials (RCTs). Recommendations are therefore based partly on research data, partly on theoretical considerations and partly on clinical experience.

Several studies supporting the efficacy of oral risperidone[1-4] and one observational study, each supporting the efficacy of quetiapine[5] and olanzapine orodispersible tablets[6] have been published. The level of behavioural disturbance exhibited by the patients in these studies was moderate at most, and all subjects accepted oral treatment (this degree of compliance would be unusual in clinical practice).

Larger, placebo-controlled RCTs support the efficacy of IM olanzapine[7,8], ziprasidone[9] and aripiprazole[10]. Again, the level of behavioural disturbance in these studies was moderate at most. One small open study supports the effectiveness of IM ziprasidone in clinical emergencies (where disturbance was severe)[11].

Two large RCTs (the TREC studies[12,13]) have investigated the efficacy of a benzodiazepine versus an antipsychotic/sedative combination (all administered IM) in 'real-life' acutely disturbed patients. TREC 1[12] found midazolam 7.5–15 mg to be more rapidly sedating than a combination of haloperidol 5–10 mg and promethazine 50 mg. TREC 2[13] found haloperidol 10 mg combined with promethazine 25–50 mg to be more rapidly sedating than lorazepam 4 mg. Although these studies are undoubtedly the best available to date, UK psychiatrists rarely prescribe IM midazolam or promethazine, and have been increasingly reluctant to prescribe IM haloperidol due to its ability to cause EPSEs. Acute EPSEs may adversely affect longer-term compliance[14]. The SPC requirement for ECG with haloperidol also limits its use. Lorazepam IM is an established treatment and TREC 2[13] supports its efficacy.

Plans for the management of individual patients should ideally be made in advance. The aim is to prevent disturbed behaviour and reduce risk of violence. Nursing interventions (de-escalation, time out), increased nursing levels, transfer of the patient to a psychiatric intensive care unit (PICU) and pharmacological management are options that may be employed. Care should be taken to avoid combinations and high cumulative doses of antipsychotic drugs. The monitoring of routine physical observations after RT is essential. Note that RT is often viewed as punitive by patients.

Special groups

The aims of RT are threefold:

1. To reduce suffering for the patient: psychological or physical (through self-harm or accidents).
2. To reduce risk of harm to others by maintaining a safe environment.
3. To do no harm (by prescribing safe regimens and monitoring physical health).

Note: *Despite the need for rapid and effective treatment, concomitant use of two or more antipsychotics (antipsychotic polypharmacy) should be avoided on the basis of risk associated with QT prolongation (common to almost all antipsychotics) (see page 115). This is a particularly important consideration in RT where the patient's physical state predisposes to cardiac arrhythmia.*

In an emergency situation (*NB: read attached notes carefully*)

Step	Intervention		
1	De-escalation, time out, placement, etc., as appropriate		
2[a,b]	Offer **oral** treatment	**Haloperidol** 5 mg or **Olanzapine**[6] 10 mg or **Risperidone**[1-4] 1–2 mg	with or without lorazepam 1–2 mg. Repeat every 45–60 min Go to step 3 if three doses fail or sooner if the patient is placing themselves or others at significant risk.
		Monotherapy with buccal midazolam, 10–20 mg may offer a useful alternative. Note that this preparation is unlicensed	
3[b-f]	Consider **IM** treatment	**Lorazepam** 1–2 mg[13,g] or **Midazolam** 7.5–15 mg[12] or **Haloperidol** 5 mg[12,13] or **Olanzapine** 5–10 mg[8,h] or **Ziprasidone** 10–20 mg[9,17,i] or **Aripiprazole** 10 mg[10]	IM olanzapine should not be combined with an IM benzodiazepine[15,16]. The safety of other SGAs combined with benzodiazepines is unknown
		Repeat up to two times at 30–60 min intervals, if insufficient effect **Promethazine**[j] 50 mg IM is an alternative in benzodiazepine-tolerant patients	
4	Consider **IV** treatment	**Diazepam**[k-m] 10 mg over at least 5 min Repeat after 5–10 min if insufficient effect (up to three times)	
5	**Seek expert advice**.	Amylobarbital[n] 250 mg IM or paraldehyde[o] 5–10 ml IM are options. Very, very few episodes of RT should reach this point	

438

Notes on the table above

a. Choice depends on current treatment. If the patient is established on antipsychotics, lorazepam may be used alone. If the patient uses street drugs or is already receiving benzodiazepines regularly, an antipsychotic may be used alone. For the majority of patients, the best response will be obtained with a combination of an antipsychotic and lorazepam.

b. Ensure that parenteral anticholinergics are available. Procyclidine 5–10 mg IM or benzatropine 1–2 mg IM may be required to reverse acute dystonic reactions (most likely with haloperidol).

c. Either an antipsychotic or benzodiazepine can be used alone as in (a), but for the majority of patients the best response will be obtained with a combination of an antipsychotic and lorazepam.

d. Have flumazenil available to reverse the effects of lorazepam or midazolam. (Monitor respiratory rate – give flumazenil if rate falls below 10/min.)

e. From this point onwards, review the patient's legal status. The requirement for enforced IM medication in informal patients should prompt the use of the Mental Health Act.

f. From this point onwards, consider consulting a senior colleague.

g. Mix lorazepam 1:1 with water for injections before injecting. Some centres use 2–4 mg.

h. Recommended by NICE only for moderate behavioural disturbance.

i. Ziprasidone is unlikely to be licensed in the UK, but is available in the USA and other countries.

j. Promethazine has a slow onset of action but is often an effective sedative. Dilution is not required before IM injection. May be repeated up to a maximum of 100 mg/day. Wait 1–2 hours after injection to assess response. Note that promethazine alone has been reported to cause NMS[18] although it is an extremely weak dopamine antagonist.

k. Use Diazemuls to avoid injection site reactions. IV therapy may be used instead of IM when a very rapid effect is required. IV therapy also ensures near immediate delivery of the drug to its site of action and effectively avoids the danger of inadvertent accumulation of slowly absorbed IM doses. Note also that IV doses can be repeated after only 5–10 min if no effect is observed.

l. Have flumazenil available to reverse the effects of diazepam. (Monitor respiratory rate – give flumazenil if rate falls below 10/min.)

m. Caution in the very young and elderly and those with pre-existing brain damage or impulse control problems, as disinhibition reactions are more likely[19].

n. Amylobarbital is a powerful respiratory depressant with no pharmacological antagonist. Have facilities for mechanical ventilation available.

o. Paraldehyde is now used extremely rarely and is difficult to obtain. It should only be used when all else has failed. In many cases, ECT may be more appropriate. Note that paraldehyde is associated with a high incidence of tachycardia and tachypnea[20]. IV diazepam may be more effective and is certainly better tolerated[20].

Rapid tranquillisation – physical monitoring

After any parenteral drug administration, monitor as follows:

Temperature

Pulse

Blood pressure

Respiratory rate

Every 5–10 min for 1 hour, and then half-hourly until patient is ambulatory. Patients who refuse to have their vital signs monitored should be observed for signs/symptoms of pyrexia, hypotension, oversedation and general physical well-being.

If the patient is asleep or **unconscious**, the use of pulse oximetry to measure oxygen saturation continuously is desirable. A nurse should remain with the patient until the patient is ambulatory again.

ECG and haematological monitoring are also strongly recommended when parenteral antipsychotics are given, especially when higher doses are used[21,22]. Hypokalaemia, stress and agitation place the patient at risk of cardiac arrhythmia[23] (see page 115). ECG monitoring is formally recommended for all patients receiving haloperidol in any formulation[24].

Remedial measures in rapid tranquillisation

Problem	Remedial measures
Acute dystonia (including oculogyric crises)	Give **procyclidine** 5–10 mg IM or IV or **benzatropine** 1–2 mg IM.
Reduced respiratory rate (<10/min) or oxygen saturation (<90%)	Give oxygen, raise legs, ensure patient is not lying face down. Give **flumazenil** if benzodiazepine-induced respiratory depression suspected (see protocol). If induced by any other sedative agent: **transfer to a medical bed and ventilate mechanically**.
Irregular or slow (<50/min) **pulse**	**Refer** to specialist medical care immediately.
Fall in blood pressure (>30 mmHg orthostatic drop or <50 mmHg diastolic)	**Have patient lie flat**, tilt bed towards head. Monitor closely.
Increased temperature	**Withhold antipsychotics:** (risk of NMS and perhaps arrhythmia). Check creatinine kinase urgently.

Guidelines for the use of flumazenil

Indication for use	If, after the administration of lorazepam or diazepam, respiratory rate falls below 10/min.
Contraindications	Patients with epilepsy who have been receiving long-term benzodiazepines.
Caution	Dose should be carefully titrated in hepatic impairment.
Dose and route of administration	*Initial:* 200 µg *intravenously* over 15 seconds – if required level of consciousness not achieved after 60 seconds, then, *Subsequent dose:* 100 µg over 10 seconds.
Time before dose can be repeated	60 seconds.
Maximum dose	1 mg in 24 hours (one initial dose and eight subsequent doses).
Side-effects	Patients may become agitated, anxious or fearful on awakening. Seizures may occur in regular benzodiazepine users.
Management	Side-effects usually subside.
Monitoring • **What to monitor?** • **How often?**	Respiratory rate. Continuously until respiratory rate returns to baseline level. Flumazenil has a short half-life (much shorter than diazepam) and respiratory function may recover and then deteriorate again. *Note: If respiratory rate does not return to normal or patient is not alert after initial doses given, assume that sedation is due to some other cause.*

Guidelines for the use of Clopixol Acuphase (zuclopenthixol acetate)

Acuphase should be used only after an acutely psychotic patient has required <u>repeated</u> injections of short-acting antipsychotic drugs such as haloperidol or olanzapine, or sedative drugs such as lorazepam.

Acuphase should be given only when enough time has elapsed to assess the full response to previously injected drugs: allow 15 min after IV injections; 60 min after IM.

*Acuphase should **never** be administered:*
- in an attempt to 'hasten' the antipsychotic effect of other antipsychotic therapy
- for rapid tranquillisation (onset of effect is too slow)
- at the same time as other parenteral antipsychotics or benzodi-azepines (may lead to oversedation which is difficult to reverse)
- as a 'test dose' for zuclopenthixol decanoate depot
- to a patient who is physically resistant (risk of intravasation and oil embolus).

*Acuphase should **never** be used for, or in, the following:*
- patients who accept oral medication
- patients who are neuroleptic naive
- patients who are sensitive to EPSE
- patients who are unconscious
- patients who are pregnant
- those with hepatic or renal impairment
- those with cardiac disease.

Onset and duration of action
Sedative effects usually begin to be seen 2 hours after injection and peak after 12 hours. The effects may last for up to 72 hours. Note: Acuphase has no place in rapid tranquillisation: *its action is not rapid*.

Dose
Acuphase should be given in a dose of 50–150 mg, up to a maximum of 400 mg over a 2-week period. This maximum duration ensures that a treatment plan is put in place. It does not indicate that there are known harmful effects from more prolonged administration, although such use should be very exceptional. There is no such thing as a 'course of Acuphase'. The patient should be assessed before each administration.

Injections should be spaced at least 24 hours apart.

Note: zuclopenthixol acetate is widely misused as a sort of 'chemical straitjacket'. In reality, it is a potentially toxic preparation with very little published information to support its use[25]. It is perhaps best reserved for those few patients who have a prior history of good response to Acuphase.

References

1. Lejeune J et al. Oral risperidone plus oral lorazepam versus standard care with intramuscular conventional neuroleptics in the initial phase of treating individuals with acute psychosis. Int Clin Psychopharmacol 2004;19:259–69.
2. Currier GW et al. Acute treatment of psychotic agitation: a randomized comparison of oral treatment with risperidone and lorazepam versus intramuscular treatment with haloperidol and lorazepam. J Clin Psychiatry 2004;65:386–94.
3. Yildiz A et al. Observational data on the antiagitation effect of risperidone tablets in emergency settings: a preliminary report. Int J Psychiatry Clin Pract 2003;7:217–21.
4. Currier GW et al. Risperidone liquid concentrate and oral lorazepam versus intramuscular haloperidol and intramuscular lorazepam for treatment of psychotic agitation. J Clin Psychiatry 2001;62:153–7.
5. Ganesan S et al. Effectiveness of quetiapine for the management of aggressive psychosis in the emergency psychiatric setting: a naturalistic uncontrolled trial. Int J Psychiatry Clin Pract 2005;9:199–203.
6. Simpson JR Jr et al. Impact of orally disintegrating olanzapine on use of intramuscular antipsychotics, seclusion, and restraint in an acute inpatient psychiatric setting. J Clin Psychopharmacol 2006;26: 333–5.
7. Wright P et al. Double-blind, placebo-controlled comparison of intramuscular olanzapine and intramuscular haloperidol in the treatment of acute agitation in schizophrenia. Am J Psychiatry 2001;158: 1149–51.
8. Breier A et al. A double-blind, placebo-controlled dose–response comparison of intramuscular olanzapine and haloperidol in the treatment of acute agitation in schizophrenia. Arch Gen Psychiatry 2002;59:441–8.
9. Brook S et al. Intramuscular ziprasidone compared with intramuscular haloperidol in the treatment of acute psychosis. Ziprasidone I.M. Study Group. J Clin Psychiatry 2000;61:933–41.
10. Andrezina R et al. Intramuscular aripiprazole for the treatment of acute agitation in patients with schizophrenia or schizoaffective disorder: a double-blind, placebo-controlled comparison with intramuscular haloperidol. Psychopharmacology 2006;188:281–92.
11. Fulton JA et al. Intramuscular ziprasidone: an effective agent for sedation of the agitated ED patient. Am J Emerg Med 2006;24:254–5.
12. TREC Collaborative Group. Rapid tranquillisation for agitated patients in emergency psychiatric rooms: a randomised trial of midazolam versus haloperidol plus promethazine. BMJ 2003;327:708–13.
13. Alexander J et al. Rapid tranquillisation of violent or agitated patients in a psychiatric emergency setting. Pragmatic randomised trial of intramuscular lorazepam v. haloperidol plus promethazine. Br J Psychiatry 2004;185:63–9.
14. van Harten PN et al. Acute dystonia induced by drug treatment. BMJ 1999;319:623–6.
15. Eli Lilly and Company Limited. Letter to Healthcare Professionals. 2004.
16. Zacher JL et al. Hypotension secondary to the combination of intramuscular olanzapine and intramuscular lorazepam. J Clin Psychiatry 2005;66:1614–15.
17. Brook S et al. Ziprasidone and haloperidol in the treatment of acute exacerbation of schizophrenia and schizoaffective disorder: comparison of intramuscular and oral formulations in a 6-week, randomized, blinded-assessment study. Psychopharmacology 2005;178:514–23.
18. Chan-Tack KM. Neuroleptic malignant syndrome due to promethazine. South Med J 1999; 92:1017–18.
19. Paton C. Benzodiazepines and disinhibition: a review. Psychiatr Bull 2002;26:460–2.
20. Thompson WL et al. Diazepam and paraldehyde for treatment of severe delirium tremens. A controlled trial. Ann Intern Med 1975;82:175–80.
21. Appleby L et al. Sudden unexplained death in psychiatric in-patients. Br J Psychiatry 2000;176:405–6.
22. Yap YG et al. Risk of torsades de pointes with non-cardiac drugs. Doctors need to be aware that many drugs can cause QT prolongation. BMJ 2000;320:1158–9.
23. Taylor DM. Antipsychotics and QT prolongation. Acta Psychiatr Scand 2003;107:85–95.
24. Janssen-Cilag Ltd. Haldol injection. http://emc.medicines.org.uk/. 2006.
25. Gibson RC et al. Zuclopenthixol acetate for acute schizophrenia and similar serious mental illnesses. Cochrane Database Syst Rev 2004;CD000525.

Further reading

Currier GW et al. Orally versus intramuscularly administered antipsychotic drugs in psychiatric emergencies. J Psychiatr Pract 2006;12:30–40.

McAllister Williams RH et al. Rapid tranquillisation: time for a reappraisal of options for parenteral therapy. Br J Psychiatry 2002;180:485–9.

Macpherson R et al. A growing evidence base for management guidelines: revisting... guidelines for the management of acutely disturbed psychiatric patients. Adv Psychiatr Treat 2005;11:404–15.

National Institute for Clinical Excellence. Violence – The short-term management of disturbed/violent behaviour in in-patient psychiatric settings and emergency departments. Guideline No 25, 2005. www.nice.org.uk.

Pilowsky LS et al. Rapid tranquillisation. A survey of emergency prescribing in a general psychiatric hospital. Br J Psychiatry 1992;160:831–5.

Special groups

Chronic behavioural disturbance in learning disability[1]

Behavioural disturbance is common in those with a learning disability. It is often very difficult to determine the aetiology. The following may be useful prompts:

1. Is there or could there be an underlying physical illness? (look for and treat).
2. Could environmental factors be contributing? (consider and alter if possible).
3. Is there an underlying psychiatric illness? (consider and treat if applicable).

Then consider:

4. Does the patient have a history of mood disturbance? (try an antidepressant/mood stabiliser).
5. Is the disturbance cyclical? (try a mood stabiliser).
6. Is/might epilepsy (be) a contributing factor? (try an anticonvulsant).
7. Is the patient aggressive? (try carbamazepine or a β-blocker).
8. Are there any signs of adrenergic overactivity, such as tachycardia or tremor? (try a β-blocker).
9. Is the patient impulsive? (try an SSRI).
10. Is the patient self-injurious? (try an antipsychotic, SSRI or naltrexone).
11. Could the behaviour be driven by psychosis? (try an antipsychotic).

Self-injurious behaviour in learning disability

Repetitive or stereotypical acts that produce self-inflicted injury (self-injurious behaviour (SIB))[2-4]:

- occur in approximately 20% of adults with learning disability (up to 50% in those requiring institutional care)
- most commonly take the form of head-banging, banging other body parts, biting, scratching, pinching, gouging, hair-pulling and pica
- occur more frequently in males; younger adults; those with impairments in hearing, vision, mobility and communication; and those with a diagnosis of autism and epilepsy. As the IQ falls, the prevalence of SIB (and multiple behaviours) increases.

SIB is a major cause of distress to carers and a major cause of institutional care.

Aetiology[5-8]

SIB is best understood as being caused by a combination of organic and environmental factors. Organic factors include rare genetic syndromes (such as Lesch–Nyhan or Smith–Magenis syndrome), developmental brain damage, neurological disorders (such as epilepsy), physical illness, psychiatric illness and communication problems. SIB may be linked to the menstrual cycle in some women. Environmental factors include lack of stimulation/overstimulation, lack of/too much affection, rejection/lack of attention and adverse life events.

Some factors may predispose to SIB (e.g. genetic syndromes), others precipitate it (e.g. depression, dysphoria) and others perpetuate it (e.g. secondary changes in neuroregulatory systems).

The prevalence of mental illness is increased in those with learning disabilities, and non-specific and atypical presentations of mental illness increase in frequency as the IQ falls. Diagnosis often has to be made from observing behaviour rather than directly eliciting symptoms.

Non-drug treatments[9-11]

It is important to try to understand why the patient self-harms (e.g. self-stimulation, relief of dysphoria, attention, social escape through being removed from communal areas, material reward). Psychological/behavioural strategies for dealing with the behaviour can then be put in place. This should always be tried before resorting to drug treatment.

Successfully preventing one form of SIB may lead to the emergence of another form. Staff may perceive SIB to be due to different causes in the same patient and may react with fear, irritation, anger, disgust or despair. Interventions based on individual belief systems will lead to inconsistent care. Effective management and support of staff is essential.

Special groups

Drug treatment options – SIB in learning disability

Drug	Rationale
Antipsychotics[12–14]	• Supersensitivity of dopamine neurons in nigro-striatal pathways may predispose to SIB. D_1 blockers (such as thioxanthines) may be more effective than D_2 blockers. Atypical antipsychotics are poorly evaluated (may have fewer severe side-effects). There is most experience with risperidone • Dopamine is involved in reward mechanisms (blocking dopamine blocks reward) • Low-dose antipsychotics reduce stereotypies
Opiate antagonists[5,8]	• SIB leads to the release of endogenous opiates (endorphins), which may lead to a rewarding mood state (positive reinforcement) • Naltrexone (an opiate antagonist) may decrease SIB acutely but is less effective in the long term (?opiate mechanisms are important in the early stages, but SIB is perpetuated via dopamine reward mechanisms)
Anticonvulsants[13]	• The prevalence of epilepsy is high in moderate/severe learning disabilities • Aggression (to others or self) can be related to seizure activity (pre-ictal, ictal or post-ictal). Note: vigabatrin and topiramate may cause behavioural problems • Rapid-cycling mood disorders and mixed affective states are more common in learning disabilities and may respond best to carbamazepine or valproate
SSRIs[5,8] Lithium[13,15] Buspirone[16]	• Drugs that increase 5HT neurotransmission have been shown to reduce SIB in some patients • These drugs may act by targeting the behaviour that precipitates SIB (e.g. fear, irritability, anxiety or depression) • Lithium is licensed for 'the control of aggressive behaviour or intentional self-harm'
Others[8,13,17]	• Other drugs may be useful in some circumstances (e.g. propranolol – probably through reducing anxiety), methylphenidate (when ADHD has been diagnosed), cyproterone (when severely problematic sexual behaviour contributes)

Most data originate from case reports and small open trials, often of heterogeneous patient groups.

Lithium is the only drug licensed for the treatment of SIB.

Prescribing and monitoring[13,18–20]

There is concern that antipsychotic drugs are prescribed excessively and inappropriately in the learning disability population and may cause undue harm. It is unclear if this patient population is more prone to side-effects. It is therefore important to document:

- The rationale for treatment (including some measure of baseline target behaviours), potential risk/benefit and consent in the patient's notes. If the patient is unable to understand the nature, purpose and side-effects of treatment, a relative or carer should be consulted.
- The impact of medication and any side-effects experienced, each time the patient is reviewed.
- Drug interactions. These should always be considered (both kinetic and dynamic) before prescribing, particularly when anticonvulsant drugs are involved.

References

1. Tyrer P. The use of psychotropic drugs. In Russell O, ed. The Psychiatry of Learning Disabilities. London: Royal College of Psychiatrists, 1997.
2. Schroeder SR et al. Self-injurious behavior: gene–brain–behavior relationships. Ment Retard Dev Disabil Res Rev 2001;7:3–12.
3. Saloviita T. The structure and correlates of self-injurious behavior in an institutional setting. Res Dev Disabil 2000;21:501–11.
4. Collacott RA et al. Epidemiology of self-injurious behaviour in adults with learning disabilities. Br J Psychiatry 1998;173:428–32.
5. Mikhail AG et al. Self-injurious behavior in mental retardation. Curr Opin Psychiatry 2001;14:457–62.
6. Moss S et al. Psychiatric symptoms in adults with learning disability and challenging behaviour. Br J Psychiatry 2000;177:452–6.
7. Deb S. Self-injurious behaviour as part of genetic syndromes. Br J Psychiatry 1998;172:385–8.
8. Clarke DJ. Psychopharmacology of severe self-injury associated with learning disabilities. Br J Psychiatry 1998;172:389–94.
9. Xeniditis K et al. Management of people with challenging behaviour. Adv Psychiatr Treat 2001;7:109–16.
10. Halliday S et al. Psychological interventions in self-injurious behaviour. Working with people with a learning disability. Br J Psychiatry 1998;172:395–400.
11. Bromley J et al. Beliefs and emotional reactions of care staff working with people with challenging behaviour. J Intellect Disabil Res 1995;39(Pt 4):341–52.
12. Branford D. Antipsychotic drugs in learning disabilities (mental handicap). Pharm J 1997;258:451–6.
13. Einfeld SL. Systematic management approach to pharmacotherapy for people with learning disabilities. Adv Psychiatr Treat 2001;7:43–9.
14. Gagiano C et al. Short- and long-term efficacy and safety of risperidone in adults with disruptive behavior disorders. Psychopharmacology 2005;179:629–36.
15. Craft M et al. Lithium in the treatment of aggression in mentally handicapped patients. A double-blind trial. Br J Psychiatry 1987;150:685–9.
16. Ratey JJ et al. Buspirone therapy for maladaptive behavior and anxiety in developmentally disabled persons. J Clin Psychiatry 1989;50:382–4.
17. Aman MG et al. Clinical effects of methylphenidate and thioridazine in intellectually subaverage children. J Am Acad Child Adolesc Psychiatry 1991;30:246–56.
18. Janowsky DS et al. Relapse of aggressive and disruptive behavior in mentally retarded adults following antipsychotic drug withdrawal predicts psychotropic drug use a decade later. J Clin Psychiatry 2006;67:1272–7.
19. Janowsky DS et al. Minimally effective doses of conventional antipsychotic medications used to treat aggression, self-injurious and destructive behaviors in mentally retarded adults. J Clin Psychopharmacol 2005;25:19–25.
20. McGillivray JA et al. Pharmacological management of challenging behavior of individuals with intellectual disability. Res Dev Disabil 2004;25:523–37.

Special groups

Further reading

Bhaumik S, Branford D. The Frith Prescribing Guidelines in Adults with Learning Disability. London: Taylor & Francis, 2005.

Deb S et al. Using medication to manage behaviour problems among adults with a learning disability. www.ld-medication.bham.ac.uk/. 2006.

Read S. Self-injury and violence in people with severe learning disabilities. Br J Psychiatry 1998;172:381–4.

Santosh PJ et al. Psychopharmacology in children and adults with intellectual disability. Lancet 1999;354:233–40.

Thompson C et al. Behavioural symptoms among people with severe and profound intellectual disabilities: a 26-year follow-up study. Br J Psychiatry 2002;181:67–71.

groups

Psychotropics and surgery

There are few worthwhile studies of the effects of non-anaesthetic drugs on surgery and the anaesthetic process[1,2]. Practice is therefore largely based on theoretical considerations, case reports, clinical experience and personal opinion. Any guidance in this area is therefore somewhat speculative. An anaesthetist's opinion should always be sought.

Stopping or continuing psychotropics

The decision as to whether or not to continue a drug during surgery and the perioperative period should take into account a number of interacting factors.

Some general considerations include:

1. Patients are at risk of aspirating their stomach contents during general anaesthesia. For this reason they are usually prevented from eating for at least 6 hours before surgery. However, clear fluids leave the stomach within 2 hours of ingestion and so fluids that enable a patient to take routine medication may be allowed up to 2 hours before surgery. A clear fluid is described as one through which newspaper print can be read[3].
2. There are a few drug interactions between drugs used during surgery and routine medication that require the drugs not to be administered concurrently. This is usually managed by the anaesthetist by their choice of anaesthetic technique.
    Significant drug interactions between medicines used during surgery and psychotropics:
    – enflurane may precipitate seizures in patients taking tricyclic antidepressants[4–6]
    – pethidine may precipitate fatal 'excitatory' reactions in patients taking MAOIs and may cause serotonin syndrome in patients taking SSRIs[4–7].
3. Major procedures induce profound physiological changes, which include electrolyte disturbances and the release of cortisol and catacholamines.
4. Postoperatively, surgical stress and some agents used in anaesthesia often lead to gastric or gastrointestinal stasis. Oral absorption is therefore likely to be compromised.

Adjustment to routine psychotropics during the perioperative period

For the most part, psychotropic drugs should be continued during the perioperative period, assuming the agreement of the anaesthetist concerned. Note, however, that psychotropic and other drugs are frequently (accidentally or unthinkingly) withheld from perioperative patients simply because they are 'nil by mouth'[1]. Patients may be labelled 'nil by mouth' for several reasons, including unconsciousness, to rest the gut or postoperatively as a result of the surgery itself. Patients may also develop an intolerance of oral medicines at any time during a stay in hospital, often because of nausea and vomiting.

Alternative routes and formulations may be sought. When changing the route or formulation, care should be taken to ensure the appropriate dose and frequency is prescribed as these may not be the same as for the oral route or previous formulation. Oral preparations may sometimes be administered via a nasogastric (NG), PEG or jejunostomy tube.

When one decides to continue a psychotropic, this needs to be explicitly outlined to appropriate medical and nursing staff.

Psychotropics and surgery

Drug or group of drug	Considerations	Safe in surgery?	Alternative formulations
Antipsychotics[4,8,9]	Generally continue to avoid relapse. If clozapine is discontinued for more than 48 hours, then re-titration is necessary. Some antipsychotics are widely used in anaesthetic practice. Increased risk of arrhythmia with most drugs. α_1 blockade may lead to hypotension and interfere with effects of epinephrine, norepinephrine. Most drugs lower seizure threshold.	Probably	Liquid preparations of some antipsychotics date are available. Some 'specials' liquids can be made for NG delivery. Before crushing tablets and mixing with water, confirm with either local guidelines or the drug company for stability information.
Antidepressants – SSRIs[4-7,10]	Danger of serotonin syndrome if administered with pethidine, pentazocine or tramadol. SSRIs increase bleeding time[11] and may be stopped before surgery. Occasional seizures have been reported. Sudden cessation may result in withdrawal syndrome.	Probably, but avoid other serotonergic agents.	Liquid escitalopram, fluoxetine and paroxetine are available. Liquid citalopram is available: 8 mg (4 drops) is equivalent to 10 mg tablet.
Antidepressants – tricyclics[4-9]	α_1 blockade may lead to hypotension and interfere with effects of epinephrine/norepinephrine Danger of serotonin syndrome if administered with pethidine, pentazocine or tramadol. Many drugs prolong QT interval so risk of arrhythmia possibly more likely.	Probably, but anaesthetic agents need to be carefully chosen.	Liquid amitriptyline is available. It is acidic and may interact with enteral feeds. Dosulepin (dothiepin) capsules can

Psychotropics and surgery (Cont.)

Drug or group of drug	Considerations	Safe in surgery?	Alternative formulations
	Most drugs lower seizure threshold. Sympathomimetic agents may give exaggerated response. Effects of tricyclics may persist for several days after cessation – if the decision is to stop the antidepressant this will need to be done at least a week before surgery.		be opened and mixed with water before flushing well. This is preferred over crushing tablets.
Antidepressants – MAOIs[4,12–15]	Dangerous, potentially fatal interaction with pethidine and dextromethorphan (serotonin syndrome or coma/respiratory depression may occur). Sympathomimetic agents may result in hypertensive crisis. MAO inhibition lasts for up to 2 weeks: early withdrawal is required. Switching to moclobemide 2 weeks before surgery allows continued treatment up until day of surgery (do not give moclobemide on the day of surgery).	Probably not, but careful selection of anaesthetic agents may reduce risks if continuation is enssential.	
Benzodiazepines[4,10,12]	Risk of withdrawal symptoms if regular benzodiazepines are suddenly stopped. Reduce requirements for induction and maintenance anaesthetics.	Probably, usually continued.	Liquid, IM, IV and rectal diazepam are available (do not use IM route). Sublingual, IM, IV and lorazepam are available.
Anticonvulsants[4,10]	Drug level monitoring may be required. CNS depressant activity may reduce anaesthetic requirements.	Probably, usually continued for epilepsy.	Carbamazepine liquid or suppositories are available: carbamazepine 100 mg tablet ≡ carbamazepine 125 mg suppository. Maximum by rectum 1 g daily in four divided doses. Phenytoin is available IV or

Psychotropics and surgery (Cont.)

Drug or group of drug	Considerations	Safe in surgery?	Alternative formulations
			liquid: IV dose ≡ oral dose Sodium valproate is available IV or liquid: IV dose ≡ oral dose. Before crushing tablets and mixing with water, confirm with either local guidelines or the drug company for stability information.
Lithium[4,8–10]	Prolongs the action of both depolarising and non-depolarising muscle relaxants. Usually discontinued 24 hours pre-operatively before major surgery and restarted once electrolytes normalise. Risk of relapse if abruptly discontinued. Surgery-related electrolyte disturbance and reduced renal function may precipitate lithium toxicity. Avoid dehydration and use of concomitant NSAIDs. Possible increased risk of arrhythmia.	Probably, safe in minor surgery but usually discontinued before major procedures and restarted once electrolytes normalise.	The bioavailability of lithium varies between brands. Care is needed with equivalent doses of salts: lithium carbonate 200 mg ≡ lithium citrate 509 mg. Liquid lithium citrate is available and is usually administered twice daily
Methadone[9,10,12]	May increase opiate requirements. Use full agonists (e.g. morphine) and not partial agonists (e.g. buprenorphine). Naloxone may induce withdrawal. Methadone prolongs QT interval.	Probably, usually continued.	IM dose ≡ oral dose

Special groups

452

References

1. Noble DW et al. Interrupting drug therapy in the perioperative period. Drug Saf 2002;25:489–95.
2. Noble DW et al. Risks of interrupting drug treatment before surgery. BMJ 2000;321:719–20.
3. Anon. Drugs in the peri-operative period: 1. Stopping or continuing drugs around surgery. Drug Ther Bull 1999;37:62–4.
4. Smith MS et al. Perioperative management of drug therapy, clinical considerations. Drugs 1996; 51:238–59.
5. Chui PT et al. Medications to withhold or continue in the preoperative consultation. Curr Anaesth Crit Care 1998;9:302–6.
6. Kudoh A et al. Antidepressant treatment for chronic depressed patients should not be discontinued prior to anesthesia. Can J Anaesth 2002;49:132–6.
7. Spivey KM et al. Perioperative seizures and fluvoxamine. Br J Anaesth 1993;71:321.
8. Kudoh A. Perioperative management for chronic schizophrenic patients. Anesth Analg 2005; 101:1867–72.
9. Desan PH et al. Assessment and management of patients with psychiatric disorders. Crit Care Med 2004;32:S166–S173.
10. De Baerdemaeker L et al. Anaesthesia for patients with mood disorders. Curr Opin Anaesthesiol 2005;18:333–8.
11. Paton C et al. SSRIs and gastrointestinal bleeding. BMJ 2005;331:529–30.
12. Rahman MH et al. Medication in the peri-operative period. Pharm J 2004;272:287–9.
13. Blom-Peters L et al. Monoamine oxidase inhibitors and anesthesia: an updated literature review. Acta Anaesthesiol Belg 1993;44:57–60.
14. Hill S et al. MAOIs to RIMAs in anaesthesia – a literature review. Psychopharmacology 1992;106 (Suppl): S43–S45.
15. Morrow JI et al. Essential drugs in the perioperative period. Curr Pract Surg 1990;90:106–9.

Special
groups

General principles of prescribing in HIV

Individuals with HIV/AIDS may experience symptoms of mental illness either as a direct consequence of (organic origin), a reaction to, or in addition to their underlying infection. In the first scenario, the focus of treatment should be the underlying infection. Where this is not feasible, or the presentation is not of organic origin, psychotropic medication will be the primary treatment.

When prescribing psychotropics, the following principles should be adhered to:

1. Start with a low dose and titrate according to tolerability and response.
2. Select the simplest dosing regimen possible.
   (Remember that the patient's drug regimen is likely to be complex already.)
3. Select an agent with the fewest side-effects/interactions. Medical co-morbidity and potential drug interactions must be considered.
4. Ensure that management is conducted in close cooperation with the HIV physicians and the rest of the multidisciplinary team.

Although most psychotropic agents are thought to be safe in HIV-infected individuals, it has been suggested that this group may be more sensitive to higher doses, adverse side-effects and interactions[1]. Patients with low CD4 counts are more likely to have exaggerated adverse reactions to psychotropic medications.

Psychosis

SGAs are usually used first line. Risperidone is the most widely studied[2] and generally appears to be safe, although idiosyncratic interactions with ritonavir have been reported[3,4]. The use of clozapine is not routinely recommended, although it may be useful in patients with higher CD4 counts who are otherwise medically stable. Although it is not known whether patients with HIV have a greater risk of agranulocytosis, extremely close monitoring of the WCC is recommended. Patients with HIV may be more susceptible to EPSEs[5], NMS[6] and TD[7].

Delirium

Organic causes should be identified and treated. Short-term symptomatic treatment may include low-dose SGAs such as risperidone[8], olanzapine[9], quetiapine[10] or ziprasidone[11]. The concomitant use of low doses of short-acting benzodiazepines such as lorazepam may also be helpful.

Depression

Depression is common in individuals with HIV, and one study estimated the prevalence in this population to be as high as 84%[12]. Of note, depression may be a risk factor for HIV[13], and it has been further suggested that much of this depression is either unrecognised or insufficiently managed[14]. First-line agents include SSRIs, especially citalopram[15] (because it does not inhibit CYP2D6 or CYP3A4), with further treatment as per standard protocols. The risk of serotonin syndrome may be increased[16]. The use of TCAs may be appropriate in some cases, although side-effects may limit efficacy and compliance[17]. MAOIs are not recommended in this population.

Bipolar affective disorder

Mania is a recognised presentation in HIV[18] and individuals with HIV may be more sensitive to the side-effects of mood stablisers such as lithium[19], especially if they have neurocognitive dysfunction[18]. Conventional agents such as lithium, valproate, lamotrigine and gabapentin may be used cautiously, but carbamazepine should be avoided because of important interactions with antiretroviral agents as well as the risk of agranulocytosis.

Anxiety disorders

Benzodiazepines have some utility in the treatment of anxiety in individuals with HIV, but caution should be exercised because of the potential for both misuse and multiple and, in rare cases, potentially serious interactions. SSRIs (remember interactions) and other antidepressants may be efficacious, and there is evidence that buspirone may be especially useful[20].

HIV neurocognitive disorders

Individuals with HIV may present with cognitive impairment at any time in the course of their illness, and this may range from mild forgetfulness to severe and debilitating dementia. The mainstay of treatment is combination antiretroviral therapy[21], with judicious, short-term use of an antipsychotic such as risperidone[22] if necessary. Treatment of these individuals is carried out primarily by HIV physicians, with liaison psychiatric input as required.

Important drug interactions

Although the majority of psychotropic agents are deemed safe for co-administration with antiretroviral agents, there are a number of clinically important interactions. These are shown in the following table. It should be noted that data are lacking, and that there is potential for other interactions not listed in the table. Although many of these interactions are not absolute contraindications to co-prescribing, extreme caution is advised. As those receiving HIV treatment may be taking medication for many different medical indications, additional interactions cannot be excluded.

A number of psychotropic agents that are potent enzyme inducers are **contraindicated** for use with antiretroviral agents of all classes, as they can compromise antiretroviral therapy; these include **carbamazepine, phenobarbital, phenytoin, primidone and St John's wort**. Enzyme inhibitors can cause severe exacerbation of side-effects (e.g. SSRIs, benzodiazepines). Caution is advised when the patient is taking ritonavir and lopinavir/ritonavir, as these drugs are potent enzyme inducers that may compromise the efficacy of psychotropic drugs.

In the table below, interactions are both specific and illustrative, but not exhaustive: reported or sample interactions are outlined; many more interactions are possible. Check the latest literature *and* estimate risk of interaction from first principles (i.e. from understanding of CYP involvement).

Table Reported and suspected interactions of antiretrovirals and psychotropics[23-25]

Antiretroviral	Psychotropic	Clinical effect
Amprenavir (CYP3A4 inhibitor)	Alprazolam, diazepam, midazolam, triazolam	↑ Sedation, confusion, respiratory depression
	Carbamazepine	↑ Carbamazepine effect; ↓ amprenavir effect
	Clozapine	↑ Clozapine effect*
	Lamotrigine	↓ Lamotrigine levels*
	Phenobarbital, phenytoin	↓ Amprenavir effect
	Pimozide	↑ Cardiac arrhythmia
	Primidone	↓ Amprenavir effect
	St John's wort	↓ Amprenavir effect
Delavirdine (inhibitor of CYP3A4, CYP2C9, CYP2C19)	Alprazolam, midalozam, triazolam	↑ Sedation, confusion, respiratory depression
	Carbamazepine	↓ Delavirdine effect
	Fluoxetine	↑ Delavirdine effect*
	Lamotrigine	↓ Lamotrigine levels*
	Phenobarbital, phenytoin	↓ Delavirdine effect
	Pimozide	↑ Cardiac arrhythmia
	Primidone	↓ Amprenavir effect
Efavirenz (inhibitor and inducer of CYP3A4)	Carbamazepine	↓ Carbamazepine effect; ↓ efavirenz effect
	Lamotrigine	↓ Lamotrigine levels*
	Phenobarbital	↓ Efavirenz effect
	Phenytoin	↓ Efavirenz effect; ↓ Phenytoin effect
	Pimozide	↑ Cardiac arrhythmia
	Primidone	↓ Efavirenz effect
	St John's wort	↓ Efavirenz effect
Indinavir (inhibitor of CYP3A4)	Carbamazepine	↓ Indinavir effect
	Lamotrigine	↓ Lamotrigine levels*
	Midazolam	↑ Sedation, confusion, respiratory depression

Table Reported and suspected interactions of antiretrovirals and psychotropics[23–25] (Cont.)

Antiretroviral	Psychotropic	Clinical effect
	Phenobarbital, phenytoin	↓ Indinavir effect
	Pimozide	↑ Cardiac arrhythmia
	Primidone	↓ Efavirenz effect
	St John's wort	↓ Indinavir effect; possible indinavir resistance
	Trazodone	↑ Sedation, confusion
Lopinavir + ritonavir (inhibitor of CYP3A4, CYP2D6) (may induce glucuronidation)	Bupropion	↑ Bupropion levels
	Buspirone	↑ Parkinsonism
	Carbamazepine	↓ Lopinavir/ritonavir effect
	Citalopram	↑ Citalopram levels*
	Clozapine	↓ Clozapine levels
	Desipramine	↑ Antimuscarinic effects*
	Fluoxetine	↑ Fluoxetine levels; possible serotonin syndrome
	Lamotrigine	↓ Lamotrigine levels*
	Midazolam, flurazepam, diazepam	↑ Sedation, confusion, respiratory depression
	Mirtazapine	↑ Mirtazapine levels*
	Olanzapine	↓ Olanzapine levels
	Phenobarbital, phenytoin	↓ Lopinavir/ritonavir effect
	Pimozide	↑ Cardiac arrhythmia
	Primidone	↓ Lopinaviv/ritonavir effect;
	Risperidone	reversible coma/↑ EPSE
	St John's wort	↓ Lopinavir/ritonavir effect
	Trazodone	↑ Trazodone levels*
Nelfinavir (inhibitor of CYP3A4, CYP142)	Bupropion	↑ Bupropion levels*
	Carbamazepine	↓ Nelfinavir effect
	Desipramine	↑ Antimuscarinic effects*
	Lamotrigine	↓ Lamotrigine levels*
	Midazolam, triazolam	↑ Sedation, confusion, respiratory depression
	Phenobarbital	↓ Nelfinavir effect
	Phenytoin	↓ Phenytoin effect
	Pimozide	↑ Cardiac arrhythmia
	Primidone	↓ Nelfinavir effect
	St John's wort	↓ Nelfinavir effect

Table Reported and suspected interactions of antiretrovirals and psychotropics[23-25] (Cont.)

Antiretroviral	Psychotropic	Clinical effect
Nevirapine (CYP3A4, ? effect)	Methadone	↑ Methadone effect
	St John's wort	↓ Nevirapine effect
Ritonavir (may inhibit and induce CYP3A4, inhibits CYP2D6, CYP2C9, CYP2C19)	Alprazolam, diazepam, midazolam, triazolam	↑ Sedation, confusion, respiratory depression
	Amitriptyline	↑ Amitriptyline levels
	Bupropion	↑ Bupropion levels
	Carbamazepine	↓ Ritonavir effect; ↑ carbamazepine effect
	Citalopram	↑ Citalopram levels*
	Clozapine	↓ Clozapine levels
	Desipramine	↑ Antimuscarinic effects*
	Disulfiram	↓ Disulphiram reaction
	Fluoxetine	↑ Fluoxetine levels; possible serotonin syndrome
	Lamotrigine	↓ Lamotrigine levels*
	Mirtazapine	↑ Mirtazapine levels*
	Olanzapine	↓ Olanzapine effect*
	Phenytoin	↑ Phenytoin effect
	Pimozide	↑ Cardiac arrhythmia
	Primidone	↓ Ritonavir effect
	Risperidone	↑ Risk of coma*
	St John's wort	↓ Ritonavir effect
	Trazodone	↑ Trazodone levels*
Saquinavir (inhibits CYP3A4)	Carbamazepine	↓ Saquinavir effect
	Lamotrigine	↑ Lamotrigine levels*
	Midazolam	↑ Sedation, confusion, respiratory depression
	Phenobarbital, phenytoin	↓ Saquinavir effect
	Pimozide	↑ Cardiac arrhythmia
	Primidone	↓ Saquinavir effect
	St John's wort	↓ Saquinavir effect

*Effects of interaction may be reduced/eliminated by reduction in psychotropic dose.

Note all antiretrovirals are metabolised via CYP3A4; some also utilise additional enzymatic routes such as CYP2D6.

Special groups

Psychotropic effects of HIV drugs

Psychosis, mania, agitation and suicidal ideation have been associated with antiretroviral treatment (see following table). Any of these conditions can appear *de novo* in HIV-positive individuals. There is, as yet, no conclusive evidence supporting an association between HIV infection and psychosis[26]. Psychosis is associated with efavirenz, zidovudine, nevirapine and, most recently, abacavir treatment[27]. In many of the reported cases, symptoms abated either when the putative offending agent was stopped or prophylactic agents were added to the medication regimen.

Although most reports suggest that these changes in mental state occur within a month of commencing antiretroviral therapy, the time frame can be highly variable, ranging from 2 days in the case of efavirenz[28] to 14 months[29] or even longer[30]. Treatment involves cessation of the putative offending agent and initiation of a suitable alternative. Inclusion of an appropriate prophylactic agent or agents can be useful, usually for a short period of time (1–3 months). It should be remembered that other drugs used to treat physical problems (apart from antiretrovirals) may also induce changes in mental state.

Table Psychotropic effects of antiretrovirals

Diagnosis	Implicated agent
Depression	Abacavir[31]
	Efavirenz[32,33]
	Indinavir[34]
	Nevirapine[35]
Mania	Didanosine[36]
	Efavirenz[29,37,38]
	Zidovudine[39–41]
Psychosis	Abacavir[27,31]
	Efavirenz[28,42–44]
	Nevirapine[35]
PTSD	Efavirenz[45]
Vivid dreams	Abacavir[46]
	Nevirapine[47]
	Efavirenz[48]
Suicidal ideation	Abacavir[31]
	Efavirenz[48,49]
Miscellaneous symptoms	Efavirenz[48]

References

1. Ayuso JL. Use of psychotropic drugs in patients with HIV infection. Drugs 1994;47:599–610.
2. Singh AN et al. Risperidone in HIV-related manic psychosis. Lancet 1994;344:1029–30.
3. Jover F et al. Reversible coma caused by risperidone–ritonavir interaction. Clin Neuropharmacol 2002;25:251–3.
4. Kelly DV et al. Extrapyramidal symptoms with ritonavir/indinavir plus risperidone. Ann Pharmacother 2002;36:827–30.
5. Hriso E et al. Extrapyramidal symptoms due to dopamine-blocking agents in patients with AIDS encephalopathy. Am J Psychiatry 1991;148:1558–61.
6. Horwath E et al. NMS and HIV. Psychiatr Serv 1999;50:564.
7. Shedlack KJ et al. Rapidly progressive tardive dyskinesia in AIDS. Biol Psychiatry 1994;35:147–8.
8. Sipahimalani A et al. Treatment of delirium with risperidone. Int J Geriatr Psychopharmacol 1997;1:24–6.
9. Sipahimalani A et al. Olanzapine in the treatment of delirium. Psychosomatics 1998;39:422–30.
10. Schwartz TL et al. Treatment of delirium with quetiapine. Prim Care Companion J Clin Psychiatry 2000; 2:10–12.
11. Leso L et al. Ziprasidone treatment of delirium. Psychosomatics 2002;43:61–2.
12. Anon. Depression is common among AIDS patients. Psych consult often is necessary. AIDS Alert 2002;17:153–4.
13. McDermott BE et al. Diagnosis, health beliefs, and risk of HIV infection in psychiatric patients. Hosp Community Psychiatry 1994;45:580–5.
14. Katz MH et al. Depression and use of mental health services among HIV-infected men. AIDS Care 1996;8:433–42.
15. Currier MB et al. Citalopram treatment of major depressive disorder in Hispanic HIV and AIDS patients: a prospective study. Psychosomatics 2004;45:210–16.
16. DeSilva KE et al. Serotonin syndrome in HIV-infected individuals receiving antiretroviral therapy and fluoxetine. AIDS 2001;15:1281–5.
17. Elliott AJ et al. Randomized, placebo-controlled trial of paroxetine versus imipramine in depressed HIV-positive outpatients. Am J Psychiatry 1998;155:367–72.
18. El-Mallakh RS. Mania in AIDS: clinical significance and theoretical considerations. Int J Psychiatry Med 1991;21:383–91.
19. Tanquary J. Lithium neurotoxicity at therapeutic levels in an AIDS patient. J Nerv Ment Dis 1993;181: 518–19.
20. Batki SL. Buspirone in drug users with AIDS or AIDS-related complex. J Clin Psychopharmacol 1990;10: 111S–15S.
21. Portegies P et al. Guidelines for the diagnosis and management of neurological complications of HIV infection. Eur J Neurol 2004;11:297–304.
22. Belzie LR. Risperidone for AIDS-associated dementia: a case series. AIDS Patient Care STDS 1996; 10:246–9.
23. HIV InSite. Database of Antiretroviral Drug Interactions. http://www.hivinsite.com/. 2006.
24. Anon. Toronto General Hospital Immunodeficiency Clinic. Drug Interaction Tables. http://www.tthhivclinic.com/. 2006.
25. Liverpool HIV Pharmacology Group. Drug Interaction Charts. http://www.hiv-druginteractions.org/. 2006.
26. Harris MJ et al. New-onset psychosis in HIV-infected patients. J Clin Psychiatry 1991;52:369–76.
27. Foster R et al. Antiretroviral therapy-induced psychosis: case report and brief review of the literature. HIV Med 2003;4:139–44.
28. de la Garza CL et al. Efavirenz-induced psychosis. AIDS 2001;15:1911–12.
29. Maxwell S et al. Manic syndrome associated with zidovudine treatment. JAMA 1988;259:3406–7.
30. Foster R. Personal communication. 2005.
31. Colebunders R et al. Neuropsychiatric reaction induced by abacavir. Am J Med 2002;113:616.
32. Lang JP et al. [Apropos of atypical melancholia with Sustiva (efavirenz)] (Article in French). Encephale 2001;27:290–3.
33. Puzantian T. Central nervous system adverse effects with efavirenz: case report and review. Pharmacotherapy 2002;22:930–3.
34. Harry TC et al. Indinavir use: associated reversible hair loss and mood disturbance. Int J STD AIDS 2000; 11:474–6.
35. Wise ME et al. Drug points: neuropsychiatric complications of nevirapine treatment. BMJ 2002; 324:879.
36. Brouillette MJ et al. Didanosine-induced mania in HIV infection. Am J Psychiatry 1994;151:1839–40.
37. Blanch J et al. Manic syndrome associated with efavirenz overdose. Clin Infect Dis 2001;33:270–1.
38. Shah MD et al. A manic episode associated with efavirenz therapy for HIV infection. AIDS 2003; 17:1713–14.
39. O'Dowd MA et al. Manic syndrome associated with zidovudine (Letter). JAMA 1988;260:3587.
40. Anon. Manic syndrome associated with zidovudine. JAMA 1988;260:3587–8.
41. Wright JM et al. Zidovudine-related mania. Med J Aust 1989;150:339–41.
42. Sabato S et al. Efavirenz-induced catatonia. AIDS 2002;16:1841–2.
43. Poulsen HD et al. Efavirenz-induced psychosis leading to involuntary detention. AIDS 2003;17:451–3.

44. Peyriere H et al. Management of sudden psychiatric disorders related to efavirenz. AIDS 2001; 15:1323–4.
45. Moreno A et al. Recurrence of post-traumatic stress disorder symptoms after initiation of antiretrovirals including efavirenz: a report of two cases. HIV Med 2003;4:302–4.
46. Foster R et al. More on abacavir-induced neuropsychiatric reactions. AIDS 2004;18:2449.
47. Morlese JF et al. Nevirapine-induced neuropsychiatric complications, a class effect of non-nucleoside reverse transcriptase inhibitors? AIDS 2002;16:1840–1.
48. Lochet P et al. Long-term assessment of neuropsychiatric adverse reactions associated with efavirenz. HIV Med 2003;4:62–6.
49. Foster R, Olajide D, Everall IP. Long-term neuropsychiatric effects of efavirenz. Case report and review of the literature. 2006.

Drug treatment of borderline personality disorder

Borderline personality disorder (BPD) is common in psychiatric settings: up to 15% of inpatients meet diagnostic criteria[1]. In BPD, co-morbid depression, anxiety spectrum disorders and bipolar illness occur more frequently than would be expected by chance association alone. The suicide rate in BPD is similar to that seen in affective disorders and schizophrenia[2,3].

Although it is classified as a personality disorder, several 'symptoms' of BPD may intuitively be expected to respond to drug treatment. These include affective instability, transient stress-related psychotic symptoms, suicidal and self-harming behaviours, and impulsivity[4].

Drug treatments are often used during periods of crisis when 'symptoms' can be severe, distressing and potentially life-threatening. By their very nature, these symptoms can be expected to wax and wane[2]. Drug therapy may then be required intermittently. It is generally easy to see when treatment is required, but much more difficult to decide when modest gains are worthwhile and whether or not continuation is likely to be necessary.

The majority of studies of drug treatment in BPD last for only 6 weeks and a large number of different outcome measures have been used, making it difficult to evaluate and compare studies. Not all RCTs report attrition data, but where this information is available, less than half of subjects tend to complete studies. Symptoms often improve in an unexpected way; for example, depressive symptoms may improve with antipsychotics and psychotic symptoms with antidepressants. The placebo response rate in RCTs of BPD is uniformly high. Caution is required when evaluating uncontrolled studies or case reports.

Antipsychotics

Open studies have found benefit for conventional antipsychotics[5], risperidone[6], olanzapine[7] and quetiapine[8] over a wide range of symptoms. In contrast, RCTs generally show only very modest benefits for active drug over placebo[9,10]. One small RCT of aripiprazole showed reductions in depression, anxiety and anger[11]. The most convincing RCT demonstrated marked reductions in suicidal behaviour with flupentixol 40 mg/month[12]. Open studies also report reductions in aggression and self-harming behaviour with clozapine[13,14]. Olanzapine, with or without fluoxetine, also seems to be effective[15].

A small study supports the efficacy of both IM olanzapine and IM ziprasidone[16].

Dysphoria and depression may develop during treatment with conventional antipsychotics[5,17].

Antidepressants

Several open studies have found that SSRIs reduce impulsivity and aggression in BPD[18–20], but controlled studies show very modest benefits[21,22]. The prevalence of so-called atypical depression is higher in people with BPD than in the general population and such patients may respond well to phenelzine[23]. Tranylcypromine[24] and amitriptyline[25] have not been shown to be effective, and both may cause behavioural disinhibition. Reboxetine has also been reported to worsen symptoms[26].

Mood stabilisers

Up to a half of people with BPD may also have a bipolar spectrum disorder[27] and mood stabilisers are commonly prescribed. Valproate semisodium[28,29] and lamotrigine[30] have both been found to reduce anger, aggression and impulsivity in open studies. A small RCT of lamotrigine supports some efficacy for this drug[31]. Valproate has also been subject to RCTs[32,33]. Both studies suggest that valproate may be superior to placebo with respect to reducing interpersonal sensitivity, anger and hostility, but the numbers in these studies were small and the attrition rate high. Larger studies are required. Topiramate has been shown in a placebo-controlled RCT to reduce aggression but the size of this effect was modest[34]. Lithium may reduce mood variation[35], anger and suicidal ideation[36]. In an open study, oxcarbazepine reduced a wide range of symptoms, including anxiety, affective instability and anger[37]. Behavioural disinhibition has been reported with carbamazepine[38].

Benzodiazepines

One case series reported on three patients who responded to alprazolam after multiple treatment failures,[39] whereas 7 of 12 patients randomised to alprazolam during an RCT developed severe behavioural disinhibition[40].

Treatment of co-morbid psychiatric illness

A diagnosis of BPD predicts a poorer outcome from treatment of depression with antidepressants[41] and ECT[42]. Symptoms of OCD may be less responsive to clomipramine[43].

References

1. Winston AP. Recent developments in borderline personality disorder. Adv Psychiatr Treat 2000;6: 211–17.
2. Links PS et al. Prospective follow-up study of borderline personality disorder: prognosis, prediction of outcome, and Axis II comorbidity. Can J Psychiatry 1998;43:265–70.
3. Paris J. Chronic suicidality among patients with borderline personality disorder. Psychiatr Serv 2002;53:738–42.
4. American Psychiatric Association. Practice guideline for the treatment of patients with borderline personality disorder. Am J Psychiatry 2001;158:1–52.
5. Teicher MH et al. Open assessment of the safety and efficacy of thioridazine in the treatment of patients with borderline personality disorder. Psychopharmacol Bull 1989;25:535–49.
6. Rocca P et al. Treatment of borderline personality disorder with risperidone. J Clin Psychiatry 2002;63:241–4.
7. Schulz SC et al. Olanzapine safety and efficacy in patients with borderline personality disorder and comorbid dysthymia. Biol Psychiatry 1999;46:1429–35.
8. Villeneuve E et al. Open-label study of atypical neuroleptic quetiapine for treatment of borderline personality disorder: impulsivity as main target. J Clin Psychiatry 2005;66:1298–303.
9. Soloff PH et al. Progress in pharmacotherapy of borderline disorders. A double-blind study of amitriptyline, haloperidol, and placebo. Arch Gen Psychiatry 1986;43:691–7.
10. Goldberg SC et al. Borderline and schizotypal personality disorders treated with low-dose thiothixene vs placebo. Arch Gen Psychiatry 1986;43:680–6.
11. Nickel MK et al. Aripiprazole in the treatment of patients with borderline personality disorder: a double-blind, placebo-controlled study. Am J Psychiatry 2006;163:833–8.
12. Montgomery SA et al. Pharmacological prevention of suicidal behaviour. J Affect Disord 1982;4:291–8.
13. Chengappa KN et al. Clozapine reduces severe self-mutilation and aggression in psychotic patients with borderline personality disorder. J Clin Psychiatry 1999;60:477–84.

14. Benedetti F et al. Low-dose clozapine in acute and continuation treatment of severe borderline personality disorder. J Clin Psychiatry 1998;59:103–7.
15. Zanarini MC et al. A preliminary, randomized trial of fluoxetine, olanzapine, and the olanzapine–fluoxetine combination in women with borderline personality disorder. J Clin Psychiatry 2004;65: 903–7.
16. Pascual JC et al. Injectable atypical antipsychotics for agitation in borderline personality disorder. Pharmacopsychiatry 2006;39:117–18.
17. Soloff PH et al. Efficacy of phenelzine and haloperidol in borderline personality disorder. Arch Gen Psychiatry 1993;50:377–85.
18. Cornelius JR et al. Fluoxetine trial in borderline personality disorder. Psychopharmacol Bull 1990;26: 151–4.
19. Markovitz PJ et al. Fluoxetine in the treatment of borderline and schizotypal personality disorders. Am J Psychiatry 1991;148:1064–7.
20. Kavoussi RJ et al. An open trial of sertraline in personality disordered patients with impulsive aggression. J Clin Psychiatry 1994;55:137–41.
21. Rinne T et al. SSRI treatment of borderline personality disorder: a randomized, placebo-controlled clinical trial for female patients with borderline personality disorder. Am J Psychiatry 2002;159:2048–54.
22. Salzman C et al. Effect of fluoxetine on anger in symptomatic volunteers with borderline personality disorder. J Clin Psychopharmacol 1995;15:23–9.
23. Parsons B et al. Phenelzine, imipramine, and placebo in borderline patients meeting criteria for atypical depression. Psychopharmacol Bull 1989;25:524–34.
24. Cowdry RW et al. Pharmacotherapy of borderline personality disorder. Alprazolam, carbamazepine, trifluoperazine, and tranylcypromine. Arch Gen Psychiatry 1988;45:111–19.
25. Soloff PH et al. Paradoxical effects of amitriptyline on borderline patients. Am J Psychiatry 1986;143: 1603–5.
26. Anghelescu I et al. Worsening of borderline symptoms under reboxetine treatment. J Neuropsychiatry Clin Neurosci 2005;17:559–60.
27. Deltito J et al. Do patients with borderline personality disorder belong to the bipolar spectrum? J Affect Disord 2001;67:221–8.
28. Stein DJ et al. An open trial of valproate in borderline personality disorder. J Clin Psychiatry 1995;56: 506–10.
29. Kavoussi RJ et al. Divalproex sodium for impulsive aggressive behavior in patients with personality disorder. J Clin Psychiatry 1998;59:676–80.
30. Pinto OC et al. Lamotrigine as a promising approach to borderline personality: an open case series without concurrent DSM-IV major mood disorder. J Affect Disord 1998;51:333–43.
31. Tritt K et al. Lamotrigine treatment of aggression in female borderline-patients: a randomized, double-blind, placebo-controlled study. J Psychopharmacol 2005;19:287–91.
32. Hollander E et al. A preliminary double-blind, placebo-controlled trial of divalproex sodium in borderline personality disorder. J Clin Psychiatry 2001;62:199–203.
33. Frankenburg FR et al. Divalproex sodium treatment of women with borderline personality disorder and bipolar II disorder: a double-blind placebo-controlled pilot study. J Clin Psychiatry 2002;63:442–6.
34. Nickel MK et al. Treatment of aggression with topiramate in male borderline patients: a double-blind, placebo-controlled study. Biol Psychiatry 2005;57:495–9.
35. Rifkin A et al. Lithium carbonate in emotionally unstable character disorder. Arch Gen Psychiatry 1972; 27:519–23.
36. Links PS et al. Lithium therapy for borderline patients: preliminary findings. J Pers Disord 1990;4: 173–81.
37. Bellino S et al. Oxcarbazepine in the treatment of borderline personality disorder: a pilot study. J Clin Psychiatry 2005;66:1111–15.
38. de la Fuente JM et al. A trial of carbamazepine in borderline personality disorder. Eur Neuropsychopharmacol 1994;4:479–86.
39. Faltus FJ. The positive effect of alprazolam in the treatment of three patients with borderline personality disorder. Am J Psychiatry 1984;141:802–3.
40. Gardner DL et al. Alprazolam-induced dyscontrol in borderline personality disorder. Am J Psychiatry 1985;142:98–100.
41. Shea MT et al. Personality disorders and treatment outcome in the NIMH Treatment of Depression Collaborative Research Program. Am J Psychiatry 1990;147:711–18.
42. DeBattista C et al. Is electroconvulsive therapy effective for the depressed patient with comorbid borderline personality disorder? J ECT 2001;17:91–8.
43. Baer L et al. Effect of axis II diagnoses on treatment outcome with clomipramine in 55 patients with obsessive-compulsive disorder. Arch Gen Psychiatry 1992;49:862–6.

Further reading

Binks CA et al. Pharmacological interventions for people with borderline personality disorder. Cochrane Database Syst Rev 2006;CD005653.
Lieb K et al. Borderline personality disorder. Lancet 2004;364:453–61.
Paton C et al. Pharmacological treatment of borderline personality disorder. J Psych Intensive Care 2005;1:105–16.

Delirium

Delirium is a common neuropsychiatric condition that presents in psychiatric, medical and surgical settings and is known by various names, including organic brain syndrome, intensive care psychosis and acute confusional state[1].

Diagnostic criteria for delirium[2]

- Disturbance of *consciousness* (reduced clarity of awareness of the environment) with reduced ability to focus, sustain or shift attention.
- A change in *cognition* (such as memory deficit, disorientation, language disturbance or perceptual disturbance) not better explained by a pre-existing or evolving dementia.
- The disturbance develops over a *short period of time* (usually hours to days) and tends to fluctuate over the course of the day.
- There is often evidence from the history, physical examination or laboratory findings that the disturbance is due to concomitant medications, a medical condition, substance intoxication or substance withdrawal.

Two distinct **clinical subtypes of delirium** are recognised:[3,4]

- Hyperactive delirium, which is characterised by increased motor activity with agitation, hallucinations and inappropriate behaviour.
- Hypoactive delirium, which is characterised by reduced motor activity and lethargy, and has a poorer prognosis.

Prevalence

Delirium occurs in 10% of hospitalised medical patients and a further 10–30% of patients develop delirium after admission[3]. Postoperative delirium occurs in 15–53% of patients and in 70–87% of those in intensive care[5].

Risk factors

Delirium is almost invariably multifactorial and it is often inappropriate to isolate a single precipitant as the cause[3].

The most important risk factors are:[3,4]

- prior cognitive impairment
- older age
- severity of illness
- psychoactive drug use
- polypharmacy
- infection with HIV
- urinary tract infections
- surgery, particularly prolonged cardiopulmonary bypass surgery.

Outcome

Patients with delirium have an increased length of stay, increased mortality and increased risk of institutional placement[1,4]. Hospital mortality rates of patients

Special groups

465

with delirium range from 6% to 18% and are twice that of matched controls[4]. The 1-year mortality rate associated with cases of delirium is 35–40%.[5] Up to 60% of individuals suffer persistent cognitive impairment following delirium and they are also three times more likely to develop dementia.[1,4]

Treatment

Preventing delirium is the most effective strategy for reducing its frequency and complications[5]. Delirium is a medical emergency and the identification and treatment of the underlying cause should be the first aim of management[6]. Provide symptomatic and supportive care until recovery.

Using pharmacological treatment to try to prevent delirium (e.g. giving haloperidol preoperatively) has not been shown to reduce the incidence of delirium[7]. However, there is evidence of it having a positive effect on the duration and severity of delirium. Common errors in managing delirium are to use antipsychotic medications in excessive doses, give them too late or over-use benzodiazepines[3].

General principles to delirium treatment:[3,4,8]

- Use one drug at a time.
- Keep the use of sedatives and antipsychotics to a minimum.
- Tailor dose according to age, body size and degree of agitation.
- Titrate dose to effect.
- Increase scheduled doses if regular 'as needed' doses are required.
- All medication should be reviewed at least every 24 hours.
- Usually medicines are discontinued 7–10 days after symptoms resolve.

Special groups

466

Table Summary of medications previously used in the treatment of delirium

Drug	Dose	Adverse effects	Notes
Haloperidol[1,4,5,9,10]	Oral 0.5–1 mg bd with additional doses every 4 hours as needed (peak effect: 4–6 hours) IM 0.5–1 mg, observe for 30–60 minutes and repeat if necessary (peak effect: 20–40 minutes)	EPSEs can occur, especially at doses above 3 mg Prolonged QT interval, particularly after IM use	Considered first-line agent Avoid in withdrawal of alcohol or sedative hypnotics, anticholinergic toxicity, hepatic failure or neuroleptic malignant syndrome Avoid in Lewy body dementia Avoid intravenous use because of effect on QT
Atypical antipsychotics[1,5,7–23]	**Quetiapine** Oral 12.5–25 mg bd This may be increased every 1–2 days to 100 mg daily if it is well tolerated **Risperidone** Oral 0.5 mg bd with additional doses every 4 hours as needed Usual maximum 4 mg/day **Olanzapine** Oral 2.5–5 mg od Usual maximum 20 mg/day **Ziprasidone** IM 10 mg every 2 hours Usual maximum 40 mg/day	EPSEs occur at a lower rate than with haloperidol Anticholinergic side effects possible with some drugs Prolonged QT interval with some drugs	Limited evidence – only in case reports or small uncontrolled studies Risperidone and olanzapine have been associated with increased risk of stroke among older patients with dementia IM olanzapine has not been assessed for the treatment of delirium Very limited evidence. Not available in the UK

Table Summary of medications previously used in the treatment of delirium (Cont.)

Drug	Dose	Adverse effects	Notes
Lorazepam[1,4,5]	Oral/IM 0.5–1 mg every 2–4 hours as needed Usual maximum 3 mg in 24 hours IV use is usually reserved for emergencies	More likely than antipsychotics to cause respiratory depression, oversedation and paradoxical excitement	Considered second-line agent Used in delirium associated with alcohol or sedative hypnotic withdrawal, in Parkinson's disease and in neuroleptic malignant symptoms Associated with prolongation and worsening of delirium symptoms
Trazodone[3,5]	25–150 mg nocte	Oversedation may be problematic	Limited experience – used only in uncontrolled studies
Rivastigmine[19]	3–9 mg od	Nausea, vomiting, loss of appetite and diarrhoea are common side-effects	Limited experience Usually used in chronic delirium as an adjunct to antipsychotics Usually used in Lewy body dementia
Sodium valproate[20]	Oral/ IM 250 mg bd increased to plasma level of 50–100 mg/l	Active liver disease is a contraindication Nausea, vomiting, gastralgia and diarrhoea are common side-effects	Some case reports of its use where antipsychotics and/or benzodiazepines are ineffective

References

1. van Zyl LT et al. Delirium concisely: condition is associated with increased morbidity, mortality, and length of hospitalization. Geriatrics 2006;61:18–21.
2. American Psychiatric Association. Diagnostic and Statistical Manual of Mental Disorders, 4th edn. Washington DC: American Psychiatric Association, 1994.
3. Nayeem K et al. Delirium. Clin Med 2003;3:412–15.
4. Potter J et al. The prevention, diagnosis and management of delirium in older people: concise guidelines. Clin Med 2006;6:303–8.
5. Inouye SK. Delirium in older persons. N Engl J Med 2006;354:1157–65.
6. Burns A et al. Delirium. J Neurol Neurosurg Psychiatry 2004;75:362–7.
7. Kalisvaart KJ et al. Haloperidol prophylaxis for elderly hip-surgery patients at risk for delirium: a randomized placebo-controlled study. J Am Geriatr Soc 2005;53:1658–66.
8. Schwartz TL et al. The role of atypical antipsychotics in the treatment of delirium. Psychosomatics 2002;43:171–4.
9. Han CS et al. A double-blind trial of risperidone and haloperidol for the treatment of delirium. Psychosomatics 2004;45:297–301.
10. Liu CY et al. Efficacy of risperidone in treating the hyperactive symptoms of delirium. Int Clin Psychopharmacol 2004;19:165–8.
11. Young CC et al. Intravenous ziprasidone for treatment of delirium in the intensive care unit. Anesthesiology 2004;101:794–5.
12. Bourgeois JA et al. Prolonged delirium managed with risperidone. Psychosomatics 2005;46:90–1.
13. Gupta N et al. Effectiveness of risperidone in delirium. Can J Psychiatry 2005;50:75.
14. Leentjens AF et al. Delirium in elderly people: an update. Curr Opin Psychiatry 2005;18:325–30.
15. Torres R et al. Use of quetiapine in delirium: case reports. Psychosomatics 2001;42:347–9.
16. Horikawa N et al. Treatment for delirium with risperidone: results of a prospective open trial with 10 patients. Gen Hosp Psychiatry 2003;25:289–92.
17. Sasaki Y et al. A prospective, open-label, flexible-dose study of quetiapine in the treatment of delirium. J Clin Psychiatry 2003;64:1316–21.
18. Skrobik YK et al. Olanzapine vs haloperidol: treating delirium in a critical care setting. Intensive Care Med 2004;30:444–9.
19. Sipahimalani A et al. Olanzapine in the treatment of delirium. Psychosomatics 1998;39:422–30.
20. Dautzenberg PL et al. Adding rivastigmine to antipsychotics in the treatment of a chronic delirium. Age Ageing 2004;33:516–17.
21. Bourgeois JA et al. Adjunctive valproic acid for delirium and/or agitation on a consultation-liaison service: a report of six cases. J Neuropsychiatry Clin Neurosci 2005;17:232–8.
22. Boettger S et al. Atypical antipsychotics in the management of delirium: a review of the empirical literature. Palliat Support Care 2005;3:227–37.
23. Duff G. Atypical antipsychotic drugs and stroke. http://www.mhra.gov.uk. 2004.

Special groups

Pharmacological treatment of Huntington's disease

Huntington's disease (HD) is a genetic disease involving slow progressive degeneration of the neurons in the basal ganglia and cerebral cortex. Neurons are damaged when the mutated Huntington protein gradually aggregates and interferes with normal metabolism and functioning. The mechanism is poorly understood[1], making it difficult to develop drugs that slow or stop progression. Choreoform movements occur in approximately 90% of patients, and between 23% and 73% of patients develop depression or psychosis during the course of their illness[2]. Dementia is inevitable.

There is very little primary literature to guide practice in this area. A summary can be found below. Clinicians who treat patients with HD are encouraged to publish reports of both positive and negative outcomes to increase the primary literature base.

The table below represents a review of the literature rather than a guide to treatment. Readers are directed to the reports cited here for details of dosage, frequency and monitoring.

Table Treatment of Huntington's disease

Symptoms	Treatment
Choreiform movements	Note that these are often more distressing for carers and healthcare professionals than they are for the patient and it should not be assumed that intervention is always in the patient's best interests.
	• Discontinue dopaminergic drugs such as piracetam, amantadine and cabergoline[3]. Consider the contribution of psychotropic drugs with dopaminergic effects such as aripiprazole and venlafaxine.
	• The use of tetrabenazine is supported by RCTs[4,5] but up to 80% of patients experience side-effects such as depression, anxiety and insomnia.
	• A small dose of a conventional antipsychotic such as haloperidol is established clinical practice[6].
	• Findings with second-generation antipsychotics are mixed. Two open studies of olanzapine 5 mg were negative[7,8] but a third using 30 mg showed improved motor function[9]. Case reports support the use of risperidone both at low[10] and higher dose[11]. Quetiapine may also be effective[12].
Hypokinetic rigidity	• Treatment is similar to that of Parkinson's disease, although response is often suboptimal. Anticholinergics and dopamine agonists are sometimes used. Note the potential to exacerbate choreiform movements and precipitate psychosis.
	• Muscle relaxants such as diazepam can also be effective in treating rigidity and are usually well tolerated[3], although aspiration secondary to sedation is a potential risk.

Table Treatment of Huntington's disease (Cont.)

Symptoms	Treatment
Psychosis	There are no RCTs to guide choice. Treatment is empirical. Note that antipsychotic drugs may exacerbate the underlying movement disorder. • Some evidence supports the efficacy of conventional antipsychotics, particularly haloperidol, when the HD is mild to moderate[6]. As HD progresses, typicals tend to be poorly tolerated due to dystonia and parkinsonism[6]. • Case reports support the efficacy of risperidone[11,13], quetiapine[14] and amisulpride[15] although EPSEs can be problematic with all of these drugs.
Depression	There are no RCTs to guide choice. Note that the suicide rate in patients with HD is 4–6 times higher than in the background population[6]. • Case reports support the efficacy of a wide range of antidepressants but TCAs are poorly tolerated (sedation, falls and anticholinergic-induced cognitive impairment) and MAOIs can worsen choreiform movements. SSRIs are preferred[16,17]. • Reviews state that lithium is best avoided; clinical experience suggests that response is likely to be poor and that toxic effects may be particularly problematic[6]. There is no primary literature. • ECT seems to be relatively well tolerated in HD patients[6].
Dementia	There are no data pertaining to the use of cholinesterase inhibitors but there is no reason to suspect that the efficacy and tolerability of these drugs would be any different in HD patients than in those with Alzheimer's disease.

References

1. Jankovic J. Huntington's disease. http://www.bcm.edu/neurology/struct/parkinson/huntington.html. 2005. Accessed 1-6-2006.
2. Petrikis P et al. Treatment of Huntington's disease with galantamine. Int Clin Psychopharmacol 2004;19:49–50.
3. Bonelli RM et al. Huntington's disease: present treatments and future therapeutic modalities. Int Clin Psychopharmacol 2004;19:51–62.
4. McLellan DL et al. A double-blind trial of tetrabenazine, thiopropazate, and placebo in patients with chorea. Lancet 1974;1:104–7.
5. Jankovic J. Treatment of hyperkinetic movement disorders with tetrabenazine: a double-blind crossover study. Ann Neurol 1982;11:41–7.
6. Rosenblatt A et al. Neuropsychiatry of Huntington's disease and other basal ganglia disorders. Psychosomatics 2000;41:24–30.
7. Squitieri F et al. Short-term effects of olanzapine in Huntington disease. Neuropsychiatry Neuropsychol Behav Neurol 2001;14:69–72.
8. Paleacu D et al. Olanzapine in Huntington's disease. Acta Neurol Scand 2002;105:441–4.
9. Bonelli RM et al. High-dose olanzapine in Huntington's disease. Int Clin Psychopharmacol 2002;17:91–3.
10. Erdemoglu AK et al. Risperidone in chorea and psychosis of Huntington's disease. Eur J Neurol 2002;9:182–3.
11. Dallocchio C et al. Effectiveness of risperidone in Huntington chorea patients. J Clin Psychopharmacol 1999;19:101–3.
12. Bonelli RM et al. Quetiapine in Huntington's disease: a first case report. J Neurol 2002;249: 1114–15.
13. Madhusoodanan S et al. Use of risperidone in psychosis associated with Huntington's disease. Am J Geriatr Psychiatry 1998;6:347–9.
14. Seitz DP et al. Quetiapine in the management of psychosis secondary to Huntington's disease: a case report. Can J Psychiatry 2004;49:413.
15. Saft C et al. Amisulpride in Huntington's disease. Psychiatr Prax 2005;32:363–6.
16. De Marchi N et al. Fluoxetine in the treatment of Huntington's disease. Psychopharmacology 2001;153:264–6.
17. Rosenblatt A et al. A Physician's Guide to the Management of Huntington's Disease, 2nd edn. New York: Huntington's Disease Society of America, 1999.

chapter 8

Miscellaneous conditions and substances

Psychotropics in overdose

Suicide attempts and suicidal gestures are frequently encountered in psychiatric and general practice, and psychotropic drugs are often taken in overdose. This section gives brief details of the toxicity in overdose of commonly used psychotropics. It is intended to help guide drug choice in those thought to be at risk of suicide and to help identify symptoms of overdose. This section gives no information on the treatment of psychotropic overdose and readers are directed to specialist poisons units. In all cases of suspected overdose, urgent referral to acute medical facilities is, of course, strongly advised.

Miscellaneous

Table Psychotropics in overdose

Drug or drug group	Toxicity in overdose	Smallest dose likely to cause death	Signs and symptoms of overdose
Antidepressants Tricyclics[1-5] (not lofepramine)	High	Around 500 mg. Doses over 50 mg/kg usually fatal.	Sedation, coma, tachycardia, arrhythmia (QRS, QT prolongation), hypotension, seizures.
Lofepramine[4,6,7]	Low	Unclear. Fatality unlikely if lofepramine taken alone.	Sedation, coma, tachycardia, hypotension.
SSRIs[6-9]	Low	Unclear. Probably above 1–2 g. Fatality unlikely if SSRI taken alone.	Vomiting, tremor, drowsiness, tachycardia, ST depression. Seizures and QT prolongation possible. Citalopram most toxic of SSRIs in overdose.
Venlafaxine[10,11]	Moderate	Probably above 5 g, but seizures may occur after ingestion of 1 g.	Vomiting, sedation, tachycardia, seizures. Very rarely QT prolongation, arrhythmia.
Moclobemide[12,13]	Low	Unclear, but probably more than 8 g. Fatality unlikely if moclobemide taken alone.	Vomiting, sedation, disorientation. QT prolongation
Trazodone[14,15]	Low	Unclear but probably more than 10 g. Fatality unlikely in overdose of trazodone alone.	Drowsiness, nausea, dizziness. Very rarely arrhythmia.
Reboxetine[10,16]	Low	Not known. Fatality unlikely in overdose of reboxetine alone.	Sweating, tachycardia, changes in blood pressure.
Mirtazapine[10,17,18]	Low	Unclear but probably more than 2.25 g. Fatality unlikely if mirtazapine taken alone.	Sedation; even large overdose may be asymptomatic.
Bupropion[10,19,20]	Moderate	Around 16 g.	Tachycardia, seizures, QRS prolongation, QT prolongation, arrhythmia.

Table Psychotropics in overdose (Cont.)

Drug or drug group	Toxicity in overdose	Smallest dose likely to cause death	Signs and symptoms of overdose
Mianserin[21]	Low	Unclear but probably more than 1 g. Fatality unlikely if mianserin taken alone.	Sedation, coma, hypertension, tachycardia.
MAOIs (not moclobemide)[1,2,4]	High	Phenelzine – 400 mg Tranylcypromine – 200 mg	Tremor, weakness, confusion, sweating, tachycardia, hypertension.
Antipsychotics Phenothiazines[22–25]	High	Chlorpromazine 5–10 g	Sedation, coma, tachycardia, arrhythmia, pulmonary oedema, hypotension, QT prolongation, seizures, dystonia, NMS.
Butyrophenones[24,26,27]	Moderate	Haloperidol – probably above 500 mg. Arrhythmia may occur at 300 mg.	Sedation, coma, dystonia, NMS, QT prolongation, arrhythmia.
Aripiprazole[28–31]	Unclear (probably low)	Unclear. Fatality unlikely when taken alone.	Sedation, lethargy, GI disturbance, drooling.
Amisulpride[32,33]	Unclear (probably low)	Unclear. Fatality unlikely when taken alone.	QT prolongation, arrhythmia.
Clozapine[34,35]	Moderate	Around 2 g.	Lethargy, coma, tachycardia, hypotension, hypersalivation, pneumonia, seizures.
Olanzapine[34,36]	Moderate	Unclear. Probably more than 200 mg.	Lethargy, confusion, myoclonus, hypotension, tachycardia, delirium.
Risperidone[34]	Low	Unclear. Fatality rare in those taking risperidone alone.	Lethargy, tachycardia, changes in blood pressure, QT prolongation.
Quetiapine[34,37–40]	Low	Unclear. Probably more than 5 g. Fatalities rare.	Lethargy, tachycardia, respiratory distress, hypotension, rhabdomyolysis.

Miscellaneous

Drug or drug group	Toxicity in overdose	Smallest dose likely to cause death	Signs and symptoms of overdose
Ziprasidone[41-43]	Unclear (probably low)	Unclear. Fatality unlikely when taken alone.	Drowsiness, lethargy. QT prolongation rarely reported.
Mood stabilisers Lithium[44,45]	Low (acute overdose)	Acute overdose does not normally result in fatality. Insidious, chronic toxicity is more dangerous.	Nausea, diarrhoea, tremor, confusion, weakness, lethargy, seizures, coma, cardiovascular collapse, arrhythmia.
Carbamazepine[46,47]	Moderate	Around 20 g, but seizures may occur at around 5 g.	Somnolence, coma, respiratory depression, ataxia, seizures, tachycardia, arrhythmia, electrolyte disturbance.
Valproate[48-50]	Moderate	Unclear. Probably more than 20 g. Doses over 400 mg/kg cause severe toxicity.	Somnolence, coma, cerebral oedema, respiratory depression, blood dyscrasia, hypotension, seizures, electrolyte disturbance.
Others Benzodiazepines[51,52]	Low	Probably more than 100 mg diazepam equivalents. Fatality unusual if taken alone. Alprazolam is most toxic.	Drowsiness, ataxia, nystagmus, respiratory depression, dysarthria, coma.
Zopiclone[51,53,54]	Low	Unclear. Probably above 100 mg. Fatality rare in those taking zopiclone alone.	Ataxia, nausea, diplopia, drowsiness, coma.
Zolpidem[55,56]	Low	Unclear. Probably above 200 mg. Fatality rare in those taking zolpidem alone.	Drowsiness, agitation, respiratory depression, tachycardia, coma.

Table Psychotropics in overdose (Cont.)

Table	Psychotropics in overdose (Cont.)		
Drug or drug group	**Toxicity in overdose**	**Smallest dose likely to cause death**	**Signs and symptoms of overdose**
Methadone[57,58]	High	20–50 mg may be fatal in non-users. Co-ingestion of benzodiazepines increases toxicity.	Drowsiness, nausea, hypotension, respiratory depression, coma, rhabdomyolysis.

High = Less than 1 week's supply likely to cause serious toxicity or death
Moderate = 1–4 weeks' supply likely to cause serious toxicity or death
Low = Death or serious toxicity unlikely even if more than 1 month's supply taken

References

1. Crome P. Antidepressant overdosage. Drugs 1982;23:431–61.
2. Henry JA. Epidemiology and relative toxicity of antidepressant drugs in overdose. Drug Saf 1997;16: 374–90.
3. Power BM et al. Antidepressant toxicity and the need for identification and concentration monitoring in overdose. Clin Pharmacokinet 1995;29:154–71.
4. Cassidy S et al. Fatal toxicity of antidepressant drugs in overdose. Br Med J 1987;295:1021–4.
5. Caksen H et al. Acute amitriptyline intoxication: an analysis of 44 children. Hum Exp Toxicol 2006; 25:107–10.
6. Henry JA et al. Relative mortality from overdose of antidepressants. BMJ 1995;310:221–4.
7. Cheeta S et al. Antidepressant-related deaths and antidepressant prescriptions in England and Wales, 1998–2000. Br J Psychiatry 2004;184:41–7.
8. Barbey JT et al. SSRI safety in overdose. J Clin Psychiatry 1998;59(Suppl 15):42–8.
9. Luchini D et al. Case report of a fatal intoxication by citalopram. Am J Forensic Med Pathol 2005; 26:352–4.
10. Buckley NA et al. 'Atypical' antidepressants in overdose: clinical considerations with respect to safety. Drug Saf 2003;26:539–51.
11. Whyte IM et al. Relative toxicity of venlafaxine and selective serotonin reuptake inhibitors in overdose compared to tricyclic antidepressants. QJM 2003;96:369–74.
12. Hetzel W. Safety of moclobemide taken in overdose for attempted suicide. Psychopharmacology 1992;106(Suppl):S127–9.
13. Myrenfors PG et al. Moclobemide overdose. J Intern Med 1993;233:113–15.
14. Gamble DE et al. Trazodone overdose: four years of experience from voluntary reports. J Clin Psychiatry 1986;47:544–6.
15. Martinez MA et al. Investigation of a fatality due to trazodone poisoning: case report and literature review. J Anal Toxicol 2005;29:262–8.
16. Baldwin DS et al. Tolerability and safety of reboxetine. Rev Contemp Pharmacother 2000;11:321–30.
17. Montgomery SA. Safety of mirtazapine: a review. Int Clin Psychopharmacol 1995;10(Suppl 4):37–45.
18. Bremner JD et al. Safety of mirtazapine in overdose. J Clin Psychiatry 1998;59:233–5.
19. Paris PA et al. ECG conduction delays associated with massive bupropion overdose. J Toxicol Clin Toxicol 1998;36:595–8.
20. Curry SC et al. Intraventricular conduction delay after bupropion overdose. J Emerg Med 2005; 29:299–305.
21. Chand S et al. One hundred cases of acute intoxication with minaserin hydrochloride. Pharma- copsychiatry 1981;14:15–17.
22. Anon. Phenothiazines. POISINDEX® System [database on CD-ROM]. Version 7.1. Greenwood Village, Colorado: Thomson Micromedex, 2004.
23. Buckley NA et al. Cardiotoxicity more common in thioridazine overdose than with other neuroleptics. J Toxicol Clin Toxicol 1995;33:199–204.
24. Haddad PM et al. Antipsychotic-related QTc prolongation, torsade de pointes and sudden death. Drugs 2002;62:1649–71.
25. Li C et al. Acute pulmonary edema induced by overdosage of phenothiazines. Chest 1992;101:102–4.
26. Levine BS et al. Two fatalities involving haloperidol. J Anal Toxicol 1991;15:282–4.
27. Henderson RA et al. Life-threatening ventricular arrhythmia (torsades de pointes) after haloperidol overdose. Hum Exp Toxicol 1991;10:59–62.

Miscellaneous

28. Lofton AL et al. Atypical experience: a case series of pediatric aripiprazole exposures. Clin Toxicol (Phila) 2005;43:151–3.
29. Seifert SA et al. Aripiprazole (Abilify) overdose in a child. Clin Toxicol (Phila) 2005;43:193–5.
30. Carstairs SD et al. Overdose of aripiprazole, a new type of antipsychotic. J Emerg Med 2005;28: 311–13.
31. Forrester MB. Aripiprazole exposures reported to Texas poison control centers during 2002–2004. J Toxicol Environ Health A 2006;69:1719–26.
32. Isbister GK et al. Amisulpride deliberate self-poisoning causing severe cardiac toxicity including QT prolongation and torsades de pointes. Med J Aust 2006;184:354–6.
33. Ward DI. Two cases of amisulpride overdose: a cause for prolonged QT syndrome. Emerg Med Australas 2005;17:274–6.
34. Trenton A et al. Fatalities associated with therapeutic use and overdose of atypical antipsychotics. CNS Drugs 2003;17:307–24.
35. Flanagan RJ et al. Suspected clozapine poisoning in the UK/Eire, 1992–2003. Forensic Sci Int 2005; 155:91–9.
36. Chue P et al. A review of olanzapine-associated toxicity and fatality in overdose. J Psychiatry Neurosci 2003;28:253–61.
37. Smith RP et al. Quetiapine overdose and severe rhabdomyolysis. J Clin Psychopharmacol 2004;24:343.
38. Langman LJ et al. Fatal overdoses associated with quetiapine. J Anal Toxicol 2004;28:520–5.
39. Hunfeld NG et al. Quetiapine in overdosage: a clinical and pharmacokinetic analysis of 14 cases. Ther Drug Monit 2006;28:185–9.
40. Strachan PM et al. Mental status change, myoclonus, electrocardiographic changes, and acute respiratory distress syndrome induced by quetiapine overdose. Pharmacotherapy 2006;26:578–82.
41. Gomez-Criado MS et al. Ziprasidone overdose: cases recorded in the database of Pfizer-Spain and literature review. Pharmacotherapy 2005;25:1660–5.
42. Arbuck DM. 12,800-mg ziprasidone overdose without significant ECG changes. Gen Hosp Psychiatry 2005;27:222–3.
43. Insa Gomez FJ et al. Ziprasidone overdose: cardiac safety. Actas Esp Psiquiatr 2005;33:398–400.
44. Tuohy K et al. Acute lithium intoxication. Dial Transplant 2003;32:478–81.
45. Chen KP et al. Implication of serum concentration monitoring in patients with lithium intoxication. Psychiatry Clin Neurosci 2004;58:25–9.
46. Spiller HA. Management of carbamazepine overdose. Pediatr Emerg Care 2001;17:452–6.
47. Schmidt S et al. Signs and symptoms of carbamazepine overdose. J Neurol 1995;242:169–73.
48. Isbister GK et al. Valproate overdose: a comparative cohort study of self poisonings. Br J Clin Pharmacol 2003;55:398–404.
49. Spiller HA et al. Multicenter case series of valproic acid ingestion: serum concentrations and toxicity. J Toxicol Clin Toxicol 2000;38:755–60.
50. Sztajnkrycer MD. Valproic acid toxicity: overview and management. J Toxicol Clin Toxicol 2002;40: 789–801.
51. Reith DM et al. Comparison of the fatal toxicity index of zopiclone with benzodiazepines. J Toxicol Clin Toxicol 2003;41:975–80.
52. Isbister GK et al. Alprazolam is relatively more toxic than other benzodiazepines in overdose. Br J Clin Pharmacol 2004;58:88–95.
53. Pounder D et al. Zopiclone poisoning. J Anal Toxicol 1996;20:273–4.
54. Bramness JG et al. Fatal overdose of zopiclone in an elderly woman with bronchogenic carcinoma. J Forensic Sci 2001;46:1247–9.
55. Gock SB et al. Acute zolpidem overdose – report of two cases. J Anal Toxicol 1999;23:559–62.
56. Garnier R et al. Acute zolpidem poisoning – analysis of 344 cases. J Toxicol Clin Toxicol 1994;32: 391–404.
57. Gable RS. Comparison of acute lethal toxicity of commonly abused psychoactive substances. Addiction 2004;99:686–96.
58. Caplehorn JR et al. Fatal methadone toxicity: signs and circumstances, and the role of benzodiazepines. Aust N Z J Public Health 2002;26:358–62.

Biochemical and haematological effects of psychotropics

Almost all psychotropics currently used in clinical practice have metabolic side-effects that may be detected using routine blood tests. While many of these changes are idiosyncratic and not clinically significant, some, such as the agranulocytosis associated with agents such as clozapine and carbamazepine, require regular monitoring of the full blood count. In general, where an agent has a high incidence of metabolic side-effects or a rare but potentially fatal effect, regular monitoring is required, as discussed in other sections.

For other agents, laboratory-related side-effects are comparatively rare (prevalence usually less than 1%), are reversible upon cessation of the putative offending agent and not always clinically significant. It should further be noted that medical co-morbidity, polypharmacy and the effects of non-prescribed agents including substances of abuse and alcohol may also influence biochemical and haematological parameters. In some cases, where a clear temporal association between starting the agent and the onset of laboratory changes is unclear, a re-challenge with the agent in question may be considered. Where there is doubt as to the aetiology and significance of the effect, the appropriate source of expert advice should always be consulted.

The following tables summarise those agents with identified biochemical and haematological effects, with information compiled from various sources[1-10]. It should be noted that in many cases the evidence for these various metabolic effects is limited, with information obtained mostly from case reports, case series and information supplied by manufacturers. For further details about each individual agent, the reader is encouraged to consult the appropriate section of the Guidelines as well as other, expert sources.

Miscellaneous

Parameter	Reference range	Agents reported to raise levels	Agents reported to lower levels
Alanine transferase (ALT)	0–45 IU/l	**Antipsychotics** Benperidol, chlorpromazine, clozapine, haloperidol, olanzapine, quetiapine, zotepine **Antidepressants** Duloxetine, mianserin, mirtazapine, moclobemide, monoamine oxidase inhibitors, SSRIs (especially paroxetine and sertraline); TCAs, trazodone, venlafaxine **Anxiolytics/hypnotics** Barbiturates, benzodiazepines, chloral hydrate, chlormethiazole, promethazine **Miscellaneous agents** Caffeine, dexamfetamine, disulfiram, opioids **Mood stabilizers** Carbamazepine, lamotrigine, valproate	None known
Albumin	3.5–4.8 g/dl	Microalbuminuria may be a feature of metabolic syndrome secondary to psychotropic use (especially phenothiazines, clozapine, olanzapine and possibly quetiapine)	None known
Alkaline phosphatase (Alk Phos)	50–120 IU/l	Carbamazepine, clozapine, disulfiram, duloxetine, galantamine, haloperidol, memantine, modafinil, nortriptyline, olanzapine, phenytoin, sertraline	None known
Amylase	<300 IU/l	Clozapine, donepezil, methadone, olanzapine, opiates, pregabalin, SSRIs (rarely), valproate	None known
Aspartate (AST) aminotransferase	10–50 IU/l	As per alanine transferase	Trifluoperazine
Bicarbonate	22–30 mmol/l	None known	None known
Bilirubin	3–20 μmol/l (total bilirubin)	Carbamazepine, chlordiazepoxide, chlorpromazine, clomethazole, disulfiram, fluphenazine, meprobamate, phenytoin, promethazine, trifluoperazine, valproate	None known
C-reactive protein	<10 μg/ml	Buprenorphine (rare)	None known
Calcium	2.2–2.6 mmol/l	Lithium (rare)	Barbiturates, haloperidol
Carbohydrate-deficient transferrin	1.9–3.4 g/l	None known	None known
Chloride	98–107 mmol/l	None known	Medications associated with

Table Summary of biochemical changes associated with psychotropics (Cont.)

Parameter	Reference range	Agents reported to raise levels	Agents reported to lower levels
			SIADH: all antidepressants, antipsychotics (clozapine, haloperidol, olanzapine, phenothiazines, pimozide, risperidone, quetiapine); carbamazepine
Cholesterol (total)	<5.2 mmol/l	Antipsychotic treatment, especially those implicated in the metabolic syndrome (phenothiazines, clozapine, olanzapine and possibly quetiapine). Rarely: aripiprazole, disulfiram, memantine, modafinil, phenytoin, rivastigmine, venlafaxine	Ziprasidone (controversial)
Creatine kinase	<90 IU/l	All drugs associated with NMS (page 102)	None known
Creatinine	60–110 μmol/l	Clozapine, lithium, thioridazine, valproate, zotepine; medications associated with rhabdomyolysis (benzodiazepines, dexamfetamine, pregabalin, thioridazine)	None known
Ferritin	Males: 40–340 μg/l Females: 14–150 μg/l	None known	None known
Gamma-glutamyl transferase (GGT)	<60 IU/l	**Antidepressants** Mirtazapine, SSRIs (paroxetine and sertraline implicated); TCAs, trazodone, venlafaxine **Anticonvulsants/mood stabilisers** Carbamazepine, lamotrigine, phenytoin, phenobarbital, valproate **Antipsychotics** Benperidol, chlorpromazine, clozapine, fluphenazine, haloperidol, olanzapine, quetiapine, zotepine **Miscellaneous** Barbiturates, clomethiazole, dexamfetamine, modafinil	None known
Glucose (blood)	Fasting: 2.8–6.0 mmol/l Random: <11.1 mmol/l	**Antidepressants** MAOI, SSRI*, TCAs* **Antipsychotics** Chlorpromazine, clozapine, olanzapine (see page 122) **Substances of abuse** Methadone, opioids *May also be associated with hypoglycaemia.	Medications associated with metabolic syndrome may result in raised or decreased glucose levels

Miscellaneous

Table Summary of biochemical changes associated with psychotropics (Cont.)

Parameter	Reference range	Agents reported to raise levels	Agents reported to lower levels
Glycated haemoglobin (HbA$_{1c}$)	3.5–5.5% (4–6% in diabetics)	All antipsychotics associated with hyperglycaemia (excluding amisulpride, ziprasidone); galantamine, methadone, morphine, TCA	Lithium, MAOIs, SSRIs
Lactate dehydro-genase	90–200 U/l	TCAs (especially imipramine), valproate	None known
Lipoproteins: HDL	>1.2 mmol/l	Carbamazepine, phenobarbital, phenytoin	Olanzapine (controversial), phenothiazines, valproate
Lipoproteins: LDL	<3.5 mmol/l	Phenothiazines, Olanzapine, quetiapine, risperidone	
Phosphate	0.8–1.4 mmol/l	Acamprosate, carbamazepine, dexamfetamine	None known
Potassium	3.5–5.0 mmol/l	Pregabalin	Haloperidol, lithium, mianserin, reboxetine, rivastigmine
Prolactin	Normal: <350 mU/l Abnormal: >600 mU/l	Antidepressants (especially MAOIs and TCAs, venlafaxine also implicated); antipsychotics, e.g. amisulpride, haloperidol, pimozide, risperidone, sulpiride, zotepine	None known
Protein (total)	60–80 g/l	None known	None known
Sodium	135–145 mmol/l	None known	Benzodiazepines, carbamazepine, chlorpromazine, donepezil, duloxetine, haloperidol, lithium, memantine, mianserin, phenothiazines, reboxetine, rivastigmine, SSRIs (especially fluoxetine), tricyclic antidepressants (especially amitriptyline) (see page 210)
Thyroid-stimulating hormone (TSH)	0.3–4.0 mU/l	Aripiprazole, carbamazepine, lithium, rivastigmine	Moclobemide
Thyroxine (T$_4$)	Free: 9–26 pmol/l	Dexamfetamine, moclobemide (rare)	Lithium (causes decreased T$_4$

Parameter	Reference range	Agents reported to raise levels	Agents reported to lower levels
	Total: 60–150 nmol/l		secretion); heroin, methadone (increase serum thyroxine-binding globulin); carbamazepine, phenytoin treatment. Rarely implicated: aripiprazole, quetiapine and rivastigmine
Triglycerides	0.4–1.8 mmol/l	Clozapine, olanzapine, quetiapine, phenothiazines, valproate, venlafaxine (see page 127)	Ziprasidone (controversial)
Triiodothyronine (T_3)	Free: 3.0–8.8 pmol/l Total: 1.2–2.9 nmol/l	Heroin, methadone; moclobemide	Free T_3: valproate Total T_3: carbamazepine, lithium
Urate (uric acid)	0.1–0.4 mmol/l	Rarely: zotepine, rivastigmine	None known
Urea	1.8–7.1 mmol/l	Rarely with agents associated with anticonvulsant hypersensitivity syndrome and rhabdomyolysis	None known

Miscellaneous

Table Summary of haematological changes associated with psychotropics

Parameter	Reference range	Agents reported to raise levels	Agents reported to lower levels
Activated partial thromboplastin time (APTT)	25–39 seconds	Phenothiazines (especially chlorpromazine)	None known
Basophils	$0.0–0.10 \times 10^9/l$	TCAs (especially desipramine)	None known
Eosinophils	$0.04–0.45 \times 10^9/l$	Amitriptyline, carbamazepine, chloral hydrate, chlorpromazine, clonazepam, clozapine, fluphenazine, haloperidol, imipramine, meprobamate, modafinil, nortriptyline, olanzapine, quetiapine, SSRIs, tryptophan, zotepine	None known
Erythrocytes	Males: $4.5–6.0 \times 10^{12}/l$ Females: $3.8–5.2 \times 10^{12}/l$	None known	Carbamazepine, phenytoin, chlordiazepoxide, chlorpromazine, meprobamate, trifluoperazine
Erythrocyte sedimentation rate	<20 mm/hour Note: levels increase with age and are slightly higher in females	Clozapine, levomepromazine, maprotiline, SSRIs, zotepine	None known
Haemoglobin (Hb)	Males: 14–18 g/dl Females: 12–16 g/dl	None known	Carbamazepine, chlordiazepoxide, chlorpromazine, duloxetine, meprobamate, phenytoin, trifluoperazine
Lymphocytes	$1.0–4.8 \times 10^9/l$	Valproate	Lithium
Mean cell haemoglobin	27–37 pg Note: levels are slightly higher in males and	Medications associated with megaloblastic anaemia, e.g. all anticonvulsants	None known

	may be raised in the elderly		None known
Mean cell haemoglobin concentration	300–350 g/l		
Men cell volume	80–100 fl		
Monocytes	$0.21–0.92 \times 10^9/l$	Haloperidol	**Agents associated with agranulocytosis** Amitriptyline, amoxapine, carbamazepine, chlordiazepoxide, chlorpromazine, clomipramine, clozapine, diazepam, fluphenazine, haloperidol, imipramine, mirtazapine, nortriptyline, tranylcypromine. **Agents associated with leukopenia** Amitriptyline, amoxapine, bupropion, carbamazepine, chlorpromazine, citalopram, clomipramine, clonazepam, clozapine, fluphenazine, haloperidol, lorazepam, mirtazapine, nefazodone, oxazepam, risperidone, tranylcypromine, venlafaxine **Agents associated with neutropenia** Trazodone, valproate
Neutrophils	$2–9 \times 10^9/l$	Carbamazepine*, citalopram, clozapine*, fluphenazine, haloperidol, lithium, olanzapine, risperidone, trazodone, venlafaxine * Rare, usually associated with leukopenia.	
Packed cell volume	Adult males: 42–52% Adult females: 35–47% (levels	None known	None known

Table Summary of haematological changes associated with psychotropics (Cont.)

Parameter	Reference range	Agents reported to raise levels	Agents reported to lower levels
	slightly lower in pregnant versus non-pregnant women)		
Platelets	150–400 × 10^9/l	Lithium	Amitriptyline, barbiturates, bupropion, carbamazepine, clomipramine, chlordiazepoxide, chlorpromazine, clonazepam, clozapine, diazepam, duloxetine, fluphenazine, imipramine, lamotrigine, meprobamate, mirtazapine, olanzapine, risperidone, sertraline, tranylcypromine, trifluoperazine, valproate
Prothrombin time/ international normalised ratio	10–13 seconds	Fluoxetine, fluvoxamine; disulfiram; bupropion	Barbiturates, carbamazepine, phenytoin
Red cell distribution width	11.5–14.5%	Agents associated with anaemia: e.g. carbamazepine, chlordiazepoxide, citalopram, clonazepam, diazepam, lamotrigine, mirtazapine, nefazodone, sertraline, tranylcypromine, trazodone, valproate, venlafaxine	None known
Reticulocyte count	0.5–1.5%	None known	Carbamazepine, chlordiazepoxide, chlorpromazine, meprobamate, phenytoin, trifluoperazine

References

1. Balon R et al. Hematologic side effects of psychotropic drugs. Psychosomatics 1986;27:119–27.
2. Bazire S. Psychotropic Drug Directory: The Professionals' Pocket Handbook and Aide Memoire. Salisbury: Fivepin Publishing, 2005.
3. British National Formularly, 52nd edn. London: British Medical Association and Royal Pharmaceutical Society of Great Britain, 2006.
4. Dukes MNG. Meyler's Side Effects of Drugs. The Encyclopedia of Adverse Reactions and Interactions, 12th edn. Amsterdam: Elsevier Science, 1992.
5. Foster R. Practical Handbook of Clinical Laboratory Medicine and Psychiatry. Oxford: Oxford University Press, 2007.
6. Laboratory Test Handbook. Hudson, Cleveland, Ohio: Lexi-Comp Inc, 1996.
7. Oyesanmi O et al. Hematologic side effects of psychotropics. Psychosomatics 1999;40:414–21.
8. Stubner S et al. Blood dyscrasias induced by psychotropic drugs. Pharmacopsychiatry 2004;37(Suppl 1): S70–8.
9. Martindale: The Complete Drug Reference, 34th edn. London: Pharmaceutical Press, 2004.
10. Tietz NW. Clinical Guide to Laboratory Tests, 3nd edn. Philadelphia: WB Saunders, 1995.

Miscellaneous

Prescribing drugs outside their licensed indications

A product licence is granted when regulatory authorities are satisfied that the drug in question has proven efficacy in the treatment of a specified disorder, along with an acceptable side-effect profile, relative to the severity of the disorder being treated and other available treatments.

The decision of a manufacturer to seek a Product Licence for a given indication is essentially a commercial one; potential sales are balanced against the cost of conducting the necessary clinical trials. It therefore follows that drugs may be effective outside their licensed indications for different disease states, age ranges, doses and durations. The absence of a formal Product Licence or labelling may simply reflect the absence of controlled trials supporting the drug's efficacy in these areas. Importantly, however, it is possible that trials have been conducted but given negative results.

The application of common sense is important here. Prescribing a drug within its licence does not guarantee that the patient will come to no harm. Likewise, prescribing outside a licence does not mean that the risk–benefit ratio is automatically adverse. Prescribing outside a licence, usually called 'off-label', does confer extra responsibilities on prescribers, who will be expected to be able to show that they acted in accordance with a respected body of medical opinion (the Bolam test)[1] and that their action was capable of withstanding logical analysis (the Bolitho test)[2].

The psychopharmacology special interest group at the Royal College of Psychiatrists has published a consensus statement on the use of licensed medicines for unlicensed uses[3]. They note that unlicensed use is common in general adult psychiatry with cross-sectional studies showing that up to 50% of patients are prescribed at least one drug outside the terms of its licence. They also note that the prevalence of this type of prescribing is likely to be higher in patients under the age of 18 or over 65, in those with a learning disability, in women who are pregnant or lactating and in those patients who are cared for in forensic psychiatry settings. The main recommendations in the consensus statement are summarised below.

Before prescribing 'off-label':

- Exclude licensed alternatives (ineffective or not tolerated).
- Ensure familiarity with the evidence base for the intended unlicensed use. If unsure, seek advice.
- Consider and document the potential risks and benefits of the proposed treatment. Share this risk assessment with the patient, and carers if applicable. Document the discussion and the patient's consent or lack of capacity to consent.
- If prescribing responsibility is to be shared with primary care, ensure that the risk assessment and consent issues are shared with the GP.
- Monitor for efficacy and side-effects.
- Consider publishing the case to add to the body of knowledge.

The more experimental the unlicensed use is, the more important it is to adhere to the above guidance.

Examples of acceptable use of drugs outside their Product Licences

The table below gives examples of common unlicensed uses of drugs in psychiatric practice. These examples would all fulfil the Bolam and Bolitho criteria in principle. An exhaustive list of unlicensed uses is impossible to prepare as:

- The evidence base is constantly changing.
- The expertise and experience of prescribers varies. A strategy may be justified in the hands of a specialist in psychopharmacology based in a tertiary referral centre but be much more difficult to justify if initiated by someone with a special interest in psychotherapy who rarely prescribes.

Drug/drug group	Established unlicensed use(s)	Further information
Second generation antipsychotics	Psychotic illness other than schizophrenia	Licences vary. All are licensed for schizophrenia, some for mania and some for prophylaxis in bipolar affective disorder
Clonidine	ADHD in children	Limited evidence supports use as a second-line treatment or augmentation strategy
Cyproheptadine	Akathisia	Some evidence to support efficacy in this distressing and difficult to treat side-effect of antipsychotics
Fluoxetine	Maintenance treatment of depression	Few prescribers are likely to be aware that this is not a licensed indication
Lamotrigine	Bipolar depression	RCTs demonstrate benefit
Methylphenidate	ADHD in children under 6	Established clinical practice
Naltrexone	Self-injurious behaviour in people with learning disabilities	Limited evidence base Acceptable in specialist hands as a treatment of last resort
Sodium valproate	Treatment and prophylaxis of bipolar disorder	Established clinical practice

Note that some drugs do not have a UK licence for any indication. Two commonly prescribed examples in psychiatric practice are melatonin (used to treat insomnia in children and adolescents) and pirenzepine (used to treat clozapine-induced hypersalivation). Awareness of the evidence base and documentation of potential benefits, side-effects and patient consent are especially important here.

Miscellaneous

References

1. Bolam v Friern Barnet Hospital Management Committee. WLR 1957;1:582.
2. Bolitho v City and Hackney Health Authority. WLR 1997;3:1151.
3. Baldwin DS. Royal College of Psychiatrists' Special Interest Group in Psychopharmacology. The use of licensed medicines for unlicensed applications in psychiatric practice. http://www.rcpsych. ac.uk/. 2006.

Observations on the placebo effect in mental illness

Target symptoms improve, to varying degrees, in approximately a third of patients given a placebo[1]. The following considerations apply when interpreting the results of placebo-controlled studies. Although the references for each point are drawn from the depression literature, the same principles apply to the treatment of other disorders. The relative importance of each point will vary depending on the disorder that is being treated.

- Placebo is not the same as no care: patients who maintain contact with services have a better outcome than those who receive no care[2].
- The placebo response is greater in mild illness[3].
- The higher the placebo response rate, the more difficult it is to power studies to show treatment effects. Where the placebo response rate exceeds 40%, studies have to recruit very large numbers of patients to be adequately powered to show differences between treatments[4].
- It is difficult to separate placebo effects from spontaneous remission. The higher the spontaneous remission rate, the more difficult it is to power studies to show treatment effects[2].
- Patients who enter RCTs generally do so when acutely unwell. Symptoms are likely to improve in the majority, irrespective of the intervention. This is so-called 'regression to the mean'[5].
- The placebo response rate in published studies is increasing over time[6]. This may be because of increasing numbers of mildly ill patients being recruited into trials because of clinicians' reluctance to risk severely ill patients being randomised into placebo arms.
- 'Breaking the blind' may influence outcome. The resultant 'expectancy effect' may explain why active placebos are more effective than inert placebos[7,8]. That is, if patients and observers note adverse effects, the placebo effect is enhanced.
- Not all placebos are the same. Patients perceive two brightly coloured tablets to be more effective than one small white one. Capsules, injections and branding also increase expectations of efficacy[1]. This may partly explain different placebo response rates in studies of similar design.
- Most psychotropic drugs have side-effects such as sedation that may improve scores on rating scales without actually treating the target illness.
- Placebo response may be short-lived: studies are usually too short to pick up placebo relapsers[9].
- Statistical significance and clinical significance are not the same thing: a study may report on a highly statistically significant difference in efficacy between active drug and placebo, but the magnitude of the difference may be too small to be clinically meaningful.
- Publication bias remains a problem[10-12]. Many negative studies are never published. Underpowered positive studies often are.
- Placebo response increases according to expectancy. For example, placebo response is greater in studies randomising 2:1 active: placebo than in those randomising 1:1 (chance of receiving active is greater).
- Note that other effects may operate: 'wish bias' probably exaggerates the efficacy of new drugs compared with established agents[13].

Miscellaneous

References

1. Rajagopal S. The placebo effect. Psychiatr Bull 2006;30:185–8.
2. Andrews G. Placebo response in depression: bane of research, boon to therapy. Br J Psychiatry 2001; 178:192–4.
3. Khan A et al. Severity of depression and response to antidepressants and placebo: an analysis of the Food and Drug Administration database. J Clin Psychopharmacol 2002;22:40–5.
4. Thase ME. Studying new antidepressants: if there were a light at the end of the tunnel, could we see it? J Clin Psychiatry 2002;63 Suppl 2:24–8.
5. McDonald CJ et al. How much of the placebo 'effect' is really statistical regression? Stat Med 1983; 2:417–27.
6. Walsh BT et al. Placebo response in studies of major depression: variable, substantial, and growing. JAMA 2002;287:1840–7.
7. Kirsch I et al. The Emperor's new drugs: An analysis of antidepressant medication data submitted to the US Food and Drug Administration. Prevention and Treatment 2002;5:10–23.
8. Moncrieff J et al. Active placebos versus antidepressants for depression. Cochrane Database Syst Rev 2004;CD003012.
9. Ross DC et al. A typological model for estimation of drug and placebo effects in depression. J Clin Psychopharmacol 2002;22:414–8.
10. Lexchin J et al. Pharmaceutical industry sponsorship and research outcome and quality: systematic review. BMJ 2003;326:1167–70.
11. Melander H et al. Evidence b(i)ased medicine – selective reporting from studies sponsored by pharmaceutical industry: review of studies in new drug applications. BMJ 2003;326:1171–3.
12. Werneke U et al. How effective is St John's wort? The evidence revisited. J Clin Psychiatry 2004;65: 611–7.
13. Barbui C et al. "Wish bias" in antidepressant drug trials? J Clin Psychopharmacol 2004;24:126–30.

Drug interactions with alcohol

Drug interactions with alcohol are complex. Many patient-related and drug-related factors need to be considered. It can be difficult to predict outcomes accurately as a number of processes may occur simultaneously.

Pharmacokinetic interactions[1,2]

Alcohol (ethanol) is absorbed from the GI tract and distributed in body water. The volume of distribution is smaller in women and the elderly where plasma levels of alcohol will be higher for a given 'dose' of alcohol than in males. Approximately 10% of ingested alcohol is subjected to first - pass metabolism by alcohol dehydrogenase (ADH). (A small proportion is metabolised by ADH in the stomach.) The remainder is metabolised in the liver by ADH and CYP2E1. CYP2E1 plays a minor role in occasional drinkers but is an important metabolic route in chronic, heavy drinkers. CYP1A2 and CYP3A4 also play a minor role[3].

CYP2E1 and ADH convert alcohol to acetaldehyde, which is the toxic substance responsible for the unpleasant symptoms of the 'antabuse reaction' (e.g. flushing, headache, nausea, malaise). Acetaldehyde is then further metabolised by aldehyde dehydrogenase to acetic acid and then to carbon dioxide and water.

All of the enzymes involved in the metabolism of alcohol exhibit genetic polymorphism. Forty percent of people of Asian origin are poor metabolisers via ADH. Chronic consumption of alcohol induces CYP2E1 and CYP3A4. The effects of alcohol on other hepatic metabolising enzymes have been poorly studied.

Metabolism of alcohol

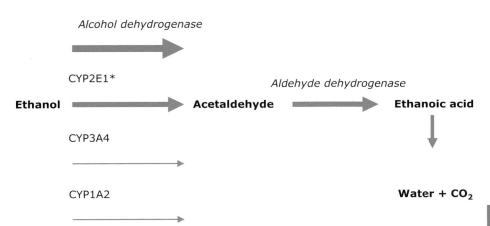

*Minor route in occasional drinkers; major route in misusers

Table Co-administration of alcohol and substrates for CYP2E1 and CYP3A4

	CYP2E1	CYP3A4
Substrates for, enzyme (note: this is not an exhaustive list)	• Paracetamol • Isoniazid • Phenobarbital	• Benzodiazepines • Carbamazepine • Clozapine • Donepezil • Galantamine • Mirtazapine • Risperidone • Tricyclics • Valproate • Venlafaxine • Z hypnotics
Effects in an intoxicated patient	Competition between alcohol and drug leading to reduced rates of metabolism of both compounds Increased plasma levels may lead to toxicity	Competition between alcohol and drug leading to reduced rates of metabolism of both compounds Increased plasma levels may lead to toxicity
Effects in a chronic, sober drinker	Activity of CYP2E1 is increased up 10-fold Increased metabolism of drugs potentially leading to therapeutic failure	Increased rate of drug metabolism potentially leading to therapeutic failure

Interactions are difficult to predict in alcohol misusers because two opposing processes may be at work: competition for enzymatic sites during periods of intoxication (increasing drug plasma levels) and enzyme induction prevailing (reducing plasma levels) during periods of sobriety. In chronic drinkers, particularly those who binge drink, serum levels of prescribed drugs may reach toxic levels during periods of intoxication with alcohol and then be subtherapeutic when the patient is sober. This makes it very difficult to optimise treatment of physical or mental illness.

Table Drugs that inhibit alcohol dehydrogenase and aldehyde dehydrogenase

Enzyme	Inhibitor of enzyme	Potential consequences
Alcohol dehydrogenase	• Aspirin • H_2 antagonists	Reduced metabolism of alcohol resulting in higher plasma levels for longer periods of time
Aldehyde dehydrogenase	• Disulfiram • Griseofulvin • Isoniazid • Metronidazole • Nitrofurantoin • Sulfamethoxazole • Isosorbide dinitrate • Chlorpropamide • Tolbutamide	Reduced ability to metabolise acetaldehyde leading to 'Antabuse' type reaction: facial flushing, headache, tachycardia, nausea & vomiting, arrhythmias and hypotension

Pharmacodynamic interactions[1,2,4]

Alcohol enhances inhibitory neurotransmission at $GABA_a$ receptors and reduces excitatory neurotransmission at glutamate NMDA receptors. It also increases dopamine release in the mesolimbic pathway and may have some effects on serotonin and opiate pathways. Alcohol, alone, would therefore be expected to cause sedation, amnesia and ataxia and give rise to feelings of pleasure (or worsen psychotic symptoms in vulnerable individuals).

Table Pharmacodynamic interactions with alcohol

Effect of alcohol	Effect exacerbated by	Potential consequences
Sedation	Other sedative drugs, e.g. • Benzodiazepines • Antipsychotics • Tricyclics, trazodone • Z-hypnotics • Antihistamines • Opiates • Lofexidine • Baclofen • Tizanidine	Increased CNS depression ranging from increased propensity to be involved in accidents through to respiratory depression and death
Amnesia	Other amnesic drugs, e.g. • Benzodiazepines • Barbiturates • Z-hypnotics	Increased amnesic effects ranging from mild memory loss to total amnesia

Miscellaneous

Table Pharmacodynamic interactions with alcohol (Cont.)

Effect of alcohol	Effect exacerbated by	Potential consequences
Ataxia	• ACE inhibitors • β-blockers • Ca channel blockers • Nitrates Adrenergic α receptor antagonists, e.g. • Clozapine • Risperidone • Tricyclics • Cartamazapine	Increased unsteadiness and falls

Alcohol can cause or worsen psychotic symptoms via increasing dopamine release in the mesolimbic pathways. The effect of antipsychotic drugs may be competitively antagonised, rendering them less effective.

Electrolyte disturbances secondary to alcohol-related dehydration can be exacerbated by other drugs that cause electrolyte disturbances such as diuretics.

Note that:
- **In the presence of pharmacokinetic interactions, pharmacodynamic interactions will be more marked.** For example, in a chronic heavy drinker who is sober, enzyme induction will increase the metabolism of diazepam which may lead to increased levels of anxiety (treatment failure). If the same patient becomes intoxicated with alcohol, the metabolism of diazepam will be greatly reduced as it will have to compete with alcohol for the metabolic capacity of CYP3A4. Plasma levels of alcohol and diazepam will rise (toxicity). As both alcohol and diazepam are sedative (via GABA$_a$ affinity), loss of consciousness and respiratory depression may occur.

Table Psychotropic drugs: choice in patients who continue to drink

	Safest choice	Best avoided
Antipsychotics	**Sulpiride & amisulpride** (non-sedative and renally excreted)	**Very sedative antipsychotics** such as chlorpromazine and clozapine
Antidepressants	**SSRI** Potent inhibitors of CYP3A4 may decrease alcohol metabolism in chronic drinkers (fluoxetine, paroxetine)	**TCAs**, because impairment of metabolism by alcohol (while intoxicated) can lead to profound hypotension, seizures, arrhythmias and coma. Cardiac effects can be exacerbated by electrolyte disturbances. Combinations of TCAs and alcohol profoundly impair psychomotor skills. **MAOIs** can cause profound hypotension. Also potential interaction with tyramine-containing drinks which can lead to hypertensive crisis
Mood stabilisers	**Valproate Carbamazepine** Note: higher serum levels achieved during periods of alcohol intoxication may be poorly tolerated	**Lithium**, because it has a narrow therapeutic index and alcohol-related dehydration and electrolyte disturbance can precipitate toxicity

NB. Be aware of the possibility of hepatic failure or reduced hepatic function in chronic alcohol misusers. See page 403. Also note risk of hepatic toxicity with some recommended drugs (e.g. valproate).

References

1. Weathermon R et al. Alcohol and medication interactions. Alcohol Res Health 1999;23:40–54.
2. Tanaka E. Toxicological interactions involving psychiatric drugs and alcohol: an update. J Clin Pharm Ther 2003;28:81–95.
3. Salmela KS et al. Respective roles of human cytochrome P-4502E1, 1A2, and 3A4 in the hepatic microsomal ethanol oxidizing system. Alcohol Clin Exp Res 1998;22:2125–32.
4. Stahl SM et al. Essential Psychopharmacology: Neuroscientific Basis and Practical Applications. Cambridge: Cambridge University Press, 2000.

Further reading

British National Formulary. No. 52, Appendix 1: Drug interactions. British Medical Association and Royal Pharmaceutical Society of Great Britain, 2006.
Stockley I. Stockley's Drug Interactions. London: The Pharmaceutical Press, 2005.

Miscellaneous

Nicotine

The most common method of consuming nicotine is by smoking cigarettes. One-third of the general population, 40–50% of those with depression and up to 90% of those with schizophrenia smoke[1]. Nicotine causes peripheral vasoconstriction, tachycardia and increased blood pressure[2]. Smokers are at increased risk of developing cardiovascular disease. As well as nicotine, cigarettes also contain tar (a complex mixture of organic molecules, many carcinogenic), a cause of cancers of the respiratory tract, chronic bronchitis and emphysema[3].

Nicotine is highly addictive. People with mental illness are 2–3 times more likely than the general population to develop and maintain a nicotine addiction[1]. Chronic smoking contributes to the increased morbidity and mortality from respiratory and cardiovascular disease that is seen in this patient group. Nicotine also has psychotropic effects. Smoking can affect the metabolism (and therefore the efficacy and toxicity) of drugs prescribed to treat psychiatric illness[4]. Nicotine use may be a gateway to experimenting with other psychoactive substances.

Psychotropic effects

Nicotine is highly lipid-soluble and rapidly enters the brain after inhalation. Nicotine receptors are found on dopaminergic cell bodies and stimulation of these receptors leads to dopamine release[1]. Dopamine release in the limbic system is associated with pleasure: dopamine is the brain's 'reward' neurotransmitter. Nicotine may be used by people with mental health problems as a form of 'self-medication' (e.g. to alleviate the negative symptoms of schizophrenia or antipsychotic-induced EPSEs or for its anxiolytic effect[5]). Drugs that increase the release of dopamine reduce the craving for nicotine. They may also worsen psychotic illness (see under smoking cessation below).

Nicotine improves concentration and vigilance[1]. It also enhances the effects of glutamate, acetylcholine and serotonin[5].

Schizophrenia

Up to 90% of people with schizophrenia regularly smoke cigarettes[1] and this increased tendency to smoke predates the onset of psychiatric symptoms[6]. Possible explanations are as follows: smoking causes dopamine release, leading to feelings of well-being and a reduction in negative symptoms[5]; to alleviate some of the side-effects of antipsychotics such as drowsiness and EPSEs[1] and cognitive slowing[7]; as a means of structuring the day (a behavioural filler); or as a means of alleviating the deficit in auditory gating that is found in schizophrenia[8]. Nicotine may also improve working memory and attentional deficits[9–11]. Nicotinic receptor agonists may have beneficial effects on neurocognition[12], although none are yet licensed for this purpose. A SPECT study has shown that the greater the occupancy of striatal D_2 receptors by antipsychotic drugs, the more likely the patient is to smoke[13]. This may partly explain the clinical observation that smoking cessation may be more achievable when clozapine (a weak dopamine antagonist) is prescribed in place of a conventional antipsychotic.

It has been suggested that people with schizophrenia find it particularly difficult to tolerate nicotine withdrawal symptoms[4].

Depression and anxiety

In 'normal' individuals a moderate consumption of nicotine is associated with pleasure and a decrease in anxiety and feelings of anger[14]. The mechanism of this anxiolytic effect is not understood. People who suffer from anxiety and/or depression are more likely to smoke and find it more difficult to stop[14,15]. This is compounded by the fact that nicotine withdrawal can precipitate or exacerbate depression in those with a history of the illness[14]. Patients with depression are at increased risk of cardiovascular disease. By directly causing tachycardia and hypertension[2], nicotine may, in theory, exacerbate this problem.

Movement disorders and Parkinson's disease

By increasing dopaminergic neurotransmission, nicotine provides a protective effect against both drug-induced EPSEs and idiopathic Parkinson's disease. Smokers are less likely to suffer from antipsychotic-induced movement disorders than non-smokers[1] and use anticholinergics less often[4]. Parkinson's disease occurs less frequently in smokers than in non-smokers and the onset of clinical symptoms is delayed[1,16]. This may reflect the inverse association between Parkinson's disease and sensation-seeking behavioural traits, rather than a direct effect of nicotine[17].

Drug interactions

Polycyclic hydrocarbons in cigarette smoke are known to stimulate the hepatic microsomal enzyme system, particularly CYP1A2[5], the enzyme responsible for the metabolism of many psychotropic drugs. Smoking can lower the blood levels of some drugs by up to 50%[5]. This can affect both efficacy and side-effects and needs to be taken into account when making clinical decisions. The drugs most likely to be affected are: clozapine[18], fluphenazine, haloperidol, chlorpromazine, olanzapine, many tricyclic antidepressants, mirtazapine, fluvoxamine and propranolol.

Withdrawal symptoms[4]

Withdrawal symptoms occur within 12–14 hours of stopping smoking and include depressed mood, insomnia, anxiety, restlessness, irritability, difficulty in concentrating and increased appetite. Nicotine withdrawal can be confused with depression, anxiety, sleep disorders and mania. It can also exacerbate the symptoms of schizophrenia.

Smoking cessation

People with mental health problems generally have low motivation to stop smoking and may find withdrawal intolerable[9]. Although the efficacy of nicotine replacement treatments in people with enduring mental illness has not been evaluated in RCTs[19], the adverse effects of smoking on physical health are so great that patients should always be encouraged to stop. Nicotine replacement is available in the form of patches, microtabs, gum, lozenges and inhalers. Full details can be found in the *BNF*. Bupropion/amfebutamone (a norepinephrine and dopamine reuptake inhibitor) and varenicline are licensed for smoking cessation[20] and may be effective in people with schizophrenia[21,22]. Nor-adrenergic antidepressants such as nortriptyline[23] and venlafaxine[24] may also be effective. SSRIs are not[25].

References

1. Goff DC et al. Cigarette smoking in schizophrenia: relationship to psychopathology and medication side effects. Am J Psychiatry 1992;149:1189–94.
2. Benowitz NL et al. Cardiovascular effects of nasal and transdermal nicotine and cigarette smoking. Hypertension 2002;39:1107–12.
3. Anderson JE et al. Treating tobacco use and dependence: an evidence-based clinical practice guideline for tobacco cessation. Chest 2002;121:932–41.
4. Ziedonis DM et al. Schizophrenia and nicotine use: report of a pilot smoking cessation program and review of neurobiological and clinical issues. Schizophr Bull 1997;23:247–54.
5. Lyon ER. A review of the effects of nicotine on schizophrenia and antipsychotic medications. Psychiatr Serv 1999;50:1346–50.
6. Weiser M et al. Higher rates of cigarette smoking in male adolescents before the onset of schizophrenia: a historical-prospective cohort study. Am J Psychiatry 2004;161:1219–23.
7. Harris JG et al. Effects of nicotine on cognitive deficits in schizophrenia. Neuropsychopharmacology 2004;29:1378–85.
8. McEvoy JP et al. Smoking and therapeutic response to clozapine in patients with schizophrenia. Biol Psychiatry 1999;46:125–9.
9. Jacobsen LK et al. Nicotine effects on brain function and functional connectivity in schizophrenia. Biol Psychiatry 2004;55:850–8.
10. Sacco KA et al. Effects of cigarette smoking on spatial working memory and attentional deficits in schizophrenia: involvement of nicotinic receptor mechanisms. Arch Gen Psychiatry 2005;62:649–59.
11. Smith RC et al. Effects of nicotine nasal spray on cognitive function in schizophrenia. Neuropsychopharmacology 2006;31:637–43.
12. Olincy A et al. Proof-of-concept trial of an alpha7 nicotinic agonist in schizophrenia. Arch Gen Psychiatry 2006;63:630–8.
13. de Haan L et al. Occupancy of dopamine D_2 receptors by antipsychotic drugs is related to nicotine addiction in young patients with schizophrenia. Psychopharmacology 2006;183:500–5.
14. Glassman AH. Cigarette smoking: implications for psychiatric illness. Am J Psychiatry 1993;150:546–53.
15. Wilhelm K et al. Clinical aspects of nicotine dependence and depression. Med Today 2004;5:40–7.
16. Scott WK et al. Family-based case-control study of cigarette smoking and Parkinson disease. Neurology 2005;64:442–7.
17. Evans AH et al. Relationship between impulsive sensation seeking traits, smoking, alcohol and caffeine intake, and Parkinson's disease. J Neurol Neurosurg Psychiatry 2006;77:317–21.
18. Derenne JL et al. Clozapine toxicity associated with smoking cessation: case report. Am J Ther 2005;12:469–71.
19. Ziedonis D et al. Management of smoking in people with psychiatric disorders. Curr Opin Psychiatry 2003;16:305–16.
20. GlaxoSmithKline UK. Zyban 150 mg prolonged release film-coated tablets. http://emc.medicines.org.uk/. 2006.
21. George TP et al. A placebo controlled trial of bupropion for smoking cessation in schizophrenia. Biol Psychiatry 2002;52:53–61.
22. Evins AE et al. A double-blind placebo-controlled trial of bupropion sustained-release for smoking cessation in schizophrenia. J Clin Psychopharmacol 2005;25:218–25.
23. Wagena EJ et al. Should nortriptyline be used as a first-line aid to help smokers quit? Results from a systematic review and meta-analysis. Addiction 2005;100:317–26.
24. Cinciripini PM et al. Combined effects of venlafaxine, nicotine replacement, and brief counseling on smoking cessation. Exp Clin Psychopharmacol 2005;13:282–92.
25. Hughes J et al. Antidepressants for smoking cessation. Cochrane Database Syst Rev 2004;CD000031.

Further reading

Aguilar MC et al. Nicotine dependence and symptoms in schizophrenia: naturalistic study of complex interactions. Br J Psychiatry 2005;186:215–21.

De Leon J et al. Schizophrenia and smoking: an epidemiological survey in a state hospital. Am J Psychiatry 1995;152:453–5.

Desai HD et al. Smoking in patients receiving psychotropic medications: a pharmacokinetic perspective. CNS Drugs 2001;15:469–94.

Lawn S et al. Smoking bans in psychiatric inpatient settings? A review of the research. Aust N Z J Psychiatry 2005;39:866–85.

Zevin S et al. Drug interactions with tobacco smoking. Clin Pharmacokinet 1999;36:425–38.

Miscellaneous

Smoking and psychotropic drugs

Tobacco smoke contains polycyclic aromatic hydrocarbons that induce (increase the activity of) certain hepatic enzymes (CYP1A2 in particular). For some drugs used in psychiatry, smoking significantly reduces drug plasma levels and higher doses are required than in non-smokers.

When smokers stop, enzyme activity reduces over a week or so. (Nicotine replacement has no effect on this process.) Plasma levels of affected drugs will then rise, sometimes substantially. Dose reduction will usually be necessary. If smoking is restarted, enzyme activity increases, plasma levels fall and dose increases are then required. The process is complicated and effects are difficult to predict. Of course, few people manage to give up smoking completely, so additional complexity is introduced by intermittent smoking and repeated attempts at stopping completely. Close monitoring of plasma levels (where useful), clinical progress and adverse-effect severity are essential.

The table below gives details of drugs most affected by smoking status. Note that other drugs not listed in the table but which may be affected by smoking include: carbamazepine[1], duloxetine[2], flupentixol[3], mirtazapine[4] and zuclopenthixol[5,6]. The effect of smoking on these drugs is usually clinically insignificant. Nonetheless, caution is advised. Note also that fluvoxamine metabolism is potently affected by smoking[7] but fluvoxamine is now rarely used.

Miscellaneous

Drug	Effect of smoking	Action to be taken on stopping smoking	Action to be taken on restarting
Clozapine[8,9]	Reduces plasma levels by up to 50% (depends on number/type of cigarettes smoked).	Take plasma level before stopping. On stopping, reduce dose gradually (over a week) until around 75% dose reached. Repeat plasma level 1 week after stopping. Consider further dose reductions.	Take plasma level before restarting. Increase dose to 'normal' smoking dose over 1 week. Repeat plasma level.
Olanzapine[10,11]	Reduces plasma levels by up to 50% (depends on number/type of cigarettes smoked).	Take plasma level before stopping. On stopping, reduce dose by 25%. After 1 week, repeat plasma level. Consider further dose reductions.	Take plasma level before restarting. Increase dose to 'normal' smoking dose over 1 week. Repeat plasma level.
Fluphenazine[12]	Reduces plasma levels by up to 50% (depends on number/type of cigarettes smoked).	On stopping, reduce dose by 25%. Monitor carefully over following 4–8 weeks. Consider further dose reductions.	On restarting, increase dose to 'normal' smoking dose.
Haloperidol[13,14]	Reduces plasma levels by around 20% (depends on number/type of cigarettes smoked).	Reduce dose by around 10%. Monitor carefully. Consider further dose reductions.	On restarting, increase dose to 'normal' smoking dose.
Chlorpromazine[1,3,15]	Plasma levels reduced. Varied estimates of exact effect.	Monitor closely, consider dose reduction.	Monitor closely, consider restarting 'normal' smoking dose.
Tricyclic antidepressants[1,15]	Plasma levels reduced by 25–50% (depends on drug and smoking status).	Monitor closely. Consider reducing dose by 10–25% over 1 week. Consider further dose reductions.	Monitor closely. Consider restarting 'normal' smoking dose.
Benzodiazapines[1,15]	Plasma levels reduced by 0–50% (depends on drug and smoking status).	Monitor closely. Consider reducing dose by up to 25% over 1 week.	Monitor closely. Consider restarting 'normal' smoking dose.

503

References

1. Desai HD et al. Smoking in patients receiving psychotropic medications: a pharmacokinetic perspective. CNS Drugs 2001;15:469–94.
2. Eli Lilly and Company Limited. Cymbalta. http://emc.medicines.org.uk/. 2006.
3. Goff DC et al. Cigarette smoking in schizophrenia: relationship to psychopathology and medication side effects. Am J Psychiatry 1992;149:1189–94.
4. Grasmader K et al. Population pharmacokinetic analysis of mirtazapine. Eur J Clin Pharmacol 2004; 60:473–80.
5. Jorgensen A et al. Zuclopenthixol decanoate in schizophrenia: serum levels and clinical state. Psychopharmacology 1985;87:364–7.
6. Jann MW et al. Clinical pharmacokinetics of the depot antipsychotics. Clin Pharmacokinet 1985;10: 315–33.
7. Spigset O et al. Effect of cigarette smoking on fluvoxamine pharmacokinetics in humans. Clin Pharmacol Ther 1995;58:399–403.
8. Haring C et al. Influence of patient-related variables on clozapine plasma levels. Am J Psychiatry 1990; 147:1471–5.
9. Haring C et al. Dose-related plasma levels of clozapine: influence of smoking behaviour, sex and age. Psychopharmacology 1989;99 (Suppl):S38–S40.
10. Carrillo JA et al. Role of the smoking-induced cytochrome P450 (CYP)1A2 and polymorphic CYP2D6 in steady-state concentration of olanzapine. J Clin Psychopharmacol 2003;23:119–27.
11. Gex-Fabry M et al. Therapeutic drug monitoring of olanzapine: the combined effect of age, gender, smoking, and comedication. Ther Drug Monit 2003;25:46–53.
12. Ereshefsky L et al. Effects of smoking on fluphenazine clearance in psychiatric inpatients. Biol Psychiatry 1985;20:329–32.
13. Jann MW et al. Effects of smoking on haloperidol and reduced haloperidol plasma concentrations and haloperidol clearance. Psychopharmacology 1986;90:468–70.
14. Shimoda K et al. Lower plasma levels of haloperidol in smoking than in nonsmoking schizophrenic patients. Ther Drug Monit 1999;21:293–6.
15. Miller LG. Recent developments in the study of the effects of cigarette smoking on clinical pharmacokinetics and clinical pharmacodynamics. Clin Pharmacokinet 1989;17:90–108.

Miscellaneous

504

Caffeine

Caffeine is probably the most popular psychoactive substance in the world. Mean daily consumption in the UK is 350–620 mg[1]. A quarter of the general population and half of those with psychiatric illness regularly consume over 500 mg caffeine/day[2]. Caffeine has *de novo* psychotropic effects and may also worsen existing psychiatric illness. It may also interact with psychotropic drugs.

Table Caffeine content of drinks	
Brewed coffee	100 mg/cup
Instant coffee	60 mg/cup
Tea	45 mg/cup
Soft drinks	25–50 mg/can

Chocolate also contains caffeine. Martindale lists over 600 medicines that contain caffeine[3]. Most are available without prescription and are marketed as analgesics or appetite suppressants.

Pharmacokinetics

Caffeine is rapidly absorbed after oral administration and has a half-life of 2.5–4.5 hours. It is metabolised by CYP1A2, a hepatic cytochrome enzyme that may exhibit genetic polymorphism. Metabolic pathways also become saturated at higher doses[4]. These factors may account for the large interindividual differences that are seen in the ability to tolerate caffeine[5].

Psychotropic effects

Caffeine is associated with CNS stimulation and increased catecholamine release[6]. Low-to-moderate doses are associated with favourable subjective effects such as elation and peacefulness[2]. Doses of >600 mg/day invariably produce anxiety, insomnia, psychomotor agitation, excitement, rambling speech (and sometimes delirium and psychosis)[7]. In sensitive people, these effects are produced by much lower doses. Caffeine has been shown to influence central dopamine binding[8] and, at high doses, it can inhibit benzodiazepine-receptor binding[6,7]. Tolerance develops to the effects of caffeine and an established withdrawal syndrome exists (headache, depressed mood, anxiety, fatigue, irritability, nausea, dysphoria and craving)[9].

Miscellaneous

Caffeine intoxication (caffeinism)

The DSM-IV[10] defines caffeinism as the recent consumption of caffeine, usually in excess of 250 mg, accompanied by five or more of the following: restlessness, nervousness, excitement, insomnia, flushed face, diuresis, GI disturbance, muscle twitching, rambling flow of thought and speech, tachycardia or cardiac arrhythmia, periods of inexhaustibility and psychomotor agitation, when these symptoms cause significant distress or impairment in social, occupational or other important areas of functioning and are not due to a general medical condition or better accounted for by another mental disorder (e.g. an anxiety disorder).

Schizophrenia

Patients with schizophrenia often consume large amounts of caffeine-containing drinks[1]. This may be to relieve dry mouth (as a side-effect of antipsychotic drugs), for the stimulant effects of caffeine (to relieve dysphoria/sedation/negative symptoms) or simply because coffee/tea drinking structures the day or relieves boredom. Excessive caffeine consumption is of concern because caffeine increases the release of catecholamines and so may theoretically precipitate or worsen psychosis. Kruger[6] found that large doses of caffeine can worsen psychotic symptoms (in particular elation and conceptual disorganisation) and result in the prescription of larger doses of antipsychotic drugs. De Freitas and Schwartz[11] found that the removal of caffeine from the diets of chronically disturbed (challenging behaviour) patients, led to decreased levels of hostility, irritability and suspiciousness. These findings have not been replicated in less disturbed populations[12].

Caffeine can also interfere with the effectiveness of drug treatment. Clozapine plasma levels can be raised by up to 60%[13], presumably through competitive inhibition of CYP1A2. Other drugs metabolised by this enzyme, such as olanzapine, imipramine and clomipramine, may be similarly affected. Large doses of caffeine taken in combination with serotonergic antidepressants may increase the risk of developing serotonin syndrome[14]. The potential effects of caffeine on the metabolism of other drugs, as well as the potential to induce a caffeine-withdrawal syndrome, should always be considered before substituting caffeine-free drinks.

Mood disorders

Caffeine may elevate mood through increasing norepinephrine release[15]. The practice of self-medication with caffeine to improve mood is common in the general population. Excessive consumption of caffeine may precipitate mania[16,17]. Depressed patients may be more sensitive to the anxiogenic effects of caffeine[18].

Caffeine can increase cortisol secretion (gives a false positive in the dexamethasone-suppression test)[19], increase seizure length during ECT[20] and increase the clearance of lithium by promoting diuresis[21]. Caffeine toxicity can be precipitated by drugs that inhibit CYP1A2. Fluvoxamine is an important example.

Anxiety disorders

Caffeine increases vigilance, decreases reaction times, increases sleep latency and worsens subjective estimates of sleep quality, effects that may be more marked in poor metabolisers. It can also precipitate or worsen generalised anxiety and panic attacks[22]. These effects are so marked that caffeine intoxication should always be considered when patients complain of anxiety symptoms or insomnia. Symptoms may diminish considerably or even abate completely if caffeine is avoided[23]. High doses of caffeine can reduce the efficacy of benzodiazepines (by reducing receptor binding[6,7]).

References

1. Rihs M et al. Caffeine consumption in hospitalized psychiatric patients. Eur Arch Psychiatry Clin Neurosci 1996;246:83–92.
2. Clementz GL et al. Psychotropic effects of caffeine. Am Fam Physician 1988;37:167–72.
3. Martindale: The Extra Pharmacopoeia, 32nd edn. London, UK: Pharmaceutical Press, 1999.
4. Kaplan GB et al. Dose-dependent pharmacokinetics and psychomotor effects of caffeine in humans. J Clin Pharmacol 1997;37:693–703.
5. Butler MA et al. Determination of CYP1A2 and NAT2 phenotypes in human populations by analysis of caffeine urinary metabolites. Pharmacogenetics 1992;2:116–27.
6. Kruger A. Chronic psychiatric patients' use of caffeine: pharmacological effects and mechanisms. Psychol Rep 1996;78:915–23.
7. Sawynok J. Pharmacological rationale for the clinical use of caffeine. Drugs 1995;49:37–50.
8. Kaasinen V et al. Dopaminergic effects of caffeine in the human striatum and thalamus. Neuroreport 2004;15:281–5.
9. Silverman K et al. Withdrawal syndrome after the double-blind cessation of caffeine consumption. N Engl J Med 1992;327:1109–14.
10. American Psychiatric Association. Diagnostic and Statistical Manual of Mental Disorders, 4th edn. Washington DC: American Psychiatric Association, 1994.
11. De Freitas B et al. Effects of caffeine in chronic psychiatric patients. Am J Psychiatry 1979;136:1337–8.
12. Koczapski A et al. Effects of caffeine on behavior of schizophrenic inpatients. Schizophr Bull 1989;15: 339–44.
13. Carrillo JA et al. Effects of caffeine withdrawal from the diet on the metabolism of clozapine in schizophrenic patients. J Clin Psychopharmacol 1998;18:311–16.
14. Shioda K et al. Possible serotonin syndrome arising from an interaction between caffeine and serotonergic antidepressants. Hum Psychopharmacol 2004;19:353–4.
15. Achor MB et al. Diet aids, mania, and affective illness. Am J Psychiatry 1981;138:392.
16. Ogawa N et al. Secondary mania caused by caffeine. Gen Hosp Psychiatry 2003;25:138–9.
17. Machado-Vieira R et al. Mania associated with an energy drink: the possible role of caffeine, taurine, and inositol. Can J Psychiatry 2001;46:454–5.
18. Lee MA et al. Anxiogenic effects of caffeine on panic and depressed patients. Am J Psychiatry 1988;145:632–5.
19. Uhde TW et al. Caffeine-induced escape from dexamethasone suppression. Arch Gen Psychiatry 1985; 42:737–8.
20. Cantu TG et al. Caffeine in electroconvulsive therapy. DICP 1991;25:1079–80.
21. Mester R et al. Caffeine withdrawal increases lithium blood levels. Biol Psychiatry 1995;37:348–50.
22. Bruce MS. The anxiogenic effects of caffeine. Postgrad Med J 1990;66 (Suppl 2):S18–S24.
23. Bruce MS et al. Caffeine abstention in the management of anxiety disorders. Psychol Med 1989; 19:211–14.

Further reading

Caffeine. In: DRUGDEX® System [database on CD-ROM]. Version 5.1. Greenwood Village, Colorado: Thomson Micromedex, 2002.
Paton C et al. Caffeine: the forgotten variable. Int J Psychiatry Clin Pract 2002;5:231–6.

Miscellaneous

Complementary therapies

A large proportion of the population currently use or have recently used complementary therapies (CTs)[1-4]. As health professionals are rarely consulted before purchase, a diagnosis is often not made and efficacy and side-effects are not monitored. The majority of those who use CTs are also taking conventional medicines[4] and many people use more than one CT simultaneously. Many do not tell their doctor[5]. The public associate natural products with safety and may be unwilling to report possible side-effects[6]. Herbal medicines, in particular, can be toxic as they contain pharmacologically active substances. Many conventional drugs prescribed today were originally derived from plants. These include medicines as diverse as aspirin, digoxin and the vinca alkaloids used in cancer chemotherapy. Herbal medicines such as St John's wort, *Ginkgo biloba* and valerian are increasingly used as self-medication for psychiatric and neurodegenerative illnesses[2,3,7]. Few CTs have been subject to randomised controlled trials, so efficacy is largely unproven[2,8,9]. For a few complementary therapies, Cochrane Reviews exist. These include the use of kava to treat anxiety (some evidence of efficacy)[10], Chinese herbal medicine as an adjunct to antipsychotics in schizophrenia (promising, more evidence required)[11], aromatherapy for behavioural problems in dementia (insufficient evidence, but worth further study)[12] and hypnosis for schizophrenia (insufficient evidence, but worth further study)[13]. Several complementary therapies are thought to be worthy of further study for the adjunctive management of substance misuse[14]. There is some preliminary, limited support for aromatherapy as an adjunct to conventional treatments in a range of psychiatric conditions[15].

There is little systematic monitoring of side-effects caused by CTs, so safety is largely unknown. There are an increasing number of published case reports of significant drug–herb interactions[16]: these include ginkgo and aspirin or warfarin, leading to increased bleeding; ginkgo and trazodone, leading to coma; and ginseng and phenelzine, leading to mania. Drug interactions with St John's wort are outlined on page 247. Some herbs are known to be very toxic[17-21].

Whatever the perceived 'evidence base' for the use of complementary therapies, the feelings of autonomy engendered by taking control of one's own illness and treatment can result in important psychological benefits irrespective of any direct therapeutic benefits of the CT[4,22,23]. There are many different complementary therapies, the most popular being homeopathy and herbal medicine with its branches of Bach's flower remedies, and Chinese and Ayurvedic medicine. Non-drug therapies such as acupuncture and osteopathy are also popular. To master one can take years of study; therefore, to ensure safe and effective treatment, referral to a qualified practitioner is recommended. Be aware, nonetheless, that scientific support for most complementary medicine is minimal and 'qualification' to practice is often dependent on wholesale acceptance of long-standing conjecture. The majority of doctors and pharmacists have no qualifications or specific training in CTs. The following table gives a brief introduction. Further reading is strongly recommended.

References

1. Fisher P et al. Medicine in Europe: complementary medicine in Europe. BMJ 1994;309:107–11.
2. Barnes J, Anderson LL, Phillipson JD. Herbal Medicines: A Guide for Healthcare Professionals. London: Pharmaceutical Press, 2002.
3. Kessler RC et al. The use of complementary and alternative therapies to treat anxiety and depression in the United States. Am J Psychiatry 2001;158:289–94.
4. Astin JA. Why patients use alternative medicine: results of a national study. JAMA 1998;279:1548–53.
5. Berry MI et al. The use of traditional Chinese medicine in Liverpool. Pharm J 1993;251:12.
6. Barnes J et al. Different standards for reporting ADRs to herbal remedies and conventional OTC medicines: face-to-face interviews with 515 users of herbal remedies. Br J Clin Pharmacol 1998;45: 496–500.
7. Pies R. Adverse neuropsychiatric reactions to herbal and over-the-counter "antidepressants". J Clin Psychiatry 2000;61:815–20.
8. Kleijnen J et al. Clinical trials of homoeopathy. BMJ 1991;302:316–23.
9. Reilly D et al. Is evidence for homoeopathy reproducible? Lancet 1994;344:1601–6.
10. Pittler MH et al. Kava extract for treating anxiety. Cochrane Database Syst Rev 2003;CD003383.
11. Rathbone J et al. Chinese herbal medicine for schizophrenia. Cochrane Database Syst Rev 2005; CD003444.
12. Thorgrimsen L et al. Aromatherapy for dementia. Cochrane Database Syst Rev 2003;CD003150.
13. Izquierdo SA et al. Hypnosis for schizophrenia. Cochrane Database Syst Rev 2004;CD004160.
14. Dean AJ. Natural and complementary therapies for substance use disorders. Curr Opin Psychiatry 2005;18:271–6.
15. Perry N et al. Aromatherapy in the management of psychiatric disorders: clinical and neuropharmacological perspectives. CNS Drugs 2006;20:257–80.
16. Hu Z et al. Herb–drug interactions: a literature review. Drugs 2005;65:1239–82.
17. Committee on Safety of Medicines. Kava Kava and hepatotoxicity. Current Problems in Pharmacovigilance 2002;28:6.
18. Committee on Safety of Medicines. Renal failure associated with traditional Chinese medicines. Current Problems in Pharmacovigilance 1999;25:18.
19. Committee on Safety of Medicines. Hypoglycaemia following the use of Chinese herbal medicine xiaoke wan. Current Problems in Pharmacovigilance 2001;27:8.
20. Ernst E. Serious psychiatric and neurological adverse effects of herbal medicines – a systematic review. Acta Psychiatr Scand 2003;108:83–91.
21. De Smet PA. Health risks of herbal remedies: an update. Clin Pharmacol Ther 2004;76:1–17.
22. Downer SM et al. Pursuit and practice of complementary therapies by cancer patients receiving conventional treatment. BMJ 1994;309:86–9.
23. Oh VM. The placebo effect: can we use it better? BMJ 1994;309:69–70.
24. Fulder S. The Handbook of Complementary Medicine, 2nd edn. London: Hodder and Stoughton, 1989.
25. NHS Centre for Reviews and Dissemination. Homeopathy. Effective Health Care Bulletin 2002;7:1–12.
26. Mills SY. The Essential Book of Herbal Medicine. London: Penguin Arkana, 1991.
27. Perharic L et al. Toxic effects of herbal medicines and food supplements. Lancet 1993;342:180–1.
28. Wong AH et al. Herbal remedies in psychiatric practice. Arch Gen Psychiatry 1998;55:1033–44.
29. Aslam M et al. Heavy metal toxicity of some Asian medicines in the UK. J Pharm Pharmacol 1980; 32:83.

Further reading

Cooke B et al. Aromatherapy: a systematic review. Br J Gen Pract 2000;455:444–5.
Ernst E et al. Complementary therapies for depression. Arch Gen Psychiatry 1998;55:1026–32.
Fugh-Berman A. Herb–drug interactions. Lancet 2000;355:134–8.
The Research Council for Complementary Medicine. Complementary and Alternative Medicine Evidence Online (CAMEOL) database. http://www.rccm.org.uk/cameol/Default.aspx. 2006. Accessed 23-8-2006.
Walter G et al. The relevance of herbal treatments for psychiatric practice. Aust NZ J Psychiatry 2000;33:482–9.
Werneke U et al. Complementary medicines in psychiatry: review of effectiveness and safety. Br J Psychiatry 2006;188:109–21.

Miscellaneous

Table An introduction to complementary therapies

	Homeopathy[12,13,24,25]	Herbal medicine (phytotherapy)[20,21,24,26–29]	Aromatherapy[24]
Health beliefs	• Treatment is selected according to the individual characteristics of the patient (hair colour and personality are as important as symptoms) • Treatment stimulates the body to restore health (there is no scientifically plausible theory to support this claim) • Like is treated with like (e.g. substances that cause a fever, treat a fever) • The more diluted the preparation, the more potent it is thought to be • Very potent preparations are unlikely to contain even one molecule of active substance	• Treatment is selected according to the individual characteristics of the patient (as with homeopathy) • Herbs are believed to stimulate the body's natural defences and enhance the elimination of toxins by increasing diuresis, defecation, bile flow and sweating • Attention to diet is important • The whole plant is used, not the specific active ingredient (this is believed to reduce side-effects) • Active ingredients vary with the source of the herb (standardisation is contrary to the philosophy of herbal medicine) • Herbalists believe that if the correct treatment is chosen, treatment will be completely free of side-effects	• Treatment is selected according to the individual characteristics of the patient (as with homeopathy and herbal medicine) • Illness is believed to be the result of imbalance in mental, emotional and physical processes, and aromatherapy is believed to promote balance • Purified oils are not used (the many natural constituents are believed to protect against adverse effects: similar to the beliefs held by herbalists) • There is no standard dose • Individual oils may be used for several unrelated indications

Used/for	• A wide range of indications (except those outlined below) • May be taken with conventional treatments • Over 2000 remedies and many dilutions are available	• Everything except as outlined • May be taken with conventional treatments but many significant interactions are possible (some have been reported) • Advertised in the lay press for a wide range of indications	• Everything except as outlined below • May be used as an adjunct to conventional treatments • Usually administered by massage onto the skin, which is known to relieve pain and tension, increase circulation and aid relaxation
Not suitable for	• Infection • Organ failure • Vitamin/mineral/hormone deficiency	• Use in pregnancy and lactation (many herbs are abortifacient)[28] • Evening primrose oil should not be used in epilepsy[28]	• Use in pregnancy (jasmine, peppermint, rose and rosemary may stimulate uterine contractions) • Rosemary should be avoided in epilepsy and hypertension
Side-effects and other information	• None known or anticipated • Inactivated by aromatherapy and strong smells (e.g. coffee, peppermint, toothpaste) • Inactivated by handling • Healing follows the law of cure: symptoms disappear down the body in the reverse order to which they appeared, move from vital to less vital organs and ultimately appear as a rash (which is a sign of cure)	• Herbal remedies are occasionally adulterated (with conventional medicines such as steroids or toxic substances such as lead[29]) • Many side-effects can be anticipated (e.g. kelp and thyrotoxicosis, St John's wort and serotonin syndrome) • Overuse, adulteration, variation in plant constituents and misidentification of plants are common causes of toxicity. Some Chinese herbs are toxic[17-19]	• Skin sensitivity • Significant systemic absorption can occur during massage • Ingestion can cause liver/kidney toxicity • All aromatherapy products should be stored in dark containers away from heat to avoid oxidation

Enhancing medication adherence

Psychotropic medication is essential in achieving the best possible health outcomes for people with a range of mental health conditions. However, approximately 50% of patients do not take medication reliably as prescribed[1]. Some authors have observed particularly high rates of non-adherence in people with schizophrenia, with up to 90% of patients stopping medication[2].

When second-generation antipsychotics and antidepressants were introduced during the 1990s it was argued by a number of researchers that patients would be more adherent with these treatments because they are better tolerated. In practice, however, adherence appears at best to be only marginally better with these newer treatments[3].

Why don't people take medication?

Studies have identified several main factors that may affect medication adherence[1]. These factors can be broadly organised into six categories:

- Illness-related factors include a lack of knowledge about treatment, denial of illness (or lack of insight) and the impact of illness on the patient's lifestyle.
- Treatment-related factors include medication side-effects, methods of medication administration and lack of treatment efficacy.
- Clinician-related factors include a lack of collaborative working and an authoritative attitude, problems accessing clinicians and infrequent medication review.
- Patient-related factors include forgetting to take medication, beliefs about treatment and perception of illness severity.
- Environmental factors include family beliefs about treatment, peer pressure and the media.
- Cultural factors include ethnic background and religious beliefs.

Strategies for improving adherence

These are 12 strategies that practitioners may find useful in working with patients to enhance medication adherence:

1. Working with the patient to find a medication that they feel helps with their problems.
2. Systematically monitoring the effects (impact on symptoms and side-effects) of medication.
3. Managing side-effects when they occur (especially movement problems, weight gain, sexual problems and tiredness).
4. Exchanging tailored medication information with patients and carers.
5. Listening, understanding and acknowledging patients' and carers' views about medication.
6. Helping patients sort out practical problems with medication (e.g. how to get repeat prescriptions).

Miscellaneous

7. Working with carers to support patients with medication taking (e.g. reminding them to take medication).
8. Helping patients and carers develop a culturally sensitive way of understanding their experiences that recognises the place for medication in enabling them to recover.
9. Working with patients and carers to elicit and explore the positive and negative things about taking or stopping medication.
10. Talking through past experiences of medication and exploring which medicines were helpful and less helpful from the patient's perspective.
11. Addressing beliefs and attitudes about medication (e.g. medication is addictive).
12. Exploring the less obvious benefits of medication (e.g. staying out of hospital, improved relationships with family).

These strategies have been organised into a structured way of working with patients: namely, adherence therapy (www.adherencetherapy.com). There have been several published trials of adherence therapy in schizophrenia[4-8] with mixed but largely positive results.

Other strategies to improve adherence include the use of long-acting injections, compensatory methods and financial incentives. Long-acting injections are commonly used to overcome non-adherence. The major advantage of long-acting injections is their improved bioavailability and the fact that if a patient relapses whilst having their depot as prescribed, the clinician can rule out non-adherence as a reason for relapse[9]. Administering long-acting injections can also help patients with cognitive deficits that may forget or are too disorganised to take oral medication. One obstacle to the use of long-acting injections is that they have over many years developed something of an image problem. However, a review of patient attitudes[10] concluded that generally patients had a positive attitude to depot antipsychotic medication. Cognitive adaptation training (CAT) uses environmental cues and modifications to compensate for the cognitive impairment associated with mental illness[11]. Following a comprehensive assessment of cognitive and adaptive functioning and the patient's environment, CAT interventions are tailored to the patient. These may include simple behavioural reminders to take medication or using more sophisticated electronic devices such as Med-eMonitor that is capable of storing a month's supply of up to five different medicines and prompts the patient if they are taking the wrong dose or at the wrong time. Finally, there is evidence from controlled trials across a number of disease areas of the potential of financial incentives to enhance medication adherence. Paying people to take their medication to enhance medication adherence in people with mental health problems is extremely controversial, though some clinicians have found it successful for improving adherence with antipsychotic medication in very high-risk patients[12].

Conclusion

People with mental health problems often stop treatment or are erratically compliant. Interventions that combine educational, behavioural and affective strategies seem to have a positive impact on adherence. Developing strategies to enhance medication adherence is an important clinical and research goal.

References

1. World Health Organisation. Adherence to Long-Term Therapies. Geneva, Switzerland: WHO Press, 2003.
2. Cramer JA et al. Compliance with medication regimens for mental and physical disorders. Psychiatr Serv 1998;49:196–201.
3. Dolder CR et al. Antipsychotic medication adherence: is there a difference between typical and atypical agents? Am J Psychiatry 2002;159:103–8.
4. Kemp R et al. Randomised controlled trial of compliance therapy. 18-month follow-up. Br J Psychiatry 1998;172:413–9.
5. O'Donnell C et al. Compliance therapy: a randomised controlled trial in schizophrenia. BMJ 2003;327:834.
6. Gray R et al. Effect of a medication management training package for nurses on clinical outcomes for patients with schizophrenia: cluster randomised controlled trial. Br J Psychiatry 2004;185:157–62.
7. Gray R et al. Adherence therapy for people with schizophrenia. European multicentre randomised controlled trial. Br J Psychiatry 2006;189:508–14.
8. Maneesakorn S et al. A RCT of adherence therapy for people with schizophrenia in Chaing Mai, Thailand. J Clin Nurs 2006;15:1–11.
9. McEvoy JP. Risks versus benefits of different types of long-acting injectable antipsychotics. J Clin Psychiatry 2006;67(Suppl 5):15–18.
10. Walburn J et al. Systematic review of patient and nurse attitudes to depot antipsychotic medication. Br J Psychiatry 2001;179:300–7.
11. Velligan DI et al. Randomized controlled trial of the use of compensatory strategies to enhance adaptive functioning in outpatients with schizophrenia. Am J Psychiatry 2000;157:1317–23.
12. Claassen D et al. Money for medication: financial incentives to improve medication adherence in assertive outreach. Psychiatr Bull 2007;31:4–7.

Communication with patients/service users

Follow the CAAT system.

Consultative

Those being prescribed medication should be consulted about their preferences with regard to adverse effects and likely outcomes with different medication. Patients' informed preferences should influence drug choice. Ideally, patients themselves should choose which medication they are prescribed. When patients are too ill to be consulted about drug choice, the opportunity for informative discussion should be provided as soon as appropriate.

Accurate

Patients have the right to factually accurate information about medicines and prescribing choices. Healthcare workers should recognise the limits of their knowledge and refer for expert advice when necessary. Consider, also, the provision of written information and patient telephone helplines.

Appropriate

Information should be presented in such a way that it can be readily understood. It is more important to tell patients how medication affects symptoms than to try to explain complex theories of drug action. It is rarely necessary to discuss, for instance, receptor theory, but likely outcomes should certainly be discussed. Everyone should be afforded the opportunity to be given more information, having first reflected on the information initially provided or after having gained first-hand experience of medication prescribed.

True

Patients have the right to be told the truth about medicines. It is morally right to impart all relevant information to those prescribed medication. Being 'economical with the truth' is unethical and likely to damage relationships and perhaps lead to litigation. Clearly, it is impossible to tell patients everything that is known about a particular medication, but it is possible to direct patients to more comprehensive, well-grounded sources of information.

Driving and psychotropic drugs

Many factors have been shown to affect driving performance. These include age, personality, physical and mental state and being under the influence of alcohol, prescribed medicines, street drugs or over-the-counter medicines[1]. Studying the effects of any of these factors in isolation is extremely difficult. Some studies have assessed the effect of medication on tests such as response time and attention[2], but these tests do not directly measure ability or inability to drive.

It has been estimated that up to 10% of people killed or injured in road traffic accidents (RTAs) may be taking psychotropic medication[3]. Patients with personality disorders and alcoholism have the highest rates of motoring offences and are more likely to be involved in accidents[3]. Driving while unfit through taking prescribed or illicit drugs is an offence and may lead to prosecution. People whose driving ability may be impaired through their illness or prescribed medication should inform their insurance company. Failure to do so is considered to be 'withholding a material fact' and may render the insurance policy void.

Table   Psychotropics and driving (see www.dvla.gov.uk)

Drug	Effect
Hypnotics and anxiolytics	Benzodiazepines cause sedation and impaired attention, information processing, memory and motor coordination. The impairment is dose-related and greater with longer half-life drugs. When used as anxiolytics, benzodiazepines have been associated with an increased risk of RTAs[4]. One study found that zopiclone (despite having a short half-life) dramatically increased the risk of RTAs[4]. Another suggests middle-of-the-night administration of zolpidem can negatively affect driving ability[5].
Antipsychotics	Sedation and EPSEs can impair coordination and response time[1]. A high proportion of patients treated with antipsychotics may have an impaired ability to drive[6,7]. One study found patients with schizophrenia taking atypical antipsychotics or clozapine performed better in tests of skills related to car-driving ability than patients with schizophrenia taking typical antipsychotics[8]. Clinical assessment is required.
Antidepressants	TCAs have been associated with an increased risk of RTAs[9], although negative studies also exist[4]. SSRIs[10] and MAOIs may be safer long term but probably not during the acute phase of the illness[11] (where impairments may be illness- rather than medication-related[12]).

Table Psychotropics and driving (see www.dvla.gov.uk) (Cont.)	
Drug	**Effect**
Anticonvulsants	Initial, dose-related side-effects may affect driving ability (e.g. blurred vision, ataxia and sedation). There are strict rules regarding epilepsy and driving.
Lithium	Lithium may impair visual adaptation to the dark[1] but the implications for driving safety are unknown. Elderly people who take lithium may be at increased risk of being involved in an injurious motor vehicle crash[13].
Alcohol	Alcohol causes sedation and impaired coordination, vision, attention and information processing. Alcohol-dependent drivers are twice as likely to be involved in traffic accidents and offences than licensed drivers as a whole[3], and a third of all fatal RTAs involve alcohol-dependent drivers[3].

Effects of psychiatric medicines

Many psychotropics can impair alertness, concentration and driving performance. Drugs that block H_1, α_1-adrenergic or cholinergic receptors may be particularly problematic. Effects are particularly marked at the start of treatment and after increasing the dose. It is important to stop driving during this time if adversely affected. The use of alcohol will further increase any impairment.

Drug-induced sedation

Many psychotropic drugs are sedative. The more sedative a drug is, the more likely it is to impair driving ability. Other medicines, either prescribed or bought over the counter, may also be sedative and/or affect driving ability (e.g. antihistamines[3]). One study found that 89% of patients taking other psychotropic drugs in addition to antidepressants failed a battery of 'fitness to drive' tests[11]. Since the degree of sedation any individual will experience is very difficult to predict, patients prescribed sedative drugs should be advised not to drive if they feel sedated.

DVLA regulations

Although the Driver and Vehicle Licensing Agency (DVLA) give quite specific guidelines regarding illness and ability to hold a driving licence (see summary of DVLA regulations), the rules regarding taking medication and driving are rather more vague.

Note 6 of the 'At a Glance' guidelines for psychiatric disorders states that 'Driving while unfit through drugs … is an offence', but what 'unfit through drugs' means appears to be at the discretion of the medical practitioner and individual concerned. The possible effects of various drugs are then listed, as in the table above.

Miscellaneous

DVLA – duty of the client

'If you have a medical condition which has become worse since your licence was issued, or you develop a new medical condition, you must write and inform the Drivers Medical Unit at the DVLA of the nature of your condition.' A list of the 'conditions' that interest the DVLA is provided, but medication used to treat these conditions is not mentioned specifically. Insurance companies should also be informed.

DVLA – duty of the prescriber

Doctors must advise patients on the effects that their illness and prescribed medication may have on their 'fitness to drive'. See also below.

The guidance also specified that patients under S17 of the MHA must be able to satisfy the standards of fitness for their respective conditions and be free from any effects of medication which would affect driving adversely, before resuming driving. Very few patients will fulfil these criteria.

GMC guidance on confidentiality[14]

If a patient lacks the capacity to understand the advice given by the doctor about 'fitness to drive' or drives contrary to that advice, it is the duty of the doctor to inform the DVLA. This duty is absolute. There is no room for discretion.

In order to persuade a patient to desist from driving, the patient's next of kin may be directly informed of the patient's lack of 'fitness to drive'.

Table Summary of DVLA regulations

Diagnosis	Group 1 entitlement (cars and motorcycles)		Group 2 entitlement (heavy goods or public service vehicles)	
	Notify DVLA?	Notes	Notify DVLA?	Notes
Uncomplicated anxiety or depression (without significant memory or agitation, behavioural disturbance or suicidal thoughts)	No	Consider effects of medication (see page XXX)	No	Very minor short-lived illnesses need not be notified to DVLA. Consider effects of medication (see page XXX).
Severe anxiety states or depressive illnesses (with significant memory or concentration problems, agitation, behavioural disturbance or suicidal thoughts)	Yes	Driving should cease pending the outcome of medical enquiry. A period of stability will be required before driving can be resumed.	Yes	Licence revoked for minimum of 6 months. Driving usually permitted if illness long-standing but controlled on medication that does not impair driving.
Acute psychotic disorders of any type	Yes	Driving must cease during the acute period. Relicensing can be considered (hypomania/mania following an isolated episode only) when the driver satisfies all of the following conditions: (a) has remained well and stable for at least 3 months (b) is compliant with treatment (c) has regained insight (hypomania/mania only)	Yes	Licence revoked for at least 3 years. Driving will only be permitted again if medication is minimal and does not interfere with driving ability and there is no significant likelihood of relapse.

Table Summary of DVLA regulations (Cont.)

Diagnosis	Group 1 entitlement (cars and motorcycles)		Group 2 entitlement (heavy goods or public service vehicles)	
	Notify DVLA?	Notes	Notify DVLA?	Notes
		(d) is free from adverse effects of medication which would impair driving (e) is subject to a favourable specialist report. Drivers with a history of instability or poor compliance will require a longer period off driving.		
Hypomania/mania	Yes	See Acute psychotic disorders of any type. Repeated changes of mood: when there have been four or more episodes of mood swing in the last 12 months, at least 6 months' stability is required under condition (a) (above).	Yes	As above.
Chronic schizophrenia	Yes	See Acute psychotic disorders of any type. Continuing symptoms even with limited insight do not necessarily preclude driving. Symptoms should be unlikely to cause significant concentration problems, memory impairment or distraction while driving.	Yes	As above.
Dementia or any organic brain syndrome	Yes	Patient should inform DVLA. Decision regarding fitness to drive based on medical subject reports. In early dementia, licence may be subject to annual review.	Yes	Licence revoked.

	Group 1		Group 2	
Learning disability (LD)	Yes	Severe LD – licence application will be refused. Mild LD – must be declared by patient on licence application form. Provisional licence may be issued: liaise with DVLA.	Yes	Only persons with minor degrees of learning disability will be considered for a licence.
Developmental disorders including autism and ADHD	No	Diagnosis not in itself a bar to licensing. Factors such as impulsivity, lack of awareness of the impact of own behaviour on self or others need to be considered.	Yes	Continuing minor symptomatology may be compatible with licensing cases considered individually.
Behavioural disorders (e.g. violent behaviour)	Yes	Court or patient should inform DVLA. Licence revoked. Licence reissued only after behaviour has been satisfactorily controlled. Medical report required.	Yes	Licence refused/revoked. Possibility of licence if person matures and psychiatric reports confirm stability.
Alcohol misuse 'Persistent misuse of alcohol confirmed by medical enquiry'	Yes	Licence refused/revoked for confirmed, persistent alcohol misuse until minimum of 6 months' controlled drinking or abstinence attained.	Yes	Same as Group 1 except **1 year's** controlled drinking or abstinence required.
Alcohol dependency	Yes	Licence refused/revoked until a 1-year period free from alcohol problems attained. Abstinence usually required. Medical reports required. Additional restrictions if seizures occur.	Yes	Licence not granted if there is a history of alcohol dependency in the past 3 years. Additional restrictions if seizures occur. Medical reports required.
Alcohol-related disorders (e.g. psychosis)	Yes	Patient should inform DVLA. Medical reports required. Licence usually refused/revoked until satisfactory recovery.	Yes	Licence refused/revoked.

Miscellaneous

Table Summary of DVLA regulations (Cont.)

Diagnosis	Group 1 entitlement (cars and motorcycles)		Group 2 entitlement (heavy goods or public service vehicles)	
	Notify DVLA?	Notes	Notify DVLA?	Notes
Drug misuse and dependency NB: Benzodiazepines prescribed above *BNF* limits for any reason constitute misuse/ dependency for DVLA purposes	Yes	Licence revoked until drug-free period shown below is attained. Assessment and urine screen arranged by DVLA may be required. **6-month drug-free period** for cannabis, amfetamines, ecstasy and other psychoactive substances. **1-year drug-free period** for heroin, morphine, methadone (there are exceptions for those on a supervised maintenance programme), cocaine and benzodiazepines. Additional restrictions if seizures occur.	Yes	Licence revocation until drug-free period attained. Assessment and urine screen arranged by DVLA will **normally** be required. **1-year drug-free period** for cannabis, amfetamines, ecstasy and other psychoactive substances. **3-year drug-free period** for heroin, morphine, methadone, cocaine and benzodiazepines. Additional restrictions if seizures occur.

Full information can be found at: www.dvla.gov.uk. on the left hand side of the page, click on "medical rules" then on the "At a Glance Guide".

References

1. Metzner JL et al. Impairment in driving and psychiatric illness. J Neuropsychiatry Clin Neurosci 1993; 5:211–20.
2. Ray WA et al. Medications and the older driver. Clin Geriatr Med 1993;9:413–38.
3. Noyes R Jr. Motor vehicle accidents related to psychiatric impairment. Psychosomatics 1985;26: 569–72,579.
4. Barbone F et al. Association of road-traffic accidents with benzodiazepine use. Lancet 1998;352:1331–6.
5. Verster JC et al. Residual effects of middle-of-the-night administration of zaleplon and zolpidem on driving ability, memory functions, and psychomotor performance. J Clin Psychopharmacol 2002;22: 576–83.
6. Grabe HJ et al. The influence of clozapine and typical neuroleptics on information processing of the central nervous system under clinical conditions in schizophrenic disorders: implications for fitness to drive. Neuropsychobiology 1999;40:196–201.
7. Wylie KR et al. Effects of depot neuroleptics on driving performance in chronic schizophrenic patients. J Neurol Neurosurg Psychiatry 1993;56:910–13.
8. Brunnauer A et al. The impact of antipsychotics on psychomotor performance with regards to car driving skills. J Clin Psychopharmacol 2004;24:155–60.
9. Currie D et al. The use of anti-depressants and benzodiazepines in the perpetrators and victims of accidents. Occup Med (Lond) 1995;45:323–5.
10. Hindmarch I et al. The effects of paroxetine and other antidepressants in combination with alcohol on psychomotor activity related to car driving. Acta Psychiatr Scand Suppl 1989;350:45.
11. Grabe HJ et al. The influence of polypharmacological antidepressive treatment on central nervous information processing of depressed patients: implications for fitness to drive. Neuropsychobiology 1998;37:200–4.
12. Gerhard U et al. Cognitive-psychomotor functions with regard to fitness for driving of psychiatric patients treated with neuroleptics and antidepressants. Neuropsychobiology 1984;12:39–47.
13. Etminan M et al. Use of lithium and the risk of injurious motor vehicle crash in elderly adults: case-control study nested within a cohort. BMJ 2004;328:558–9.
14. Morgan JF. DVLA and GMC guidelines on 'fitness to drive' and psychiatric disorders: knowledge following an educational campaign. Med Sci Law 1998;38:28–33.

Further reading

Niveau G et al. Psychiatric disorders and fitness to drive. J Med Ethics 2001;27:36–9.

Miscellaneous

Use of antibiotics in psychiatry

Antibiotics are possibly the most frequently prescribed non-psychotropics in psychiatric institutions. Their use in psychiatry is often complicated by a number of factors: the absence of in-house specialist microbiologist advice; lack of experience or knowledge of modern antibiotic therapy; and restrictions on possible routes of administration because nursing staff are unlikely to hold necessary certification.

The following table sets out broad guidelines for the use of antibiotics in some commonly encountered conditions. In using this table, some general guidance should be noted:

- Take samples for microbiological examination before starting treatment.
- Start with oral therapy unless patient is very unwell or if condition requires a parenteral-only agent.
- Consult microbiology (where available) sooner rather than later – certainly if treatment has had no effect after 48 hours, ideally before starting treatment.
- Always check allergy status before giving any antibiotic. Check case notes, the prescription chart and ask the patient.
- Be aware of the risk of antibiotic-associated colitis. Consult microbiology if this is suspected.

Infection/ condition	First-line treatment	Second-line treatment
Ears – e.g. otitis externa, otitis media	Consult microbiologist if otitis media suspected Chloramphenicol 0.5% drops, four times daily	Neomycin or polymyxin drops
Fungal infections	**Mouth/pharynx** Nystatin suspension (100,000 IU/ml), 1 ml four times daily **Skin** Clotrimazole 1% cream three times daily **Systemic or resistant skin infection** Fluconazole 50 mg daily for 7-14 days **Nail** Terbinafine 250 mg daily (see *BNF* for duration)	Fluconazole Fluconazole Consult microbiology Consult microbiology
Gastroenteritis	Not usually indicated – consult microbiology	
Pelvic inflammatory disease	Collect high vaginal swab; if *Neisseria gonococcus* excluded: metronidazole 400 mg three times daily for 7 days plus doxycycline 100 mg twice daily for 2 weeks. Give after food	Consult microbiology
Respiratory tract infections	Amoxicillin 250 mg three times daily or erythromycin 500 mg three times daily	Co-amoxiclav 375 mg three times daily or Clarithromycin 250 mg twice daily
Throat infection	Usually has viral cause. Consult microbiology; if *Streptococcus* confirmed: phenoxymethylpenicillin 250 mg four times daily or cefadroxil 500 mg twice daily or erythromycin 500 mg three times daily	Consult microbiology
Tuberculosis	Consult microbiology	
Urinary tract infections	Trimethoprim 200 mg twice daily or amoxicillin 250 mg three times daily	Nalidixic acid 1 g four times daily or co-amoxiclav 375 mg three times daily

Table (Cont.)

Infection/ condition	First-line treatment	Second-line treatment
		or ciprofloxacin 250 mg twice daily
Vaginal candidiosis	Oral fluconazole 150 mg as a single dose or clotrimazole 500 mg vaginal pessary	Consult microbiology
Wounds, ulcers, pressure sores	Do not use topical agents If cellulitis present – consult microbiology	

Index

528

529

531

537